Litman's Basics of Pediatric Anesthesia

Litman's Basics of Pediatric Anesthesia

Third Edition

Ronald S. Litman, DO, ML

Professor of Anesthesiology and Critical Care Medicine, Pediatrics
Children's Hospital of Philadelphia
Perelman School of Medicine at the University of Pennsylvania

Aditee P. Ambardekar, MD, MSEd

Residency Program Director
Associate Professor and Distinguished Teaching Professor
Department of Anesthesiology and Pain Management
Children's Health, Dallas
UT Southwestern Medical Center

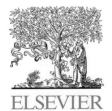

ELSEVIER

Elsevier
1600 John F. Kennedy Blvd.
Ste 1800
Philadelphia, PA 19103-2899

LITMAN'S BASICS OF PEDIATRIC ANESTHESIA, THIRD EDITION ISBN: 978-0-323-82902-1

Content Strategist: Sarah Barth
Content Development Manager: Somodatta Roy Choudhury
Content Development Specialist: Akanksha Marwah
Publishing Services Manager: Shereen Jameel
Project Manager: Janish Paul
Design Direction: Brian Salisbury

Printed in India

Last digit is the print number: 9 8 7 6 5 4 3 2 1

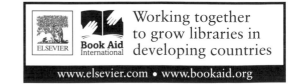

In Memoriam

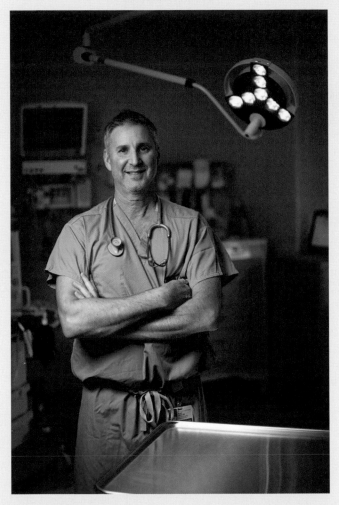

This edition of Litman's Basics of Pediatric Anesthesia *honors the physician, mentor, colleague, and friend that Dr. Litman was to many of us. His curiosity of all things medical and nonmedical, his inclination to challenge all things status quo, and his enduring commitment to training and mentoring the next generation of pediatric anesthesiologists defined his professional and personal life. So many colleagues benefited from his sponsorship, myself included, as evidenced by my coeditorship of this book. May Dr. Litman's enthusiasm for pediatric anesthesia and support for our learners live on in readers of this book for years to come.*

List of Contributors

Adam C. Adler, MD, MS, FAAP, FASE
Associate Professor
Department of Anesthesiology, Perioperative and Pain
    Medicine
Baylor College of Medicine
Texas Children's Hospital
Houston, TX

Aditee P. Ambardekar, MD, MSEd
Associate Professor and Distinguished Teaching Professor
Department of Anesthesiology and Pain Management
UT Southwestern Medical Center and Children's Health
Dallas, TX

Naomi Balamuth, MD
Associate Professor of Clinical Pediatrics
Department of Pediatrics
Division of Oncology
The Perelman School of Medicine at the University of
    Pennsylvania
Children's Hospital of Philadelphia
Philadelphia, PA

Alexandra Berman, MD
Resident
Department of Anesthesiology
New York Presbyterian Weill Cornell Medicine
New York, NY

Tarun Bhalla, MD, MBA, FASA, FAAP
Chair
Department of Anesthesiology and Pain Medicine
Akron Children's Hospital
Professor
Anesthesiology and Surgery
Northeastern Ohio Medical University (NEOMED)
Akron, OH

Donald L. Boyer, MD, MSEd
Associate Professor of Clinical Anesthesiology and Critical
    Care
The Perelman School of Medicine at the University of
    Pennsylvania
Department of Anesthesiology and Critical Care Medicine
Division of Critical Care Medicine
Children's Hospital of Philadelphia
Philadelphia, PA

Andrew J. Costandi, MD, MMM
Clinical Associate Professor of Anesthesiology
Department of Anesthesiology Critical Care Medicine
Division of Pain Management
Keck School of Medicine of USC
Children's Hospital of Los Angeles
Los Angeles, CA

C. Hunter Daigle, MD
Assistant Professor
Department of Pediatrics
Division of Critical Care Medicine
The University of Texas at Austin
Dell Medical School
Dell Children's Medical Center
Austin, TX

Gregory Dodson, DO
Assistant Professor
Department of Anesthesiology
Cooper Medical School of Rowan University
Camden, NJ

Jeffrey M. Feldman, MD, MSE
Professor of Anesthesiology and Critical Care
The Perelman School of Medicine at the University of
    Pennsylvania
Department of Anesthesiology and Critical Care Medicine
Children's Hospital of Philadelphia
Philadelphia, PA

John E. Fiadjoe, MD
Assistant Professor of Anesthesiology
Harvard Medical School
Boston Children's Hospital
Boston, MA

Jessica Foster, MD
Instructor and Attending Physician
Department of Pediatrics
Division of Oncology
Perelman School of Medicine at the University of
    Pennsylvania
Children's Hospital of Philadelphia
Philadelphia, PA

Susan Gallagher, RN
Hemophilia Nurse Coordinator
Children's Hospital of Philadelphia
University of Pennsylvania
Philadelphia, PA

F. Jay Garcia, MD
Resident
Department of Pediatrics
The Perelman School of Medicine at the University of
    Pennsylvania
Children's Hospital of Philadelphia
Philadelphia, PA

Thierry Girard, MD
Deputy Chair
Anesthesiology
University Hospital Basel
Switzerland

Anastasia D. Grivoyannis, MD
Assistant Professor
Department of Anesthesiology & Critical Care Medicine
Johns Hopkins University School of Medicine
Baltimore, MD

Harshad Gurnaney, MBBS, MPH
Associate Professor of Anesthesiology and Critical Care
The Perelman School of Medicine at the University of
    Pennsylvania
Department of Anesthesiology and Critical Care Medicine
Children's Hospital of Philadelphia
Philadelphia, PA

Fatimah Habib, MD
Assistant Professor of Anesthesiology
Assistant Professor
Department of Anesthesiology
Cooper Medical School of Rowan University
Camden, NJ

Grace Hsu, MD
Clinical Associate Professor of Anesthesiology
Department of Anesthesiology Critical Care Medicine
Division of Pain Management
Keck School of Medicine of USC
Children's Hospital of Los Angeles
Los Angeles, CA

Samuel Hunter, MD
Assistant Professor of Anesthesiology and Critical Care
    Medicine
The Perelman School of Medicine at the University of
    Pennsylvania
Department of Anesthesiology and Critical Care Medicine
Children's Hospital of Philadelphia
Philadelphia, PA

Rebecca S. Isserman, MD
Assistant Professor of Anesthesiology and Critical Care
    Medicine
The Perelman School of Medicine at the University of
    Pennsylvania
Department of Anesthesiology and Critical Care Medicine
Children's Hospital of Philadelphia
Philadelphia, PA

Jeremy Jones, MD
Resident
Department of Pediatrics
The Perelman School of Medicine at the University of
    Pennsylvania
Children's Hospital of Philadelphia
Philadelphia, PA

Ji Yeon Jemma Kang, MD
Assistant Professor
Department of Anesthesia
University of Cincinnati College of Medicine
Cincinnati Children's Hospital Medical Center
Cincinnati, OH

Michael R. King, MD
Assistant Professor
Northwestern University Feinberg School of Medicine
Ann and Robert H. Lurie Children's Hospital of Chicago
Chicago, IL

F. Wickam Kraemer III, MD
Associate Professor of Clinical Anesthesiology and Critical
    Care Medicine
The Perelman School of Medicine at the University of
    Pennsylvania
Department of Anesthesiology and Critical Care
Children's Hospital of Philadelphia
Philadelphia, PA

Grace E. Linder, MD
Assistant Professor
Department of Pathology and Laboratory Medicine
The Perelman School of Medicine at the University of
    Pennsylvania
Children's Hospital of Philadelphia
Philadelphia, PA

Ronald S. Litman, DO, ML
Professor of Anesthesiology and Critical Care Medicine
    and Pediatrics
The Perelman School of Medicine at the University of
    Pennsylvania
Department of Anesthesiology and Critical Care
Children's Hospital of Philadelphia
Philadelphia, PA

Katherine H. Loh, MD
Assistant Professor
Department of Anesthesiology
Division of Pediatric Anesthesiology
Vanderbilt School of Medicine
Monroe Carell Jr. Children's Hospital at Vanderbilt
Nashville, TN

Petar Mamula, MD
Professor of Pediatrics
Department of Pediatrics
Division of Gastroenterology, Hepatology, and Nutrition
The Perelman School of Medicine at the University of
    Pennsylvania
Children's Hospital of Philadelphia
Philadelphia, PA

Annery Garcia-Marcinikiewicz, MD
Assistant Professor of Clinical Anesthesiology and Critical
    Care Medicine
The Perelman School of Medicine at the University of
    Pennsylvania
Department of Anesthesiology and Critical Care
Children's Hospital of Philadelphia
Philadelphia, PA

Lynne G. Maxwell, MD
Emeritus Professor of Clinical Anesthesiology and Critical
    Care Medicine
The Perelman School of Medicine at the University of
    Pennsylvania
Department of Anesthesiology and Critical Care
Children's Hospital of Philadelphia
Philadelphia, PA

Wallis T. Muhly, MD
Assistant Professor of Clinical Anesthesiology and Critical
    Care Medicine
The Perelman School of Medicine at the University of
    Pennsylvania
Department of Anesthesiology and Critical Care
Children's Hospital of Philadelphia
Philadclphia, PA

Olivia Nelson, MD
Assistant Profcssor of Clinical Anesthesiology and Critical
    Care Medicine
The Perelman School of Medicine at the University of
    Pennsylvania
Department of Anesthesiology and Critical Care
Children's Hospital of Philadelphia
Philadelphia, PA

Asha Nookala, MD
Pediatric Anesthesiologist
Children's Minnesota
Minneapolis, MN

Vanessa A. Olbrecht, MD, MBA, FASA
Associate Professor
Department of Anesthesiology and Pain Medicine
Nationwide Children's Hospital
Columbus, OH

Shikha Patel, BS
Medical Student
Drexel University College of Medicine
Philadelphia, PA

Alison Perate, MD
Assistant Professor of Clinical Anesthesiology and Critical
    Care Medicine
The Perelman School of Medicine at the University of
    Pennsylvania
Department of Anesthesiology and Critical Care
Children's Hospital of Philadelphia
Philadelphia, PA

Laura A. Petrini, MD
Assistant Professor of Clinical Anesthesiology and Critical
    Care Medicine
The Perelman School of Medicine at the University of
    Pennsylvania
Department of Anesthesiology and Critical Care
Children's Hospital of Philadelphia
Philadelphia, PA

Teeda Pinyavat, MD
Assistant Professor
Department of Anesthesiology
Division of Pediatric Anesthesiology
Columbia University
New York, NY

Andrew Renuart, MD, MSc
Assistant in Perioperative and Critical Care Medicine
Department of Anesthesiology
Critical Care and Pain Medicine
Boston Children's Hospital
Instructor of Anaesthesia
Harvard Medical School
Boston, MA

Susan R. Rheingold, MD
Professor of Clinical Pediatrics
The Perelman School of Medicine at the University of
Pennsylvania
Children's Hospital of Philadelphia
Philadelphia, PA

Samuel Rosenblatt, MD, MSEd
Assistant Professor of Clinical Anesthesiology and Critical
Care Medicine
The Perelman School of Medicine at the University of
Pennsylvania
Department of Anesthesiology and Critical Care
Children's Hospital of Philadelphia
Philadelphia, PA

Julia Rosenbloom, MD
Assistant Professor
Mass General Anesthesia and Pain Medicine
Boston, MA

William Ryan, BS
Medical student
Drexel University College of Medicine
Philadelphia, PA

Deborah Ann Sesok-Pizzini, MD, MBA
Chief, Blood Bank and Transfusion Medicine
Pathology and Laboratory Medicine
Children's Hospital of Philadelphia
Philadelphia, PA

Christopher Setiawan, MD
Assistant Professor
Department of Anesthesiology and Pain Management
UT Southwestern Medical Center and Children's Health
Dallas, TX

Allan F. Simpao, MD, MBI
Associate Professor of Clinical Anesthesiology and Critical
Care Medicine
The Perelman School of Medicine at the University of
Pennsylvania
Department of Anesthesiology and Critical Care
Children's Hospital of Philadelphia
Philadelphia, PA

Paul A. Stricker, MD
Associate Professor of Clinical Anesthesiology and Critical
Care Medicine
The Perelman School of Medicine at the University of
Pennsylvania
Department of Anesthesiology and Critical Care
Children's Hospital of Philadelphia
Philadelphia, PA

Ari Y. Weintraub, MD
The Perelman School of Medicine at the University of
Pennsylvania
Department of Anesthesiology and Critical Care
Children's Hospital of Philadelphia
Philadelphia, PA

Char M. Witmer, MD, MSCE
Associate Professor of Clinical Pediatrics
Department of Pediatrics
The Perelman School of Medicine at the University of
Pennsylvania
Children's Hospital of Philadelphia
Philadelphia, PA

Theoklis Zaoutis, MD, MSCE
Professor of Pediatrics and Epidemiology
Division of Infectious Diseases
The Perelman School of Medicine at the University of
Pennsylvania
Children's Hospital of Philadelphia
Philadelphia, PA

Karen B. Zur, MD
Professor and Chief
Division of Otolaryngology
Department of Otolaryngology
Head and Neck Surgery
The Perelman School of Medicine at The University of
Pennsylvania
Children's Hospital of Philadelphia
Philadelphia, PA

Preface

When I sat down to write the preface of this book, I spent a fair bit of time wondering, "What was Ron thinking?" Not in a critical way; rather, I wondered how I could best represent the thoughts and energy that Ron put into this without the pleasure of having a colorful conversation with him. Although I had very little role in assembling the content and authors, I felt a huge responsibility for completing this in the way Ron had intended, ultimately to honor his work. In the best way I knew how, I hobbled together something based on past prefaces, my review of the book in its entirety, and my knowledge of Ron. Well, Ron must not have been thrilled with the way it sounded because, as we were preparing the book for copyediting, he made sure we found the file of the preface he intended for this edition of the book. What a treat to hear his voice in the words on this page. Enjoy!

Aditee P. Ambardekar, MD, MSEd

I caved. After a very successful run self-publishing *Basics of Pediatric Anesthesia* in 2013, I didn't have the energy to self-publish again. It takes a lot of work and focus worrying about the cover, layout, tables, photos, and figures. And that godawful index! Then there's the marketing, distribution, author-chasing, and wondering who, if anyone, will ever buy it after all that effort. So, in 2020, when I knew that some of the concepts in *Basics* were getting seriously out of date, I caved. I sent book proposals to publishers of anesthesia textbooks and was lucky enough to connect with Sarah Barth of Elsevier, who, along with Ellen Wurm-Cutter, stewarded this next edition through to completion. So, there are a few less jokes. It was time to grow up anyway.

Many aspects of the practice of clinical pediatric anesthesia that have changed since the first edition are now addressed in this third edition. They include opioid sparing, sugammadex, changes in fasting intervals, difficult intubation protocols, and pediatric advanced life support algorithms, to name just a few. Don't worry: anesthesia circuits are still absent. I'm sticking with the basics. Many of the original chapter authors have been replaced with motivated and energetic junior pediatric anesthesiologists (and sometimes even brilliant medical students) to fact-check the chapters and add additional material where appropriate.

One new aspect of *Basics* is the inclusion of special sections called "Deeper Dive," designed for readers that want a more nuanced and granular perspective on a particular topic. Most of these Deeper Dives consist of detailed examination of published research studies that have not only advanced knowledge in pediatric anesthesia but have also influenced its practice. These sections are scattered throughout the book. Some chapters have none, while some have more than one.

Notably absent from this revision is any mention of the anesthetic management of children with SARS COVID-19. As I write this, we are in the midst of two of the worst public health crises in US history, notably, the viral pandemic and continuing racial injustice. Fortunately, I am confident that by the time *Basics* is published, we will have emerged from the pandemic with many lessons learned about the public health implications of the management of children with severe viral disease or the cytokine storm that follows. There is no doubt that dangerous pandemics will recur in most of our lifetimes, but this material is not suitable in a book on the basics.

Unfortunately, I am not confident that racial injustice will be similarly relegated to the past. That's why I've asked Julia Rosenbloom, a pediatric anesthesiologist, to write a section on racial inequities in pediatric anesthesia and pain management. Julia is currently on the faculty of Harvard Medical School and has devoted her career to this crucially important topic. Every anesthesia provider should be intimately familiar with our unacceptable track record of treating children of color and how to advocate for and protect those children and their families.

Ronald S. Litman, DO, ML

Acknowledgements

Editorship of this edition fell into my lap in April 2021 under extenuating circumstances as Ron spent some of his last moments with his sweet family. Ron had spent the better part of 2020 planning his third edition, recruiting young authors to update the content, and editing the chapters as they came in... all the while fighting cancer and getting stronger. What had been a small commitment from me in November 2020 to update the pediatric burn chapter morphed into one of the biggest honors of my professional career. Ron and Daphne, thank you for the opportunity to honor Ron's legacy in pediatric anesthesia as the coeditor of this book.

It would have been ideal to have done this alongside Ron, as had originally been planned down the road, rather than in his absence. However, this was not meant to be. Through Ron's sponsorship and the mentorship of several individuals, however, I felt empowered to take the baton and cross the finish line. To Ron and the many others who served and continue to serve in a role of mentor to me, I thank you. I hope I can be as impactful of a mentor to others as you have been to me. You know who you are.

All of this is for naught without the medical students, residents, and fellows we have the honor and responsibility to teach. It is your inquisitiveness, compassion, and dedication to our field that energizes those of us in academic medicine. Thank you for the privilege to be part of this exciting journey.

Finally deepest gratitude to my family. To my mother and father, who instilled in me the desire to work hard and make a difference with humility and grace, I thank you. As Dr. Schwartz would say, I "picked the right parents." To my husband, Sumeet, who believes in me and encourages me with any new academic endeavor, I thank you. Your support means the world to me. To my sons, Arjun and Aarav, thank you for sharing your mommy with her patients, her residents and fellows, and her work. Although some days feel like cacophony rather than harmony, your unconditional love and beautiful souls make it all worth it.

Aditee P. Ambardekar, MD, MSEd

Contents

Section V: Pain Management

Section VI: Critical Care

Litman's Basics of
Pediatric Anesthesia

1

Transition From Fetal to Pediatric Anesthesia

VANESSA OLBRECHT, ANDREW RENUART
AND RONALD S. LITMAN

We begin this journey into the magical world of pediatric anesthesia by describing fetal cardiopulmonary physiology and the physiologic changes that occur during birth. Knowledge of these changes is important for understanding the pathophysiologic conditions that occur in neonates when these changes do not occur normally.

First, for clarity and consistency across the pediatric anesthesia literature, and to make sure we are all on the same page, there are a few universal definitions that you need to know.

- A **neonate** is a child in the first 28 days (or 1 month) of life, regardless of gestational age.
- An **infant** is a child from birth to 12 months of life.
- The **gestational age** is the number of weeks between conception and birth.

The following definitions are relatively new[1]:

- **Early term** delivery refers to birth during the period between 37 and 38 6/7 weeks' gestation.
  - **Full term** refers to delivery between 39 and 40 6/7 weeks' gestation.
- **Late term** refers to delivery between 41 and 41 6/7 weeks' gestation.
  - **Postterm** refers to delivery after 42 weeks' gestation.
- **Extremely preterm** infants are born before 28 weeks' gestation.
- **Very preterm** infants are born between 28 and 31 6/7 weeks' gestation.
- **Moderate to late preterm** infants are born between 32 and 36 6/7 weeks' gestation.

Sometimes, newborn infants are classified by their weight relative to their gestational age. For example:

- **Appropriate for gestational age (AGA)** describes an infant with a birth weight between the 10th and 90th percentiles.
- **Small for gestational age (SGA)** describes an infant with a birth weight below the 10th percentile.
- **Large for gestational age (LGA)** describes an infant with a birth weight above the 90th percentile.

Intrauterine growth restriction (IUGR) is an abnormal pattern of restricted fetal growth for gestational age. It is mainly an obstetric term that is used to describe a pattern of growth over a period of time *in utero*, whereas *SGA* is a term used by pediatricians to describe the infant at or shortly after birth.

Lung Growth and Development

During gestation, the fetal lungs grow and develop but are not responsible for oxygenation and ventilation. We normally rely on the lungs to provide oxygenation and ventilation, but in fetal life, that is the placenta's responsibility. The intrauterine environment allows the alveoli and bronchial tree of the lungs to develop. The fetal lungs are filled with fluid and transition to their role as the organ of gas exchange shortly before, during, and after the birth process.

Fetal lung development is divided into four stages of progressive lower airway and alveolar growth (Table 1.1). In the embryonic stage, primitive lung tissue is developed and vascular connections are made. In the pseudoglandular stage, the bronchial tree begins to form lumens, and in the canalicular stage at 16 to 26 weeks' gestation, alveoli begin to form. It is also during this period that blood and lymphatic vessels begin to develop in parallel to the bronchial tree, and surfactant production begins. Finally, during the saccular stage, the fetal lung completes the physiologic processes that allow it to accomplish respiration in the extrauterine environment. This includes maturation of the alveolar-vascular interface and development of a full complement of surfactant, which will reduce surface tension within the alveoli and prevent their collapse after transition to the outside world. During gestation, the fetal airways and alveoli become distended by secreted lung fluid, which becomes a component of the amniotic fluid and allows for proper development of the lungs.

As the peripheral chemoreceptors and the respiratory center of the brain mature, the fetus develops stronger and more

TABLE 1.1	Stages of Fetal Lung Development	
Stage	**Gestation**	**Events**
Embryonic	4–17 weeks	Formation of primitive lung tissue and vascular connections.
Pseudoglandular	5–17 weeks	Development of a bronchial tree that begins to form lumens.
Canalicular	16–26 weeks	Alveoli begin to form. Vascular and lymphatic systems develop alongside the bronchial tree. Differentiation of type 1 and type 2 pneumocytes with beginning of surfactant production. Extrauterine life possible at later weeks.
Saccular	24 weeks–birth	Peripheral bronchiole branching. Maturation of surfactant system. Breathing efforts begin. 30–50 million alveoli at birth.
Alveolar	Birth–3+ years	Continued alveolar growth to adult level of approximately 500 million. Reduction of interstitial tissues.

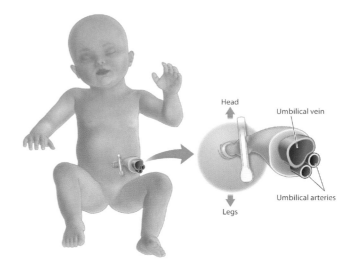

• **Fig 1.1.** Umbilical cord anatomy. *(Illustration by Rob Fedirko.)*

regular breathing patterns throughout development. After the 30th week of gestation, the fetus is seen to "practice" breathing at about 60 times per minute, approximately 40% of the time. There are conflicting reports as to the number of years into childhood that it takes for the alveoli to finish growing. In the past, it was thought that alveolar growth terminated somewhere between 3 and 8 years; but more recent data indicate that it could be even later into childhood.

Development of the Circulatory System

The primary difference between the fetal and adult circulatory systems is that the fetal circulation consists of two parallel circulations (right and left), whereas the adult system exists in series. Fetal circulation is also characterized by the presence of several right-to-left shunts that result from the high pulmonary vascular resistance of the fetal lungs and the low vascular resistance of the placenta. The main purpose of having a fetal circulation is to distribute oxygen, glucose, and

other nutrients from the placenta (which receives about 40% of mom's cardiac output) to the developing brain and vital organs of the fetus.

Let us describe the pattern of fetal circulation by starting with blood returning to the placenta. Deoxygenated blood from the fetus travels to the placenta via the two umbilical arteries that are encased by the umbilical cord (Fig. 1.1). In the placenta, the fetal blood picks up oxygen, releases carbon dioxide, and is returned to the fetus via the single umbilical vein (also contained in the umbilical cord). With a PO_2 that may reach as high as 55 mm Hg, fetal blood is at its highest oxygen level in the umbilical vein. This may seem low compared with the developed human, but there are several reasons why the fetus is able to successfully maintain adequate tissue oxygenation with such a low PO_2. These include:

- Fetal hemoglobin (Hgb F) has a higher affinity for oxygen than maternal hemoglobin, which facilitates movement of oxygen from the maternal to the fetal blood via diffusion. This increased affinity of Hgb F for oxygen causes a leftward shift of the oxyhemoglobin dissociation curve.
- Release of oxygen from Hgb F to fetal tissues is facilitated by the relatively higher temperature and lower pH of the fetus, both of which shift the oxyhemoglobin dissociation curve to the right.
- A relatively low PO_2 is better suited to the metabolic needs of the fetus, which has relatively lower oxygen consumption.
- Evolutionary forces influenced the fetal circulation such that blood flow with a relatively higher degree of oxygen saturation preferentially perfuses vital organs such as the liver, heart, and brain.

Oxygenated blood is carried through the umbilical vein to the liver, where approximately half of the blood flow joins the hepatic circulation to supply oxygen and nutrients to the hepatic tissue, while the other half bypasses the liver through the ***ductus venosus***, a structure present only in fetal life. The ductus venosus carries the oxygenated blood into the inferior vena cava (IVC). Here, the oxygen-rich blood mixes with poorly oxygenated blood returning from the fetal lower extremities and the newly acquainted circulations travel together to the right atrium.

Inside the fetal right atrium, oxygenated blood from the IVC is preferentially directed across the ***foramen ovale*** and into the left atrium, while deoxygenated blood returning from the head via the superior vena cava (SVC) is preferentially directed to the tricuspid valve into the right ventricle. This circulation pattern allows preferential perfusion of oxygen-rich blood to vital organs.

The deoxygenated blood that enters the right ventricle is ejected into the pulmonary artery, but because pulmonary vascular resistance is high, only a small portion (about 10%) actually gets into the pulmonary arterial system. Most (90%) is directed through the ***ductus arteriosus***, a connection between the pulmonary artery and the aorta, where it joins aortic blood flow returning to the placenta via the umbilical arteries. The ductus arteriosus usually enters the aorta just distal to the origin of the left subclavian artery.

The oxygenated blood that has crossed into the left atrium passes through the mitral valve into the left ventricle and is ejected out through the ascending aorta where it provides oxygen and glucose to the developing brain via the carotid arteries. Although the PO_2 is now about 27 mm Hg, the fetus still receives sufficient oxygen for fetal organ growth.

Cardiopulmonary Changes at Birth

The birth process entails several complicated physiologic transitions to an extrauterine existence that all seem to occur at once (Fig. 1.2). Alveolar and bronchial fluid must be

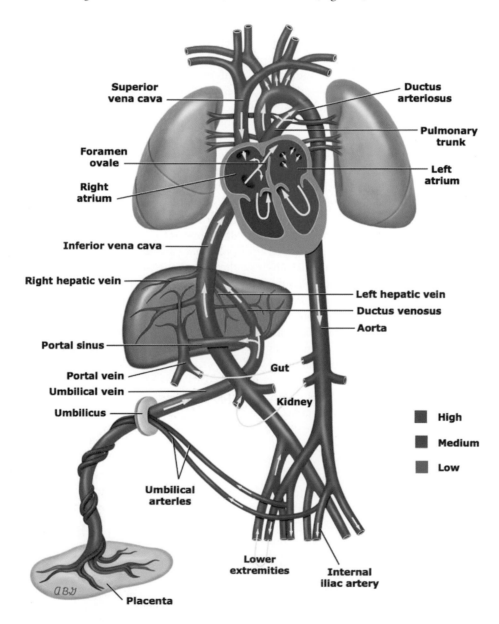

• **Fig 1.2.** Fetal circulation. (Reproduced with permission from: Fernandes CJ. Physiologic transition from intrauterine to extrauterine life. In: Post TW, ed., *UpToDate* (website). Accessed on 20.9.22. Available from: www.uptodate.com.)

expunged, the lungs must expand, and the circulatory conduits that serve as right-to-left shunts must quickly close. When these occur, the lungs officially become the organ of respiration and the cardiovascular system converts from two parallel circulations to two circulations in series. If any of these fails to occur, hypoxemia may result from residual right-to-left shunting.

Several mechanisms facilitate the clearance of alveolar fluid from the fetal lungs. During labor, a state of physiologic stress that is induced in the fetus causes the lung epithelium to convert from one that secretes liquid into the air spaces to one that actively reabsorbs salt and fluid. This change is further enhanced when the lung epithelium is exposed to oxygen after delivery. During the newborn's first breaths, air is drawn into the lungs because of a large negative inspiratory force, and lung fluid is absorbed or expelled. Intrathoracic pressures are estimated to range from -60 cmH_2O during inhalation and approximately $+70$ cmH_2O during exhalation. This large fluctuation in intrathoracic pressure helps force fluid from the air spaces into the interstitium and then ultimately back into the intravascular space. The pressure required for lung expansion becomes increasingly less negative over several breaths. These initial breaths establish the residual volume (RV) and functional residual capacity (FRC) of the newborn's lungs. These volumes are maintained by the newborn's expiratory braking maneuver (see Chapter 2) that also prevents the expunged fluid from reentering the lungs. Pressure exerted on the chest from contractions during delivery is thought to play only a minor role in this transition.

Also important in this transition is the shift in vascular resistance that occurs when the umbilical cord is clamped as the newborn takes its first breaths. Clamping the umbilical cord causes a dramatic increase in systemic vascular resistance (SVR) and immediate loss of preload from the umbilical vein. At the same time, as the lungs expand, the increase in pulmonary PO_2 causes pulmonary vascular resistance (PVR) to decrease; pulmonary blood flow increases and reestablishes preload to the left ventricle. Arterial blood gas values normalize within the first 24 hours of life.

The combined increase in SVR and decrease in PVR cause resistance to blood flow through the ductus arteriosus. Increasing left atrial pressure causes the "flap-valve" foramen ovale (which connects the right and left atria) to close, thus establishing for the first time a circulation in series. The umbilical arteries form a portion of the internal iliac and superior vesical arteries, and the ductus venosus (previously supplied by the umbilical vein) will atrophy and form a remnant known as the ***ligamentum venosum***.

Over the first several hours of life, the ductus arteriosus functionally closes as a result of constriction of specialized contractile tissue within its arterial wall. This constriction is caused by a number of factors, including withdrawal from placenta-derived prostaglandin E2, an increase in arterial oxygen tension, and an increase in blood pH. Over the next several weeks, the ductus arteriosus becomes anatomically closed; its remnant is called the ***ligamentum arteriosum***.

Persistent Pulmonary Hypertension of the Newborn

Although the majority of neonates undergo this transition to extrauterine life successfully, approximately 10% will have difficulty and will require some level of neonatal resuscitation. Several factors are associated with an increased risk of requiring assistance. These include maternal conditions (e.g., advanced maternal age, maternal substance abuse), fetal conditions (e.g., prematurity, congenital anomalies), and delivery complications (e.g., breech presentation, peripartum infection). Any of these could result in hypoxia, hypercarbia, and/or acidosis, all of which predispose to the newborn's inability to transition out of fetal circulation.

A particularly hazardous outcome from this transition failure is the development of **persistent pulmonary hypertension of the newborn (PPHN).** This disorder leads to persistence of pulmonary vasoconstriction, which causes pulmonary hypertension. PPHN primarily occurs in term or late preterm infants over the age of 34 weeks' gestation, and its prevalence is estimated to occur in approximately 2 per 1000 live births.

Because of the abnormally high PVR, the fetal pattern of circulation continues: blood flows through a patent ductus arteriosus (PDA) or foramen ovale in a right-to-left direction and hypoxemia worsens, thus creating a vicious cycle that can be overcome only by aggressive therapy for the underlying disorder and reversal of hypoxemia, hypercarbia, and acidosis. The management of PPHN focuses on supportive measures, including the use of 100% oxygen, with the goal of decreasing PVR compared with SVR. Other more aggressive treatment measures include the use of inhaled nitric oxide (iNO) and extracorporeal membrane oxygenation (ECMO).

References

1. ACOG Committee Opinion No 579: Definition of term pregnancy. *Obstet Gynecol.* 2013;122(5):1139–1140. https://doi.org/10.1097/01.AOG.0000437385.88715.4a.

Suggested Readings

Hooper SB, Polglase GR, Roehr CC. Cardiopulmonary changes with acration of the newborn lung. *Paediatr Respir Rev* 2015;16(3):147–150. https://doi.org/10.1016/j.prrv.2015.03.003.

van Vonderen JJ, Te Pas AB. The first breaths of life: imaging studies of the human infant during neonatal transition. *Paediatr Respir Rev.* 2015;16(3):143–146. https://doi.org/10.1016/j.prrv.2015.03.001.

2

Developmental Physiology and Pharmacology

SHIKHA PATEL AND RONALD S. LITMAN

Developmental physiology describes the bodily changes that take place during early development. Anesthesiologists must be familiar with these changes as they pertain to the different organ systems. Developmental pharmacology describes the changes in pharmacokinetics and pharmacodynamics during early life. In pediatric anesthesia, this is especially important because it influences the administration of intravenous and inhaled anesthetic agents in young children.

Respiratory Physiology

A term newborn will have near full functionality of the lungs within several hours after birth. Its lung contains approximately 50 million alveoli, which grow during early childhood until reaching the adult level of approximately 500 million sometime before adolescence.

Healthy term newborns have a well-developed biochemical and reflex control of ventilation. Although they may demonstrate episodes of periodic breathing that last 5 seconds or more, in the healthy infant, these episodes of central apnea are self-limited and are not associated with clinically significant bradycardia, which may occur in preterm infants. Periodic breathing after the first month of life is not normal and should warrant further investigation.

One of the ways that respiratory physiologists measure ventilatory drive is to note the increase in ventilation when a subject inhales carbon dioxide (CO_2). The newborn's ventilatory response to breathing CO_2 will be less than that of older children. The newborn's response to breathing a hypoxic mixture is more unique and includes an immediate increase in ventilation that lasts about 1 minute, followed by a decrease in ventilation that lasts about 5 minutes. This reflects carotid body immaturity, and differs from older children in whom the initial protective phase of ventilatory stimulation has a longer duration. This shortened phase of ventilatory depression is even more prominent during hypercarbia, acidosis, or hypothermia.

Newborns demonstrate maladaptive respiratory depression (including apnea) in response to certain provocations that would normally result in stimulation of respiratory function in older infants. These stimuli may include lung inflation (Hering-Breuer reflex), stimulation of the carina or superior laryngeal nerve, and upper airway obstruction. Taken together, all these observations demonstrate the relatively weaker ability of newborns to adapt to acute hypoxemia.

The most important differences in respiratory function between children and adults are anatomically based, related to the growth and maturity of the chest wall during the first 2 years of life. These differences directly influence the mechanism by which functional residual capacity (FRC) is maintained. The newborn infant's FRC is established in the first several breaths after birth. In unanesthetized infants and adults, FRC is approximately the same, although the mechanisms by which FRC is attained are different in these two populations. However, when anesthetized, these differences impart substantial effects on FRC.

In neonates and small infants, the orientation of the ribs is more parallel than angled (Fig. 2.1). This results in a relative inefficiency of movement because the volume of the rib cage is not increased by raising the ribs as in older children and adults. At about 2 years of age, when the child spends more time in the upright position, the effect of gravity causes the ribs to be angled downward, and the rib cage then becomes more adult-like, thus providing an advantage to maintaining FRC while anesthetized. During early childhood development, the structure of the ribs becomes bonier and less cartilaginous and provides an inherent stiffness to the thoracic cavity. This stiffness imparts a tendency for the chest wall to expand outward, which counteracts the tendency for the lungs to collapse inward. The opposing tendencies between lungs and chest wall generate a slightly negative intrapleural pressure at the end of exhalation, and serve to maintain FRC in older children and adults, but this mechanism does not exist in infants.

The chest wall of neonates and small infants is primarily cartilaginous because it has not yet developed its bony components. It is highly compliant and tends to collapse

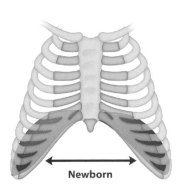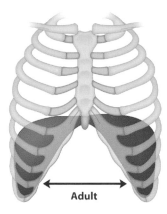

Newborn   **Adult**

• **Fig 2.1** Developmental changes of the rib cage and diaphragm from birth to adulthood. Adults can increase lung volume by raising the ribs and contracting the diaphragm. Early in development, the configuration of the rib cage and muscular attachments of the diaphragm place the newborn at a mechanical disadvantage because the ribs are already "raised," and contraction of the diaphragm results in a relatively smaller increase in thoracic cavity volume. (Illustration by Rob Fedirko.)

inward along with the lungs. As a consequence, infants must maintain their negative intrathoracic pressure (and negative intrapleural pressure) by active recruitment of accessory muscles of respiration, such as the intercostal muscles. In addition, the adductor muscles of the larynx of the neonate act as a valve; they contract during exhalation to maintain positive end-expiratory pressure and contribute to the maintenance of FRC. This phenomenon is called *laryngeal braking*. Newborns commonly demonstrate prominent abdominal excursions during normal breathing because of their reliance on diaphragmatic contraction for development of a sufficiently negative intrapleural pressure during inspiration. Despite the above-mentioned intrinsic mechanisms that attempt to maintain lung volumes, neonates may develop small airway collapse during normal tidal breathing.

These differences explain the marked changes in FRC in infants after the onset of general anesthesia that is normally not observed in older children and adults. After the administration of sedatives or anesthetics, older children and adults tend to maintain FRC. However, sedated or anesthetized infants will rapidly develop hypoxemia because their tonic muscular contraction that maintains FRC is lost. This loss of FRC can be remedied by application of continuous positive airway pressure (CPAP) or institution of positive-pressure breathing.

The unique anatomic insertion of the infant diaphragm affects respiratory function. At the initiation of inhalation, the newborn diaphragm is relatively flat. Its anterior insertion onto the internal surface of the rib cage confers a mechanical disadvantage during inspiration compared with the high-domed structure of the adult diaphragm. The muscular composition of the newborn's diaphragm is also unique. In contrast to the adult diaphragm, which has a high proportion (50%–60%) of slow-twitch, high-oxidative, fatigue-resistant (type 1) fibers, the newborn diaphragm is made up of only 10% to 30% type 1 fibers. This characteristic predisposes the newborn diaphragm to fatigue, and may contribute to the inherent instability of

the chest wall and apnea and respiratory failure in the face of increased ventilatory demands or work of breathing.

On a per-kilogram basis, tidal volume is the same for both neonates and adults and ranges from 7 to 9 mL/kg. Because oxygen consumption is relatively high in neonates and small infants (7–9 mL/kg versus 3 mL/kg for the adult), minute ventilation must be increased to deliver a sufficient amount of oxygen into the lungs (nearly three times that of the adult). As a consequence, small children have a relatively increased ratio of minute volume to FRC. This results in more rapid oxyhemoglobin desaturation during ventilatory depression or apnea.

The generalities are mentioned for discussion purposes only. Research studies demonstrate that respiratory function indices in children are primarily influenced by age, height, gender, stage of puberty, ethnicity, and coexisting disease. Therefore, it would be impossible to predict with any accuracy a given child's tidal volume, FRC, or any other ventilatory function without sophisticated testing.

Hematologic Physiology

At birth, the hemoglobin concentration is approximately 19 g/dL, of which 70% is fetal hemoglobin (Hgb F). This relatively high hemoglobin concentration is needed to offset the leftward shift of the oxyhemoglobin dissociation curve, which causes oxygen to be held tightly by Hgb F. During the first year of life Hgb F is progressively replaced by adult hemoglobin (Hgb A). Production of erythropoietin is absent until hemoglobin levels drop to the physiologic nadir of about 9 to 11 g/dL, between approximately 6 to 9 weeks of age. This is referred to as *physiologic anemia of infancy*. Although this relative anemia may decrease oxygen delivery to the peripheral tissues, it is offset by the increased production of Hgb A and increase in red-cell 2,3-diphosphoglycerate, both of which shift the oxyhemoglobin dissociation curve to the right, which facilitates unloading of oxygen to the peripheral tissues.

TABLE 2.1   Effect of Age on Coagulation Tests[a]

Test	25–31 Weeks Gestation	30–36 Weeks Gestation	Full-Term Newborn	1–10 Years	11–18 Years
Prothrombin time (s)	15.4 (15–17)	13 (11–16)	15 (14–16)	12 (11.4–13.7)	12.6 (11.4–13.8)
Partial thromboplastin time (s)	108 (80–168)	54 (28–79)	41 (32–47)	37 (31–44)	36 (30–43)
Bleeding time (s)	207 ± 105	157 ± 68	107 ± 38	420 (180–780)	300 (180–480)

[a]Values are mean, approximate normal range in parentheses, and standard deviations for bleeding times for neonatal ages

Coagulation factors are relatively low at birth and normalize within the first year of life (Table 2.1).

Cardiovascular Physiology

Substantial cellular and structural changes occur in the heart in the first several months of life. Neonatal cardiac muscle cells contain all the normal structural elements of the adult heart but are qualitatively and quantitatively different. The pattern of myofilaments is described as chaotic, compared with the long parallel rows of the mature heart. More specifically, the elements of the myocyte that are responsible for contraction are less able to function properly when challenged with a resistive load. Thus, force development is impaired compared with the adult heart, and cardiac output is relatively less in response to changes in preload and afterload. This makes intuitive sense when one considers that during fetal life the left side of the heart had little responsibility against a low-pressure systemic circuit, but in the postnatal period must adapt to a higher stroke volume and increased wall tension.

The postnatal left ventricle develops into a thick organ capable of contracting against higher systemic pressures by increasing the size and number of myocytes. In addition, the shape of the myocyte changes from spheroidal to one with more tapered edges, to increase efficiency of contraction. Factors that increase systemic vascular resistance (e.g., acidosis, cold, pain) in the newborn may lead to a decrease in cardiac output. Therefore, it is possible that intraoperative cardiovascular stability can be enhanced in the newborn by preventing hypothermia and adequately blunting the stress response[1] by titration of opioids. Indeed, a well-publicized, yet controversial, study[2] in newborn cardiac anesthesia suggested that an opioid-based anesthetic technique is associated with improved postoperative cardiac function.

One of the most important clinical correlations of these morphologic differences in the neonate is a decrease in compliance of the left ventricle. The newborn, therefore, is more prone to development of congestive heart failure during periods of fluid overload because the left ventricle is less able to stretch in response to this increase in stroke volume. Also, because of this stiffness, distention of either ventricle will result in compression and dysfunction of the contralateral ventricle, thus further decreasing cardiac function. Newborns with respiratory disease who require high inspiratory pressures may develop left ventricular dysfunction with right ventricular overload. Perhaps more importantly, the newborn left ventricle has an impaired ability to shorten normally, and the heart is less able to increase left ventricular stroke volume during periods of hypovolemia or bradycardia. Thus, episodes of hypovolemia or bradycardia can significantly decrease cardiac output in the neonate, and will endanger end organ perfusion.

Because of these differences in neonatal cardiac function it is often taught that increases in heart rate are needed to increase cardiac output. This should be done with caution, however. Cardiac output will fail to increase substantially if heart rate is increased to levels significantly above normal. Volume expansion also remains an effective method to increase blood pressure and cardiac output during, especially periods of hypovolemia.

Sympathetic innervation of the heart and production of catecholamines, which are not fully developed at birth, increase during postnatal maturation. In contrast, the parasympathetic system appears to be fully functional at birth. Thus, neonates and small infants will demonstrate an imbalance whereby seemingly minor stimuli (e.g., suctioning of the pharynx) result in an exaggerated parasympathetic or vagal response that results in bradycardia. For this reason, pediatric anesthesiologists may administer atropine before airway manipulation in small infants. The belief that bradycardia will result from too small a dose of atropine (<0.1 mg) was ultimately proven erroneous.[3]

These structural and physiologic differences in the cardiovascular system explain why neonates and infants under 6 months of age appear to be more sensitive to the depressant effects of volatile anesthetics. Isoflurane, sevoflurane, and desflurane appear to depress myocardial contractility equally.

The normal heart rate of the newborn ranges from 120 to 160 beats per minute (bpm). Lower rates (e.g., 85 bpm) are frequently observed during sleep, and higher rates

(>200 bpm) are common during anxiety or pain. Heart rates tend to decrease with age and parallel decreases in oxygen consumption. Many children have a noticeable variation in heart rate that varies with respiration (i.e., sinus arrhythmia).

Blood pressure increases gradually throughout childhood[4] and has a positive relationship with height. Taller children have higher blood pressure. These reference values have been retrospectively determined[5] for anesthetized children. Blood pressure ranges in premature infants have been defined[6] and will vary depending on the health status of the infant and mother. One of the most important current topics in pediatric anesthesia is defining the safe limits of blood pressure in young infants. As Mary Ellen McCann points out in her important paper[7] on the topic, these limits have not been delineated. However, there is accumulating evidence that low blood pressures may not be as safe as once thought.

In most children, careful auscultation of the heart reveals a soft, vibratory, systolic flow murmur. A heart murmur is considered abnormal when it is louder than II/VI or has a diastolic component. Peripheral pulses in children of all ages should be clearly palpable. Absence of femoral pulses may indicate an aortic arch abnormality. Capillary refill in the distal extremities should be brisk (less than 2 seconds), but may be slightly delayed in the first few hours of life. Distal limb cyanosis (acrocyanosis) is normal in the first few hours of life.

As described in Chapter 1, the fetal heart is characterized by right-sided dominance that gradually abates in the first few months of life as pulmonary pressures decrease toward normal adult values. The normal newborn ECG (Fig. 2.2) demonstrates a preponderance of right-sided forces with a mean QRS axis of +110 degrees (range +30 to +190

degrees), and decreasing R wave size from leads V1 to V6. T waves are normally inverted in lead AVR and the right-sided precordial leads. This gradually shifts to left-sided dominance during early childhood as the left ventricle hypertrophies to its normal size and the ECG becomes more like that of an adult.

The newborn cardiac output (about 350 mL/kg/min) falls over the first 2 months of life to about 150 mL/kg/min and then more gradually to the normal adult cardiac output of about 75 mL/kg/min.

Renal Physiology

By the 36th week of gestation, the formation of nephrons in the kidney is complete. However, the nephrons are small, and the glomerular filtration rate (GFR) is only 25% of adult values at birth. GFR reaches adult levels gradually during the first year of life. Tubular function is also immature; there is a decreased ability to concentrate and dilute the urine in the immediate newborn period. The maximal concentrating ability of the full-term newborn is 400 mOsm/L; the adult value of 1200 mOsm/L is attained by 1 year of age. Therefore, intraoperative evaporative fluid losses may result in development of hypernatremia in the neonate.

In newborn infants, daily fluid intake is gradually increased from 80 mL/kg on the first day of life to 150 mL/kg by the third or fourth day of life. It is adjusted based on additional factors, such as extreme prematurity or use of a radiant warmer, in which evaporative losses from the skin are increased. Neonates who are unable to ingest enteral feeds should receive supplementation of electrolytes (sodium, potassium, and calcium) on the second day of life (Table 2.2).

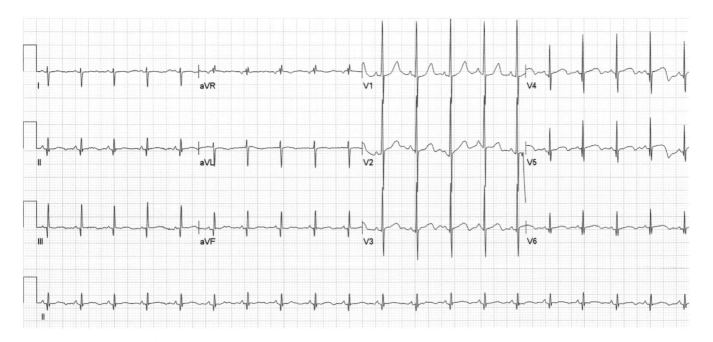

• **Fig 2.2** Normal newborn ECG. The normal newborn ECG demonstrates a preponderance of right-sided forces, as evidenced by a QRS axis greater than 90 degrees, and decreasing R wave size from right to left in the precordial leads. T waves are normally inverted in lead AVR and the right-sided precordial leads. (ECG courtesy Akash Patel.)

TABLE 2.2 Normal Newborn Daily Electrolyte Requirements

Electrolyte	Average Daily Requirement[a]
Sodium	2–3 mEq/kg
Potassium	1–2 mEq/kg
Calcium[b]	150–200 mg/kg

[a]Adjusted to normal values on a daily basis.
[b]In premature infants under 2,000 g.

Central Nervous System Physiology

The skull and CNS undergo substantial postnatal maturation. At birth, the brain is encased within several pieces of the skull that are separated by strong, fibrous, elastic tissues called *cranial sutures*. The anterior fontanel, located at the junction of the frontal and parietal bones, is formed by the intersection of the metopic, coronal, and sagittal sutures. Fusion of these sutures and closure of the anterior fontanel normally closes by 20 months of age. The posterior fontanel, located at the junction of the parietal and occipital bones, is formed by the intersection of the lambdoid and sagittal sutures. The posterior fontanel usually closes by 3 months of age.

The metabolic demand of the brain increases throughout the first year of life and then decreases gradually throughout childhood. The average cerebral metabolic rate of oxygen consumption ($CMRO_2$) of the child's brain (5.2 mL/min of oxygen per 100 g of brain tissue) is greater than the adult's brain (3.5 mL/min/100 g) and greater than that of anesthetized newborns and infants (2.3 mL/min/100 g).

Cerebral blood flow (CBF) is closely coupled to the $CMRO_2$. Whereas in adults the CBF is 50 to 60 mL/min per 100 g of brain tissue, the CBF of term newborns is approximately 40 mL/min/100 g and may be <5 mL/min/100 g in premature infants; in older children the CBF may reach 100 mL/min/100 g.

Autoregulation of CBF is based on systemic blood pressure. While it is thought that autoregulation does occur in newborns its limits are unknown. Extrapolation from animal studies indicates an approximate range of 20 to 80 mm Hg, in contrast to the adult whose autoregulatory limits lie between 60 and 150 mm Hg. Extremely premature infants may have largely pressure-passive CBF that predisposes to brain injury in the face of hypotension or hypertension.

Developmental Pharmacology

The broad subject of pharmacology encompasses the study of pharmacokinetics (the body's influence on the drug) and pharmacodynamics (the drug's influence on the body). Each of these two components is influenced by age and developmental stage. Major differences in pharmacology between adults and children exist because of differences in body composition that influence pharmacokinetics and pharmacodynamics. This section will review the ways in which these factors influence the pharmacology of intravenous and inhaled anesthetics in children.

Pharmacokinetics of Intravenous Anesthetics

The term *pharmacokinetics* describes the physiologic processes that alter a drug's disposition after entering the body. Pharmacokinetic processes determine the amount of drug that arrives at the effect site (the central nervous system for general anesthetic agents) at a given point in time (i.e., the "effect site" concentration) and the speed at which it arrives. The two general pharmacokinetic processes of interest are those that determine the rate and amount of drug that initially reaches the effect site, and those that determine the rate and amount of drug that leave the effect site. These two processes, which are of prime importance to anesthesiologists, are determined by a drug's unique combination of pharmacokinetic parameters: volume of distribution, distribution clearance, protein binding, and elimination clearance (metabolism and excretion). Each of these parameters will be discussed, with an emphasis on the changes that occur during development.

Volume of Distribution

The total (or steady-state) volume of distribution is the calculated amount of plasma into which the drug appears to have distributed at a specified interval after administration. It is not a discrete body compartment but rather is calculated by dividing the dose administered by the plasma concentration. Put another way, the dose of an intravenously administered drug is determined by multiplying the volume of distribution and the desired effect site concentration:

$$Dose\left(\tfrac{mg}{kg}\right) = Volume\ of\ Distribution\left(\tfrac{L}{kg}\right) \times Desired\ Effect\ Site\ Concentration\left(\tfrac{mg}{L}\right)$$

The relative percentage of extracellular and total body water is greatest at birth and declines with advancing age during childhood.[8] Because younger children have a relatively greater amount of extracellular body water and possess adipose stores with a relatively higher ratio of water to lipid than adults, the volume of distribution for water-soluble drugs, such as neuromuscular blockers, will be greater. A larger volume of distribution will be reflected as a larger loading (bolus) dose to achieve the desired plasma concentration and, if clearance is unchanged, a longer half-life.

Protein Binding

Parenterally administered medications are bound primarily to two proteins that are manufactured in the liver: albumin and alpha 1-acid glycoprotein. Albumin binds weak acids (e.g., aspirin), while alpha 1-acid glycoprotein binds weak bases (e.g., local anesthetics). Albumin levels are only slightly reduced in the newborn period but may have some qualitative immaturity. Alpha 1-acid glycoprotein is not fully produced until sometime in the first year of life. Therefore, drugs such as local anesthetics that are normally bound to alpha 1-acid glycoprotein may have a larger free fraction in the blood of young infants, which predisposes to systemic toxicity.

Metabolism

Most intravenously administered anesthetic drugs are lipid soluble and are metabolized in the liver or in the bloodstream. In general, children have more rapid clearance of drugs because of the relatively high proportion of blood traversing the liver. However, in neonates, the phase I (cytochrome-dependent) reactions—oxidation, reduction, and hydrolysis—are not fully developed. Therefore, some anesthetic-related drugs that rely on hepatic metabolism for termination of their action (e.g., vecuronium) may last longer than anticipated. These processes are usually fully functional within the first week

TABLE 2.3	Anesthetic-Related Drugs Metabolized by CYP2D6

- Codeine
- Dexamethasone
- Diphenhydramine
- Lidocaine
- Methadone
- Metoclopramide
- Ondansetron
- Ranitidine

after birth. However, the activities of some cytochromes, such as CYP3A4 and CYP3A5 (which metabolize midazolam, for example), continue to increase during the first 3 months of life. It appears that chronologic age, not postconceptional age, is important for development of these metabolic pathways.

Another important example of a cytochrome involved with metabolism of anesthetic drugs is CYP2D6 (Table 2.3 and Fig. 2.3). Levels of this cytochrome

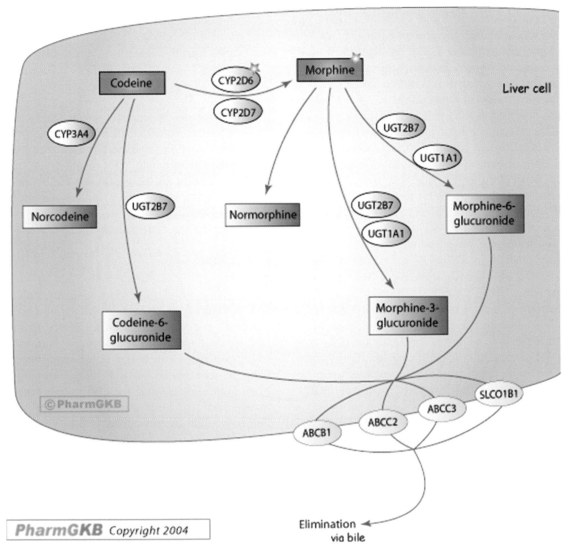

• **Fig 2.3** Codeine metabolism pathway. (Permission from PharmGKB and Stanford University.)

increase greatly and approach adult levels in the first 2 weeks of life. There is a great deal of genetic polymorphism variability of CYP2D6, which renders enzymatic activity from being nearly absent to substantially greater than average. As a result, an individual's metabolic activity can be categorized as *ultrarapid, extensive, intermediate* (the predominant phenotype), and *poor* (absence of enzyme activity). Poor metabolizers are at risk for drug accumulation and toxicity if the drug cannot be metabolized to its inactive form. Conversely, some drugs, such as codeine and tramadol, require metabolism to a beneficial active form, and thus, these poor metabolizers will not experience a drug effect. Ultrarapid metabolizers, on the other hand, are at risk for opioid toxicity. For these reasons, codeine should not be used to treat postoperative pain (in any aged child) because of the unpredictability of its effect. In fact, the FDA has issued several safety bulletins[9] that addressed this issue. Up to 10% of Caucasians are poor metabolizers, while up to 30% of Middle Easterners and North Africans are thought to be ultrarapid metabolizers.

The phase II reactions consist primarily of conjugation with sulfate, acetate, glucuronic acids, and amino acids. These reactions convert the parent drug to a more polar metabolite by introducing or unmasking a functional group (-OH, NH_2, -SH). These reactions are limited at birth but mature within the first few weeks of age, and may differ between classes of drugs.

Excretion

Excretion of intravenous anesthetic drugs is primarily via the kidney. In the first several weeks of life, especially in infants born at less than 34 weeks' gestation, GFR is below normal values, so excretion of drugs may be delayed. After the first several weeks of life, GFR and tubular secretion rise steadily during the first year of life.

Elimination Clearance

Clearance is the volume of plasma that is cleared of drug (by metabolism or excretion) per unit of time. Like the volume of distribution, it is a calculated value that is obtained by dividing the continuous infusion dose of a drug by the resulting plasma concentration:

$$Clearance\,(L/kg/h) = \frac{Dose\,(mg/kg/h)}{Plasma\,Concentration\,(mg/L)}$$

Infants and children tend to have a more rapid clearance of drugs than adults, and for drugs metabolized in the liver, there is an age-dependent increase in plasma clearance up to approximately 10 years of age. The mechanism of this is largely unknown, but it may be related to the fact that the liver receives a proportionately higher fraction of cardiac output in children than in adults.

Pharmacodynamics of Intravenous Anesthetics

Pharmacodynamics refers to the processes that affect the drug's action at a given plasma (or effect site) concentration. Developmental pharmacodynamic differences for most intravenous anesthetic agents are not well studied. However, it appears that neonates may be more sensitive to drugs that act in the central nervous system. This may be due, in part, to an age-dependency for passive diffusion into the brain (i.e., an immature blood-brain barrier) and to relatively greater central nervous system blood flow in neonates and small infants.

Pharmacokinetics of Inhaled Anesthetics

A variety of pharmacokinetic factors can influence the concentration of inhaled anesthetics in the brain and the speed at which this process occurs (i.e., uptake and distribution). The rate of rise of an inhaled anesthetic into the lungs is determined by the delivered concentration of the anesthetic and the minute ventilation of the patient, and is quantitatively described as the alveolar to inspired concentration ratio (F_A/F_I). Compared with adults, children demonstrate a higher minute ventilation per bodyweight and a higher tidal volume to FRC ratio, so the F_A/F_I ratio rises faster during an inhaled induction.

Once in the lungs, uptake of the anesthetic into the bloodstream is determined by the cardiac output, the blood-gas coefficient of the anesthetic agent, and the arterial-to-venous (A-V) concentration difference. All of these factors are influenced by the developmental age of the child.

Cardiac output per bodyweight is relatively higher in children than in adults. A higher cardiac output will tend to slow inhaled induction of anesthesia by removing anesthetic from the alveoli at a more rapid rate.

The blood-gas partition coefficient will determine the speed at which the inhaled anesthetic equilibrates between the alveolar gas and the blood. Although blood-gas partition coefficients have been shown to be lower in small children, it is to an insignificant degree, without clinical importance.

Anesthetic breathed into the alveoli moves into the bloodstream based on the concentration gradient difference between the alveolus and the blood in the pulmonary artery. Therefore, the larger the pulmonary A-V concentration difference, the more rapid the anesthetic will leave the alveoli, slowing the speed of induction. Upon initial uptake of inhaled anesthetic from the alveoli into the bloodstream, the anesthetic will be distributed to the various body tissues. As anesthetic partial pressures in tissues equilibrate with those in the blood, the concentration of the agent that returns to the lungs in the pulmonary artery increases. Consequently, the A-V difference decreases, which reduces the amount of anesthetic agent that is removed from the alveoli. This increases the partial pressure of the anesthetic agent in the alveolus and speeds loss of consciousness. Children demonstrate a faster decrease in the A-V difference because of their

TABLE 2.4	Effect of Age on Body Compartment		
	Vessel-Rich		
Age Group	Group	Muscle Group	Fat Group
Newborn	22.0%	38.7%	13.2%
1 year	17.3%	38.7%	25.4%
4 years	16.6%	40.7%	23.4%
8 years	13.2%	44.8%	21.4%
Adult	10.2%	50.0%	22.4%

proportionately larger vessel-rich group that equilibrates anesthetic relatively faster than in adults. As children grow, they increase their content of muscle and fat and take longer to equilibrate inhaled anesthetic (Table 2.4).

The combination of these differences in factors that affect uptake and distribution of inhaled anesthetics results in children demonstrating a more rapid inhaled induction compared with adults.

Pharmacodynamics of Inhaled Anesthetics

The relative potency of inhaled anesthetics, which is quantitatively described as the minimum alveolar concentration (MAC), changes with age.[10] MAC is relatively low for premature infants and gradually increases with age until approximately 6 months of age, after which it tends to decrease with advancing age. The reasons for these changes with age are unknown.

References

1. Anand KJ, Sippell WG, Aynsley-Green A. Randomised trial of fentanyl anaesthesia in preterm babies undergoing surgery: effects on the stress response. *Lancet*. 1987;1(8524):62–66. doi:10.1016/S0140-6736(87)91907-6.

2. Anand KJ, Hickey PR. Halothane-morphine compared with high-does sufentanil for anesthesia and postoperative analgesia in neonatal cardiac surgery. *N Engl J Med*. 1992;326(1):1–9. doi:10.1056/NEJM199201023260101.

3. Eisa L, Passi Y, Lerman J, Raczka M, Heard C. Do small doses of Atropine (<0.1 mg) cause bradycardia in young children? *Arch Dis Child*. 2015;100(7):684–688. doi:10.1136/archdischild-2014-307868.

4. Report of the Second Task Force on Blood Pressure Control in Children—1987 Task force on blood cressure Control in children. National Heart, Lung, and Blood Institute, Bethesda, Maryland. *Pediatrics*. 1987;79(1):1–25.

5. De Graaff JC, Pasma W, van Buuren S, et al. Reference values for noninvasive blood pressure in children during anesthesia: A multicentered retrospective observational cohort study. *Anesthesiology*. 2016;125(5):904–913. doi:10.1097/ALN.0000000000001310.

6. Hegyi T, Anwar M, Carbone MT, et al. Blood pressure ranges in premature infants: II. The first week of life. *Pediatrics*. 1996;97(3):336–342.

7. McCann ME, Lee JK, Inder T. Beyond anesthesia toxicity: anesthetic considerations to lessen the risk of neonatal neurological injury. *Anesth Analg*. 2019;129(5):1354–1364. doi:10.1213/ANE.0000000000004271.

8. Kearns GL, Abdel-Rahman SM, Alander SW, Blowey DL, Leeder JS, Kauffman RE. Developmental pharmacology — drug disposition, action, and therapy in infants and children. *N Engl J Med*. 2003;349:1157–1167. doi:10.1056/NEJMra035092.

9. U.S. Food & Drug Administration. (2020). *Codeine Information*. Updated May 26, 2020. https://www.fda.gov/drugs/drug-safety-and-availability/postmarket-drug-safety-information-patients-and-providers. Accessed Accessed 21.10.5.

10. Nickalls RW, Mapleson WW. Age-related iso-MAC charts for isoflurane, sevoflurane and desflurane in man. *Br J Anaesth*. 2003;91(2):170–174. doi:10.1093/bja/aeg132.

Suggested Reading

Lambrechts L, Fourie B. How to interpret an electrocardiogram in children. *BJA Educ*. 2020;20(8):266–277. doi:10.1016/j.bjae.2020.03.009.

3

Congenital Heart Disease

ADAM C. ADLER AND RONALD S. LITMAN

The overall incidence of **congenital heart disease (CHD)** is approximately 8 per 1000 live births and is usually divided into two categories: cyanotic (the defect contains a right-to-left shunt) and acyanotic (the defect may contain a left-to-right shunt). The most common cyanotic lesions, in order of decreasing frequency, are **pulmonary stenosis (PS)**, **transposition of the great arteries (TGA)**, **tetralogy of Fallot** (ToF), tricuspid atresia (TA), and pulmonary atresia with intact ventricular septum (PA/IVS). The most common acyanotic lesions, in order of descending frequency, are **ventricular septal defect (VSD)**, **atrial septal defect (ASD)**, aortic stenosis (AS), **coarctation of the aorta (CoA)**, persistent ductus arteriosus (PDA), and complete common atrioventricular canal (CCAVC).

Pathophysiology of Congenital Heart Disease

Anesthesia providers caring for children with CHD must fully understand the anatomic components of the lesion and how the blood flows through the heart and lungs. Because of the complexity of the lesions and subsequent repairs, this can often be confusing. Therefore, a structured approach should be used, with a focus on determining the relative ratios of pulmonary and systemic blood flow. These ratios may ultimately determine the important aspects of anesthetic management. This structured approach involves the following steps:

1. Determine whether blood flow is obstructed in any part of the heart. Right-sided obstructions decrease blood flow to the lungs and result in low PaO_2. Left-sided obstructions decrease blood flow to the body, resulting in decreased tissue perfusion, metabolic acidosis, and shock.
2. Determine whether blood is being shunted from one side of the heart to the other. If blood is shunted from the right side to the left side (e.g., ToF), it does not go through the lungs and results in cyanosis. Left-to-right shunting (e.g., VSD) will result in volume and pressure overload on either or both ventricles and may lead to CHF. In its advanced form, overcirculation of the pulmonary bed leads to pulmonary hypertension and, if untreated, irreversible pulmonary vascular obstructive disease. This results in a reversal of the shunt (to right-to-left) and causes hypoxemia and cyanosis (sometimes known as *Eisenmenger syndrome*). On a basic level, it may seem that the direction of shunting is determined by the location of the defect and obstruction. However, in many cases the resistance in the pulmonary and systemic circuits will determine the direction of shunt. Specialists in CHD like to refer to the ratio of pulmonary vascular resistance (PVR) to systemic vascular resistance (SVR), also expressed as pulmonary blood flow (Qp) and systemic blood flow (Qs), respectively. This ratio will determine whether the patient has a right-to-left shunt (Qp:Qs <1), a left-to-right shunt (Qp:Qs >1), or both at different times during the cardiac cycle. Other factors, such as ventricular failure or dilation and severe valvulopathy, may also contribute to shunting.
3. Determine whether there is a volume load or a pressure load on the heart. When a ventricle is overburdened by excessive volume overload (e.g., large VSD) or obstruction to forward flow (e.g., right ventricular outflow tract obstruction), the ventricle can begin to fail. In general, the right ventricle responds with dilatation, and the left ventricle with concentric hypertrophy. In either case, when the load exceeds the ventricular capacity, CHF develops. Left-sided CHF often results in pulmonary manifestations and/or systemic hypoperfusion while right-sided CHF can lead to hypoperfusion, hepatomegaly, liver dysfunction, and peripheral edema.

Once these three key points are determined, the anesthesia provider can begin to formulate a plan to safely anesthetize the child with CHD with respect to choice of anesthetic drugs, ventilation strategy and plan for responding to intraoperative cyanosis or hypotension. In the next section, we will take a closer look at the anatomy and physiology of some of the more common causes of CHD, starting with the acyanotic defects.

Acyanotic CHD

Ventricular Septal Defect

The most common congenital heart defect (approximately 25% of all congenital cardiac lesions) is the ventricular septal defect (VSD). There are five types of VSD, based on the anatomic location of the defect:

- **Muscular:** occurs in the posterior, apical, or anterior muscular portion of the septum and can be single or multiple.
- **Inlet:** occurs in the part of the septum underneath the septal leaflet of the tricuspid valve.
- **Conoseptal:** occurs in the outflow tract of the right ventricle beneath the pulmonary valve.
- **Conoventricular:** occurs in the membranous portion of the septum.
- **Malalignment:** results from a malalignment of the infundibular part of the septum.

A VSD may be isolated or occur in conjunction with other lesions (Fig. 3.1). The type of VSD does not usually influence anesthetic management; however, when it is

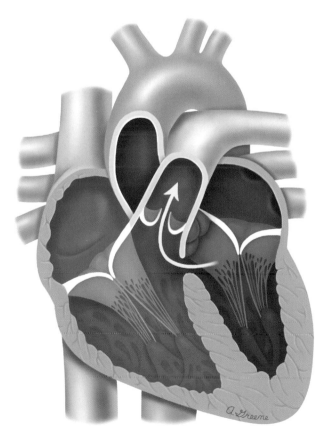

• **Fig 3.1.** Ventricular septal defect. (Reproduced with permission from: Fulton DR. Isolated ventricular septal defects in infants and children: anatomy, clinical features, and diagnosis. In: Post TW, ed. UpToDate (website). Accessed on 20.9.22. Available from: www.uptodate.com.)

excessively large or when associated with other anatomic defects, hemodynamic changes may occur during anesthesia.

The clinical features of a VSD are determined by its size and direction of blood flow. If the VSD is relatively small, there are usually no clinical symptoms. A large VSD allows unrestricted blood flow, the direction depending on the PVR to SVR ratio. In almost all children with a VSD, SVR is higher than PVR, and blood flows from left to right through the VSD. If untreated, over time this will result in CHF as the right ventricle becomes overloaded (from the normal venous return plus the extra volume from the left ventricle returning through the VSD). The excessive pulmonary blood flow eventually leads to pulmonary hypertension and reversal of the shunt (right-to-left flow leading to cyanosis).

Treatment of CHF may include digoxin, diuretics, and an angiotensin-converting enzyme (ACE) inhibitor while waiting for natural or surgical closure. Small muscular and conoventricular VSDs close naturally (40% by age 3 years, 75% by age 10 years); however, large VSDs should be closed surgically before pulmonary vascular changes become irreversible. Children with a previous VSD repair may occasionally demonstrate myocardial dysfunction, arrhythmias, or right bundle-branch block.

Atrial Septal Defect

Atrial septal defect (ASD) accounts for about 7.5% of CHD. There are multiple types based on the anatomic location of the defect (Fig. 3.2).

- **Ostium secundum:** occurs in the midportion of the atrial septum and is the most common form of ASD.
- **Ostium primum:** occurs low in the atrial septum.
- **Sinus venosus:** occurs at the junction of the right atrium and the SVC or IVC.
- **Coronary sinus:** refers to a hole in the wall of the coronary sinus as it traverses the left atrium.
- **Patent foramen ovale (PFO):** occurs when there is inadequate fusion of the septum secundum and the septum primum.

Nearly all small secundum type ASDs close spontaneously during the first year of life. However, large secundum ASDs, or those with significant shunting, will require surgical repair or placement of a closure device via cardiac catheterization.

Ostium primum, sinus venosus, and coronary sinus ASDs do not close spontaneously and must be closed surgically. PFOs occur in about 20% to 30% of the general population. Children are usually asymptomatic after ASD repair. Although there are no unique anesthetic considerations for noncardiac surgery, careful attention must be paid to de-bubbling the intravenous lines. Air bubbles that enter into the venous system may cross over to the arterial system and cause a clinically significant air embolus in the cardiac or cerebral arteries. The specific type of ASD does not influence anesthetic management unless it causes physiologic abnormalities.

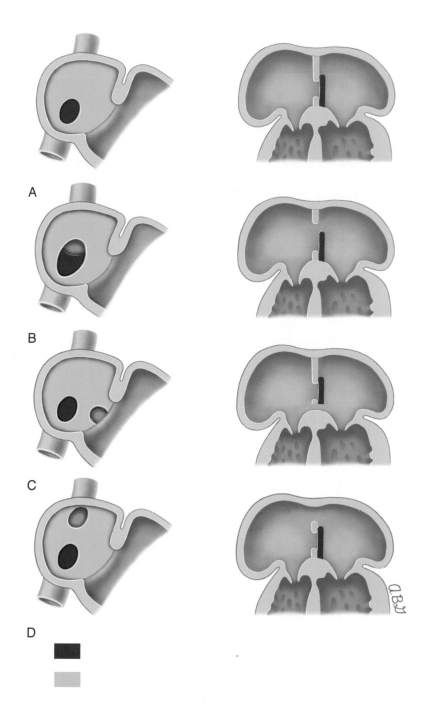

• **Fig 3.2.** Arterial septal defects. (Panel A) The normal atrial septum and various types of atrial septal defects (ASD) are shown. (Panel B) Secundum ASD is formed by the poor growth of the septum secundum or excessive absorption of the septum primum. (Panel C) Primum ASD is formed by the failure of the septum primum to fuse with the endocardial cushions. The fossa ovalis is normal. The frontal view of the primum ASD shows the caudal location of the ASD just above the endocardial cushion. (Panel D) Sinus venosus ASD is caused by the malposition of the insertion of the superior or inferior vena cava and is outside the area of the fossa ovalis. (Reproduced with permission from: Wick GW, Bezold LI. Isolated atrial septal defects (ASDs) in children: classification, clinical features, and diagnosis. In: Post TW, ed. *UpToDate* (website). Accessed on 20.9.22. Available from: www.uptodate.com.)

Complete Common Atrioventricular Canal

Complete common atrioventricular canal (CCAVC, also referred to as an *endocardial cushion defect*) consists of an ostium primum ASD and a nonrestrictive inlet VSD, and often occurs in children with trisomy 21. There is usually a left-to-right shunt at the atrial and ventricular levels which can result in CHF during infancy. Pulmonary hypertension may develop from the increase in pulmonary blood flow.

Surgical repair of CCAVC is usually performed in the first year of life. Complete heart block occurs in 5% of patients undergoing repair, and residual mitral insufficiency may be seen.

Patent Ductus Arteriosus

Before birth, blood bypasses the lungs and travels from the main pulmonary artery to the descending aorta through the ductus arteriosus (Fig. 3.3). Normally, there is *physiologic* ductus closure in the first days of life (because of pressure differences in the aorta and pulmonary artery) and *anatomic* closure in the first months of life. In certain conditions such as prematurity, the ductus remains patent indefinitely and serves as a source of left-to-right shunt and right-sided pulmonary overcirculation. **Patent ductus arteriosus (PDA)** represents approximately 7.5% of congenital heart disease.

A variety of factors tend to contribute to patency of the ductus arteriosus, such as hypoxemia, respiratory or metabolic acidosis, and persistent pulmonary hypertension of the newborn. The direction of shunted blood through a large PDA depends on the ratio of PVR to SVR. In a nonrestrictive PDA, a left-to-right shunt occurs if SVR is greater than PVR. Newborns with a large PDA and left-to-right shunt may show signs of pulmonary overcirculation and CHF, which include a widened pulse pressure, a continuous murmur, and an inability to wean ventilatory parameters. Treatment usually consists of diuretics until the PDA can be closed either medically, with administration of indomethacin, or surgically with an open or video-assisted catherization device closure (coil embolization).

It is crucial to identify ductal-dependent lesions in the newborn, in which patency of the ductus arteriosus is not only favorable but required for survival. These include cyanotic lesions such as pulmonary atresia/stenosis, tricuspid atresia/stenosis, and transposition of the great arteries, and some acyanotic lesions, such as coarctation of the aorta, hypoplastic left heart syndrome, critical aortic stenosis, and interrupted aortic arch. As soon as a ductal-dependent lesion is discovered, a prostaglandin E1 (PGE1; alprostadil) infusion is started at 0.05 to 0.1 mcg/kg/min. Infants should be monitored for apnea during administration of PGE1, and are maintained at relatively low concentrations of oxygen to encourage ductal patency.

Aortic Stenosis

Aortic stenosis (AS) represents up to 5% of CHD. It ranges in severity from mild to severe, or complete aortic atresia as seen in hypoplastic left heart syndrome (see below). The neonate with critical AS relies on their PDA for systemic blood flow; if the PDA closes, circulatory shock will occur. Most cases of mild AS are detected later in childhood by the presence of a murmur.

The clinical manifestations of AS will depend on the degree of stenosis and the ventricular function. Significant stenosis produces a large pressure gradient between the left ventricle and the aorta resulting in left ventricular hypertrophy with subsequent decreased ventricular compliance and function.

Hemodynamically significant AS requires surgical intervention, which is accomplished by balloon valvuloplasty or open surgical valvotomy. In some cases, treatment of AS causes aortic regurgitation, which may eventually require aortic valve replacement. In some children, a Ross procedure (pulmonary autograft) is performed, in which the child's own pulmonary valve is moved into the aortic position, and a right ventricle-to-pulmonary artery homograft conduit is placed.

Coarctation of the Aorta

Coarctation of the aorta (CoA) represents about 8% of all congenital heart defects, of which approximately 80% also have a bicuspid aortic valve. It usually occurs distal to the origin of the left subclavian artery at the insertion site of the ductus arteriosus. The coarctation narrows the aorta, thus increasing left ventricular afterload. CHF develops in about 10% of cases in infancy. There is a 15% to 20% risk for having CoA in girls with Turner syndrome (45, XO).

Neonates with severe CoA need their PDA to provide blood to the systemic circulation. If the PDA closes, the infant goes into circulatory shock. Therefore, PGE1 is administered to keep the ductus open until the CoA is repaired. More commonly, CoA presents during childhood.

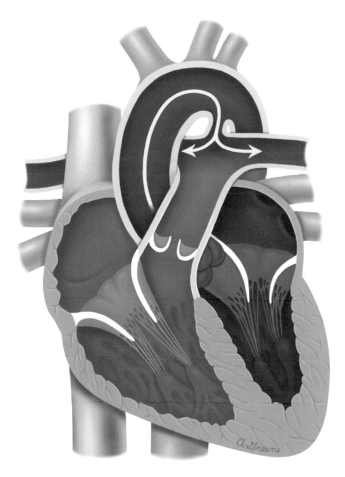

• **Fig 3.3.** Patent ductus arteriosus. (Reproduced with permission from: Doyle T, Kavanaugh-McHugh A. Clinical manifestations and diagnosis of patent ductus arteriosus in term infants, children, and adults. In: Post PW. *UpToDate* (website). Available from: www.uptodate.com.)

Typically, it is diagnosed during investigation of a new heart murmur, accompanied by hypertension of the upper extremities and decreased or absent femoral pulses. Left ventricular hypertrophy and CHF can result from chronic pressure overload.

The CoA can be treated by balloon dilation angioplasty, stent placement, surgical end-to-end anastomosis, subclavian flap repair, or graft placement. In many patients hypertension persists throughout childhood; the duration of postoperative hypertension correlates with the duration of hypertension before the repair.

Cyanotic Congenital Heart Diseasae

D-Transposition of the Great Arteries

D-transposition of the great arteries (TGA) accounts for about 5% of CHD and is the most common form of cyanotic CHD in the neonatal period. In TGA, the great vessels are transposed, which means that the aorta arises from the right ventricle, and the pulmonary artery rises from the left ventricle. Thus, circulation exists as two separate parallel circuits unless a communication (PDA, VSD, or PFO) can mix the blood to maintain survival. Infants with TGA will appear cyanotic shortly after birth when the PDA functionally closes. As soon as the diagnosis is made by echocardiogram (or even before), PGE1 is administered to maintain ductal patency, and the infant is considered for emergent balloon atrial septostomy in the cardiac catheterization lab to allow more complete mixing at the atrial level through an unrestricted communication.

Treatment for TGA requires the arterial switch operation[1] usually within the first 2 weeks of life. Survival exceeds 95%. Left ventricular function usually remains good throughout childhood, although supravalvular pulmonary stenosis may remain and require intervention. Occasionally, children will demonstrate atrial and ventricular tachyarrhythmias.

Hypoplastic Left Heart Syndrome

Hypoplastic left heart syndrome (HLHS) is the second most common type of cyanotic CHD. It presents in the first week of life, and is the most common cause of death from CHD in the first month of life. HLHS consists of hypoplasia of the left ventricle, aortic valve stenosis or atresia, mitral valve stenosis or atresia, and hypoplasia of the ascending aorta with a discrete CoA. The result is the lack of blood flow through the left heart, causing an obligatory left-to-right shunt at the atrial level and a right-to-left shunt through a PDA. Systemic flow becomes completely dependent on the PDA, and coronary perfusion is retrograde in the presence of aortic atresia or critical aortic stenosis. The diagnosis of HLHS is often made *in utero* or in the first few days of life when the PDA closes and the infant presents in heart failure and shock. Clinical signs include tachycardia, tachypnea, pulmonary rales (from pulmonary edema), hepatomegaly, and poor peripheral pulses with diminished distal capillary

refill. PGE1 is started immediately upon diagnosis to maintain ductal patency, and the infant is prepared for urgent surgery.

In most centers, treatment consists of a three-stage surgical correction performed over the first several years of life. In the first week of life, a Norwood procedure is performed to create a "neo-aorta" to establish unobstructed systemic blood flow. This allows the majority of neonates with HLHS to survive infancy. The single right ventricle provides systemic blood flow, and pulmonary blood flow is provided by placement of a modified Blalock–Taussig (subclavian-to-pulmonary artery) shunt (see below) or a right ventricle-to-PA conduit (Sano shunt). An atrial septectomy (or permanent ASD creation) is performed to create an unobstructed atrial communication to allow oxygenated blood flow to return from the lungs and reach the systemic circulation. After this initial stage the patient's oxygen saturation is usually 60% to 75%.

The second stage is usually performed between 4 and 6 months of age. The procedure is known as a hemi-Fontan (also called *bidirectional Glenn* or *Norwood 2*). The SVC is anastomosed to the right PA, so that blood returning from the head bypasses the right ventricle and flows passively into the pulmonary circulation. This procedure is delayed until the patient's PVR, which continues to drop after birth, decreases to the point at which the lungs are able to accept the additional blood flow. The second stage also decreases the effective blood flow load on the single ventricle. At this age, the patient does not require their BT shunt, as the newly created SVC-to-PA anastomosis serves as the source of pulmonary blood flow. After this stage, the patient's oxygen saturation is usually 70% to 85%.

The third stage, performed at approximately 2 to 3 years of age, is the completion Fontan, in which the IVC is joined directly to the pulmonary artery. After this procedure, all venous blood returning to the heart bypasses the single ventricle heart and flows passively into the lungs, while the single right ventricle serves to pump oxygenated blood returning from the lungs to the body. After this stage, the patient's oxygen saturation now approaches normal values for the first time. Patients with a fenestrated Fontan (a small hole or connection between the IVC-PA connection and the atrium) may serve as a source of right-to-left shunt reducing the patient's normal saturation. Shunting across the fenestration occurs during times of elevated pulmonary pressure.

The circulation that remains is referred to as *Fontan physiology*. Blood flow to the lungs becomes dependent on the transpulmonary gradient, which is the pressure difference between the Fontan circuit (systemic veins and pulmonary arteries) and the pulmonary venous atrium. Thus, any condition that increases PVR will decrease blood flow through the lungs and cause hypoxemia (Table 3.1).

A number of perioperative factors can decrease pulmonary blood flow. After a Fontan procedure, patients may develop atrial arrhythmias or complete heart block. These arrhythmias are poorly tolerated because of the relatively large contribution of atrial contraction to ventricular filling.

TABLE 3.1	Determinants Of Pulmonary Blood Flow	
Factors that Increase Pulmonary Blood Flow	**Factors that Decrease Pulmonary Blood Flow**
• Decreased PVR • Hyperoxia • Hypocarbia • Alkalosis • Hypertension or increased SVR (e.g., inotropic therapy) in patients with single-ventricle physiology • Low mean airway pressure	• Increased PVR • Hypoxia • Hypercarbia • Acidosis • Hypotension or lowering of SVR (e.g., inhaled anesthetics) in patients with single-ventricle physiology • Positive end-expiratory pressure (PEEP)

Adult patients with Fontan physiology may progressively develop myocardial failure, which sometimes manifests as ventricular arrhythmias.

Inhaled anesthetics decrease SVR by dilating arteriolar and venous beds, resulting in a decrease in venous return. This may critically limit pulmonary blood flow by decreasing the transpulmonary gradient. In a patient with Fontan physiology, positive-pressure ventilation can also decrease pulmonary blood flow. Positive end-expiratory pressure (PEEP) and elevated mean airway pressures can impede venous return and decrease pulmonary blood flow. These patients may become hypotensive during induction of anesthesia, or with prolonged NPO duration or gastrointestinal (GI) illnesses. Patients with Fontan circulation require judicious fluid monitoring and the shortest possible NPO times. Spontaneous ventilation is preferred in these patients as negative intrathoracic pressure increases the gradient between extrathoracic and intrathoracic pressures and results in increased flow through the pulmonary circulation. Preferred anesthetic techniques in the Fontan patient include use of a face mask or supraglottic airway with spontaneous ventilation, or a regional technique with IV sedation. However, atelectasis is likely in longer cases, in which controlled ventilation may be the most prudent option, with the goal of immediate tracheal extubation at the completion of the procedure.

Pulmonary Stenosis

Pulmonary Stenosis (PS) accounts for approximately 8% of all CHD and usually occurs at the level of the valve, although subvalvular and supravalvular stenoses may occur. It can also occur as a component of other heart defects, especially tetralogy of Fallot. The clinical manifestations of PS depend on the degree of valve restriction. Right ventricular hypertrophy occurs as the ventricle attempts to maintain cardiac output. Symptoms of severe PS include CHF and cyanosis.

Moderate and severe PS (gradient ≥50 mm Hg) are treated with balloon valvuloplasty. Open surgical repair may be necessary in some cases. Once dilated or repaired, children with isolated PS are relatively healthy and usually present no further anesthetic considerations.

PS should not be confused with peripheral pulmonic stenosis, which is a benign condition of the newborn that produces a murmur as a result of the acute angle of bifurcation of the main pulmonary artery.

Tetralogy of Fallot

After the immediate newborn period, tetra of Fallot (ToF) (Fig. 3.4) is the leading cause of cyanotic CHD. ToF encompasses four defects: typically, infundibular hypoplasia (the area between the aortic and pulmonary valves) results in a shift of tissue to the right compressing the right ventricular outflow tract to varying degrees. The right ventricular outflow tract obstruction results in compensatory right ventricular hypertrophy. This movement also includes a portion of the ventricular septum resulting in an anterior malalignment VSD together with the aorta which overrides the VSD. Cyanosis results from right-to-left shunting across the VSD and decreased pulmonary blood flow caused by the right ventricular outflow tract obstruction. The degree of right ventricular outflow tract obstruction determines the overall severity of the defect.

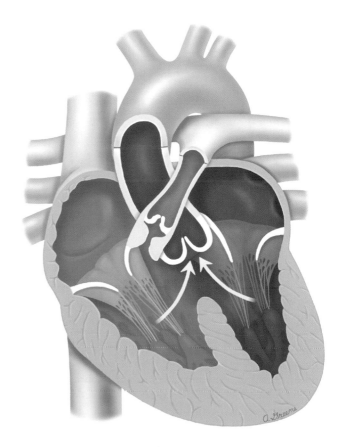

• **Fig 3.4.** Tetralogy of Fallot. (Reproduced with permission from: Doyle T, Kavanaugh-McHugh A, Graham, Jr, TP. Pathophysiology, clinical features, and diagnosis of tetralogy of Fallot. In: Post PW. *UpToDate* (website). Available from: www.uptodate.com. Accessed 04/29/2022)

If ToF is not corrected during infancy, the child may experience sudden episodes of cyanosis secondary to infundibular spasm that worsens right ventricular outflow tract obstruction. These are commonly known as *Tet spells*, and they may last minutes to hours. They usually resolve spontaneously but might lead to syncope, progressive hypoxia, or death. Tet spells can occur at any time in the perioperative period and can be treated by diminishing right-to-left shunting by increasing SVR and decreasing PVR. They are treated by a stepwise approach, consisting of placing the child in the knee-chest position, administration of a sedative, such as an opioid or benzodiazepine, administration of a beta-blocker, such as propranolol or esmolol, or administration of phenylephrine.

ToF is usually repaired within the first 6 months of life, depending on the anatomic variation. Pulmonary stenosis and right ventricular outflow tract obstruction are managed initially by balloon angioplasty followed by patch VSD closure. Postoperatively, these infants commonly exhibit some degree of residual pulmonary insufficiency and right bundle-branch block. Ventricular arrhythmias may occur in adolescence when there is pulmonary insufficiency and right ventricular dilatation or dysfunction.

Tricuspid Valve Atresia

Tricuspid valve atresia (TA) leads to hypoplasia or absence of the right ventricle. An associated VSD is found in 90% of TA cases. Blood passes from the right atrium to the left atrium and into the systemic circulation via the aorta or the lungs via the ductus arteriosus. The VSD allows blood to pass from the left ventricle to the right ventricle and into the pulmonary artery, however, the majority of patients with TA also have pulmonary stenosis. Newborns with TA manifest cyanosis, poor feeding, and tachypnea within the first 2 weeks of life. Cyanosis in the neonatal period is correlated with the amount of restriction of pulmonary blood flow. PGE1 is administered to maintain ductal patency and pulmonary flow, and a balloon atrial septostomy is performed if the atrial defect is not adequate. Surgical management involves placing a modified Blalock–Taussig shunt to maintain pulmonary blood flow. Later in infancy, a cavopulmonary anastomosis (hemi-Fontan or bidirectional Glenn) is performed to provide stable pulmonary blood flow. In most centers, a modified Fontan procedure is performed to redirect the inferior vena cava and hepatic vein flow into the pulmonary circulation. Compared with HLHS patients, these children usually benefit from having the left ventricle remain the primary pumping chamber for the systemic circulation.

Anesthetic Management of Children With CHD

Preoperative Assessment

The extent of the preoperative evaluation depends on the underlying diagnosis, degree of hemodynamic stability, and coexisting medical conditions. The anatomic and hemodynamic function of the child's heart should be mapped out, and previous anesthetics reviewed. Children that are currently under the care of a cardiologist should have an updated consult that includes a description of the child's cardiac anatomy.

The best way to determine the child's functional status is to assess limitations of daily activities and exercise. The feeding patterns of infants may provide a clue to cardiac function because of the physical effort involved to coordinate suck and swallow. Cardiac reserve is likely reduced if an infant is unable to finish a feed without tiring, or develops cyanosis, diaphoresis, or respiratory distress during feeding. Smaller children with limited cardiac output and increasing oxygen consumption will demonstrate failure to thrive or decreased normal activity. Older children may become more sedentary. Syncope, palpitations, and chest pain are additional symptoms of cardiac limitation that should be investigated before elective surgery.

Medications administered to children with CHD include diuretics, afterload reduction agents, antipulmonary hypertensives, antiarrhythmics, antiplatelet or anticoagulation drugs, and possibly inotropic or immunosuppressant agents in heart transplant recipients. All scheduled medications should be taken on the day of surgery, except for diuretics, which are usually withheld, depending on the clinical condition of the child. Children taking diuretics should have a preoperative evaluation of electrolytes.

Preoperative laboratory or diagnostic testing will depend on the nature of the child's disease and recent manifestations. A hemoglobin level may be indicated for children with cyanotic CHD who compensate for chronic hypoxemia by developing polycythemia. A hematocrit that approaches 65% will increase blood viscosity and interfere with tissue microcirculation, contribute to tissue hypoxia, increase SVR, and predispose to venous thrombosis and strokes. A normal or low hematocrit may indicate relative anemia, and is usually caused by iron deficiency. Iron-deficient red blood cells are less deformable and increase blood viscosity. Anemia or polycythemia should be evaluated and corrected before elective surgery. This is often done in consultation with the patient's cardiologist and/or hematologist.

Preoperative vital signs, including room air SpO_2, are used as a baseline to determine intraoperative norms. Baseline heart sounds, and the presence of cyanosis or pallor should be noted. The presence of tachypnea or rales on lung auscultation may indicate pneumonia or CHF. An upper respiratory tract infection warrants particularly careful evaluation and possible cancellation, as it may lead to complications in children with CHD, especially when caused by respiratory syncytial virus (RSV).

CHD may be accompanied by tracheobronchial anomalies, such as shortening or stenosis, and may remain unrecognized until endotracheal intubation is required. This is particularly true for children with trisomy 21. A history of prolonged intubation after CHD surgery raises the possibility of an airway abnormality. Inspiratory stridor is an indication of airway narrowing because of subglottic stenosis or a vascular malformation that causes compression of the lower airway.

Neurologic abnormalities are not uncommon in children with CHD. The presence of a right-to-left shunt with polycythemia may predispose to an embolic stroke. Cardiopulmonary bypass is associated with microemboli that travel to the brain and cause vascular occlusion.

Preoperative dehydration may be hazardous in children with cyanotic CHD and polycythemia. Attention to preoperative oral or IV hydration is especially important for children with ToF, cyanotic patients with polycythemia, and children with Fontan physiology. Dehydration may cause ToF patients to have a hypercyanotic Tet spell. Fontan patients are dependent on venous return for pulmonary blood flow; thus, dehydration may lead to decreased central venous pressure and subsequent decreased pulmonary blood flow and poor cardiac output. These patients may benefit from preoperative admission for overnight hydration. Fasting intervals should be no different for children with CHD than for healthy children and drinking clear liquids 1 to 2 hours before planned induction of general anesthesia should be encouraged.

Premedication with oral midazolam is useful to allay preoperative anxiety, and even hemodynamically unstable children can receive carefully titrated IV midazolam. The advantages of preoperative anxiolysis in children with CHD include easy separation from parents, less crying, decreased oxygen consumption, and decreased levels of intraoperative anesthetics. Some anesthesiologists fear that even minimal respiratory depression caused by sedatives may cause significant oxyhemoglobin desaturation in children with cyanotic CHD whose resting oxyhemoglobin saturations lie on the steep portion of the hemoglobin dissociation curve. However, several investigations that assessed this risk demonstrated that preoperative anxiolysis resulted in less oxyhemoglobin desaturation during induction of anesthesia.

Subacute Bacterial Endocarditis (SBE) Prophylaxis

The American Heart Association published updated guidelines[2] in 2015 on administration of prophylactic antibiotics to prevent infective endocarditis (IE), an infection of the endocardial surface of the heart, in susceptible children. The mechanism of IE involves endothelial damage with platelet and fibrin deposition, which allow for bacterial colonization. "Subacute" refers to the slow and often ambiguous onset and detection of the infection in patients with preexisting heart disease, and is associated, generally, with good outcomes. Perioperative antibiotics are recommended for dental procedures that involve manipulation of gingival tissue or perforation of oral mucosa in the following types of high-risk patients who have cardiac conditions that include the following:

- Prosthetic cardiac valves
- Previous endocarditis
- Unrepaired cyanotic CHD, including palliative shunts and conduits
- Completely repaired CHD repaired with prosthetic material or device, whether placed surgically or by catheter intervention, during the first 6 months after the procedure
- Repaired CHD with residual defects at the site or adjacent to the site of a prosthetic patch or prosthetic device
- Cardiac transplant recipients with valve regurgitation because of a structurally abnormal valve

Antibiotic prophylaxis for IE is no longer recommended for patients (without an active infection) undergoing GI and genitourinary (GU) procedures, transesophageal echocardiograms, and respiratory tract procedures, unless there is an incision of the mucosa. Respiratory procedures that should be covered include tonsillectomy, adenoidectomy, bronchoscopy, nasotracheal intubation, and any other procedure that involves an incision of the respiratory mucosa. Note that the recommended SBE prophylaxis dose is typically greater than the standard dose for surgical site infection prophylaxis and dose adjustments should be made accordingly (Table 3.2).

Anesthetic Techniques in Children With CHD

By virtue of their propensity to cause hemodynamic compromise in susceptible CHD patients, there is no anesthetic regimen that is inherently safer than any other. All volatile anesthetics can alter PVR, SVR, myocardial contractility, heart rhythm, heart rate, and shunt flow. In healthy patients, isoflurane produces a drop in SVR by vasodilation, which may decrease mean arterial pressure. In children with CHD, isoflurane slightly increases heart rate and tends to maintain cardiac index. In normal children and in those with CHD, sevoflurane decreases SVR and can decrease the LV shortening fraction, yet cardiac index and heart rate are maintained. Sevoflurane can also produce diastolic dysfunction. Nitrous oxide produces minimal myocardial depression, and although it is associated with increased PVR in adults, it produces minimal changes in infants with both normal and increased PVR. Nitrous oxide can, however, increase the size of an air embolus.

In children with right-to-left shunts, inhaled induction may result in an increased shunt fraction and cyanosis secondary to a decrease in SVR. In these children, a slow titration of agent is necessary with frequent measurements of blood pressure. The occurrence of hypoxemia that is not the result of respiratory causes should be attributed to systemic vasodilation and right-to-left shunting and should be treated with a direct vasoconstrictor such as phenylephrine.

Intracardiac shunts can affect the rate of anesthetic induction. In the presence of a right-to-left shunt, dilution of anesthetic agent in the left ventricle by venous blood that bypasses the lung results in a decreased concentration

TABLE 3.2	Regimens for Antimicrobial Prophylaxis for a Dental Procedures

Regimen: Single Dose 30–60 min Before Procedure

Situation	Agent	Children	Adults
Oral	Amoxicillin	50 mg/kg	2 g
Unable to take oral medication	Ampicillin	50 mg/kg, IM or IV	2 g, IM or IV
Allergic to penicillins or oral ampicillin	Cephalexin[b,c]	50 mg/kg	2 g
	OR		
	Clindamycin	20 mg/kg	600 mg
	OR		
	Azithromycin or clarithromycin	15 mg/kg	500 mg
Allergic to penicillins or ampicillin and unable to take oral medication	Cefazolin or ceftriaxone[e]	50 mg/kg, IM or IV (cefazolin); 50 mg/kg, IM or IV (ceftriaxone)	1 g, IM or IV
	OR		
	Clindamycin	20 mg/kg, IM or IV	600 mg, IM or IV

IM, intramuscular; *IV*, intravenous.

[a]Pediatric dosage should not exceed recommended adult dosage.

[b]Or other first- or second-generation oral cephalosporin in equivalent pediatric or adult dosage.

[c]Cephalosporins should not be used in a person with a history of anaphylaxis, angioedema, or urticaria with penicillins or ampicillin.

[From: Baltimore RS, Gewitz M, Baddour LM, et al; American Heart Association Rheumatic Fever, Endocarditis, and Kawasaki Disease Committee of the Council on Cardiovascular Disease in the Young and the Council on Cardiovascular and Stroke Nursing. Infective endocarditis in childhood: 2015 update: a scientific statement from the American Heart Association. *Circulation*. 2015;132(15):1487–1515.)

of agent reaching the brain. This will, theoretically, slow the rate of induction of anesthesia. Conversely, left-to-right shunts may speed induction of anesthesia by rapidly decreasing the arterial-to-venous difference of agent in the lungs. In clinical practice, these effects are hardly noticeable.

Small amounts of air trapped in IV tubing that enters the circulation can cause complications in children with CHD. Therefore, IV lines must be de-aired before connection. With a right-to-left shunt, an injected air bubble can cross into the systemic circulation and cause a stroke if it passes from the aorta to the brain via a carotid or vertebral artery or result in other end organ damage. With a left-to-right shunt, air bubbles pass into the lungs and are absorbed.

High oxygen concentrations decrease PVR and increase SVR; hypoxemia increases PVR and decreases SVR. These changes may significantly alter pulmonary blood flow by changing the PVR to SVR ratio in the presence of a large, unrestrictive intracardiac shunt.

Intravenous induction of general anesthesia with propofol can be accomplished by titrating the drug judiciously, depending on the patient's tolerance for changes in heart rate and blood pressure. In theory, a left-to-right shunt will slow IV induction and a right-to-left shunt will speed the time of induction by shunting more anesthetic agent to the brain without passing first through the lungs. But as with inhaled induction, these effects are difficult to appreciate clinically.

Ketamine, etomidate, and dexmedetomidine may provide greater hemodynamic stability in children with CHD. The sympathomimetic effects of ketamine tend to maintain heart rate, contractility, and SVR. There are theoretical concerns with ketamine's ability to cause an increase in PVR, especially in patients with Fontan physiology. However, this has not been substantiated in clinical studies performed in children with CHD. For the most part, opioids and benzodiazepines are safe in children with CHD as long as clinically significant bradycardia is avoided.

Regional anesthesia should be encouraged in children with CHD but with several caveats:

1. The child with longstanding CoA and dilated tortuous intercostal arteries is at risk for arterial puncture or excessive absorption of local anesthetic during intercostal blockade.
2. Because the lungs may absorb up to 80% of the local anesthetic on first passage, the risk for local anesthetic toxicity is theoretically increased in a patient with a right-to-left shunt because the brain will be exposed to a higher concentration than usual.
3. Vasodilatation resulting from central axis blockade may be hazardous in patients with left-sided obstructive lesions. Vasodilatation may also cause a decrease in oxyhemoglobin saturation in children with a right-to-left shunt. On the other hand, peripheral vasodilatation in patients with polycythemia may have the benefit of improved microcirculatory flow and decreased venous thrombosis.
4. Children with chronic cyanosis are at risk for coagulation abnormalities and should be adequately evaluated before initiation of regional anesthesia.

Monitoring Children with CHD

Pulse oximetry reliably predicts oxyhemoglobin saturation in the range that is normally encountered in children with cyanotic CHD (SpO_2 70%–90%). However, it may have limited accuracy at oxyhemoglobin saturations below 70%, and should be verified by blood gas analysis when in question.

Intraoperative $P_{ET}CO_2$ monitoring can be unreliable in children with CHD. $P_{ET}CO_2$ will tend to underestimate $PaCO_2$ because abnormal pulmonary ventilation/perfusion ratios result in increased dead space and/or shunt, which alter the arterial-to- $P_{ET}CO_2$ difference.

Blood pressure monitoring accuracy in children with CHD will depend on the presence of arterial tree malformations and anatomic alteration by previous surgical corrections. For example, a modified Blalock–Taussig shunt or left subclavian flap procedure for CoA repair may render the blood pressure reading in the respective extremity inaccurate or difficult to obtain. Before CoA repair, lower-extremity blood pressure readings will differ from upper extremity pressures.

Postoperative Management of Children With CHD

Hypoventilation or mildly decreased oxyhemoglobin saturation are particularly hazardous in children with CHD. After tracheal extubation, oxygen should be administered during transport to the PACU (or ICU) and gradually weaned based on the patient's clinical condition. In patients with single ventricle or stage I physiology, oxygen saturation should be titrated to 85% for fear of decreasing PVR, increasing pulmonary blood flow, and decreasing systemic blood flow. Postoperatively, an anesthesiologist or intensivist familiar with their specific cardiac disease should follow these children closely. Analgesics and commonly used antiemetics are well tolerated in children with CHD.

References

1. Arterial Switch Operation for Transposition of the Great Arteries. Cincinnati Children's. Accessed on June 23, 2021. https://youtu.be/QNUnZqoeBTo.
2. Baltimore RS, Gewitz M, Baddour LM, et al. Infective Endocarditis in Childhood: 2015 Update: A Scientific Statement From the American Heart Association. *Circulation*. 2015;132(15):1487–1515. https://doi.org/10.1161/CIR.0000000000000298.

Suggested Readings

Marjot R, Valentine SJ. Arterial oxygen saturation following premedication for cardiac surgery. *Br J Anaesth*. 1990;64(6):737–740.

4

Respiratory Diseases

LAURA PETRINI AND RONALD S. LITMAN

Upper Respiratory Infection

Upper respiratory infection (URI) is common in children presenting for anesthesia and the most common infection overall in children. The average child will have 6 to 8 URIs per year. Thus, it is important to understand the pathogenesis, clinical features, risk stratification, and anesthetic management of children with a URI.

URIs are almost always viral. Rhinoviruses are the most common, but influenza, parainfluenza, respiratory syncytial virus (RSV), adenovirus, and coronavirus are also seen. Although the specific virus can be identified by laboratory testing, this is rarely performed.

Viral transmission most commonly occurs via mucosal contact from hands contaminated with infectious material, inhalation of airborne particles, or droplet contact with mucosa (e.g., sneezing). For this reason, patients with a URI will likely be on both contact and droplet type precautions when hospitalized, mainly to protect staff. Symptoms are caused by the child's immune response to the virus. For example, the influx of polymorphonuclear (PMN) cells in response to cytokine signals results in increased nasal secretions.

The symptoms of a URI vary based on the age of the patient and the specific virus. Most commonly, patients will present with nasal congestion, rhinorrhea, cough, and sneezing. Fever is less common (reported in approximately 15% of cases) and, if persistent, may be the sign of a bacterial infection such as otitis media, *Streptococcal* tonsillitis, or pneumonia. The color of nasal secretions is not indicative of severity of infection; rather, color is dictated by the number and activity of the PMN cells in the immune response.

A current or recent URI increases the risk for a perioperative respiratory adverse event (PRAE). These events range from benign coughing to serious laryngospasm, bronchospasm, or hypoxia that results in the need for escalation of care. Some clues to the risks of URI can be gleaned by the results of a 2010 study[1] in over 9000 patients. A positive respiratory history (nocturnal dry cough, wheezing during exercise, wheezing more than three times in the past 12 months, or a history of present or past eczema) in a child with a URI was associated with an increased risk for intraoperative bronchospasm, laryngospasm, and perioperative cough, desaturation, or airway obstruction. In addition, a history of at least two family members having asthma, atopy, or smoking increased the risk for PRAEs.

The risk for a PRAE decreases with time after initial infection, although controversy exists about the duration of time required for reduction of risk (ranging from 2 to 6 weeks). Because of this uncertainty, there is also no consensus when to schedule elective surgery after an acute URI. In a 1979 publication[2] that described the development of lower respiratory symptoms during general anesthesia in children with a URI, McGill and colleagues from National Children's Hospital wrote: "the optimal period of recovery from the URI that should be allowed before considering the patient a candidate for an elective surgical procedure has not been defined." More than 40 years later, this is still true. Subclinical pathology, such as airway edema, atelectasis, and bronchial reactivity may remain for up to several weeks after the symptoms of the acute URI have resolved, depending on the specific type of viral agent. Three to 4 weeks seems to be a reasonable waiting time, but for many children this merely represents the period between successive infections.

With these possible complications in mind, when a child presents with a URI, it is intuitive that an elective procedure requiring general anesthesia should be canceled. But, because so many children have a concurrent URI at the time of their scheduled surgery and long-term negative outcomes have not been demonstrated, this decision process is complex. How should the anesthesia provider decide when to cancel an elective procedure in a child with a URI? First, one should assess the severity of the child's illness. The child with a runny nose without additional findings may be suffering from vasomotor or allergic rhinitis, which is usually not associated with perioperative airway complications. If it is likely that the illness is viral, one must then identify the factors that increase perioperative complications. These include the following:

- Significant coexisting medical disease (especially cardiac, pulmonary, or neuromuscular disease)
- History of prematurity
- Lower respiratory tract signs (e.g., wheezing, rales)
- High fever (>102°F)
- Productive cough

- Major airway, abdominal, or thoracic surgery
- Parent is worried about proceeding
- Surgeon is worried about proceeding (That'll be the day!)

If any of these risk factors are present, it may be prudent to perform the procedure when the child is in better health.

On the other hand, there are a variety of additional factors that may influence your decision to proceed with surgery. The most common reason for proceeding with a case even though risk factors are present is the presence of a URI that will likely continue without surgical intervention. This occurs when children require adenoidectomy or myringotomy to relieve chronic middle ear fluid collections. Nonmedical factors that might sway you to proceed with the case are logistical family concerns, such as the parents taking a day off from work, difficulty obtaining day care, traveling a long distance at a great inconvenience, and so forth. Because outcomes are not proven to be worse after surgery in children with a URI, these factors may play a role in the decision of whether or not to proceed. Most children who present with a URI have neither extremely mild symptoms nor severe symptoms. For these in-between children we must use our judgment to determine the proper course of action based on what we believe is best for the child.

Racial identity may influence risk. In a 2018 publication[3] from the University of Texas, African American children were shown to have significantly higher odds of PRAEs compared with a Caucasian group.

For urgent or emergent procedures, a discussion with the patient and family about the risk for PRAEs is prudent. In these situations, surgery will often need to proceed because of the risk for delaying. To optimize the patient preoperatively, additional treatments can be considered including:

- Inhaled beta agonist therapy (e.g., albuterol) is useful in patients with a history of asthma, although may also be of benefit to those with no prior diagnosis who present with wheezing secondary to a URI.
- Anticholinergics (e.g., glycopyrrolate) can be given to dry secretions but their use has not been proven effective.
- Steroids are rarely beneficial for a simple URI, except when the patient is presenting with a concomitant asthma exacerbation.

The risk for a PRAE can be approximately determined by clues from the preoperative evaluation. A history of fever, increased work of breathing, productive cough, wheeze, shortness of breath, copious secretions, or lethargy are important symptoms that may increase risk. Passive exposure to cigarette smoke and a history of atopy are additional risk factors. On physical exam, a toxic appearance or abnormal lung sounds, such as wheezing or rales, are also important predictors of increased risk. Additional evaluation with imaging or laboratory information is rarely needed.

Anesthetic management of the child with an active URI should be tailored to minimize airway irritability. Administration of a neuromuscular blocker to facilitate tracheal intubation will prevent laryngospasm. Humidification[4] of airway gases may prevent the thickening of secretions that is commonly encountered in these children. Some authors suggest administration of an anticholinergic agent, such as atropine or glycopyrrolate, to attenuate vagally mediated airway complications; however, this remains untested.

The anesthesiologist should also carefully consider the appropriate type of airway management based on the patient's history and the surgical procedure. When possible, airway instrumentation and placement of an endotracheal tube should be avoided as multiple studies have shown an increased risk for PRAEs (bronchospasm, desaturation, cough, and breath holding) in these patients. A natural airway or use of a laryngeal mask airway may decrease risk, but even LMA placement may be associated with complications in children with a URI.[5] Ventilation should be carefully tailored with judicious positive end–expiratory pressure (PEEP) to avoid the development of atelectasis. Anesthesia providers should expect PRAEs such as bronchospasm or laryngospasm and be prepared to treat these immediately.

In infants and children with a URI, apneic oxygenation is less effective; thus, oxyhemoglobin desaturation may occur faster than usual during rapid sequence induction when the child may not be receiving positive-pressure ventilation.

Postoperatively, the majority of patients with a URI will have an uneventful recovery without need for additional respiratory management. Patients with underlying pulmonary or cardiac comorbidities, however, are at higher risk for PRAEs.

Transient postoperative hypoxemia, postintubation croup, and postoperative pneumonia are probably more likely to occur in children with a URI. Long-term complications and true outcomes are difficult to define and quantify and may not differ between normal children and those with a current or recent URI.

Asthma

Asthma, or reactive airway disease, is an acute-on-chronic inflammatory disease of both larger and smaller airways. With a prevalence of 8%, it is the most common chronic illness in children in the United States and in other resource-rich countries and is concentrated in urban geographic areas that have a predominantly African American or Hispanic population. There is a strong genetic component and a correlation to other allergic-type conditions such as seasonal allergies and eczema. The majority of children present early in life (80% by age 5), although the presentation is often earlier and more severe in children with underlying pulmonary conditions such as bronchopulmonary dysplasia or respiratory syncytial virus infection.

The pathophysiology of asthma consists of the classic triad of bronchial hyperreactivity, inflammation, and mucous secretion. Triggers such as inhaled allergens (e.g., dust, pet dander, pollen, etc.), viruses, smoke, exercise, or even administration of nonsteroidal antiinflammatory drugs (NSAIDs) result in activation of an immunoglobulin E-mediated and nonimmunologic response in the airway. Specifically, mast cells located in the airway mucosa release mediators such as histamine, tryptase, leukotrienes, and prostaglandins that result in contraction of airway smooth muscle (i.e., bronchoconstriction). These mediators also result in the hypersecretion of mucous, infiltration of inflammatory cells, and airway edema. Because of the continued immune response with the infiltration of more and more inflammatory cells, the airway remains hyperreactive. In addition to the immune response, the parasympathetic nervous system also plays a role in maintaining airway tone; when activated because of histamine release or other stimuli such as inhaled cold air or airway instrumentation, increased parasympathetic output via the vagus nerve results in an intracellular signaling cascade and ultimately, bronchoconstriction. Depending on the type and duration of exposure to the trigger, and the patient's immune and parasympathetic responses, exacerbations of asthma can last for hours or days, some resolving spontaneously whereas others require aggressive medical therapy.

Clinically, patients with asthma classically present with wheeze because of the narrowing of their airways from dynamic bronchoconstriction. Children may also demonstrate a persistent cough (often worse at night) and dyspnea on exertion. During an acute exacerbation, marked respiratory distress occurs, which may include chest wall retractions and a prolonged expiratory phase secondary to lower airway obstruction. The degree of audible wheeze, which is directly related to the amount of airflow in the airways, can fluctuate during an acute exacerbation. As the severity of an asthma exacerbation worsens and bronchoconstriction increases, the degree of audible wheeze may first increase because of airway narrowing but ultimately can decrease as the severity of bronchospasm results in lack of air flow. Thus, lack of wheeze can actually be a sign of impending respiratory failure.

The treatment of children with asthma targets the underlying pathophysiology, specifically bronchoconstriction and the hyperactive airway immune response. For patients with known triggers such as allergens and irritants, avoidance is key. Further chronic treatments are stratified based of the frequency of symptoms (Table 4.1) and the type of treatment used (Table 4.2).

Acute exacerbations are managed with escalated use of beta-agonist therapy and addition of other classes of medications. Inhaled anticholinergics targeting the parasympathetic nervous system, such as ipratropium bromide, combined with beta-agonist therapy has been shown to decrease the rate of hospital admission and thus will often be used in the acute management of these patients. Systemic steroids (prednisone, methylprednisolone, or dexamethasone), given orally or IV, are used to dampen the underlying immune response and decrease airway inflammation, although the initial effect is delayed and not seen until several hours after administration. For severely ill children, other treatment modalities include IV magnesium sulfate (direct smooth-muscle relaxation secondary to inhibition of calcium uptake), IV or subcutaneous epinephrine (direct beta-agonist), IV or subcutaneous terbutaline (direct beta-agonist), IV ketamine (sympathomimetic bronchorelaxation), intubation with

TABLE 4.1 Stratification and Treatment of Asthma Based on Symptom Frequency

Classification	Symptom Frequency	Treatment
Mild Intermittent	≤2 days/week or ≤2 nights/month	No daily treatment Short-acting bronchodilator as needed
Mild Persistent	>2 days/week but not daily or >2 nights/month	Inhaled steroid (low dose)
Moderate Persistent	Daily or 1 night/week	Inhaled steroid (low dose) plus long-acting inhaled beta agonist or Inhaled steroid (medium dose)
Severe Persistent	Continual or Frequent nighttime	Inhaled steroid (high dose)

delivery of inhaled anesthetic agents (bronchodilation), and finally extracorporeal membrane oxygenation (ECMO) for the most severe life-threatening cases.

Anesthetic Management of Children With Asthma

A thorough history and physical examination will inform the anesthesia provider about the child's current or recent control of their asthma and indicate their relative risk for complications.

We recommend focusing on the following preoperative details to estimate the child's current risk of receiving general anesthesia:
- What is the child's category of asthma severity (see Table 4.1)?
- When was the child's last exacerbation that required use of a rescue inhaler or treatment with oral steroids?
- How frequently do the exacerbations occur?
- What typically triggers the child's exacerbation (e.g., environmental allergens, URI, smoke, etc.)?
- Has the child ever been hospitalized for asthma and if so, when was the last hospitalization?
- Has the child ever required ICU admission for asthma or noninvasive support or tracheal intubation for an asthma exacerbation?

The physical examination should focus on detecting expiratory wheeze, a prolonged expiratory time, and the child's use of accessory muscles of respiration. A pulse oximetry reading less than 96% in room air should prompt additional evaluation.

TABLE 4.2	Treatment of Asthma Based on Drug Class		
Drug Class	**Examples**	**Mechanism of Action**	**Things To Remember**
Beta-agonist	Albuterol (short acting) Salmeterol (long acting)	Relaxation of airway smooth muscle by direct activation of the beta-2 receptor	Most commonly used for acute exacerbations Can be given with a metered-dose inhaler (MDI) or nebulization
Inhaled glucocorticoid	Fluticasone Budesonide Beclomethasone Triamcinolone	Antiinflammatory effects	Part of the controller therapy for asthma Can have systemic effects
Leukotriene receptor antagonist	Montelukast	Interferes with the pathway of metabolism of arachidonic acid, thus blocking inflammation	
Mast cell membrane stabilizer	Cromolyn	Prevents release of inflammatory mediators	Decreases the likelihood of acute exacerbations
Methylxanthine	Theophylline	Causes bronchodilation by inhibiting phosphodiesterase	Very narrow therapeutic range and safety concerns Fallen out of favor for chronic asthma management

Based on the information gathered in the history and physical examination, the anesthesia provider must determine whether the patient is appropriate for an elective procedure. If the patient does not appear to be optimized for elective surgery, they should be rescheduled at a later date. Optimized, however, does not necessarily mean that the child is symptom free. For example, mild wheezing may be serious in a child who never wheezes between acute exacerbations, as opposed to the child who continually has a baseline wheeze, and is considered to be optimized at the time of surgery. Preoperatively, the patient should be continued on all asthma medications. Prophylactic inhaled beta-agonists should be considered, given both at home before arrival and in the preoperative period.

The anesthetic management of children with asthma[6] is primarily aimed at preventing PRAEs. Bronchoconstriction may be triggered by airway manipulation; if possible, a face mask or supraglottic airway is preferred. If tracheal intubation is required, a cuffed endotracheal tube will facilitate higher peak inspiratory pressures should bronchospasm develop. Before tracheal tube placement, airway reflexes should be suppressed with a sufficiently deep level of general anesthesia. All inhaled anesthetic agents will accomplish this goal, in addition to providing direct bronchodilation. Desflurane should be avoided because of its irritative effects on the upper and lower airways. Propofol decreases respiratory events when used during induction, and in adults, propofol is associated with less bronchospasm than etomidate. Ketamine is also frequently used in asthmatic patients because of its ability to cause bronchodilation by releasing endogenous adrenergic agonists, but there appears to be no advantage over propofol. Use of neuromuscular blockade has been shown to reduce the risk of perioperative respiratory events, although caution must be used to avoid those that cause histamine release (e.g., atracurium). Similarly, some opioids (e.g., morphine) are associated with histamine release.

Regional anesthesia is encouraged as an alternative or supplement to general anesthesia in patients with asthma. Although regional anesthesia alone eliminates the use of airway manipulation, it is rarely feasible in younger children. Blunting of the sympathetic response as a result of central regional blockade is not likely to initiate or exacerbate bronchospasm in an asthmatic child because there is no direct adrenergic innervation to human airway smooth-muscle.

Artificial ventilation may differ in children with asthma because of the inherent obstructive physiology in these patients. The anesthesiologist should ensure an appropriate expiratory time to allow for adequate exhalation and prevent breath stacking, which may result in air trapping and hyperinflation. Obstruction will be evident on capnography as a delayed or up-sloping rise of the end tidal carbon dioxide tracing. The ventilation strategy should be modified by decreasing minute ventilation (decreasing respiratory rate or tidal volume) with resultant permissive hypercapnia, or reducing the inspiratory/expiratory ratio to allow for more time for complete exhalation.

Children with preexisting asthma do not often develop exacerbation of their disease during an anesthetic. When it does, bronchospasm often presents as wheezing, increased peak inspiratory pressures, decreased tidal volume, obstructive pattern on capnography, and oxyhemoglobin desaturation. The anesthesiologist should first rule out other causes of that constellation of signs. The circuit and endotracheal tube should be checked to be sure there are no obvious obstructions, including kinks or mucous plugs. Endotracheal tube depth should be assessed and breath sounds confirmed to ensure lack of caudad tube migration (main bronchial intubation) or pneumothorax. If upon further investigation bronchospasm is still assumed, several steps in management should occur simultaneously. First, the patient should be transitioned to 100% inspired oxygen. Next, assuming hemodynamic stability, the anesthetic

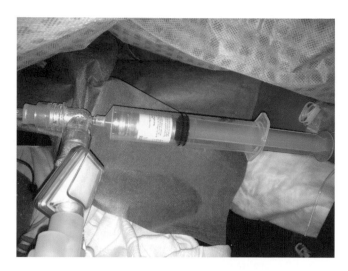

• **Fig 4.1.** The albuterol canister is placed within the barrel of a 60-mL syringe, which is connected directly to the elbow in the breathing circuit. The plunger of the syringe is used to actuate the canister. (Photo credit to Ronald S. Litman)

should be deepened by administering an intravenous agent such as propofol or increasing the concentration of inhaled agent. Often, the deepening of anesthesia will be sufficient to resolve the episode of bronchospasm, which is frequently secondary to stimulation of the tracheal mucosa during a period of light anesthesia.

When bronchospasm is not amenable to deepening the anesthetic, further bronchodilatory strategies are warranted. The first line treatment is administration of an inhaled beta-agonist. Practically, this can be accomplished intraoperatively by using a metered-dose inhaler connected to the anesthesia breathing circuit between the inspiratory limb and patient Y-piece (Fig. 4.1). This is performed by inserting the drug canister into a 60 mL syringe barrel and using the plunger to actuate the medication, or by directly inserting the canister into the breathing circuit using a specialized adapter (Fig. 4.2, Medicomp, part 1423, Princeton, MN 55371). Access into the circuit is attained through a removable cap, through which the spray is actuated just before a positive-pressure breath. In practice, however, a very low percentage of the bronchodilator actually reaches the lungs[7] because of adherence to the circuit and endotracheal tube. The smaller the diameter of the endotracheal tube, the less actuated medication will actually reach the lungs. Therefore, multiple administrations of albuterol are delivered (usually between 10 and 20) until bronchospasm is relieved, or until the patient develops tachycardia from absorption of the adrenergic agonist. Conversely, an infusion of low-dose epinephrine can also be used for refractory bronchospasm.

Cystic Fibrosis

With a frequency of approximately 1 in 3000 live births, cystic fibrosis (CF) is the most common fatal autosomal recessive disease in Caucasians. The disease can occur because of any of more than 2000 pathogenic variants in the cystic

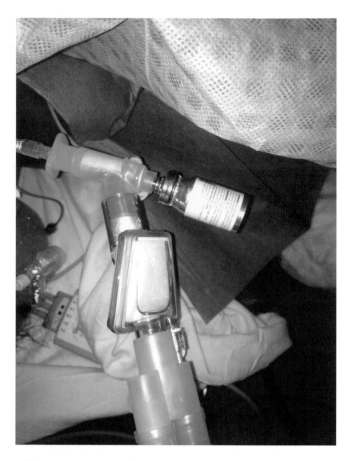

• **Fig 4.2.** The albuterol canister is connected to the breathing circuit via a specialized adaptor and actuated by pushing on the bottom of the canister.

fibrosis transmembrane conductance regulator (CFTR[8]) gene, which encodes a regulatory protein found in exocrine tissue. Because of the vast number of possible mutations, many individuals are carriers for the disease, with frequencies as high as 1 in 25 in some Caucasian populations. The most common pathogenic variant in the Northern European Caucasian population and the United States is F508del, accounting for up to 90% of patients with CF.

The CFTR gene is located on the long arm of chromosome 7 and codes for an ion channel which transports chloride ions down the electrochemical concentration gradient across epithelial cell membranes. When chloride ions move across the cell membrane, sodium ions follow passively to counterbalance the ionic charge. This results in an increased electrolyte concentration, which in turn draws water by osmosis. When the gene is altered, the ion channel is unable to conduct chloride ions appropriately, resulting in abnormalities in water movement. Without this water, secretions become thick and viscous which limits clearance and causes progressive obstruction. Static insipid secretions create a prime culture medium for bacteria, leading to bacterial colonization and overgrowth with chronic inflammation and destruction of extracellular architecture. Multiple organs contain the CFTR protein, including the respiratory tract, pancreas, liver, gallbladder, intestine, and reproductive tract.

This pathophysiology leads to a variety of clinical manifestations that take the form of a chronic life-threatening illness throughout an affected person's life. Patients often present with cough in early childhood because of difficulty clearing secretions. As the build-up of secretions results in smaller and then larger airway blockage, further symptoms such as atelectasis, bronchospasm, pneumothoraces, and frequent antibiotic-resistant bacterial infections occur. Chronic hypoxia may result in clubbing of the digits and right-heart failure. Destruction of the architecture of the respiratory tree puts patients at risk for bronchiectasis and hemoptysis, which can cause anemia. Pansinusitis and nasal polyps are common. In the gastrointestinal tract, thickened secretions result in large malabsorptive stools. This can present in the newborn period as a meconium ileus. Older children may have constipation, vomiting, and abdominal distention. Pancreatic insufficiency occurs in about two-thirds of CF patients from birth and about 85% into adulthood. This results in malabsorption and fat-soluble vitamin (A, D, E, and K) deficiencies. Progressive pancreatic insufficiency results in bouts of pancreatitis and islet cell damage, which leads to abnormal glucose homeostasis and diabetes mellitus.

The diagnosis of CF is confirmed by history, physical examination, and laboratory analysis. In the United States, all newborns are tested for CF in the routine newborn screen. If positive, the child is referred for further testing with either a sweat test (elevated sweat chloride levels are a diagnostic hallmark) or genetic testing. Children with confirmed CF are followed with periodic chest radiographs, pulmonary function tests, and blood markers consistent with the pathophysiology of the disease (e.g., glucose and Hb A_{1c} for endocrine pancreatic function, prothrombin time for signs of vitamin K deficiency, sputum cultures for bacterial overgrowth, etc.).

Medical management of CF improves continuously, and patients now often live well into adulthood. Treatment strategies include chest physiotherapy, exercise, and frequent coughing to mobilize secretions. Bronchodilators and antiinflammatory medications decrease airway reactivity. Bacterial pneumonia requires aggressive antibiotic therapy. Nebulized hypertonic saline and dornase (Pulmozyme) break down thick DNA complexes that accumulate in mucus from cell destruction and bacterial infection. Normal growth is often achieved with pancreatic enzyme replacement, fat-soluble vitamin supplements, and high-caloric high-protein diets.

Common reasons that children with CF require surgery include meconium ileus in the newborn period, intestinal obstruction, nasal polypectomy, and endoscopic sinus surgery. Older or more severely ill children may require anesthesia for placement of indwelling central line access or gastrostomy tube insertion. Preoperative evaluation of pulmonary function may include chest radiography or pulmonary function tests; arterial blood gas analysis is rarely useful. Optimization of infection control and physiotherapy for secretion clearance are priorities and should be coordinated with the child's pulmonologist.

There is no best anesthetic technique for patients with CF. Some advocate use of ketamine because of its minimal effects on ventilatory function; however, others cite ketamine's ability to increase airway secretions. Some pediatric anesthesiologists prefer a liberal fluid strategy to decrease viscosity of bronchial secretions while others advocate minimization of fluids to decrease airway secretions at the expense of increased viscosity. It seems that avoidance of either overhydration or dehydration is the most prudent course of action. There are no modern clinical studies on anesthetic management of children with CF.

In children with significant pulmonary disease and poor nutritional status, placement of an endotracheal tube and application of mechanical ventilation often entails postoperative transfer to the ICU and the difficult decision-making process concerning the timing and appropriateness of tracheal extubation. Postoperative management should be proactively planned in conjunction with the intensive care physicians and with the input of the patient and family. When possible, the least invasive form of ventilatory support should be chosen.

References

1. von Ungern-Sternberg BS, Boda K, Chambers NA, et al. Risk assessment for respiratory complications in paediatric anaesthesia: a prospective cohort study. *Lancet*. 2010;376(9743):773–783. https://doi.org/10.1016/S0140-6736(10)61193-2.
2. McGill WA, Coveler LA, Epstein BS. Subacute upper respiratory infection in small children. *Anesth Analg*. 1979;58(4):331–333. https://doi.org/10.1213/00000539-197907000-00017.
3. Tariq S, Syed M, Martin T, Zhang X, Schmitz M. Rates of perioperative respiratory adverse events among Caucasian and African American children undergoing general anesthesia. *Anesth Analg*. 2018;127(1):181–187. https://doi.org/10.1213/ANE.0000000000003430.
4. Tait AR, Malviya S. Anesthesia for the child with an upper respiratory tract infection: still a dilemma? *Anesth Analg*. 2005;100(1):59–65. https://doi.org/10.1213/01.ANE.0000139653.53618.91.
5. von Ungern-Sternberg BS, Boda K, Schwab C, Sims C, Johnson C, Habre W. Laryngeal mask airway is associated with an increased incidence of adverse respiratory events in children with recent upper respiratory tract infections. *Anesthesiology*. 2007;107(5):714–719. https://doi.org/10.1097/01.anes.0000286925.25272.b5.
6. Lauer R, Vadi M, Mason L. Anaesthetic management of the child with co-existing pulmonary disease. *Br J Anaesth*. 2012;109(Suppl 1):i47–i59. https://doi.org/10.1093/bja/aes392.
7. Taylor RH, Lerman J. High-efficiency delivery of salbutamol with a metered-dose inhaler in narrow tracheal tubes and catheters. *Anesthesiology*. 1991;74(2):360–363. https://doi.org/10.1097/00000542-199102000-00024.
8. Cystic fibrosis transmembrane conductance regulator (CFTR) gene. MassGenomics. Accessed October 5, 2021. http://www.massgenomics.org/wp-content/uploads/2011/02/cftrdiagramlarge.gif.

Suggested Reading

Huffmyer JL, Littlewood KE, Nemergut EC. Perioperative management of the adult with cystic fibrosis. *Anesth Analg*. 2009;109(6):1949–1961. https://doi.org/10.1213/ANE.0b013e3181b845d0.

5

Neurologic and Neuromuscular Diseases

JAY GARCIA AND RONALD S. LITMAN

Cerebral palsy and seizure disorders are very common in the pediatric population, thus anesthesia providers should be familiar with their clinical characteristics and the pharmacologic agents used for their treatment. Although less common, myopathies are associated with significant morbidity in children, and are noteworthy because of their potential association with malignant hyperthermia and the potentially catastrophic[1] hyperkalemic response to administration of succinylcholine (and in some cases, volatile anesthetics).

Cerebral Palsy

Cerebral palsy (CP) is a static motor encephalopathy that affects tone, coordination, and movement of the musculoskeletal system. It is a collection of motor system disorders caused by perinatal or early childhood neurologic insult. The cumulative incidence rate of CP at the age of 5 to 7 years is 2.4 cases per 1000 live births. The contribution of very low birth weight infants to this population of children is significant: about 52,000 very low birth weight infants (<1500 g) are born annually. These infants make up more than 25% of children diagnosed with CP.

Children with CP exhibit a wide variety of clinical manifestations that range from mild (e.g., slight lower extremity spasticity and normal cognitive function) to severe (e.g., spastic quadriplegia and marked intellectual disability). Respiratory system dysfunction usually parallels the overall severity of the disease. Bulbar motor dysfunction causes a loss of airway protective mechanisms (impaired cough, gag, etc.) and leads to chronic pulmonary aspiration, recurrent pneumonia, reactive airway disease, and parenchymal lung damage. Other airway considerations include abnormal dentition, temporomandibular joint dysfunction, and positioning difficulties. Gastrostomy tubes are often placed during infancy to optimize nutritional status.

Prematurely born infants may develop areas of brain ischemia secondary to cerebral hemorrhages in the early newborn period. The area of infarction is termed *periventricular leukomalacia* (white matter atrophy surrounding the ventricles) and is associated with development of varying degrees of limb spasticity (Fig. 5.1).

Chronic absence of motor input results in progressive development of limb contractures during childhood that worsen with age. Baclofen, a gamma-aminobutyric acid (GABA) agonist, reduces pain associated with muscle spasms and slows development of contractures. Side effects are common with oral baclofen,[2] thus intrathecal baclofen has become popular for children of any age.[3] This requires surgical intervention for catheter placement and implantation of the baclofen pump in the anterior abdominal wall. Side effects of baclofen include urinary retention and lower extremity weakness, which usually abate when the dose is reduced. Abrupt withdrawal from oral or intrathecal baclofen may cause seizures, hallucinations, disorientation, and dyskinesias, and when severe may be fatal. If intrathecal baclofen is discontinued because of infection of local structures or cerebrospinal fluid (CSF), close observation of the patient for withdrawal symptoms is necessary. On occasion, when withdrawal is severe enough, a temporary intrathecal catheter may be placed to provide baclofen. Two case reports[4,5] highlight the successful use of dexmedetomidine to manage acute, severe withdrawal in two patients.

Children with CP may undergo various surgical interventions during childhood. Orthopedic procedures are the most common and include scoliosis repair and a variety of limb procedures to improve range of motion and decrease progression of contractures. Dorsal rhizotomy may be required to control painful lower limb spasticity. Nissen fundoplication is performed to control chronic gastroesophageal reflux and may include a feeding gastrostomy, which is increasingly performed by laparoscopy.

Surgical complications are relatively common. In a review of 19 children[6] with CP undergoing scoliosis surgery, 9 had at least one major complication, most commonly blood loss or the need for postoperative mechanical ventilation. Risk factors included the presence of two or more comorbidities and thoracotomy.

Preoperative assessment includes defining and optimizing all systemic medical illnesses. Concurrent upper

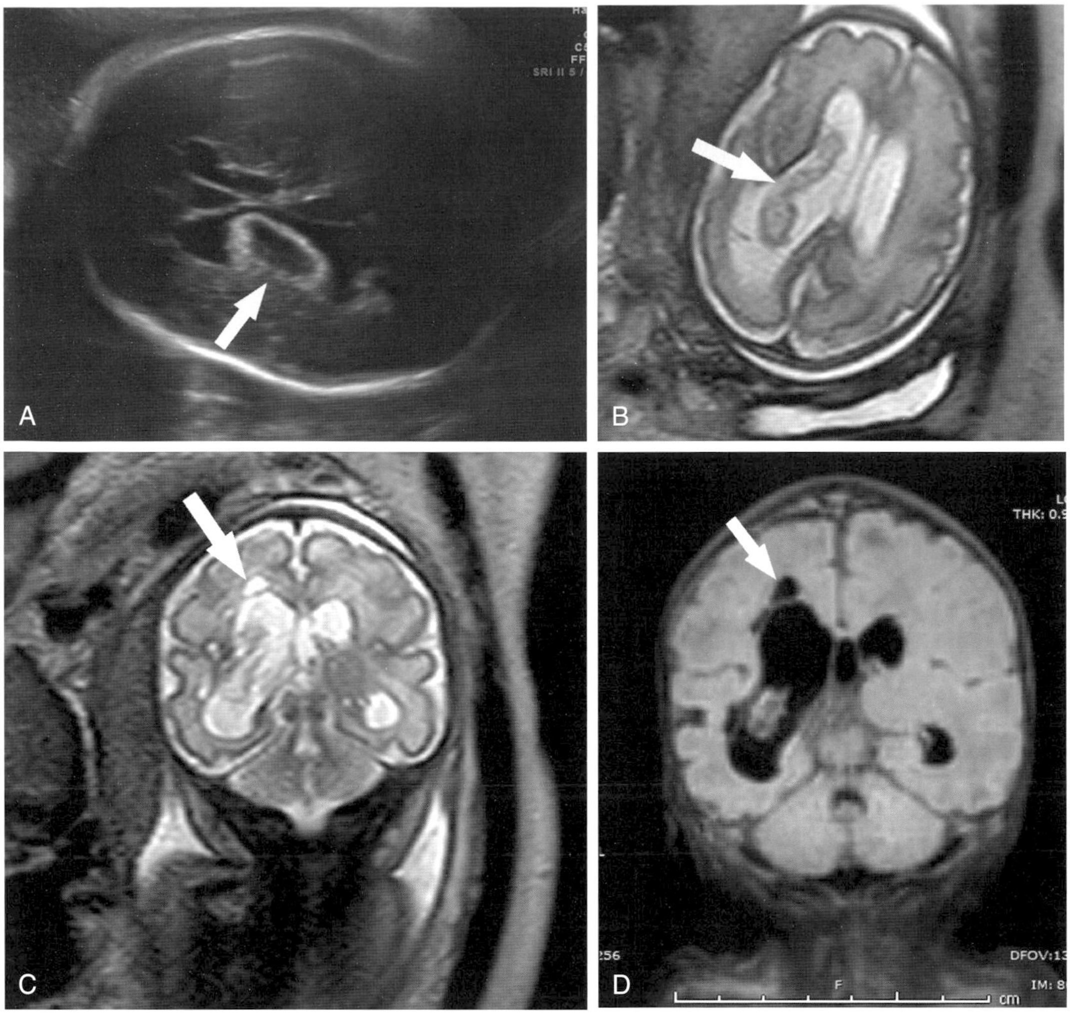

• **Fig 5.1.** Periventricular leukomalacia. (A) Axial fetal ultrasound through the brain shows enlargement of the right choroid plexus (arrow). (B) Axial fetal magnetic resonance imaging shows blood products within the choroid plexus (arrow). (C) Coronal T2-weighted, and (D) coronal FLAIR images show cystic lesions in the periventricular region (arrow) consistent with periventricular leukomalacia. (From Berlin, Sheila C, Meyers Mariana L. Neonatal imaging. In: *Klaus and Fanaroff's Care of the High-Risk Neonate.* 18th ed. Elsevier; 2020:409–436.)

respiratory infections are poorly tolerated and will exacerbate preexisting respiratory disease. Preoperative anxiolysis should be administered to children when appropriate, although some children with CP are prone to upper airway obstruction with mild sedation and should be closely monitored. Administration of an anticholinergic agent may decrease pooling of oropharyngeal secretions, but this is not evidence-based. Routine preoperative echocardiography for cardiovascular evaluation in the absence of signs or symptoms suggestive of cardiac dysfunction is not necessary.[7]

There are no special considerations when choosing an agent for induction or maintenance of general anesthesia because children with CP usually tolerate all anesthetic agents well. If a gastrostomy tube is present, suctioning or leaving it open before induction of general anesthesia may help decompress the stomach. Because of possible malformation of facial structures, mask ventilation may be difficult, but endotracheal intubation should be straightforward in most cases. Presence of gastroesophageal reflux and increased oropharyngeal

secretions may encourage the anesthesia provider to secure intravenous (IV) access earlier during induction of anesthesia and secure the airway using IV induction agents.

Children with CP demonstrate increased sensitivity to succinylcholine[8]; approximately 30% of children with CP have abnormal distribution of acetylcholine receptors. Succinylcholine-induced hyperkalemia in CP has not been studied to the extent that is required to capture such a rare event. We are aware of a child with CP that experienced cardiac arrest upon receiving succinylcholine; therefore, succinylcholine should be used only to treat life-threatening airway emergencies in CP patients. Nondepolarizing muscle relaxants are less potent and have a relatively shorter duration of action in children with CP. This may be related to chronic anticonvulsant administration or underlying spasticity.

Sevoflurane is relatively more potent (i.e., lower minimum alveolar concentration) in children with CP. Increased opioid sensitivity should be assumed in all but mild forms of CP. Doses should be reduced, and greater vigilance at the time of extubation is necessary to ensure the child's ability to maintain a patent upper airway. Hypothermia is a common intraoperative problem in children with CP. Impaired temperature regulation is caused by hypothalamic dysfunction and the relative absence of muscle and subcutaneous fat. A child with spastic quadriplegic CP may have an esophageal temperature of 34°C to 35°C within a few minutes of induction of anesthesia. Therefore the ambient temperature should be 21°C to 24°C (70°F–75°F) in the operating room while the patient is relatively exposed during induction and line placement. Line placement will also become increasingly more difficult as the child becomes increasingly hypothermic. Forced-air warming is effective and should be used starting in the preoperative holding area, if possible.

Regional analgesia may benefit children with CP who have difficulty communicating the severity of their pain. Epidural catheter placement via lumbar or caudal approach is commonly used for lower extremity orthopedic procedures. Addition of epidural clonidine[9] to local anesthesia may help reduce postoperative lower limb spasticity, which can be a significant component of their postoperative discomfort. Oral diazepam[10] may help alleviate muscles spasms.

Seizures are present in about 30% of patients with cerebral palsy. Anticonvulsants should be continued until the morning of surgery and reinstituted as quickly as possible during the postoperative period. When it is not feasible to continue enterally administered anticonvulsants, some can be administrated rectally (phenytoin, valproic acid, carbamazepine, levetiracetam) and some intravenously (phenytoin, valproic acid, phenobarbital, levetiracetam). If the surgical procedure causes significant blood loss, anticonvulsant levels should be checked postoperatively, and doses should be adjusted to reestablish optimal levels.

Seizure Disorders

Seizures are clinical manifestations of a variety of disorders. Febrile seizures are the most common type, affecting 5% of children. Idiopathic epilepsy, primarily seen in older children, is less common with an estimated incidence of 0.6% of the population. Trauma, hypoxia, and infection are the primary pathologic causes of seizures in infants. Additional causes include metabolic disease, hypoglycemia, electrolyte abnormalities, toxic ingestions, and congenital or developmental defects. However, in about 50% of children, the etiology of the seizure is unknown.

The currently accepted international classification[11] of epileptic seizures divides these disorders into three etiologic categories and three types of seizures (Table 5.1). Etiologic categories include genetic, structural/metabolic, and unknown. Seizure types are divided by onset location: focal, generalized, or unknown.

Focal onset seizures are akin to partial seizures, in which the initial clinical and electroencephalogram (EEG) changes indicate activation of a system of neurons limited to part of one cerebral hemisphere. Focal seizures may or may not

TABLE 5.1	International Classification of Seizures

Focal Onset Seizures
- Aware or impaired awareness
- Motor onset or non motor onset
- Focal to bilateral tonic-clonic

Generalized Onset Seizures
- Motor
  - Tonic-clonic
  - Other motor
- Non motor (absence)

Unknown Onset Seizures
- Motor
  - Tonic-clonic
  - Other motor
- Non motor (absence)
- Infantile spasms (West syndrome)
- Unclassified Seizures

have impaired awareness. Focal seizures can be subdivided by clinical presentation and EEG characteristics into motor, sensory, autonomic, or higher cortical/aura symptoms. There may not be a postictal state. Focal onset seizures may spread bilaterally and progress to a "focal to bilateral" tonic-conic seizure.

Generalized onset seizures involve bilateral cerebral hemispheres with clinical and EEG changes from the onset and accompanied with impaired awareness. Motor manifestations, if present, are also bilateral. Generalized seizures may be convulsive or nonconvulsive.

Generalized tonic-clonic seizures consist of an initial tonic contraction phase, during which it is common for patients to become apneic and cyanotic from the tonic rigidity of the thoracic cavity. This is followed by the clonic, repetitive twitching phase, where breathing resumes but can be shallow and irregular.

Nonmotor "absence" seizures are nonconvulsive generalized seizures. They are further subdivided into typical (staring spells during which the patient is not responsive, and last a few seconds), atypical (less abrupt onset/offset, some loss of muscle tone), myoclonic, or eyelid myoclonia.

Motor seizures are subdivided by the presence or absence of three characteristics:
1. Tone
2. Clonus (regular and rhythmic twitch)
3. Myoclonus (irregular, arhythmic)

Generalized motor seizures range from **atonic** (where atonia is the only prominent feature) to **myoclonic-tonic-clonic** (where all three abnormalities are alternatively present).

Epileptic spasms, which include infantile spasms, are of poorly understood origin and classified as "unknown."

Infantile spasms (West syndrome) consist of the triad of unique salaam-like seizure movements, arrest of psychomotor development, and a characteristic EEG pattern called

hypsarrhythmia. The onset peaks between 4 and 7 months of age and almost always occurs before 12 months. It can be associated with a known underlying neurologic disorder, or it can be idiopathic and associated with a poor neurodevelopmental outcome. Lennox-Gastaut syndrome consists of different types of seizures that occur frequently and are difficult to control. It manifests itself in the 3- to 5-year age group and is associated with severe intellectual disability. Both infantile spasms and Lennox-Gastaut syndrome are difficult to control with anticonvulsant agents.

Anesthetic concerns for children with seizure disorders depend on coexisting morbidities and are individualized depending on the mental status of the child. If necessary, children who require strict pharmacologic control of their seizure disorder should have their oral anticonvulsants converted to the IV forms (or equivalent medications if IV forms are not available) during the preanesthetic fasting interval and during the postoperative period if oral intake is not possible. In most cases, preanesthetic anticonvulsant levels are not necessary. Anesthesiologists should be aware of the most common side effects of anticonvulsants.[12]

Most anesthetic and analgesic agents can be safely administered to children with seizure disorders. A possible exception is multiple doses of meperidine. Its metabolite, normeperidine, possesses proconvulsant properties. Nitrous oxide, sevoflurane, etomidate, propofol, and all opioids have been anecdotally associated with seizure-like movements or lowering of the seizure threshold[13] in both healthy and epileptic patients, without serious sequelae. In most of these cases these movements were a benign form of myoclonus. Virtually all general anesthetic agents except ketamine have anticonvulsant properties in doses associated with loss of consciousness but lower doses have been associated with an increase in EEG spike activity.[14] Higher doses and shorter dosing intervals of neuromuscular blockers are required in patients taking anticonvulsants. The precise mechanism of this is unknown. However, this resistance is not as prominent for neuromuscular blockers that are metabolized in the plasma (i.e., atracurium), so it may be related to a pharmacokinetic effect based in the liver. Levetiracetam may prolong neuromuscular blockade. Anticonvulsants may also cause some resistance to opioids. Although definitive data are lacking, it does not appear that general anesthesia impacts the postoperatively subsequent frequency or severity of seizures.

Neuromuscular Diseases

Neuromuscular diseases can be broadly divided into disorders of the muscle or of neuromuscular transmission (Table 5.2). Muscle diseases can be further categorized into developmental myopathies, muscular dystrophies, and metabolic myopathies. Disorders of neuromuscular transmission can be further categorized into diseases of the neuromuscular junction and diseases of anterior horn cells. This list is extensive and only the most common and most important in pediatric anesthesia will be reviewed here.

TABLE 5.2	Classification of Neuromuscular Diseases of Childhood

Muscle Diseases

Developmental
- Nemaline myopathy
- Central core myopathy
- Myotubular myopathy

Muscular Dystrophies
- Duchenne muscular dystrophy
- Becker muscular dystrophy
- Myotonic dystrophy
- Limb-girdle muscular dystrophy
- Facioscapulohumeral muscular dystrophy
- Congenital muscular dystrophy

Metabolic Dystrophies
- Potassium-related periodic paralysis
- Glycogenoses
- Mitochondrial myopathies
- Lipid myopathies

Diseases of Neuromuscular Transmission

Neuromuscular Junction Disorders
- Myasthenia gravis
- Organophosphate poisoning botulism
- Tick paralysis

Anterior Horn Cell Diseases
- Spinal muscular atrophy (SMA)
- Poliomyelitis

Muscle diseases, or myopathies, are characterized by muscle weakness and atrophy. Many children are symptomatic at birth, although others are normal in early infancy only to develop weakness in the first few years of life. The myopathies are of interest to anesthesiologists for two major reasons. First, some are associated with an increased risk for malignant hyperthermia; second, all myopathies have at least a theoretical risk for developing life-threatening hyperkalemia after administration of succinylcholine (and, rarely, inhalational anesthetics). Children with myopathies often require multiple surgical procedures throughout childhood. These include a muscle biopsy as a component of the diagnostic workup, insertion of a gastrostomy or tracheostomy as weakness worsens, and a variety of orthopedic procedures for alleviation of contractures and scoliosis. A retrospective 20-year review[15] of 877 consecutive neuromuscular disorder patients undergoing muscle biopsies found no incidents involving hyperkalemia or malignant hyperthermia (MH), providing further evidence of the rarity of these events and of the safety of modern anesthetics.

As with neurologic diseases, anesthetic considerations for children with muscle diseases[16] largely depend on the medical condition of the child because there is a wide spectrum of affliction, even between children with the same diagnosis. Although only central core disease and a handful of other rare ryanodine receptor-related myopathies have been genetically linked to MH,[17] many pediatric anesthesiologists choose a nontriggering anesthetic technique for all children with myopathies. Use of nondepolarizing muscle relaxants depends on the baseline strength of the child. Careful titration of the neuromuscular blocker based on train-of-four monitoring is recommended. Children with muscle weakness are at increased risk for requiring postoperative mechanical ventilation; therefore, this possibility should be proactively addressed with the parents and child if appropriate.

Developmental Myopathies

The developmental myopathies consist of a heterogeneous group of congenital myopathies that are mostly nonprogressive, although some patients show slow clinical deterioration. Most of these conditions are hereditary, but some are sporadic. These include nemaline rod myopathy, central core disease (CCD), and myotubular myopathy. CCD is an autosomal dominant disease characterized by hypotonia and proximal weakness at birth. Unlike other muscle diseases, there appears to be a predisposition of CCD patients to malignant hyperthermia susceptibility in the form of a pathogenic variant for the ryanodine receptor on chromosome 19 (*RYR1*). However, the literature is conflicting, and the subject of myopathies and MH susceptibility continues to evolve. However, any patient with a myopathy associated with an *RYR1* pathogenic variant should be considered MH susceptible. Current best practices[18] favor regional anesthesia whenever possible, supplemented with total intravenous anesthesia. Inhaled anesthetics are considered safe in conditions not associated with MH susceptibility, such as mitochondrial myopathy. Most important, in all myopathic patients is attention to the cardiopulmonary system, the degree of muscular paralysis, and the core temperature. When significant muscle atrophy is present, these children are predisposed to hypothermia and hypoglycemia.

Muscular Dystrophies

Although the muscular dystrophies are a group of unrelated disorders, there are four obligatory criteria that distinguish them from other neuromuscular diseases:

1. They are primary myopathies.
2. They have a genetic basis.
3. Their course is progressive.
4. Degeneration and death of muscle fibers occur at some stage in the disease.

Duchenne muscular dystrophy (DMD) is an X-linked recessive disease that, although present at birth, usually presents in early childhood as weakness and motor delay. Additional clinical manifestations include pseudohypertrophy of the calves and elevated baseline creatine phosphokinase. Because weakness is greatest in the proximal muscle groups, the child must rise from the sitting position in two steps: first leaning on the hypertrophied calves and then pushing the trunk up with the arms. This is referred to as *Gower sign* and is nearly pathognomonic for DMD. Eventually, progressive and severe muscle atrophy and weakness cause loss of the ability to ambulate. The most serious aspects of DMD include a progressive cardiomyopathy and respiratory failure secondary to ventilatory pump failure. A retrospective review[19] of 12 DMD patients who underwent gastrostomy found that 9 had a forced vital capacity $\leq 36\%$ of predicted, with 8 being dependent on non-invasive positive pressure ventilation (NIPPV). Cognitive abnormalities are usually mild, if present at all. Most children become wheelchair-bound early in the second decade, with death in early adulthood from either respiratory failure or cardiomyopathy.

Adverse myocardial changes arise before overt cardiac dysfunction, and guidelines[20] recommend yearly cardiac screening beginning at diagnosis. Anesthesiologists are involved in the multidisciplinary consideration[21] and approach to left ventricular assist device (LVAD) placement, implantable cardioverter-defibrillator (ICD) placement, or heart transplantation in patients with advanced cardiac dysfunction.

Although there is no genetic link to MH susceptibility for these patients, many pediatric anesthesiologists perform a nontriggering technique because of the increased risk for rhabdomyolysis upon exposure to succinylcholine or inhaled agents. Some authors refer to it as *anesthesia-induced rhabdomyolysis*. However, careful use of inhaled agents for a relatively short period of time to secure an IV line is likely safe. Nondepolarizing muscle relaxants should be used with caution: administration of rocuronium to patients with DMD results in a delayed time to onset and delayed time to recovery. Use of succinylcholine in dystrophinopathies is contraindicated because of the risk for life-threatening hyperkalemia. A word of caution: there exists a report of a child[22] with DMD who had a stable cardiovascular profile preoperatively but unexpectedly developed acute heart failure when exposed to a propofol-sufentanil anesthetic for spinal fusion.

A less severe (yet debilitating) disease is Becker-type muscular dystrophy. Similar features to DMD include calf pseudohypertrophy, cardiomyopathy, and elevated serum levels of CK. However, the onset of weakness in Becker-type dystrophy is later in life than with DMD, and death usually occurs at a later age than with DMD. The anesthetic considerations are identical to those for DMD. Life-threatening rhabdomyolysis has been reported immediately after isoflurane anesthesia.

Spinal Muscle Atrophy

Spinal muscle atrophy (SMA) is an inherited autosomal recessive disorder characterized by anterior horn cell degeneration and is found as one of three clinical syndromes. Type 1 (Werdnig-Hoffman, disease) is the most severe, beginning in early infancy. It is characterized by significant muscle weakness and atrophy, except for diaphragmatic sparing which occurs later in life. Type 2 (Dubowitz disease) presents between 6 and 12 months of age and has a more prolonged, slightly milder course. Type 3 (Kugelberg-Welander disease) is the least debilitating. Cognitive abilities remain unaffected in all forms of the illness. Life expectancies vary with the severity of the disease and are improving with the emergence of targeted therapies; death occurs from repeated aspiration or lung infections.

As of 2016, there is a Food and Drug Administration (FDA)-approved treatment for SMA: intrathecal nusinersen.[23] Adverse events of intrathecal therapy such as headache and postlumbar puncture syndrome occur about 32% of the time and appear to be more common when the procedure involves older children, SMA type 3 patients, or larger (21- or 22-gauge) needles.

References

1. Larach MG, Rosenberg H, Gronert GA, Allen GC. Hyperkalemic cardiac arrest during anesthesia in infants and children with occult myopathies. *Clin Pediatr (Phila)*. 1997;36(1):9–16. https://doi.org/10.1177/000992289703600102.

2. Ertzgaard P, Campo C, Calabrese A. Efficacy and safety of oral baclofen in the management of spasticity: A rationale for intrathecal baclofen. *J Rehabil Med*. 2017;49(3):193–203. https://doi.org/10.2340/16501977-2211.

3. Hagemann C, Schmitt I, Lischetzki G, Kunkel P. Intrathecal baclofen therapy for treatment of spasticity in infants and small children under 6 years of age. *Childs Nerv Syst*. 2020;36(4):767–773. https://doi.org/10.1007/s00381-019-04341-7.

4. Gottula AL, Gorder KL, Peck AR, Renne BC. Dexmedetomidine for Acute Management of Intrathecal Baclofen Withdrawal [published online ahead of print, 2019 Nov 20]. *J Emerg Med*. 2019;S0736-4679(19),30827-3.https://doi.org/10.1016/j.jemermed.2019.09.043.

5. Morr S, Heard CM, Li V, Reynolds RM. Dexmedetomidine for acute baclofen withdrawal. *Neurocrit Care*. 2015;22(2):288–292. https://doi.org/10.1007/s12028-014-0083-8.

6. Bendon AA, George KA, Patel D. Perioperative complications and outcomes in children with cerebral palsy undergoing scoliosis surgery. *Paediatr Anaesth*. 2016;26(10):970–975. https://doi.org/10.1111/pan.12981.

7. DiCindio S, Arai L, McCulloch M, et al. Clinical relevance of echocardiogram in patients with cerebral palsy undergoing posterior spinal fusion. *Paediatr Anaesth*. 2015;25(8):840–845. https://doi.org/10.1111/pan.12676.

8. Theroux MC, Akins RE. Surgery and anesthesia for children who have cerebral palsy. *Anesthesiol Clin North Am*. 2005;23(4):733–743, ix. https://doi.org/10.1016/j.atc.2005.08.001.

9. Chalkiadis GA, Sommerfield D, Low J, et al. Comparison of lumbar epidural bupivacaine with fentanyl or clonidine for postoperative analgesia in children with cerebral palsy after single-event multilevel surgery. *Dev Med Child Neurol*. 2016;58(4):402–408. https://doi.org/10.1111/dmcn.12930.

10. Delgado MR, Hirtz D, et al. Practice Parameter: Pharmacologic treatment of spasticity in children and adolescents with cerebral palsy (an evidence-based review): Report of the Quality Standards Subcommittee of the American Academy of Neurology and the Practice Committee of the Child Neurology Society. *Neurology*. 2010;74(4):336–343. https://doi.org/10.1212/WNL.0b013e3181cbcd2f.

11. Fisher RS, Cross JH, French JA, et al. Operational classification of seizure types by the International League Against Epilepsy: Position Paper of the ILAE Commission for Classification and Terminology. *Epilepsia*. 2017;58(4):522–530. https://doi.org/10.1111/epi.13670.

12. Bloor M, Nandi R, Thomas M. Antiepileptic drugs and anesthesia. *Paediatr Anaesth*. 2017;27(3):248–250. https://doi.org/10.1111/pan.13074.

13. Chao JY, Legatt AD, Yozawitz EG, Adams DC, Delphin ES, Shinnar S. Electroencephalographic Findings and Clinical Behavior During Induction of Anesthesia With Sevoflurane in Human Infants: A Prospective Observational Study. *Anesth Analg*. 2020;130(6):e161–e164. https://doi.org/10.1213/ANE.0000000000004380.

14. Tanaka S, Oda Y, Ryokai M, et al. The effect of sevoflurane on electrocorticographic spike activity in pediatric patients with epilepsy. *Paediatr Anaesth*. 2017;27(4):409–416. https://doi.org/10.1111/pan.13111.

15. Shapiro F, Athiraman U, Clendenin DJ, Hoagland M, Sethna NF. Anesthetic management of 877 pediatric patients undergoing muscle biopsy for neuromuscular disorders: a 20-year review. *Paediatr Anaesth*. 2016;26(7):710–721. https://doi.org/10.1111/pan.12909.

16. Lerman J. Perioperative management of the paediatric patient with coexisting neuromuscular disease. *Br J Anaesth*. 2011;107(Suppl 1):i79–i89. https://doi.org/10.1093/bja/aer335.

17. Litman RS, Griggs SM, Dowling JJ, Riazi S. Malignant Hyperthermia Susceptibility and Related Diseases. *Anesthesiology*. 2018;128(1):159–167. https://doi.org/10.1097/ALN.0000000000001877.

18. Schieren M, Defosse J, Böhmer A, Wappler F, Gerbershagen MU. Anaesthetic management of patients with myopathies. *Eur J Anaesthesiol*. 2017;34(10):641–649. https://doi.org/10.1097/EJA.0000000000000672.

19. Boivin A, Antonelli R, Sethna NF. Perioperative management of gastrostomy tube placement in Duchenne muscular dystrophy adolescent and young adult patients: A role for a perioperative surgical home. *Paediatr Anaesth*. 2018;28(2):127–133. https://doi.org/10.1111/pan.13295.

20. Duchenne Muscular Dystrophy Care Considerations. National Center on Birth Defects and Developmental Disabilities, Centers for Disease Control and Prevention. Updated on October 27, 2020. Accessed on October 6, 2021. https://www.cdc.gov/ncbddd/musculardystrophy/care-considerations.html.

21. Buddhe S, Cripe L, Friedland-Little J, et al. Cardiac Management of the Patient With Duchenne Muscular Dystrophy. *Pediatrics*. 2018;142(Suppl 2):S72–S81. https://doi.org/10.1542/peds.2018-0333I.

22. Schmidt GN, Burmeister MA, Lilje C, Wappler F, Bischoff P. Acute heart failure during spinal surgery in a boy with Duchenne muscular dystrophy. *Br J Anaesth*. 2003;90(6):800–804. https://doi.org/10.1093/bja/aeg116.

23. Haché M, Swoboda KJ, Sethna N, et al. Intrathecal Injections in Children With Spinal Muscular Atrophy: Nusinersen Clinical Trial Experience. *J Child Neurol*. 2016;31(7):899–906. https://doi.org/10.1177/0883073815627882.

Suggested Reading

Schummer W, Schummer C, Hayes JA, Ames WA, et al. Acute heart failure during spinal surgery in a boy with Duchenne muscular dystrophy. *Br J Anaesth*. 2004;92(1):149–150.

6

Gastrointestinal Diseases

REBECCA ISSERMAN, PETAR MAMULA AND RONALD S. LITMAN

Gastroesophageal Reflux

Gastroesophageal reflux (GER) is a term used to describe a leaky lower esophageal sphincter that causes a child to regurgitate recently ingested meals. It is common in the first year of life, especially in children born premature, and usually resolves during early childhood. Children with GER related to neuromuscular disorders, such as cerebral palsy, will continue to reflux throughout childhood. Because of weakened airway protective mechanisms, these children often demonstrate chronic pulmonary aspiration that results in repeated episodes of pneumonitis and hypoxemia. Some children require a Nissen fundoplication, a surgical "tightening" of the lower esophageal sphincter, to prevent GER.

Many anesthesiologists assume that children with GER are at risk for pulmonary aspiration on induction of anesthesia and will opt for a rapid sequence induction. But to do so, an IV catheter must be placed preoperatively, which is not a routine procedure in many pediatric centers. This practice also obligates the placement of an endotracheal tube instead of a face mask or a supraglottic airway (SGA). No data exist to justify this practice. Studies that assessed residual gastric volumes after a normal preanesthetic fast have demonstrated no differences between children with GER and normal controls. The authors' opinion is that GER occurs only when there is food in the stomach of susceptible children. When these children are fasted normally, gastric volumes at induction of anesthesia are low and do not pose an increased risk for pulmonary aspiration.

There are additional valid reasons for not performing a rapid sequence induction in children with GER. First, the performance of cricoid pressure[1] reflexively decreases lower esophageal pressure, thus promoting passive regurgitation of gastric contents. Second, paralysis or relaxation of the cricopharyngeus muscle (a striated skeletal muscle) that forms the upper esophageal sphincter may allow passively regurgitated gastric contents to reach the larynx. Lastly, acid reflux into the lower third of the esophagus reflexively causes an increase in upper esophageal sphincter tone, which would not occur in the presence of neuromuscular blockade.

Inflammatory Bowel Disease

Inflammatory bowel disease[2] (IBD) primarily consists of Crohn disease and ulcerative colitis (UC). Crohn disease is a chronic inflammatory bowel disease that is seen in children and young adults, but it is also increasingly seen in very young children. (This "very early onset"[3] IBD is seen primarily in children with IBD associated with genetic syndromes.) Clinical manifestations, among others, include diarrhea, abdominal pain, rectal bleeding, anal fistulas, anemia, and weight loss. Extraintestinal manifestations include joint pain and swelling, growth failure, and delayed puberty. Therapy includes administration of 5-aminosalicylic acid (5-ASA) preparations, nutritional therapy, corticosteroids, immunosuppressants like methotrexate and 6-mercaptopurine, and biologic medications (i.e., monoclonal antibodies such as infliximab, vedolizumab, and ustekinumab).

Ulcerative colitis is characterized by inflammation of the large intestine that manifests clinically as abdominal cramping, diarrhea, and bloody stools. Associated systemic findings include anorexia, weight loss, low-grade fever, and anemia. Severe cases of colitis can result in severe anemia requiring blood transfusion, hypoalbuminemia, and toxic megacolon. Approximately 20% of cases of UC occur during childhood. As with Crohn disease, the primary therapeutic options are antiinflammatory therapy with 5-ASA preparations, corticosteroids, and biologic therapy, depending on disease severity.

Children with IBD require repeated esophagogastroduodenoscopies and colonoscopies during the course of their disease, for which general anesthesia is usually required. In Crohn disease surgery is indicated in select cases when medical therapy has failed. For example, when microperforations have resulted in a phlegmon, in cases of intestinal strictures which result in obstruction, or with perforation. Intestinal or colonic resections are palliative but not curative. Surgery is indicated for intractable colitis and toxic megacolon with peritonitis. Because UC is confined to the large intestine, colectomy is considered curative.

There are no unique anesthetic considerations for children with IBD. Anecdotal data indicate that these children require higher than usual amounts of opioids. This may be related to tolerance from intermittent or chronic opioid use.

Neonatal Hyperbilirubinemia

Some neonates manifest jaundice in the first week of life. Unconjugated (indirect) hyperbilirubinemia[4] occurs because of the breakdown of fetal erythrocytes in combination with low activity of glucuronyl transferase, the enzyme responsible for conjugation of bilirubin to glucuronic acid. It manifests clinically as jaundice of the skin and sclera and is most prominent after the third day of life, especially in prematurely born infants and in term breast-fed infants. Concomitant medical disorders that cause hemolysis and contribute to hyperbilirubinemia in an additive fashion include hemolytic disease of the newborn, spherocytosis, G-6-PD deficiency, and presence of a cephalohematoma.

Treatment is indicated when serum bilirubin levels are excessively high. The potential for neurotoxicity of the developing brain (kernicterus) is historically associated with bilirubin levels greater than 20 mg/dL in full-term infants. Prematurity, hypoxemia, acidosis, and hypothermia increase the likelihood of kernicterus in the presence of hyperbilirubinemia. Phototherapy is the initial treatment; exchange transfusions are required in accelerated cases. Bilirubin values that trigger phototherapy or exchange transfusion vary between institutions.

Chronic Liver Disease

Chronic liver disease is associated with congenital biliary atresia for which a Kasai procedure or liver transplant is required. Other possible causes include α_1-antitrypsin deficiency, cystic fibrosis, tyrosinemia, and Wilson disease, among others. Clinical manifestations will depend on the remaining degree of liver function and will include ascites, portal hypertension (with esophageal varices), and coagulopathy. Respiratory insufficiency in children with advanced liver disease is caused by loss of functional residual capacity from the mass effect of ascites or hepatomegaly, and creation of intrapulmonary shunts (hepatopulmonary syndrome).

Fulminant hepatic failure is associated with encephalopathy and increased intracranial pressure.

Principles of anesthetic management for children with liver disease include avoidance of medications that are metabolized in the liver (e.g., steroidal neuromuscular blockers) that will have an increased duration of action. All inhaled agents have minimal liver metabolism and reduce hepatic blood flow to a similar extent.

Achalasia

Achalasia[5] is a rare esophageal motor disorder characterized by loss of organized peristalsis in the body of the esophagus, along with elevated lower esophageal sphincter (LES) tone, both of which lead to esophageal stasis. The annual incidence is estimated at 1.6 in 100,000 individuals, with less than 5% of those occurring in children. It is caused by a loss of inhibitory ganglion cells in the myenteric plexus in the esophageal wall. Symptoms include dysphagia for both solids and liquids, chest pain, regurgitation, poor weight gain, and respiratory symptoms such as cough and breathing difficulties, especially when supine. Diagnosis is confirmed by esophagram, which shows a dilated esophagus that tapers at the LES, and by esophageal manometry.

The initial management of achalasia in children includes endoscopy with pneumatic dilation of the LES and is repeated if symptoms recur. Advanced surgical management, after one or more dilations, consists of peroral endoscopic myotomy, or Heller myotomy via laparoscopy.

Induction of anesthesia in these children carries a significant risk of pulmonary aspiration as a result of esophageal stasis and requires strategies to mitigate this risk. Prolonged fasting times may decrease the food burden in the esophagus but do not guarantee an empty esophagus. Awake (or sedated) nasogastric tube placement with esophageal evacuation before induction can further decrease esophageal content. Nebulized lidocaine beforehand can help facilitate this process. Rapid sequence induction should be performed by an experienced laryngoscopist with the head of the bed elevated.

A DEEPER DIVE

Almost all anesthetics for children with GI disease include **esophagogastroduodenoscopy (EGD)** and/or **colonoscopy**. Common pediatric indications for EGD include evaluation of reflux, chronic abdominal pain, periodic biopsies for eosinophilic esophagitis, evaluation and treatment of esophageal varices in chronic liver disease, unexplained weight loss, and diagnosis/evaluation of Crohn disease or ulcerative colitis. Common indications for colonoscopy in children include evaluation of chronic diarrhea, inflammatory bowel disease, and familial polyposis, among others. EGD is performed in the supine or lateral position, depending on the preference of the endoscopist.

Colonoscopy is almost always performed in the lateral position, though the supine position is preferred by some.

There are a variety of anesthetic techniques for these procedures, and every anesthesia provider (at least at the Children's Hospital of Philadelphia) will tell you that their technique is the best and safest of them all, and the patient is in grave danger if anyone else's technique is used. The techniques discussed assume the patient is an outpatient without IV access. If the child has an IV, propofol is usually used for induction. Let us take a deeper dive into the different anesthetic techniques used for EGD and colonoscopy.

(Continued)

A DEEPER DIVE—cont'd

Esophagogastroduodenoscopy (EGD)

- Many different techniques have been successfully used, including deep sedation with a natural airway, or general anesthesia with a supraglottic airway (SGA) or endotracheal tube.
- The most important consideration is maintenance of upper airway patency during shifting levels of stimulation as the endoscopist maneuvers the scope from mouth to duodenum, and back.
- These procedures tend to end abruptly with little advance warning.
- Some anesthesiologists use the natural airway approach with propofol (bolus and continuous infusion) and monitoring of end-tidal CO_2 via nasal cannula, which also supplies supplemental oxygen. This approach is unappealing because it is difficult to keep the patient motionless with pure propofol and you end up toggling between calm, and apneic with a lot of chin lifts, jaw thrusts, and transient hypoxemia. Remember, the apneic dose of propofol is lower than the analgesic dose.
- Some anesthesiologists try intermittent face mask airway with sevoflurane, but if the procedure is prolonged, the sevoflurane will inevitably escape into the room. If the endoscopist is quite skilled, however, one could anesthetize the child with sevoflurane at a high level, and then turn it off completely when the procedure begins, and the procedure will be done before the sevoflurane has worn off.
- The most perfect anesthetic technique for EGD is the SGA/sevoflurane method. The child is induced with sevoflurane, and an SGA is inserted when an appropriate level of unconsciousness is achieved (Fig. 6.1). Occasionally, a small bolus of propofol is needed for teenagers. Ondansetron is administered as prophylaxis for postoperative nausea and vomiting PONV. The child breathes spontaneously throughout the procedure and the SGA is removed along with the endoscope. The child is then ready for discharge about 15 to 20 minutes later, nausea-free.
- Opioids are rarely used because pain is not a prominent concern during and after upper endoscopy, and their administration may delay awakening and contribute to the usual opioid side effects.
- Tracheal intubation is occasionally preferred for EGD because of an underlying condition that puts the patient at risk for pulmonary aspiration, such as achalasia,

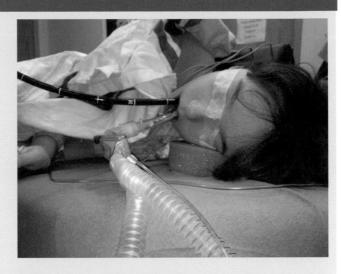

• Fig 6.1. Laryngeal mask anesthesia for upper endoscopy. (Photo credit to Petar Mamula)

severe reflux, or ablation of esophageal varices, which carries the possibility of significant bleeding.

Colonoscopy

- Most children require extensive fasting and bowel cleansing before colonoscopy, and we have found a small incidence of hypoglycemia upon admission to the endoscopy unit. For this reason, finger stick glucose determinations are performed on all children after induction of general anesthesia.
- Colonoscopy can often be stimulating because there may be numerous twists and turns of the colonoscope to reach the cecum.
- These children do not require tracheal intubation unless they are susceptible to pulmonary aspiration of gastric contents because of a preexisting medical condition.
- After induction of general anesthesia with sevoflurane, as for EGD, a sevoflurane-based technique with an SGA is the preferred technique; however, a propofol-based anesthetic technique with a natural airway and nasal cannula is a reasonable alternative.

References

1. Lerman J. On Cricoid Pressure: "May the force be with you." *Anesth Analg.* 2009;109(5):1363–1366. https://doi.org/10.1213/ANE.0b013e3181bbc6cf.
2. Matsuoka K, Kobayashi T, Ueno F, et al. Evidence-based clinical practice guidelines for inflammatory bowel disease. *J Gastroenterol.* 2018;53(3):305–353. https://doi.org/10.1007/s00535-018-1439-1.
3. Moran CJ. Very early onset inflammatory bowel disease. *Semin Pediatr Surg.* 2017;26(6):356–359. https://doi.org/10.1053/j.sempedsurg.2017.10.004.
4. Dennery PA, Seidman DS, Stevenson DK. Neonatal hyperbilirubinemia. *N Engl J Med.* 2001;344(8):581–590. https://doi.org/10.1056/NEJM200102223440807.
5. Islam S. Achalasia. *Semin Pediatr Surg.* 2017;26(2):116–120. https://doi.org/10.1053/j.sempedsurg.2017.02.001.

7

Hematologic Diseases

CHAR WITMER, SUSAN GALLAGHER, AND RONALD S. LITMAN

Inherited Coagulation Disorders

Hemophilia

The **hemophilias**[1] are a group of X-linked recessive bleeding disorders characterized by insufficient production of coagulation factor VIII (hemophilia A) or factor IX (hemophilia B). Formation of the platelet plug (primary hemostasis) is normal; however, stabilization of the plug by fibrin (secondary hemostasis) is defective because an insufficient amount of factor VIII or IX results in ineffective thrombin generation.

Hemophilia A results from a deficiency of factor VIII and occurs in approximately 1 in 5000 males. Hemophilia B results from a deficiency of factor IX and occurs in 1 in 30,000 males. Approximately 20% to 30% of female carriers produce low factor concentrations within the hemophilia range with associated bleeding tendencies. Clinically, adequate clotting usually occurs with 40% of normal factor levels.

The diagnosis of hemophilia is confirmed by demonstration of a prolonged partial thromboplastin time (PTT) plus low functional concentrations of either factor VIII or factor IX. Genetic testing is available for both hemophilia A and B. Approximately 98% of patients with either form of hemophilia will have an identifiable pathogenic variant.

The clinical manifestations of hemophilia A and B are indistinguishable. The severity is determined by the patient's pathogenic variant and their baseline factor level and is categorized as severe (<1%), moderate (1%–5%) or mild (>5 to <40%). Mild hemophilia may go undiagnosed for many years, whereas severe hemophilia may manifest during early infancy as a result of a traumatic delivery (intracranial hemorrhage), bleeding after circumcision, or intramuscular injections. If bleeding does not occur in early infancy, the remainder of children with severe hemophilia are typically asymptomatic until they begin to crawl or walk. Severe hemophilia is characterized by spontaneous or traumatic hemorrhages, which can be subcutaneous (palpable bruising), intramuscular, or within joints (hemarthroses). Acute hemarthroses are exquisitely painful and if repeated over time will result in progressive joint damage and subsequent disability.

Hemophilia is treated by IV administration of the appropriate coagulation factor. These factors are produced by either plasma-derived or recombinant technology. Advances have been made in prolonging the half-life of factor products through the addition of different moieties (e.g., Fc protein fragment, albumin, or PEGylation) to the factor VIII or IX molecule.

A novel antibody therapy was approved for prophylaxis in patients with factor VIII deficiency with[2] and without[3] an inhibitor. Emicizumab (Hemlibra) is a recombinant monoclonal antibody that bridges activated factor IX and factor X to replace the function of the missing activated factor VIII. Emicizumab improves but does not normalize baseline hemostasis. The estimated hemostatic effect is thought to be similar to a patient with mild hemophilia (equivalent factor VIII level of 10%–20%). Emicizumab has a long half-life of 28 days and takes approximately 1 month to reach steady state with initiation of therapy. Factor VIII concentrate or bypassing therapy with recombinant factor VIIa can be used concurrently with emicizumab therapy.

Emicizumab will shorten the activated prothrombin complex concentrate (aPTT) and activitated clotting time ACT. Therefore, these tests cannot be used intraoperatively to monitor a patient's ongoing coagulation status. This drug effect may last for up to 6 months after stopping the medication. In addition, any one-stage aPTT-based factor assays are also unreliable.

Factor-Replacement Therapy

Factor-replacement dosing is based on the type of product and individual pharmacokinetics. The plasma half-life of unmodified and plasma derived factor VIII is approximately 12 hours, and the plasma half-life for unmodified and plasma derived factor IX is approximately 24 hours. The prolonged factor VIII products have an estimated extended half-life of approximately 18 hours and the prolonged factor IX products have an extended half-life of 85 to 90 hours. Peak plasma factor concentration is reached 30 minutes to 1 hour after an intravenous infusion. Table 7.1 provides formulas for factor correction.

In the United States, the majority of children with severe hemophilia are treated with prophylactic therapy, which consists of either IV factor administration at regular intervals to prevent spontaneous bleeding or subcutaneous injections of emicizumab (see Table 7.1). Patients with mild or moderate hemophilia are treated as needed to prevent

TABLE 7.1	Calculation of Factor Doses

Dose of Recombinant Factor VIII (Units) = Desired Rise in % Factor Activity × Weight (kg) × 0.5[a]

Dose of Plasma-derived Factor IX (Units) = Desired Rise in % Factor Activity × Weight (kg)

Pediatric dose of Recombinant Factor IX (Units) = Desired Rise in % Factor Activity × Weight (kg) × 1.4

Adult dose of Recombinant Factor IX (Units) = Desired Rise in % Factor Activity × Weight (kg) × 1.2

Prolonged Recombinant Factor IX (Units) = Desired Rise in % Factor Activity × Weight (kg)

[a]Dosing can vary based on the patient's individual pharmacokinetics.

bleeding before surgical procedures. For nonlife-threatening bleeding episodes, such as hemarthroses, coagulation factor activity should be raised to 40% to 50% of normal. For life-threatening bleeding, coagulation factor activity is raised to 80% to 100% of normal.

The goal of treatment in a patient with hemophilia undergoing a surgical procedure[4] is to obtain a factor level of 0.8 to 1.0 units/mL (80%–100%) before the procedure. Factor replacement is continued into the postoperative period to prevent excessive bleeding and promote adequate healing. Factor replacement is usually continued for 2 to 3 days after a minor procedure and 10 to 14 days after major procedures. Intermittent dosing or continuous infusion factor replacement can be used to accomplish this goal. Preoperative evaluation for elective procedures in a patient with hemophilia should include measurement of an inhibitor titer and assessment of factor recovery and half-life.

Adjuvant hemostatic therapies include antifibrinolytics, such as aminocaproic acid and tranexamic acid, that inhibit clot lysis. Antifibrinolytic agents are particularly beneficial for surgeries that involve the oral mucosa (i.e., adenotonsillar procedures or dental extractions) because of a high concentration of fibrinolytic enzymes in saliva. Aminocaproic acid can be administered orally or IV, 100 mg/kg (maximum 6 grams) every 6 hours. Tranexamic acid is administered IV 10 mg/kg every 6 to 8 hours. A range of dosing has been reported for oral tranexamic from 10 to 25 mg/kg orally every 6 to 8 hours (maximum of 3900–6000 mg/day) has been reported.

An alternative hemostatic option for some patients with mild hemophilia A is desmopressin acetate (DDAVP). DDAVP is a synthetic vasopressin analog that causes release of factor VIII and von Willebrand factor from endothelial cells. In patients with mild hemophilia A, there is a significant variation in individual response to DDAVP, and it should not be used in severe or moderate hemophilia A. A trial administration to demonstrate an adequate rise in factor VIII levels is recommended before using DDAVP in the operative setting. (See von Willebrand disease section for more detailed information regarding DDAVP.)

Up to 30% of patients with severe hemophilia A and 3% to 5% of patients with hemophilia B develop an immune response to administered coagulation factors, with the development of IgG antibodies against factor VIII or IX. These antibodies are called *inhibitors*, and their development is the most significant treatment complication in hemophilia. High titer inhibitors interfere with the infused factor concentrates rendering them ineffective and necessitating the use of costlier and less effective alternative hemostatic agents. Alternative hemostatic agents for patients with an inhibitor include an aPCC or recombinant factor VIIa. The efficacy of these bypassing agents has significant inter-patient variation and treatment is complicated with a lack of a clinical dose response relationship and ineffective laboratory methods to monitor efficacy. Because of these limitations, surgical interventions in patients with hemophilia and a high titer inhibitor should be limited to only those procedures deemed medically necessary.[5]

For patients without an inhibitor who are receiving emicizumab prophylaxis, concurrent factor can be used in the setting of surgery to ensure adequate hemostasis. Minor procedures can be completed without additional therapy. Patients with inhibitors who are on emicizumab for prophylaxis and are having surgery should receive rFVIIa. The use of aPCC in combination with emicizumab has been associated with thrombotic events (venous and arterial) and thrombotic microangiopathy. This is hypothesized to be secondary to excessive FIXa from the aPCC that promotes abnormal clotting. In general, aPCC should not be used with emicizumab. If there is a poor clincial response to rFVIIa then aPCC can be used cautiously with recommended dosing <100 U/kg/24 hours.

Ideally, a hematologist should be involved in the perioperative management of patients with hemophilia to help develop an individualized hemostatic plan, consultation for intraoperative hemorrhage complications, and postoperative management.

Von Willebrand Disease

von Willebrand disease (vWD) is the most common hereditary bleeding disorder, present in up to 1% of the population. It results from a quantitative and/or qualitative defect of von Willebrand factor (vWF), a glycoprotein synthesized by endothelial cells and megakaryocytes. In the process of primary hemostasis, vWF acts as an adhesive bridge between the platelets and damaged subendothelium at the site of vascular injury. In the process of secondary hemostasis, it functions as the carrier protein for factor VIII.

There are different types of vWD:

- Type 1 (>85% of cases) is associated with quantitative reductions in all multimeric sizes of vWF. There is a wide variation of clinical manifestations, even for members of the same family. Children with type 1 vWD may be asymptomatic, or may have a history of frequent nosebleeds, mucosal bleeding, and easy bruising. A history of excessive bleeding during menses, or after mucosal surgery such as tonsillectomy or wisdom tooth extraction, is common. These patients are usually responsive to treatment with DDAVP.

- Type 2 is associated with quantitative and qualitative abnormalities of vWF and accounts for about 10% of cases. There are four subtypes of type 2 vWD: 2A, 2B, 2M, and 2N. Type 2A includes genetic defects that impact multimer formation or processing. Type 2B includes gain of function variants with vWF platelet binding and can be associated with mild thrombocytopenia. Type 2M includes variants that result in decreased binding to platelets. Type 2N results from pathogenic variants in the vWF FVIII binding region and results in low FVIII levels and can be mistaken for hemophilia A. Many patients with type 2 variants will not be responsive to DDAVP therapy, and require vWF replacement.
- Type 3 is the rarest and severest form, and results in a severe quantitative vWF deficiency associated with low factor VIII levels. It is associated with major bleeding requiring treatment with vWF and FVIII-containing concentrates.

Laboratory screening in patients with vWD may reveal a PTT, but many children with vWD have normal coagulation screening tests. More directed tests for vWD include a quantitative assay for vWF antigen, vWF (ristocetin cofactor) activity, plasma factor VIII activity, determination of vWF structure (vWF multimers), and a platelet count (decreased in type 2B vWD).

Treatment of vWD[6] can be accomplished by using either DDAVP to stimulate the release of endogenous stores of vWF and factor VIII or through the use of either plasma-derived factor VIII-vWF concentrates (e.g., Humate-P) or recombinant vWF (e.g., Vonvendi). Treatment decisions are based on a patient's type of vWD and their individual response to DDAVP.

Most commonly, children with type 1 vWD are responsive to DDAVP and are pretreated 30 minutes before surgery with IV DDAVP, 0.3 μg/kg. Additional doses can be administered every 12 to 24 hours postoperatively, but the response diminishes with repeated treatments as a result of tachyphylaxis. In general, DDAVP can be repeated for up to three to four consecutive doses. DDAVP has a known antidiuretic effect with resultant free water retention. Excessive fluid intake after DDAVP administration can result in hyponatremia and seizures. To minimize the risk for hyponatremia, fluid intake should be limited to two-thirds maintenance for 24 hours after DDAVP is given. This fluid limit includes the intraoperative period and should direct your anesthetic of choice and use of fluids. Even the use of isotonic fluids in the OR can still result in significant hyponatremia.

DDAVP is not used in patients who are nonresponders, type 3 vWD and some type 2 variants. In these patients, plasma-derived factor VIII concentrate with vWF or recombinant vWF is administered pre- and postoperatively. Plasma-derived vWF products should be dosed using ristocetin units and the half-life is approximately 12 hours. Recombinant vWF has a half-life of approximately 20 hours and contains ultra large multimers that do not exist in plasma-derived products.

Dosage formulae for recombinant and plasma derived FVIII vWF products (Humate P or Alphanate):

$$\text{Dose (ristocetin units)} = \% \text{ Desired Rise} \times \text{Weight} \times 0.5$$

As in hemophilia, antifibrinolytics can be used as a hemostatic adjuvant therapy in mucosal surgeries.

Hemoglobinopathies

The understanding of hemoglobinopathies requires knowledge of the structure and function of the hemoglobin molecule. All normal forms of hemoglobin contain a tetramer consisting of two alpha-polypeptide (globin) chains and two non-alpha chains. The non-alpha chains vary by the stage of maturation. For example, fetal hemoglobin (hemoglobin F) is composed of two alpha chains and two gamma chains, whereas adult hemoglobin (hemoglobin A) consists of two alpha and two beta chains. Each globin chain binds one heme group. A heme group consists of a porphyrin ring and a ferrous atom that binds to an oxygen molecule.

Sickle Cell Disease

Sickle cell disease (SCD) is an autosomal recessive disorder secondary to pathogenic variants in the beta-globin gene, and occurs in approximately 1 in 650 (0.15%) African Americans. Common forms of SCD include homozygous S or a combination of hemoglobin S with other hemoglobinopathies, commonly either hemoglobin C or beta thalassemia mutations. In all forms of SCD, the red cell containing the abnormal hemoglobin can assume an abnormal sickled shape, which predisposes the cells to impaired motility characteristics and hemolysis. Specifically, the sickled red cell membrane more easily adheres to the capillary endothelium resulting in occlusion of small capillaries and resultant reduction of perfusion to the peripheral tissues. The formation of sickled cells is promoted by hypoxemia, acidosis, hypothermia, dehydration, and hypotension.

The heterozygous state in which a child inherits a single affected beta globin gene is called *sickle cell trait* and is found in approximately 7% to 8% of African Americans. It does not cause anemia or red cell fragility. Rarely, an individual with sickle trait will exhibit painless hematuria and the inability to properly concentrate the urine (isosthenuria). They are also at increased risk for rhabdomyolosis from excessive exertion.

Clinical Syndromes in Sickle Cell Disease

Children with SCD exhibit a number of clinical syndromes, all of which are caused by aggregation of sickled red cells in small vessels, hemolysis, and decreased survival of abnormal red cells.

Painful vaso-occlusive events are the hallmarks of SCD. Pain results from vascular occlusion and resultant ischemia and can be seen in bony or soft tissues. Precipitating factors include infection, fever, cold exposure, dehydration, venous stasis, and acidosis. Dactylitis, or hand–foot syndrome, is painful swelling of the dorsal surface of the hands and feet caused by vaso-occlusion of the metacarpal and metatarsal bones. It is often the initial clinical manifestation of SCD in the first year of life. Older children typically develop pain crises in the long bones of the arms, legs, vertebral column, and sternum. Pain episodes typically last up to a week and may warrant hospitalization for administration of nonsteroidal antiinflammatory drugs (NSAIDs) and IV opioid analgesics.

Hemolytic anemia becomes apparent at approximately 4 to 6 months of age when the percentage of hemoglobin F diminishes and that of hemoglobin S increases. The anemia of SCD is chronic and well compensated. The chronic hemolysis is responsible for an increased risk for gallstone formation. In general, red cell transfusion is used during life-threatening complications such as aplastic crises, splenic sequestration, ACS, severe symptomatic anemia, or in preparation for major surgery. Chronic transfusion therapy is indicated for patients with severe SCD complications including stroke or recurrent ACS.

Splenic sequestration of sickled red blood cells leads to splenomegaly, acute exacerbation of anemia, and possibly hypovolemic shock. Splenic dysfunction occurs from repeated episodes of splenic infarction during childhood and results in susceptibility to sepsis from encapsulated organisms such as *Streptococcus pneumoniae*, *Neisseria meningitidis*, and *Haemophilus influenzae*. Children with SCD should receive vaccination against these organisms and daily penicillin prophylaxis and prompt evaluation for any fever >38.5°C.

Aplastic crises are typically caused by temporary cessation of red blood cell production in the bone marrow and are most often associated with parvovirus B-19 infection. Symptomatic anemia is treated with hospitalization and red cell transfusion. In addition, during an acute parvovirus infection, patients can have increase SCD complications including pain, splenic sequestration, and acute chest syndrome.

Acute chest syndrome (ACS) is a clinical diagnosis characterized by a new pulmonary infiltrate on chest radiograph associated with one or more clinical symptoms including fever, cough, tachypnea, dyspnea, or hypoxia. The pathophysiology of ACS in SCD is complex and multifactorial and includes infection (bacterial or viral), *in situ* vaso-occlusion, pulmonary edema, fat embolism, or thromboembolism. General anesthesia is a known risk factor for the development of ACS; therefore, preoperative transfusions are used to reduce this risk. Treatment of ACS includes supplemental oxygen, analgesia, antibiotics, and red cell transfusion to maximize respiratory function and minimize further pulmonary damage. Pulmonary complications account for a large proportion of morbidity and mortality in patients with SCD. During childhood, a substantial number of children with SCD will develop reactive airway disease and progressive pulmonary dysfunction. Up to 40% of adult patients develop moderate to severe pulmonary hypertension, which is associated with an increased mortality rate.

Stroke is one of the most disabling complications of SCD and occurs in approximately 11% of patients before the age of 20 years without screening interventions. The predominant etiology is a large vessel vasculopathy with proliferative intimal hyperplasia. Presenting signs and symptoms include mental status changes, seizures, and focal paralysis (e.g., hemiparesis). Stroke prevention is possible through routine transcranial Doppler imaging, which measures the velocity of cerebral blood flow and detects those children at increased risk for a first stroke. Children with persistently elevated transcranial Doppler measurements are placed on chronic prophylactic red cell transfusions. Children who have a stroke are also placed on a chronic red cell transfusion protocol to minimize the risk for future strokes.

Additional complications of SCD include priapism, retinopathy, leg ulcers, and progressive renal failure. By adolescence the effects of chronic myocardial microvascular obstruction and anemia result in ventricular hypertrophy. Microvascular obstruction of the intestinal circulation results in abdominal crises that manifest as signs and symptoms of an acute abdomen.

The treatment of sickle cell complications includes volume support, administration of antimicrobial agents, and prevention or reversal of anemia, hypothermia, hypoperfusion, acidosis, and pulmonary dysfunction. Hydration decreases blood viscosity and helps prevent capillary stasis. Red cell transfusion is an important aspect of sickle cell treatment because it increases the amount of hemoglobin A, while reducing the proportion of the patient's own hemoglobin S, which is responsible for sickling. Red cell transfusions are targeted to a hemoglobin level of 10 to 11 g/dL; higher hemoglobin levels will unnecessarily increase blood viscosity. Exchange transfusion to reduce the hemoglobin S level to less than 30% is used in the context of life-threatening episodes such as stroke or severe ACS with pending respiratory failure that does not resolve with simple red cell transfusion.

Hydroxyurea is currently the main drug therapy that is used to prevent SCD complications. Hydroxyurea is thought to mitigate SCD complications through the induction of hemoglobin F production which stabilizes the red cell and prevents sickling. Hydroxyurea should be started at 9 to 12 months of age for all patients with SS or S-Beta-0-thalassemia. A monoclonal antibody (crizanlizumab tmca, Adakveo[7]) that functions as a p-selectin inhibitor may prevent recurrent pain in patients with all forms of SCD. In a clinical trial of 198 patients, crizanlizumab decreased the annual rate of pain crises by 45% (1.63 versus 2.98) and the duration of hospitalization by 42% (4 versus 6.87 days).

Perioperative Management of Children With Sickle Cell Disease

Historically, patients with SCD have not fared well in the perioperative period. Development of hypoxemia, hypotension, hypothermia, hypovolemia, and acidosis are associated with exacerbation of vaso-occlusive events, and should be prevented. All ongoing medical problems should be optimized before elective surgery. We follow the current

National Institute of Health guidelines[8] for perioperative management. Except for short and minor procedures, red cells should be administered to achieve a hemoglobin level of 10 g/dL.[9] If the patient's baseline hemoglobin is close to 10 g/dL exchange transfusion can be used. Patients with cerebral vasculopathy should have special consideration for anesthesia that maximizes cerebral perfusion. The use of a tourniquet during limb surgery is discouraged because of the possibility of precipitating distal limb hypoxia, hypothermia, and acidosis; however, poor outcomes after tourniquet use have not been reported. When appropriate, regional analgesic techniques are recommended for management of postoperative pain to reduce acute painful crises, to enhance respiratory function, and to minimize opioid use in the postoperative period. Postoperative mortality is often related to development of severe ACS.

Thalassemia

The **thalassemias** (from the Greek *thalassa;* thalassemia means blood as watery as the sea) encompass a group of inherited disorders of hemoglobin synthesis that involve decreased or defective synthesis of one or more globin chains. Thalassemias are named after the affected globin chain, with alpha and beta thalassemia being the most common and clinically important types. When one globin chain is ineffectively produced, the unaffected chains are overproduced, causing red cell abnormalities that lead to immature red cell destruction and a subsequent microcytic, hypochromic, hemolytic anemia.

Alpha Thalassemias[10]

Hemoglobin Bart's hydrops fetalis syndrome is the homozygous form of the disease that results in the absence of all four alpha globin chains. This condition results in the fetal overproduction of gamma globin chains (hemoglobin Bart's) that are incapable of releasing oxygen to the tissues. Severe fetal anemia (hydrops fetalis) develops and is not compatible with intrauterine life unless intrauterine transfusions are instituted. After birth, life-long transfusions are necessary and bone marrow transplantation is curative.

Alpha thalassemia intermedia (hemoglobin H disease) results when three globin chains are absent. Hemoglobin H is the beta-4 tetramer that forms as a result of decreased alpha globin production and relative overproduction of beta globin chains. It is characterized by a mild to moderate microcytic anemia. Patients may develop splenomegaly but only rarely require splenectomy. Alpha thalassemia trait (alpha thalassemia minor) is the heterozygous form of the disease that results in the absence of two globin chains. It is present in approximately 3% of African Americans, and manifests as a microcytic anemia (rarely less than 9 g/dL) that is often confused with mild iron deficiency.

Silent-carrier alpha thalassemia is characterized by the absence of only one globin chain. The hemoglobin concentration and red cell indices are normal.

Beta Thalassemias

Beta thalassemia major (Cooley anemia) is the homozygous form of the disease characterized by the absence of beta globin chains. These children develop a severe anemia and splenomegaly during the first year of life. If the condition is left untreated, bone marrow hyperplasia and extramedullary hematopoiesis produce characteristic features such as tower skull, frontal bossing, maxillary hypertrophy with prominent cheekbones, and an overbite. In the absence of chronic blood transfusions, death occurs within the first few years of life owing to progressive congestive heart failure. A typical treatment regimen will consist of 10 to 15 mL/kg of leukodepleted red blood cells every 3 to 5 weeks to maintain the hemoglobin above 9 to 10 g/dL. Transfusion therapy prevents the clinical manifestations of the anemia but requires concomitant chelation therapy to reverse transfusion-related iron overload.

Thalassemia intermedia is a compound heterozygous state and results in a moderate anemia that does not usually require regular blood transfusions. These patients usually present later in childhood, and may develop clinical manifestations of chronic anemia as seen in thalassemia major. Transfusion therapy is reserved for acute illnesses. Beta thalassemia trait is caused by the absence of one beta chain, and is characterized by an asymptomatic mild microcytic anemia with a hemoglobin level rarely less than 9 g/dL.

Anesthetic management of patients with severe forms of thalassemia (i.e., beta thalassemia major) should focus on ensuring an adequate hemoglobin level before the procedure. Patients with iron overload complicated by cardiac disease (i.e., dilated cardiomyopathy) and/or endocrinopathies (i.e., diabetes, hypothyroidism, hypoparathyroidism) require subspecialty consultation to aid in perioperative management. Patients with alpha or beta thalassemia trait do not require any additional hematologic interventions before surgery.

References

1. Carcao MD. The diagnosis and management of congenital hemophilia. *Semin Thromb Hemost.* 2012;38(7):727–734. https://doi.org/10.1055/s-0032-1326786.
2. Oldenburg J, Mahlangu JN, Kim B, et al. Emicizumab prophylaxis in hemophilia A with inhibitors. *N Engl J Med.* 2017;377(9):809–818. https://doi.org/10.1056/NEJMoa1703068.
3. Mahlangu J, Oldenburg J, Paz-Priel I, et al. Emicizumab prophylaxis in patients who have hemophilia A without inhibitors. *N Engl J Med.* 2018;379(9):811–822. https://doi.org/10.1056/NEJMoa1803550.
4. Ljung RC, Knobe K. How to manage invasive procedures in children with haemophilia. *Br J Haematol.* 2012;157(5):519–528. https://doi.org/10.1111/j.1365-2141.2012.09089.x.
5. Kulkarni R. Comprehensive care of the patient with haemophilia and inhibitors undergoing surgery: practical aspects [published correction appears in Haemophilia. 2013 Jul;19(4):642. Dosage error in article text]. *Haemophilia.* 2013;19(1):2–10. https://doi.org/10.1111/j.1365-2516.2012.02922.x.

6. Mazzeffi MA, Stone ME. Perioperative management of von Willebrand disease: a review for the anesthesiologist. *J Clin Anesth*. 2011;23(5):418–426. https://doi.org/10.1016/j.jclinane.2011.02.003.

7. Ataga KI, Kutlar A, Kanter J, et al. Crizanlizumab for the prevention of pain crises in sickle cell disease. *N Engl J Med*. 2017;376(5):429–439. https://doi.org/10.1056/NEJMoa1611770.

8. Evidence based management of sickle cell disease. Expert Panel Report, 2014. U.S. Department of Health and Human Services, National Institute of Health. Accessed on October 5, 2021. https://www.nhlbi.nih.gov/sites/default/files/media/docs/sickle-cell-disease-report%20020816_0.pdf.

9. Vichinsky EP, Haberkern CM, Neumayr L, et al. A Comparison of Conservative and Aggressive Transfusion Regimens in the Perioperative Management of Sickle Cell Disease. The Preoperative Transfusion in Sickle Cell Disease Study Group. *N Engl J Med*. 1995;333(4):206–214. https://doi.org/10.1056/NEJM199507273330402.

10. Piel F, Weatherall DJ. The α-Thalassemias. *N Engl J Med*. 2014;371(20):1908–1916. https://doi.org/10.1056/NEJMra1404415.

Suggested Reading

Akrimi S, Simiyu V. Anaesthetic management of children with sickle cell disease. *BJAEduc*. 2018;18(11):331–336. https://doi.org/10.1016/j.bjae.2018.08.003.

8

Oncologic Diseases

JESSICA FOSTER, NAOMI BALAMUTH, SUSAN RHEINGOLD, AND RONALD S. LITMAN

Common Oncologic Disorders

Leukemia

The leukemias, which result from malignant transformation of early hematopoietic stem cells, are some of the most common malignancies of childhood (Table 8.1). Acute lymphoblastic leukemia (ALL) accounts for 75% of all childhood acute leukemia, acute myelogenous leukemia (AML) accounts for 20%, and chronic myelogenous leukemias (CML) accounts for the other 5% of childhood leukemias.

Clinical manifestations of the leukemias are similar and consist primarily of lethargy, malaise, fever, and signs of bone marrow failure such as pallor, ecchymoses, or petechiae. Bone pain related to marrow infiltration from tumor cells is also a common presenting symptom. Infiltration by leukemic blasts can also cause lymphadenopathy, hepatosplenomegaly, testicular enlargement, and respiratory symptoms from a mediastinal mass or leukostasis. Initial laboratory findings usually include signs related to bone marrow failure, such as anemia, neutropenia, and thrombocytopenia. A white blood cell (WBC) count greater than 50,000 uL/mL is also highly suspicious for leukemia.

The treatment strategy for a newly diagnosed patient with leukemia is to stabilize the patient acutely (i.e., transfusions, antibiotics) and begin definitive treatment as soon as the diagnosis has been made. Delay in treatment initiation can lead to disease progression and critical complications including respiratory failure and stroke from leukostasis.

Patients with ALL are risk-stratified based upon age and WBC at presentation, pre-B versus T-ALL subtype, cytogenetics, and minimal residual disease response testing that can identify 1 in 100,000 leukemia cells. ALL therapy has several distinct phases, each with specific objectives. These phases are as following:

Induction: Four weeks of chemotherapy to induce a morphologic remission. Leukemia cell killing is highest in this month and patients are at very high risk for developing tumor lysis syndrome (see TLS section).

Consolidation: The goal in this 8-week period is to consolidate the remission but also to provide prophylaxis or treat the CNS, a common sight of recurrence.

Interim Maintenance: An 8-week cycle of intensified methotrexate, sometimes requiring inpatient admission.

Delayed Intensification: A reinduction and reconsolidation to intensify therapy one more time before moving to maintenance therapy.

Maintenance: Low-dose chemotherapy for 2–3 years, primarily taken orally at home to maintain a remission and eradicate any remaining leukemia cells.

Approximately 85% of pediatric patients with ALL are cured with the above therapy.

Chemotherapy for AML is more intensive than for ALL and results in significant myelosuppression. The prognosis for AML is worse than that for ALL, although subtypes of AML have been associated with better (NPM + and CEBPα +) and worse (FLT3-ITD) outcomes. Children with the best prognosis get four of five cycles of intensive chemotherapy. Those with a worse prognosis move to allogeneic bone marrow transplant after three cycles of intensive chemotherapy. Current cure rates for pediatric AML patients are 55% to 60%. CML is treated with an oral tyrosine kinase inhibitors (e.g., imatinib or dasatinib), possibly for life.

Lymphoma

Lymphomas are the third-most common malignancy of childhood. Approximately 60% of pediatric lymphomas consist of non-Hodgkin lymphoma (NHL), and the remainder is Hodgkin disease (Table 8.2).

TABLE 8.1	Incidence of Childhood Cancer by Diagnosis
TYPE OF CANCER	**INCIDENCE PER 1,000,000**
CNS (Central Nervous System)	42.2
ALL (Acute Lymphocytic Leukemia)	39.9
Neuroblastoma	10.1
Non-Hodgkin Lymphoma	10.1
AML (Acute Myelogenous Leukemia)	7.7
Wilms Tumor	7.5
Hodgkin Lymphoma	6.4
Rhabdomyosarcoma	5.3
Osteosarcoma	4.2
Retinoblastoma	4.1
Ewing Sarcoma	2.4
CML (Chronic Myelogenous Leukemia)	1.5

(Data (2005–2009) from the Surveillance, Epidemiology, and End Result program [National Cancer Institute] and based on the International Classification of Childhood Cancer.)

TABLE 8.2	Common Subtypes of Pediatric Lymphoma
NON-HODGKIN LYMPHOMA (60%)	
Lymphoblastic Lymphoma (T & B-cell) Mature B-cell	

Mature B-cell
- Burkitt Lymphoma
- Diffuse Large B-cell Lymphoma
- Primary Mediastinal B-cell Lymphoma

Mature T-cell
- Anaplastic Large-cell Lymphoma
- Peripheral T-cell Lymphoma
- NK/T-cell Lymphoma

Post Transplant Lymphoproliferative Disease

HODGKIN LYMPHOMA (40%)

(From WHO Classification of Lymphoid Malignancies, 2008.)

Non-Hodgkin Lymphoma

NHL encompasses a heterogeneous group of diseases caused by neoplastic proliferation of immature lymphoid cells, which, unlike the malignant lymphoid cells of ALL, accumulate outside the bone marrow. Unlike adults, most cases of NHL in children are highly malignant and proliferate rapidly. The most common subtypes of NHL in children and adolescents are lymphoblastic lymphoma (30%); the mature B-cell lymphomas, including Burkitt's and diffuse large B-cell lymphoma (50%); and the mature T-cell lymphomas, including anaplastic large cell lymphoma (20%). Distant noncontiguous metastases to the CNS and bone marrow are common.

Initial clinical manifestations may include fever, weight loss, prominent lymphadenopathy, and other nonspecific constitutional symptoms. Anterior mediastinal masses are associated with cough, wheeze, airway compromise, pleural and pericardial effusions, and superior vena cava syndrome (see anterior mediastinal mass, below). Gastrointestinal involvement, especially in Burkitt's lymphomas, can result in rapid abdominal enlargement, pain, or ascites; intestinal obstruction occurs when the lymphoma serves as the lead point for an intussusception.

Each NHL subtype is treated differently but all involve aggressive multidrug chemotherapy. Radiation is avoided unless needed emergently or with recurrence. The therapy for lymphoblastic lymphoma is similar to that used for ALL. Therapy for Burkitt's and diffuse large B-cell lymphoma is more intensive but of shorter duration.

Hodgkin Disease

Hodgkin disease accounts for 4% of all childhood cancer. Histopathologic subtypes are similar to those in adults: 40% to 60% nodular sclerosis, 10% to 20% lymphocyte predominance, 20% to 40% mixed cellularity, and 10% lymphocyte depleted. Its incidence has a bimodal distribution with peaks occurring at 15 to 30 years of age and after the age of 50 years. The most common presentation is painless firm lymphadenopathy involving either the supraclavicular or cervical nodes. Two-thirds of patients will also have mediastinal lymphadenopathy. Fever, night sweats, and weight loss, also termed "B" symptoms, occur in 30% of children. Staging and therapy is based upon histologic subtype, localized versus diffuse disease, presence of B symptoms, bulk of disease, and rapidity of response to initial therapy.

Most pediatric treatment protocols consist of multiagent chemotherapy, which may be combined with low-dose radiation therapy. The addition of radiation improves disease-free survival in children with bulk disease, those who present with B symptoms, and slow responders to initial chemotherapy but is avoided in females because of the risk for secondary breast cancer. Prognosis varies from a 90% to 95% cure of stage I disease to a 70% cure of stage IV disease.

Central Nervous System Tumors

Central nervous system (CNS) tumors are the most common solid tumors in children and are second to leukemia in overall incidence of malignant diseases. In contrast to adults, brain tumors in children are located predominantly infratentorial in the cerebellum and brainstem but can occur anywhere in the brain and spinal cord. Childhood brain tumors are usually low-grade astrocytomas or malignant neoplasms such as medulloblastoma. Infratentorial tumors may present with signs of increased intracranial pressure

(ICP) (headache, nausea, emesis, lethargy, impaired upward gaze), nystagmus, ataxia, or cranial nerve deficits. Children with supratentorial tumors commonly present with signs of ICP, seizures, hemiparesis, or visual-field deficits. The treatment regimen depends on the histology, location, and staging of the tumor and the age of the patient. Surgery is undertaken to establish a diagnosis (biopsy), attempt maximal safe resection, and treat obstructive hydrocephalus. Radiation dose and volume (e.g., focal to the tumor bed, craniospinal, etc.) depend on tumor type and age (e.g., whole brain radiation is avoided in children less than 3 years of age). Many brain tumors are responsive to chemotherapy, which may even obviate the need for radiotherapy. Inhibitors of angiogenesis, molecularly targeted therapies, and immune-based therapeutics are being increasingly used and evaluated.

Neuroblastoma

Neuroblastoma accounts for 6% of all childhood cancers and in children is the most common solid tumor outside the central nervous system. Neuroblastoma is a malignancy of the primitive neural crest cells that form the adrenal medulla and the paraspinal sympathetic ganglia. Abdominal tumors account for 70% of cases, one-third of which arise from the retroperitoneal sympathetic ganglia and two-thirds from the adrenal medulla itself. Thoracic masses, accounting for 20% of the tumors, tend to arise from paraspinal ganglia in the posterior mediastinum. Neuroblastoma of the neck occurs in 5% of cases and often involves the cervical sympathetic ganglion.

Neuroblastoma represents a broad spectrum of disease. Although low-risk patients are often incidentally diagnosed, patients with high-risk disease are often ill, appearing with bone and bone marrow involvement. Symptoms depend on the location and spread of the tumor. Hypertension can result from compression of the renal vasculature by a large calcified abdominal mass or from tumor secretion of catecholamines. Thoracic or abdominal tumors may invade the epidural space posteriorly in a dumbbell fashion and cause back pain and symptoms of spinal cord compression. Children with neuroblastoma may be volume depleted secondary to chronic hypertension or diarrhea resulting from tumor production of vasoactive intestinal peptides.

The treatment of high-risk neuroblastoma is among the most intensive in pediatric oncology. The multidisciplinary approach includes chemotherapy, surgery, radiation therapy, stem cell transplant, and immunotherapy. Patients with low and intermediate risk disease may be treated with less intensive chemotherapy, surgery alone, or simply observation. Prognosis is dependent on age, stage, and histologic and molecular characteristics.

Wilms Tumor

Wilms tumor, a cancer of embryonal renal cells, accounts for 5% of all childhood cancers and predominantly occurs in the first 5 years of life. Wilms tumor occurs frequently in the setting of additional genitourinary tract anomalies. Most children are diagnosed after incidental detection of an asymptomatic abdominal mass. Associated findings include microscopic or gross hematuria, and hypertension. Hypertension may occur from renin secretion by tumor cells or compression of the renal vasculature by the tumor. Local extension of the tumor often involves the renal vein and inferior vena cava, with occasional extension to the level of the right atrium. The lung is the most common site of distant metastases.

Unilateral Wilms tumors are treated, when possible, with surgical resection of the affected kidney followed by chemotherapy. Unresectable tumors are treated with neoadjuvant chemotherapy. Radiotherapy may also be added for patients with higher stage disease. When the tumor is bilateral, presurgical chemotherapy is performed to shrink the tumors in an attempt to salvage some renal function, after which local tumor excision is attempted. Tumors with favorable histology, such as classic nephroblastoma, have a better than 90% overall survival rate. Tumors with unfavorable histology, such as anaplastic or sarcomatous variants, have a much lower survival rate.

Bone Tumors

Primary malignant bone tumors account for 4% of childhood cancer and consist primarily of Ewing sarcoma and osteogenic sarcoma.

Ewing Sarcoma

Ewing sarcoma, an undifferentiated sarcoma that arises primarily in bone, occurs mostly in adolescents. The most common presenting symptoms include pain and swelling at the site of the tumor. The most commonly involved sites are the femur (20%), pelvis (20%), fibula (12%), humerus (10%), and tibia (10%). Systemic manifestations are more common with metastases and include fever, weight loss, and fatigue.

Treatment consists of chemotherapy, surgery, and/or radiation therapy to provide local control of the primary tumor. If the tumor affects an expendable bone (proximal fibula, rib, or clavicle), complete surgical excision may be indicated. Patients with Ewing sarcoma are presumed to have micrometastatic disease at the time of diagnosis. As a result, chemotherapy is used not only to reduce the size of the primary tumor, but also to eradicate micrometastases. The prognosis is generally good (~75% survival) for patients with distal-extremity nonmetastatic tumors. Children with metastatic disease at diagnosis or tumors of the pelvic bones or proximal femur have less favorable outcomes.

Osteogenic Sarcoma

Osteogenic sarcoma (or osteosarcoma), a malignant tumor of the bone-producing osteoblasts, arises in the medullary cavity or the periosteum. The primary tumor is usually located at the metaphyseal portion of bones associated with maximum growth velocity (e.g., distal femur, proximal tibia, and proximal humerus) and occurs mostly during early adolescence. Similar to Ewing sarcoma, pain and localized swelling are the most common presenting complaints; but in contrast to Ewing's sarcoma, systemic manifestations are rare. At diagnosis, 20% of patients have clinically detectable metastatic disease and most of the remaining patients have microscopic metastatic disease. Neoadjuvant and postoperative chemotherapy increases disease-free survival to greater than 70%. Osteogenic sarcomas are not radiation sensitive tumors, so complete resection of all known sites of disease is critical for cure. When feasible, limb-salvage surgical procedures are performed to limit resection to the tumor-bearing portion of the bone.

Chemotherapeutic Agents

A variety of classes of chemotherapeutic agents are used in children, depending on the particular type of malignancy and its progression. All chemotherapeutic agents have adverse effects. In particular, the anthracyclines—doxorubicin and daunorubicin—are associated with cardiac toxic effects. Atrial and ventricular conduction disturbances may occur acutely, and left ventricular failure may occur in chronically treated children. Heart failure is associated with a cumulative dose in excess of $300\,\mathrm{mg/m^2}$, age less than 4 years, the use of additional chemotherapeutic agents, and mediastinal irradiation. Children who receive these drugs are assessed by echocardiography before initiation of treatment and at regular intervals during treatment. Other significant chemotherapy toxicities include pulmonary toxicity with bleomycin and renal toxicity with cisplatin. Methotrexate when given in high doses can lead to neurotoxicity, and acute liver or renal failure. Intrathecal chemotherapy can cause seizures and neurotoxicity. Antiangiogenic agents (e.g. bevacizumab) increase the risk for bleeding and delay wound healing; therefore, such agents should be discontinued for an appropriate interval before any major surgical procedure. The preanesthetic evaluation should include a review of all chemotherapeutic agents used, as well as the results of toxicity studies, such as echocardiograms.

Miscellaneous Problems in Children With Cancer

Bone Marrow Dysfunction

Bone marrow dysfunction is a common occurrence in children with cancer as a result of the tumor's effect on the bone marrow or as an effect of chemotherapeutic agents. Most children's hospitals have prophylactic transfusion guidelines for patients receiving chemotherapy, often permitting the hemoglobin level to fall to 7 to $8\,\mathrm{g/dL}$ and the platelet count to about $10,000/\mu L$. Although well-tolerated by patients for daily activities, these guidelines are not appropriate for invasive procedures. The presence of mild to moderate anemia is not normally hazardous to otherwise healthy children, but it may pose a threat to oxygen delivery when chemotherapy-induced cardiac toxicity is also present. Clinically significant thrombocytopenia is usually considered to be a platelet count $<50,000/\mu L$ and should be corrected before major surgery. Many oncologists perform routine minor procedures such as bone marrow aspirates with platelet counts as low as 20 to $30,000/\mu L$. Thrombocytopenia is considered a contraindication to central regional anesthesia or peripheral nerve blocks in the area of large blood vessels.

Neutropenic children are at increased risk for serious infections. Anesthesiologists should take extreme care to perform procedures and handle intravenous lines with meticulous sterile technique in these children. All members

---

A DEEPER DIVE

Guidelines for Handling Central Lines to Prevent Central Line-Associated Bloodstream Infection

The prevention of central line-associated bloodsteam infection (CLABSI) is of utmost importance in hospitalized children with central lines because CLABSI contributes to patient morbidity and mortality. This is the protocol we use to prevent CLABSI when a patient with a central line or centrally placed peripheral line (PIC) presents for anesthetic care.

- If the patient arrives with an infusion running via the central line, it is continued if it is appropriate for the patient's care, but the sterile connection of the infusion to the catheter must be maintained.
- If the existing infusion line is changed, or if the line is accessed for medication administration, special procedures for central line access must be followed.
- Administration of any IV medication should be preceded by a 15-second hub scrub with alcohol and a 15-second pause to allow the alcohol to dry.

- When administering medications in a rapid series, there is no need to rescrub the hub assuming that the injection site sterility is maintained by holding it in one's hand without touching the site or allowing it to rest on any surface. Once the injection site is no longer held in your hand it should be reprepped with a 15-second hub scrub and 15-second drying period before use.
- If a central venous line is changed during a procedure, infusions that were running through the line before it was changed should not be used with the new line. A new infusion setup must be used.
- An infusion set with two stopcocks should be used to facilitate injection of more than one drug rapidly. The stopcocks must be introduced into the line in sterile fashion, and accessed for injection using an injection hub or similar permanent cap that maintains a closed system.
- It is not acceptable to access central lines via a stopcock port that is open (i.e., not capped with a closed injection hub).

of the anesthesia team should rigorously follow central line care-and-use standards for their institution.

Anterior Mediastinal Mass

An anterior mediastinal mass may be present in children with a variety of malignancies, most commonly T-cell ALL, NHL, and Hodgkin disease, but also neuroblastoma, intrathoracic germ cell tumors, and thymomas. These masses may be sufficiently large as to cause tracheal and/or bronchial compression that leads to airway obstruction. Great vessel or atrial compression may lead to obstruction of blood flow into or out of the heart (superior vena cava syndrome). In severe cases, the negative intrathoracic pressure generated by spontaneous ventilation precariously maintains the patency of the lower airway and great vessels. Reduction of respiratory drive by narcotics, sedatives, and induction of general anesthesia or neuromuscular blockade can cause loss of negative intrathoracic pressure as a result of weakening of the chest wall muscles and is associated with life-threatening airway obstruction and great vessel compression. This obstruction cannot always be alleviated by administration of positive-pressure ventilation.

Typical symptoms of an anterior mediastinal mass in children include new onset of wheeze, dyspnea, cough, or stridor, gradually worsening or more obvious when supine. Children with more advanced tumors may have begun to sleep in an upright position. Any child with presumed malignant lymphadenopathy of the neck or a new diagnosis of leukemia should be evaluated radiologically for an anterior mediastinal mass, regardless of respiratory symptoms, before administration of general anesthesia. Cases of life-threatening airway obstruction or death during induction of general anesthesia have occurred in children without classic symptomatology.

When a mediastinal mass is suspected, an immediate diagnostic evaluation is indicated. Chest radiography may reveal a widened mediastinum and pleural effusion, but computed tomography (CT) is best suited for demonstrating the extent of spread of the mediastinal mass and the severity of tracheal compression. Echocardiography is necessary to evaluate the severity of great vessel compression

and the presence of a pericardial effusion. Because tumor growth is often rapid, these studies should be performed immediately before any planned procedure requiring general anesthesia or sedation.

Many papers have tried to correlate preoperative evaluations and anesthetic outcomes but no perfect algorithm exists for predicting poor anesthetic outcome. Intra- and postoperative complications have been associated with positional dyspnea, stridor or orthopnea, presence of superior vena cava syndrome tracheal airway compression of >50% by CT[1] and compression of cardiac vasculature or large pericardial effusions identified by echocardiogram. When general anesthesia is required, a detailed evaluation and plan should be formulated preoperatively, including having a cardiopulmonary bypass team available if the patient is at risk for hemodynamic compromise.

In some cases, the risk for anesthesia outweighs the need for an immediate tissue diagnosis. In patients with critical respiratory or vascular compromise an attempt should be made to obtain tissue for diagnosis in a minimally invasive manner without sedation or general anesthesia. If a patient is at a significant risk for a catastrophic airway obstruction and/or cardiovascular collapse[2], steroids, chemotherapy and/or radiation can be used to decrease the size of the mediastinal mass before diagnostic procedures requiring sedation or general anesthesia.

The principles of anesthetizing children[3] with an anterior mediastinal mass are similar to those of the difficult airway secondary to upper-airway obstruction and are based on maintenance of negative intrathoracic pressure provided by continuous spontaneous ventilation (see Chapter 18). However, there are several important differences. Children with mediastinal masses with tracheal compression may require induction of anesthesia in the sitting or semisitting position to avoid gravity-induced tracheal compression by the mass. Furthermore, in the event of life-threatening airway obstruction, there are several unique maneuvers that may alleviate the obstruction caused by the mass. These include advancing the endotracheal tube (or rigid bronchoscope) distal to the site of the tracheal obstruction, placing the patient in the lateral position, and instituting emergency extracorporeal membrane oxygenation (ECMO) when no other option exists.

A DEEPER DIVE

Anesthetic Technique for Patients With an Anterior Mediastinal Mass

Patients with an anterior mediastinal mass require a meticulous preoperative assessment to evaluate the location and severity of intrathoracic airway obstruction or interference with cardiovascular function before any procedure requiring general anesthesia or sedation. In any patient where an increased potential for such obstruction is noted preoperatively, provision should be made for the availability of a rigid bronchoscope, the ability to easily move the operating room table to effect position changes, and the ability to immediately institute

cardiopulmonary bypass or extracorporeal membrane oxygenation (ECMO) if necessary.

Computed tomography (CT) of the chest is helpful in planning the anesthetic induction technique and in evaluating the potential for airway compromise during anesthetic care. Compression of greater than 50% of the cross-sectional area of the trachea on CT imaging has been suggested[4] to indicate a risk for airway collapse during induction of general anesthesia. In patients with this degree of tracheal compression, preoperative therapeutic options include radiation therapy, and/or administration of corticosteroids or chemotherapy to shrink the mass

(Continued)

and decrease the severity of the tracheal obstruction. Except in situations in which the size and/or location of the mass is truly life-threatening, many oncologists prefer to refrain from the use of such preoperative treatments because of their effect on the histopathology or tumor markers in the specimen. In patients who have additional tissue sites from which a biopsy can be obtained (e.g., cervical, axillary, or inguinal lymph nodes), it may be safer to proceed with the patient in a semisitting position using local anesthesia and carefully titrating sedation so that spontaneous ventilation is preserved. Dexmedetomidine infusion in combination with ketamine may be a useful sedation strategy with maintenance of spontaneous ventilation for peripheral lymph node biopsy or fine needle biopsy of a mediastinal mass. If general anesthesia is essential for biopsy of the chest mass, patients with a significant degree of upper-airway obstruction require an induction technique that preserves spontaneous ventilation.

With a large mediastinal mass, there may not be airway compromise but rather obstruction of blood inflow to the right atrium[2] and/or outflow tract obstruction from the right or left ventricle. This may be responsible for the cardiorespiratory collapse that has been described during anesthetic induction with or without loss of spontaneous ventilation. Preoperative echocardiography is suggested to rule out compression of the heart or great vessels by the tumor mass.

Preoperative

- Carefully delineate size and effect of mass on surrounding tissues (i.e., tracheal compression, great vessel compression) with CT scan and echocardiography, respectfully.
- In older children, attempt tissue diagnosis of peripheral blood, lymph nodes, bone marrow or effusion without the use of deep sedation or general anesthesia.
- If the mediastinal mass dangerously obstructs the trachea or inflow of blood to the heart, attempt to reduce the size of the mass using chemotherapy and/or radiation

before proceeding with a procedure that requires sedation or general anesthesia. This is rare.
- A rigid bronchoscope and a physician with expertise in its use should be immediately available before and during induction of general anesthesia.
- Some centers advocate immediate availability of ECMO.

Intraoperative

- Induction of general anesthesia should be performed while maintaining spontaneous ventilation. CPAP may help maintain upper-airway patency and preserve functional residual capacity (FRC).
- Some children may require induction of general anesthesia in the semisitting or lateral position to keep the mass from compressing the trachea.
- Tracheal intubation or supraglottic airway placement (if required) should be accomplished during deep anesthesia and spontaneous ventilation.
- It is preferable to avoid neuromuscular blockade for fear of losing airway muscle tone and exacerbating airway obstruction.

Management of Airway Obstruction

- In the event of airway obstruction during induction of general anesthesia, the standard algorithm for difficult ventilation (see Chapter 18) should be applied.
- If ventilation cannot be accomplished despite tracheal tube placement, perform the following steps:
  - Push the endotracheal tube distally past the tracheal obstruction or into the right main bronchus.
  - If the endotracheal tube cannot be advanced past the obstruction, rigid bronchoscopy should be performed.
  - Alleviate gravity-induced tracheal or great vessel compression by placing the patient in the sitting, lateral, or prone position.
- If the above measures are unsuccessful in restoring oxygenation or circulation, institute ECMO immediately.

Tumor Lysis Syndrome

Tumor lysis syndrome (TLS) describes a constellation of metabolic abnormalities resulting from spontaneous or treatment-induced tumor cell death, leading to rapid release of cellular contents into the bloodstream. This leads to hyperphosphatemia, hyperkalemia, and hyperuricemia. Hyperkalemia can cause cardiac arrhythmias. Phosphate, especially at high serum levels, binds to calcium, resulting in precipitation of calcium phosphate in renal tubules, hypocalcemia, and tetany. Purines are processed to uric acid, and hyperuricemia can result in precipitation of uric acid in renal tubules with subsequent renal failure.

Tumors with high growth rates such as T-cell ALL or Burkitt's lymphoma are at highest risk for TLS. High WBC counts ($>100,000/\mu L$) and evidence of high disease burden (hepatosplenomegaly or lymphadenopathy) also increase the likelihood of developing TLS. Complications of TLS include renal insufficiency, cardiac dysrhythmias, and uncontrollable metabolic abnormalities.

The risk for tumor lysis is greatest during the first 3 days of chemotherapy. At admission, management includes vigorous hydration with nonpotassium-containing fluids and diuresis, sometimes requiring diuretic therapy with furosemide. Uric acid reduction with allopurinol can be initiated immediately, but if a patient already has a very elevated uric acid, requires intensive care unit (ICU) level care, or is at very high risk for TLS, rasburicase is recommended for its more efficient onset. Temporary dialysis is sometimes required to manage fluid overload, metabolic abnormalities, and/or renal insufficiency.

Infection

Neutropenia that results from administration of chemotherapeutic agents predisposes to the development of bacterial and fungal infections, especially at the site of indwelling central venous catheters. Neutropenic patients presenting with fever of unknown origin are hospitalized, cultured, and placed on broad-spectrum antibiotics. Removal of an indwelling central venous catheter may be necessary if blood cultures do not clear or if a fungal infection is found. All anesthesia providers should follow hospital guidelines for central line management to prevent central line-related infections.

References

1. Shamberger RC. Preanesthetic evaluation of children with anterior mediastinal masses. *Semin Pediatr Surg*. 1999;8(2):61–68. https://doi.org/10.1016/s1055-8586(99)70020-x.
2. Keon TP. Death on induction of anesthesia for cervical node biopsy. *Anesthesiology*. 1981;55(4):471–472.
3. Stricker PA, Gurnaney HG, Litman RS. Anesthetic management of children with an anterior mediastinal mass. *J Clin Anesth*. 2010;22(3):159–163. https://doi.org/10.1016/j.jclinane.2009.10.004.
4. Shamberger RC, Holzman RS, Griscom NT, Tarbell NJ, Weinstein HJ. CT quantitation of tracheal cross-sectional area as a guide to the surgical and anesthetic management of children with anterior mediastinal masses. *J Pediatr Surg*. 1991;26(2):138–142. https://doi.org/10.1016/0022-3468(91)90894-y.

Suggested Readings

Malik R, Mullassery D, Kleine-Brueggeney M, et al. Anterior mediastinal masses - A multidisciplinary pathway for safe diagnostic procedures. *J Pediatr Surg*. 2019;54(2):251–254. https://doi.org/10.1016/j.jpedsurg.2018.10.080.
Mcleod M, Dobbie M. Anterior mediastinal masses in children. *BJA Educ*. 2019;19(1):21–26. https://doi.org/10.1016/j.bjae.2018.10.001.

9

Genetic and Inherited Diseases

ALEXANDRA BERMAN* AND RONALD S. LITMAN

Trisomy 21 (Down Syndrome)

With an incidence of approximately1 in 700 live births[1], trisomy 21[2] is the most common chromosomal abnormality and the most common cause of intellectual disability associated with genetic disease. These children are characterized by their distinctive facial appearance (Fig. 9.1) and a variety of possible disorders.

Surgical intervention is required for a number of disease entities that occur in children with trisomy 21 (Table 9.1). Furthermore, a number of associated congenital anomalies may cause unique anesthetic-related challenges.

Preoperative evaluation should focus on delineation of associated comorbidities. Many children with trisomy 21 have only mild intellectual disability and will benefit from a full explanation of the perioperative process. An anxiolytic premedication such as oral midazolam should be ordered unless there are concerns about severe obstructive sleep apnea (OSA). Older children with trisomy 21 tend to have a large body mass index (BMI) which, along with developmental delay or autism, may present as a preoperative behavioral management problem. Administration of intramuscular ketamine 2 to 3 mg/kg is occasionally required in this patient population to facilitate parental separation and mask induction of anesthesia or intravenous (IV) line placement.

Children with trisomy 21 have inherently smaller upper airways, tonsillar hypertrophy,[3] and frequent OSA. Upper airway obstruction during inhalation induction of general anesthesia is common and is probably caused by a combination of a large tongue, large adenoidal and tonsillar tissue, an abnormally small pharynx, and hypotonia of the pharyngeal dilator muscles. Almost always, placement of an oral airway device provides satisfactory relief of the obstruction.

Children with trisomy 21 have an increased incidence of tracheal anomalies,[4] which are more likely in the presence of congenital heart disease. Therefore whenever tracheal intubation is performed, one should ensure that the endotracheal tube is not too large, and that the endotracheal tube is normally positioned above the carina.

*Many thanks to Mary Theroux, the creator of the original version of the chapter. Her vision and original thoughts form the backbone of the chapter.

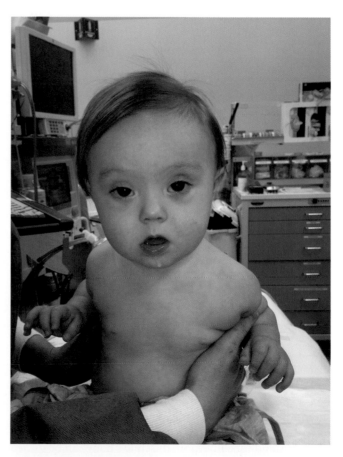

• **Fig. 9.1** The distinctive facies of trisomy 21 (Down syndrome). Courtesy of Ronald S. Litman.

TABLE 9.1	Common Medical Diseases and Surgical Procedures in Children With Trisomy 21	
Medical Disease	**Surgical Procedure**	
Leukemia	Lumbar puncture, bone marrow aspiration and biopsy	
Narrowed eustachian tube and frequent middle ear infections	Myringotomy and tube insertion, tympanomastoidectomy	
Obstructive sleep apnea	Tonsillectomy and adenoidectomy	
Poor dentition	Oral rehabilitation	
Congenital heart disease	Cardiac surgery	
Hirshprung disease	Colonic biopsy, often with resection and pull-through procedures	
Imperforate anus	Neonatal colostomy with definitive repair later in infancy	
Duodenal atresia	Repair in the neonatal period	

Lower airway anomalies[5] are also common in children with trisomy 21. These include tracheomalacia and bronchomalacia, which predispose to intrathoracic tracheal and bronchial collapse during forced expiration, and extrathoracic tracheal collapse during forced inspiration. Pulmonary abnormalities may also occur in this population.

One of the most important anesthetic considerations in children with trisomy 21 is the potential presence of atlantoaxial instability (AAI).[6] Children with trisomy 21 tend to have generalized ligamental laxity, which includes the transverse ligament that holds the dens of the axis (C2) in place against the posterior surface of the anterior arch of the atlas (C1) (Fig. 9.2). Normally, this ligament holds the dens tightly against the anterior arch of the atlas to facilitate rotatory neck motion, and maintains cervical stability during flexion, extension, and side-bending of the neck. However, when the ligament is lax, the dens may separate from the anterior arch of the atlas and encroach upon the spinal cord during motion away from the neutral position.

There have been a number of reported cases of children with trisomy 21 who exhibited new signs and symptoms of spinal cord damage upon awakening from general anesthesia or sedation, presumed because of excessive neck movement while unconscious. Most pediatric centers do not require preoperative cervical radiographs but assume that all children with trisomy 21 may be susceptible to AAI while sedated or anesthetized. The head and neck should be kept in as neutral a position as clinically feasible, and it should be documented in the anesthesia record that these safety precautions were observed. For example, during myringotomy and tube insertion, the child's body can be turned along with the neck while the tubes are being placed; during

tonsillectomy, instead of neck extension, the table can be placed in the Trendelenburg position.

Approximately 40% of children with trisomy 21 have congenital heart disease, including (in descending order of incidence) atrial septal defect, ventricular septal defect, tetralogy of Fallot, and endocardial cushion defects. Pulmonary hypertension may occur in up to 5% patients with trisomy 21, even in the absence of heart disease. Optimization of cardiac status is essential before elective surgery, and prophylaxis against infective endocarditis may be necessary. Bradycardia[7] during sevoflurane induction occurs often in children with trisomy 21, even in the absence of structural heart disease. Although unsubstantiated, it appears that resting heart rates during sevoflurane anesthesia seem to be lower in this population.

Additional medical problems in children with trisomy 21 that may impact anesthetic management include obesity, immunodeficiency, hypothyroidism, autism, hearing and vision deficits, epilepsy, and moyamoya disease, to name a few. An exaggerated response to atropine has been reported but has not been clinically proven. Children with trisomy 21 do not have different analgesic requirements.[8,9]

Phakomatoses

The phakomatoses encompass a group of inherited neuroectodermal diseases, several of which are important in pediatric anesthesia because they are associated with anomalies that require surgical intervention, and may predispose to anesthetic-related complications. This section reviews neurofibromatosis, tuberous sclerosis, Sturge-Weber syndrome, and Parkes Weber syndrome.

The two most common types of neurofibromatosis (NF) in children are type 1 (von Recklinghausen disease) and type 2 (bilateral acoustic neurofibromatosis). The clinical presentation of type 1 disease is variable and may include multiple café-au-lait spots, nodular neurofibromas in the skin, upper airway, and nervous system, Lisch nodules in the iris, optic gliomas, bony dysplasias, tumors of the brain or spine that cause neurologic symptoms (e.g., seizures, increased intracranial pressure) or lead to kyphoscoliosis, and variable degrees of developmental delay or intellectual disability. Patients with NF-2 may demonstrate hearing loss and vestibular disorientation. Neurofibromas, meningiomas, schwannomas, and astrocytomas are also associated with NF-2. Surgical debulking is indicated for NF-2 when hearing becomes substantially impaired.

Children with NF require general anesthesia for a variety of reasons, the most common being surveillance MRI to detect or monitor the growth of central nervous system (CNS) tumors. There are few discrete anesthetic risks in these children, and little data in the anesthesia literature to indicate any type of unique anesthetic management in the pediatric population. In general, anesthetic considerations[10] concern the degree of disruption to organ systems affected by the tumors. In rare cases, patients with NF-1

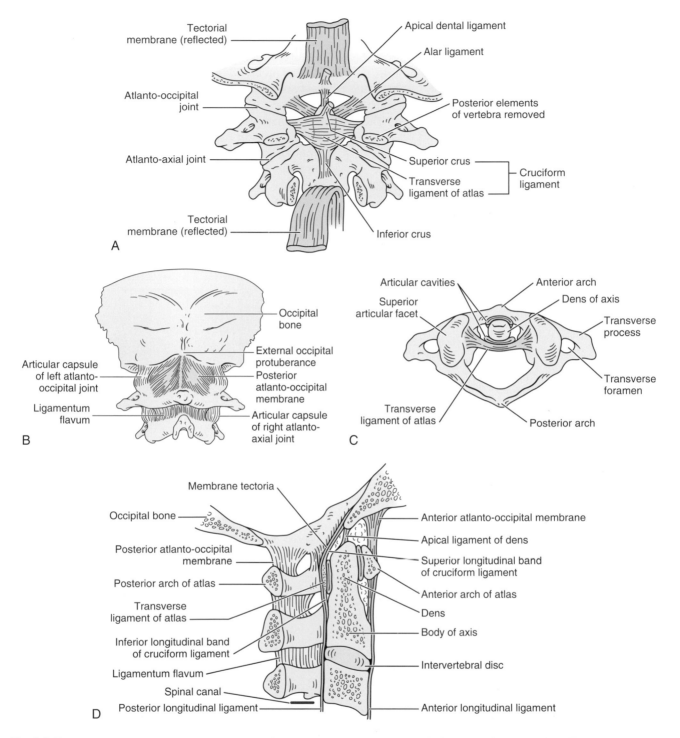

• **Fig. 9.2** Transverse ligament holding dens against anterior arch of atlas. Panel A through D show the relationship of the Transverse ligament of the atlas to the dens and anterior arch of the atlas from various perspectives. A and B posteriorly, C is viewed above, and D is a sagittal view. (From Magee David J, Manske Robert C. Cervical spine. In: *Orthopedic Physical Assessment*. 7th ed. Elsevier; 2021:164–242.)

will demonstrate hypertension caused by either renal artery stenosis[11] or a pheochromocytoma. Laryngeal involvement with a tumor that impedes airflow has been reported but is also rare (Fig. 9.3).

Tuberous sclerosis[12] is a progressive, multisystemic disorder characterized by angiofibromas of the face (Fig. 9.4), intellectual disability, hyperactivity, seizures, tuberous nodules in the brain, rhabdomyomas of the heart, a variety of congenital heart disease defects, renal cysts and tumors, and bone and lung cysts. As with NF-1, these children most often present for MRI examination under general anesthesia. If the child is intellectually disabled and not amenable to mask or IV induction, intramuscular ketamine is a useful alternative. If cardiac tumors are present, a recent echocardiogram is indicated to confirm their anatomic location and effect on cardiovascular physiology.

Sturge-Weber syndrome[13] (encephalofacial angiomatosis) is a progressive neurologic disorder associated with unilateral capillary hemangiomas (port-wine stains) of the face over the area innervated by the first division of the trigeminal nerve (V1) (Fig. 9.5). They may rarely involve CNS structures with accompanying neurologic symptoms such as intellectual disability, seizures, and visual impairment. These children commonly undergo laser removal of the hemangioma, which often requires several treatments over time. As with NF-1 and tuberous sclerosis, anesthetic considerations depend on location of the hemangiomas, particularly in the oral cavity or upper airway.

Parkes Weber syndrome (formerly called Klippel-Trenaunay-Weber syndrome) is a disorder defined by a large capillary malformation with soft tissue and boney hypertrophy on an extremity (most commonly a lower limb) and multiple, microscopic arteriovenous fistulae (Fig. 9.6). In particular, these arteriovenous fistulas (AVFs) may cause abnormal bleeding, anemia, thrombocytopenia, or high-output congestive heart failure.

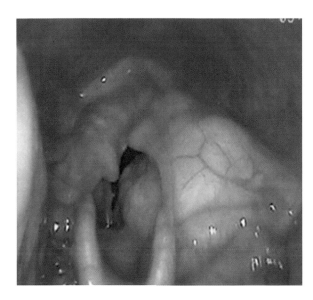

• **Fig. 9.3** Flexible laryngoscopy imaging shows a large neurofibroma on the left arytenoid cartilage that is nearly obliterating the larynx. (From Chinn SB, Collar RM, McHugh JB, et al. Pediatric laryngeal neurofibroma: case report and review of the literature. *Int. J. Pediatr. Otorhinolaryngol*. 2014; 78(1):142-147. doi: https://doi.org/10.1016/j.ijporl.2013.10.047.)

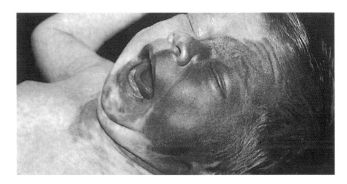

• **Fig. 9.5** Port-wine stain of Sturge-Weber syndrome. A nonelevated purple cutaneous vascular malformation is seen in a trigeminal distribution, including the ophthalmic division. (From Varma R., Williams Shelley D. Neurology. In: Zitelli Basil J, Mcintire Sara C, Nowalk Andrew J, eds. *Zitelli and Davis' Atlas of Pediatric Physical Diagnosis*. 7th ed. Elsevier; 2018:562–592.)

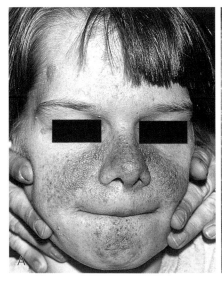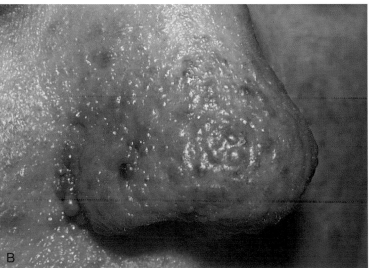

• **Fig. 9.4** Tuberous sclerosis (TS). (A) This adolescent boy had adenoma sebaceum in a characteristic malar distribution and chin lesions. (B) A close-up view of the angiofibromas of tuberous sclerosis. (From Varma R., Williams Shelley D. Neurology. In: Zitelli Basil J, Mcintire Sara C, Nowalk Andrew J, eds. *Zitelli and Davis' Atlas of Pediatric Physical Diagnosis*. 7th ed. Elsevier;2018: 562–592.)

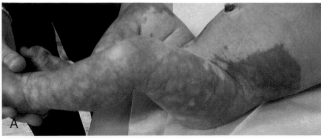

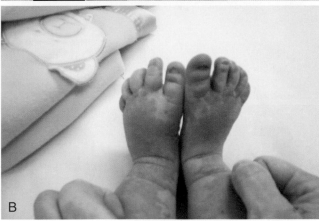

• **Fig. 9.6** This infant with Parkes Weber syndrome is unusual in that he has vascular malformations involving both lower extremities (Panel B), which extend upward over the lateral aspects of the abdominal wall (Panel A). (From Varma R., Williams Shelley D. Neurology. In: Zitelli Basil J, Mcintire Sara C, Nowalk Andrew J, eds. *Zitelli and Davis' Atlas of Pediatric Physical Diagnosis*. 7th ed. Elsevier; 2018:562–592.)

Dwarfism (Osteochondrodystrophy)

Short stature is a relative term that refers to individuals that are more than two standard deviations below the average height for a person of the same age and sex. Children with severe short stature are generally divided into two categories: (1) proportionate growth with a normal ratio of trunk length to limb length, and (2) disproportionate development characterized by short limbs (often deformed) or short trunk. The latter group are referred to as *dwarfs*. Achondroplasia is the most common form of dwarfism, with an incidence of 1 in 20,000 live births (Fig. 9.7). Significant anesthetic concerns[14] in dwarfs include abnormalities of the cervical spine, upper airway, cardiopulmonary system, and neuromuscular and skeletal systems.

Perioperatively, an abnormal cervical spine, with or without instability, necessitates careful positioning. Induction of general anesthesia will increase ligamental laxity and may worsen cervical spine alignment. Surgical intervention for cervical instability should precede other elective surgeries. Spinal cord injury has been reported after an otherwise minor surgical procedure in such a patient.

When cervical spine instability is suspected in a child that will not remain cooperative during sedated tracheal intubation, monitoring of evoked potentials can be performed during intubation in the anesthetized child.

Unique airway difficulties are common in children with skeletal dysplasia and differ from the more common craniofacial anomalies that are characterized by micrognathia and an anterior larynx. Children with skeletal dysplasia have narrow nasopharyngeal passages, a large and redundant tongue, thickened pharyngeal mucosa, short neck, and decreased mobility of the neck and temporomandibular joints. Like children with trisomy 21, the neck should be maintained in the neutral position as much as possible because of the possibility of cervical spine instability. Many of these patients may have had prior cervical spine fusion resulting in difficulty with head and neck motion.

Regional anesthetics have been used, mainly for labor and delivery, in adults with skeletal dysplasia. Spinal canal abnormalities predispose to difficult lumbar puncture and epidural catheter placement. When children with dwarfism require an epidural catheter for pain management, a caudally placed catheter poses less difficulty with placement and a decreased risk[15] of spinal cord damage.

Skeletal dysplasia with dwarfism is associated with restrictive airway disease and thoracic dystrophy. In severe cases respiratory insufficiency leads to chronic hypoxemia and cor pulmonale.

Cardiac valvular lesions and cardiomyopathy occur in many types of dwarf syndromes, such as the mucopolysaccharidoses.

Neurologic abnormalities include hydrocephalus and compressive spinal cord and nerve root syndromes. Macrocephaly is caused by accelerated head growth but is not associated with elevated intracranial pressure. Kyphoscoliosis, lumbar lordosis, and a stenotic spinal canal may impede effective neuraxial regional anesthesia techniques.

Osteogenesis imperfecta, a form of dwarfism (Fig. 9.8), has been associated with hyperthermia during general anesthesia. The etiology is unknown, and no association with malignant hyperthermia has been established. The elevated temperature is not associated with muscle cell injury or with metabolic or respiratory acidosis. Temperature should be monitored in these patients to attain normothermia. Hyperthermia accompanied by hypercapnia that does not respond to an increase in minute ventilation is suggestive of malignant hyperthermia.

Mucopolysaccharidoses

The mucopolysaccharidoses are lysosomal storage disorders characterized by the accumulation of glycosaminoglycans (heparan, keratan, and dermatan sulfates) in the connective tissue (Fig. 9.9). Accumulation of these substances causes progressive skeletal and soft tissue deformities during childhood and is associated with early death secondary to cardiopulmonary dysfunction. The most important anesthetic-related considerations[14] include difficult airway management because of anatomic abnormalities[16] and cervical spine instability. Because of soft tissue infiltration

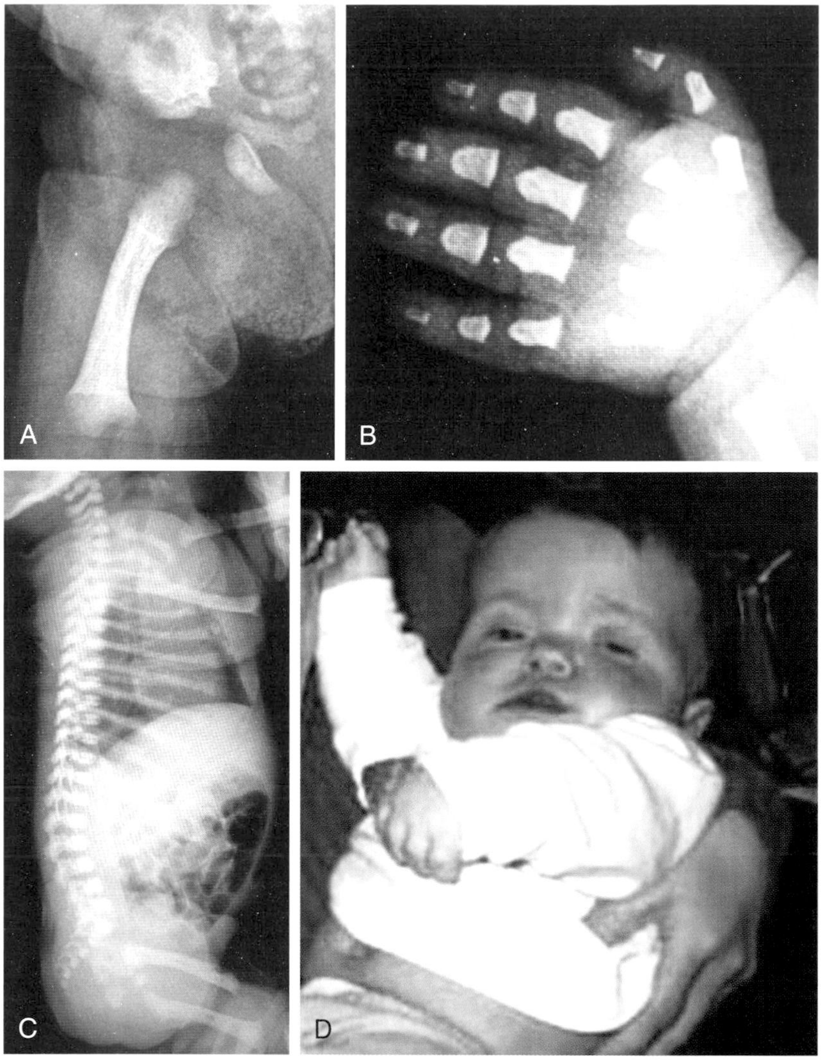

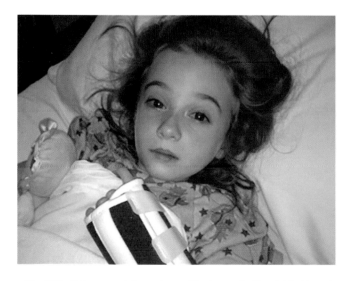

• **Fig. 9.7** Achondroplasia. (A) Radiograph of the femur in an infant with achondroplasia. The proximal ends of the femurs are relatively club-like with metaphyseal flaring and shortening of the lower extremities. (B) Radiograph of the hand, showing shortened metacarpals and phalanges. (C) Radiograph of the spine, showing thoracic lumbar kyphoscoliosis. (D) A 4-month-old female with distinctive facial features: upturned nose, flat nasal bridge, and large forehead. (From Deeney Vincent F, Arnold J. Orthopedics. In: Zitelli Basil J, Mcintire Sara C, Nowalk Andrew J, eds. *Zitelli and Davis' Atlas of Pediatric Physical Diagnosis*. 7th ed. Elsevier; 2018:759–844.)

• **Fig. 9.8** Osteogenesis imperfecta. (Photo credit: Ronald S. Litman)

of the upper airway and adenotonsillar hypertrophy, bag-mask ventilation and tracheal intubation may be difficult; thus a laryngeal mask should be immediately available during airway management. Difficult ventilation may also occur after tracheal extubation. Patients with Morquio syndrome (type IV) can have atlantoaxial instability with spinal cord compression. Therefore these patients need preoperative evaluation and screening for neurologic signs of spinal cord compression, including radiologic assessment. Some children with these disorders are treated with bone marrow transplantation, so immunosuppression becomes another perioperative consideration. Respiratory and cardiac comorbidities result in an increased incidence of postoperative mortality[17] in patients with Hurler syndrome (type I).

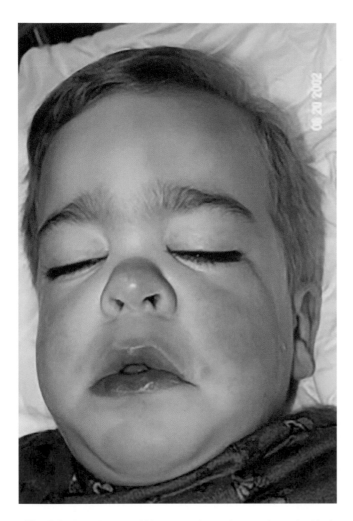

• **Fig. 9.9** Typical facies of Hunter syndrome (mucopolysaccharidosis type II). (Photo credit: Ronald S. Litman)

References

1. Data and Statistics on Down Syndrome National Center on Birth Defects and Developmental Disabilities, Centers for Disease Control and Prevention. *Birth Defects.* October 5, 2021 Reviewed on October 23, 2020. Accessed on 5.3.2022. https://www.cdc.gov/ncbddd/birthdefects/downsyndrome/data.html.

2. Mitchell V, Howard R, Facer E. Down's syndrome and anaesthesia. *Paediatr Anaesth.* 1995;5(6):379–384. https://doi.org/10.1111/j.1460-9592.1995.tb00331.x.

3. Jacobs IN, Gray RF, Todd NW. Upper airway obstruction in children with Down Syndrome. *Arch Otolaryngol Head Neck Surg.* 1996;122(9):945–950. https://doi.org/10.1001/archotol.1996.01890210025007.

4. Hansen DD, Haberkern CM, Jonas RA, Davis PJ, McGowan Jr. FX. Case 1—1991. Tracheal stenosis in an infant with Down's syndrome and complex congenital heart defect. *J Cardiothorac Vasc Anesth.* 1991;5(1):81–85. https://doi.org/10.1016/1053-0770(91)90100-8.

5. Bertrand P, Navarro H, Caussade S, Holmgren N, Sánchez I. Airway anomalies in children with Down syndrome: endoscopic findings. *Pediatr Pulmonol.* 2003;36(2):137–141. https://doi.org/10.1002/ppul.10332.

6. Litman RS, Perkins FM. Atlantoaxial subluxation after typanomastoidectomy in a child with trisomy 21. *Otolaryngol Head Neck Surg.* 1994;110(6):584–586. https://doi.org/10.1177/019459989411000619.

7. Kraemer W, Stricker PA, Gurnaney HG, et al. Bradycardia during induction of anesthesia with sevoflurane in children with Down Syndrome. *Anesth Analg.* 2010;111(5):1259–1263. https://doi.org/10.1213/ANE.0b013e3181f2eacf.

8. Walker SM. Perioperative care of neonates with Down's syndrome: should it be different? *Br J Anaesth.* 2012;108(2):177–179. https://doi.org/10.1093/bja/aer452.

9. Valkenburg AJ, van Dijk M, de Leeuw TG, Meeussen CJ, Knibbe CA, Tibboel D. Anaesthesia and postoperative analgesia in surgical neonates with or without Down's syndrome: is it really different? *Br J Anaesth.* 2012;108(2):295–301. https://doi.org/10.1093/bja/aer421.

10. Hirsch NP, Murphy A, Radcliffe JJ. Neurofibromatosis: clinical presentations and anaesthetic implications. *Br J Anaesth.* 2001;86(4):555–564. https://doi.org/10.1093/bja/86.4.555.

11. Fossali E, Signorini E, Intermite RC, et al. Renovascular disease and hypertension in children with neurofibromatosis. *Pediatr Nephrol.* 2000;14(8-9):806–810. https://doi.org/10.1007/s004679900260.

12. Shenkman Z, Rockoff MA, Eldredge EA, Korf BR, Black PM, Soriano SG. Anaesthetic management of children with tuberous sclerosis. *Paediatr Anaesth.* 2002;12(8):700–704. https://doi.org/10.1046/j.1460-9592.2002.00917.x.

13. Khanna P, Ray BR, Govindrajan SR, Sinha R, Chandralekha Talawar P. Anesthetic management of pediatric patients with Sturge-Weber syndrome: our experience and a review of the literature. *J Anesth.* 2015;29(6):857–861. https://doi.org/10.1007/s00540-015-2042-8.

14. Berkowitz ID, Raja SN, Bender KS, Kopits SE. Dwarfs: pathophysiology and anesthetic implications. *Anesthesiology.* 1990;73(4):739–759.

15. Sasaki-Adams DM, Campbell JW, Bajelidze G, Assis MC, Mackenzie WG, Ritter AM. Level of the conus in pediatric patients with skeletal dysplasia. *J Neurosurg Pediatr.* 2010;5(5):455–459. https://doi.org/10.3171/2009.12.PEDS09364.

16. Theroux MC, Nerker T, Ditro C, Mackenzie WG. Anesthetic care and perioperative complications of children with Morquio syndrome. *Paediatr Anaesth.* 2012;22(9):901–907. https://doi.org/10.1111/j.1460-9592.2012.03904.x.

17. Arn P, Whitley C, Wraith JE, et al. High rate of postoperative mortality in patients with mucopolysaccharidosis I: findings from the MPS I Registry. *J Pediatr Surg.* 2012;47(3):477–484. https://doi.org/10.1016/j.jpedsurg.2011.09.042.

Suggested Readings

De Lausnay M, Verhulst S, Boel L, Wojciechowski M, Boudewyns A, Van Hoorenbeeck K. The prevalence of lower airway anomalies in children with Down syndrome compared to controls. *Pediatr Pulmonol.* 2020;55(5):1259–1263. https://doi.org/10.1002/ppul.24741.

Hamilton J, Yaneza MMC, Clement WA, Kubba H. The prevalence of airway problems in children with Down's syndrome. *Int J*

Pediatr Otorhinolaryngol. 2016;81:1–4. https://doi.org/10.1016/j.ijporl.2015.11.027.

Mayhew JF, Katz J, Miner M, Leiman BC, Hall ID. Anaesthesia for the achondroplastic dwarf. *Can Anaesth Soc J.* 1986;33(2):216–221. https://doi.org/10.1007/BF03010834.

Zhang S. The Last Children of Down Syndrome. *The Atlantic.* December 2020 Accessed on October 5, 2021. https://www.theatlantic.com/magazine/archive/2020/12/the-last-children-of-down-syndrome/616928/.

10

Endocrine Diseases

ARI Y. WEINTRAUB AND RONALD S. LITMAN*

Diabetes Mellitus

The endocrine condition most frequently encountered in the perioperative period in children is diabetes mellitus. Diabetes mellitus is the result of an absolute or functional deficiency of insulin production by the pancreas. In type 1 diabetes, this deficiency is caused by an autoimmune process, mediated by autoantibodies including anti-GAD (glutamic acid decarboxylase) and insulinoma-associated antibody. Insulin deficiency results in abnormalities of glucose transport and storage and of lipid and protein synthesis. Over time, these metabolic derangements result in the vascular pathology that leads to end-stage complications of renal, cardiac, and eye disease; diseases that typically do not occur in childhood. The anesthetic implications of type 1 diabetes in children differ from those in adults with the same disease, for whom the primary concern is the type and severity of end organ disease. Perioperative insulin administration is essential to control glucose and to promote an anabolic state, which is most conducive to speedy healing and metabolic homeostasis.

Type 2 diabetes, insulin resistance without evidence of autoimmunity, has been increasing in the pediatric population by 4.8% per year.

Children with insulin-dependent diabetes may be treated with various types of insulin on a daily basis to maintain tight blood glucose control, with the aid of frequent or constant blood glucose monitoring. Currently, all Food and Drug Administration (FDA)-approved insulin preparations are produced using recombinant DNA technology with laboratory-cultivated bacteria or yeast. Animal-sourced insulin has not been produced in the United States since the manufacturers voluntarily discontinued production of beef insulin in 1998 and porcine insulin in 2006. Insulin products called *insulin analogs* are produced so the structure differs slightly from human insulin (by one or two amino acids) to change onset and peak of action. Examples of analogs include lispro (Humalog), aspart (Novolog), and glulisine (Apidra), ultrashort-acting insulins that may be given only 15 minutes before a meal or even within 20 minutes of beginning a meal (Table 10.1). The peak and duration of action of these analogs parallel the glucose rise that results from carbohydrate ingestion.

Glargine (Lantus, Basaglar) and detemir (Levemir), which almost mimic an insulin pump's basal infusion, provide a 24-hour, continuous low background level of insulin with only one subcutaneous daily injection. Twice-daily injections may be superior to once-daily with detemir. Both of these agents are used in combination with ultrashort-acting analogs to mimic endogenous insulin secretion seen in nondiabetics.

An increasing number of children are being managed with continuous subcutaneous insulin infusion (CSII) via an external insulin pump, which provides a background (basal) infusion of insulin and the ability to give boluses before meals and for correction of hyperglycemia. The newest insulin pumps incorporate feedback from continuous glucose monitoring systems (CGMS) to adjust insulin delivery according to the patient's blood sugar using a hybrid closed-loop system (HCLS).

Type 2 diabetes in children and adolescents may be controlled with diet and exercise, but these children also may be taking metformin (Glucophage).

Preoperative Optimization

Because of the effects of surgical stress on glucose homeostasis, insulin-dependent diabetic children are at risk for acute fluctuations in blood glucose, even when their preoperative

*Portions of this chapter were reprinted from Bruins BB, Kilbaugh TJ, and Weintraub AY. Endocrine Disorders, In Smith's Anesthesia for Infants and Children, 10th Edition, Eds. Davis PJ and Cladis FP, 2021.

TABLE 10.1	Kinetics of Commonly Used Insulin Analogs					
Insulin	Trade Name	Route	Onset (h)	Peak (h)	Effective Duration (h)	
Rapid-Acting						
Lispro	*Humalog*	SC	0.25	0.5–1.5	3–4	
Aspart	*Novolog*	SC	0.25	1–3	3–5	
Glulisine	*Apidra*	SC	0.25–0.5	0.5–1	4	
Short-Acting						
Regular	*Humulin, Novolin*	IV/SC	0.5–1.0	2–3	3–6	
Long-Acting						
Glargine	*Lantus*	SC	1.0	2–3	24	
Detemir	*Levemir*	SC	1.0	3–6	20*	

IV, Intravenous; *SC*, subcutaneous; *NPH*, neutral protamine Hagedorn.

glucose control is good. Poorly controlled or noncompliant diabetic patients have additional problems, including an increased risk for perioperative hypoglycemia or hyperglycemia, osmotic diuresis with resultant hypovolemia, and altered mental status. Coordination and cooperation among the patient, parents, pediatrician, endocrinologist, and anesthesiologist are essential to prepare for the perioperative period.

Preoperative anesthesia evaluation for elective procedures, informed by contemporaneous endocrine assessment of adequacy of glucose control, should be completed 7 to 10 days before the scheduled date of surgery to allow adjustment of treatment regimen or delay of procedure if control is not optimal. The International Society for Pediatric and Adolescent Diabetes published a comprehensive review[1] of concerns and perioperative management of pediatric diabetic patients; it features useful clinical practice guidelines, incorporating both preoperative assessment and perioperative insulin regimens.

The preoperative evaluation should include a review of recent measurements of glucose levels over a period of days or weeks because a single, isolated value does not indicate the adequacy or quality of glycemic control. A hemoglobin A_{1C} level (i.e., glycosylated hemoglobin assay), although a useful index of long-term (i.e., over the preceding 2–3 months) glucose control, is unlikely to affect the anesthetic plan and is not an essential preoperative test. With the rise of continuous glucose monitoring systems, time in range (TIR) has become a useful and clinically meaningful metric and outcome measure. TIR has been defined as the percentage of blood glucose readings in the target range of 70 to 180 mg/dL per unit of time. Compared with Hb A_{1C}, TIR captures all glucose levels, including hypoglycemia and hyperglycemia, over a given time frame and is more likely to reveal the impact of acute interventions and changes in diabetes management.

Perioperative Management

Various regimens for managing insulin therapy perioperatively have been proposed, including frequent blood sugar monitoring without altering the patient's usual regimen and relying upon either a long-acting insulin analog or the patient's subcutaneous infusion insulin pump to provide a basal level of insulin, intravenous (IV) insulin infusion, and the "classic" regimen (Table 10.2).

Regardless of the regimen chosen, it is ideal to schedule elective surgery for the diabetic child as early as possible in the day to minimize fasting times and thus reduce the risk for hypoglycemia. The fasting interval should be the same as that recommended for nondiabetic patients: no solid food or milk for 6 hours (or 8 hours, depending on institutional practice and policy). Children with diabetes should be encouraged to continue to drink clear liquids up until the time allowed by institutional policy. The sugar content of the clear liquid will depend on the chosen perioperative insulin regimen. With type 2 diabetes, metformin should be stopped 48 hours before surgery based on reports of lactic acidosis in patients who remain on the drug and are in a fasting state perioperatively.

Although some investigators have recommended the withholding of preoperative sedation from diabetic patients to better monitor for signs of hypoglycemia, premedication is recommended in children. The use of agents such as benzodiazepines, opioids, or barbiturates does not alter glucose metabolism, and a mild rise in blood sugar (caused by the catecholamine response to anxiety) might actually occur with avoidance of these agents.

Based on blood glucose level determined on arrival to the preoperative facility and before implementation of the regimens discussed below, glucose and/or insulin should be administered according to a sliding scale scheme (Table 10.3). With the proliferation of long-acting insulin

TABLE 10.2   Protocols for Perioperative Insulin Therapy in Patients Using Multiple Daily Insulin Injections

Regimen	Morning of Surgery Procedure
Classic regimen	• Start IV infusion of 5% dextrose in 0.45% saline or Ringer lactate solution at maintenance rate (GIR ~1.66 mg/kg/min). • Administer half of usual morning insulin dose as regular insulin. • Check blood glucose before induction and during and after anesthesia
Continuous insulin infusion	• Start IV infusion of 5% dextrose in 0.45% saline or Ringer lactate solution at maintenance rate (GIR ~1.66 mg/kg/min). • Add 1–2 units of insulin per 100 mL of 5% dextrose. • Starting insulin dose should be 0.02 units/kg/h. • Check blood glucose before induction and during and after anesthesia.
Insulin- and glucose-free regimen (for operative procedures of short duration)	• Withhold morning insulin dose. • If indicated for procedure, give glucose-free solution (e.g., Ringer lactate) at maintenance rate. • Check blood glucose before induction and during and after anesthesia. • Give usual insulin dose postoperatively with first meal.

TABLE 10.3   Preoperative Glucose and Insulin Management for Diabetic Patients

Blood Glucose Level	Management
<80 mg/dL	2 mL/kg D10W followed by glucose infusion
80–250 mg/dL	D5/0.45 NS or D10/0.45 NS solution at maintenance if IV insulin is to be administered; 0.9 NS if short case without insulin infusion
>250 mg/dL	Administer rapid-acting (lispro) or short-acting (regular) insulin SC to reduce blood sugar; use correction factor from patient's endocrine provider or 0.2 unit/kg SC
>350 mg/dL	Consider canceling or postponing surgery, especially if ketonuria is present

NS, Normal saline; *SC*, subcutaneously.

analogs and subcutaneous insulin infusion pumps, perioperative insulin therapy often does not require major deviation from the patient's usual regimen.

Long-Acting Insulin Analogs and Subcutaneous Infusion Insulin Pumps

Patients who are maintained on a home regimen involving once- (or twice-) daily subcutaneous injections of a long-acting analog (e.g., glargine or detemir) can take their normal dose the night before and/or on the morning of surgery. Insulin pump basal infusions can be maintained at their normal rate. If morning hypoglycemia is an issue or concern, the dose or basal rate can be reduced slightly (up to one-third of normal), but this carries the risk for hyperglycemia and ketosis that may be more problematic than

mild hypoglycemia. Parents should be advised to check their child's blood sugar upon arising that morning and correct hyperglycemia according to their usual routine, and blood sugar should be rechecked upon arrival to the hospital or surgical facility. Hypoglycemia should be treated with clear, glucose-containing fluids (e.g., apple juice, white grape juice, Pedialyte) to avoid delaying the anesthetic, because clear liquids may be allowed up until 1 hour before the induction of anesthesia.

Increasing numbers of pediatric patients with type 1 diabetes are being managed with external insulin pumps capable of subcutaneous administration of both continuous and bolus doses of insulin. Such pumps afford excellent control, with changes in administration coordinated with eating, exercise, and stress. The increasing adoption of CSII technology is an indication of the added convenience and quality of glucose control for patients in the outpatient setting, and these benefits can be observed in the inpatient and hospital setting as well. The use of insulin pumps throughout the perioperative period, including intraoperatively, has become widely accepted as standard practice, regardless of the anticipated duration of the procedure or anesthetic. The use of insulin pumps in the MRI suite or magnetoencephalography (MEG) is contraindicated, but for short studies (under 1–2 hours), the pump can be disconnected with little effect on blood glucose levels and reconnected immediately at the cessation of the study; any hyperglycemia can be corrected at that time. Most manufacturers recommend against the use of insulin pumps in the setting of ionizing radiation (e.g., x-rays, fluoroscopy, computed tomography [CT] scan), but many practitioners will use lead aprons to shield the pump in those cases. In surgical cases requiring electrocautery, either bipolar cautery should be used or the grounding pad should be placed between the surgical site and the infusion set.

Because of the rapid development and advances in technology, CGMS and HCLS (Fig. 10.1) have not yet been studied extensively in the perioperative setting. Nevertheless, these systems likely will provide superior perioperative glucose management compared with intermittent finger-sticks and/or fixed basal infusion rates, in conjunction with frequent monitoring of the CGM values and close attention to pump alarms.

Anesthetic Management

Regional and general anesthesia are both appropriate for the child with diabetes mellitus. Plasma glucose concentrations should be maintained between 100 and 180 mg/dL. This target range is chosen because mild to moderate hyperglycemia (without ketosis) usually does not present a serious problem to the child, whereas hypoglycemia may have devastating consequences. Hyperglycemia greater than 250 mg/dL should be avoided because of associated mental status changes, diuresis, and subsequent dehydration, which can occur because of the hyperosmolar state. Hyperglycemia has been associated with poorer outcomes in patients at risk for central nervous system (CNS) ischemia, including those undergoing cardiopulmonary bypass. Hyperglycemia has also been shown to impair wound healing and has adverse effects on neutrophil function in vitro.

The most serious perioperative complication that can occur in the diabetic child is hypoglycemia. Common signs of low blood glucose levels include tachycardia, diaphoresis, and hypertension. In the anesthetized patient, these signs may be misinterpreted as indications of inadequate anesthesia. Because the clinical signs of hypoglycemia are masked by sedation or anesthesia, frequent (hourly) measurement of

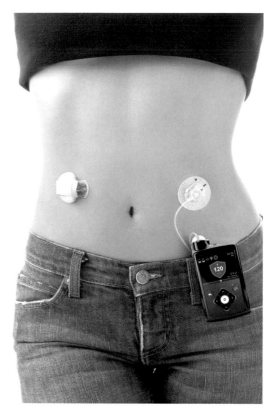

• **Fig. 10.1** Insulin pump and integrated CGMS system. CGM sensor and transmitter (left), insulin pump displaying CGM sensor value and connected to infusion set (right). (Copyright © 2020 Medtronic. All rights reserved. Used with the permission of Medtronic Minneapolis, Minnesota.)

A DEEPER DIVE

In this Deeper Dive, we provide sample protocols adapted from our own institution for the perioperative management of children on continuous insulin pump or intermittent injections.

Perioperative Management of Patients on Insulin Pump

- Information from family or endocrinologist:
  - What is the patient's basal rate?
  - What is the bolus (insulin to carb) ratio?
  - How much will 1 unit insulin typically decrease blood glucose?
  - What is the patient's target for corrections?
  - Does the patient use a continuous glucose monitoring sensor (CGMS) device?

Preoperative Home Instructions:

- Continue usual basal rates and boluses for carbohydrates and correction of high blood sugars up until the time of admission.
- Check blood sugar upon waking up in the morning.
- Treat hypoglycemia with clear carb-containing fluid (e.g., apple juice).
- Treat hyperglycemia using usual correction boluses; can give every 3 hours as needed.

Preoperative Hospital Instructions:

Based on use of aspart insulin (Novolog); clinically equivalent insulin formulations are lispro (Humalog) and glulisine (Apidra).
- Blood glucose checked immediately upon arrival to the hospital or surgical facility.

- For hyperglycemia (>240 mg/dL), treat with insulin bolus with pump or subcutaneous injection and check for urine ketones.
- Correct to a goal of 150 mg/dL.
- If moderate to large urine ketones present, contact the diabetes consult service for management recommendations.
- Consider rescheduling elective procedures in the presence of elevated, persistent ketonuria AND blood glucose greater than 350 mg/dL.
- For hypoglycemia (<80 mg/dL or symptomatic), treat with intravenous dextrose (2–3 mL/kg D10W) and recheck blood sugar in 20 minutes.
- Disconnect the insulin pump before MRI scans or at anesthesia/sedation team request. Consider disconnecting the pump for CT scans, interventional radiology procedures, and radiation therapy. Pump can safely be disconnected for 1 hour without giving Novolog. Disconnecting for longer than 2 hours without Novolog will result in hyperglycemia and possibly ketones.

Perioperative Management

- Check blood sugars after inducing anesthesia/sedation and after airway is secured. Continue to check blood sugars hourly.
- For hyperglycemia (>240 mg/dL): Give Novolog insulin every 2 hours as needed; refer to dose recommendation for hyperglycemia above.

(Continued)

- For hypoglycemia (<80 mg/dL): Give IV dextrose bolus (2–3 mL/kg D10W) and recheck blood sugar in 20 minutes.
- Recurrent or refractory hypoglycemia should be treated with additional IV boluses of dextrose or initiation of dextrose infusions (D5W at maintenance rates).
- If the insulin pump is accidentally or unexpectedly dislodged or removed:
  - Give subcutaneous injections every 2 hours. Use the correction factor recommendation for hyperglycemia (see Section 2) above; or
  - Start a continuous regular insulin infusion. See below for dosing recommendations for insulin infusion; titrate hourly for goal blood sugars 100 to 150.

Postoperative Management

- Allow child to take fluids/food postoperatively per surgical protocol.
- Initiate continuous dextrose-containing fluids IV (D5 and 1/2NS at maintenance) if child is unable to meet maintenance oral intake.
- Once child is able to tolerate PO intake, family may resume home insulin regimen unless otherwise directed by the Diabetes Consult service.
- Check blood sugars every 2 hours. May give Novolog insulin correction every 3 to 4 hours as needed for hyperglycemia according to dose guidelines in Section 2 above.
- Call Diabetes Consult service for:
  - Urine ketones
  - Vomiting
  - Persistent low blood sugars (below 80 mg/dL)
  - Persistent high blood sugars requiring more than two corrections with Novolog as described above
  - All patients requiring an overnight hospital admission

At Time of Discharge, Advise Family to:

- Check blood sugar every 2 hours for first 4 hours. After the first 4 hours, family may resume checking blood sugars according to usual routine.
- Bolus via pump to correct for high blood sugar readings using usual correction factor.
- Bolus via pump to cover all meals and snacks using usual insulin: CHO ratio.
- Check for and treat ketones as per usual protocol.

Perioperative Management of Patients on Insulin Injections

Information From Family or Endocrinologist:

- What is the patient's normal daily insulin regimen?
- What is the bolus (insulin to carb) ratio?
- How much will 1 unit insulin typically decrease blood glucose?
- What is the patient's target for corrections?
- Does the patient use a continuous glucose monitoring sensor (CGMS) device?

Preoperative Home Instructions

- Follow preoperative feeding instructions provided by surgical team.
- Check blood sugar upon waking up in the morning.
- Continue usual boluses for carbohydrates and correction of high blood sugars up until the time of admission.
- CGMS: If advised by procedure team, remove sensor and reinitiate system after procedure is complete.
- Treat hypoglycemia with clear carb-containing fluid (e.g., apple juice).

- Treat hyperglycemia using usual correction boluses; can give every 3 hours as needed.

Preoperative Hospital Instructions

Based on use of aspart insulin (Novolog); clinically equivalent insulin formulations are lispro (Humalog) and glulisine (Apidra).

- Blood glucose checked immediately upon arrival to the hospital or surgical facility.
- For hyperglycemia (>240 mg/dL), treat with subcutaneous injection of Novolog insulin (or equivalent) and check for urine ketones.
- Correct to a goal of 150 mg/dL.
- If moderate to large urine ketones present, contact the diabetes consult service for management recommendations.
- Consider rescheduling elective procedures in the presence of elevated, persistent ketonuria AND blood glucose greater than 350 mg/dL.
- For hypoglycemia (<80 mg/dL or symptomatic), treat with intravenous dextrose (2–3 mL/kg of D10W) and recheck blood sugar in 20 minutes.

Perioperative Management

- Check blood sugar after inducing anesthesia/sedation and airway is secured; continue to check blood sugars hourly.
- For hyperglycemia (>240 mg/dL): Give Novolog insulin every 2 hours as needed; refer to dose recommendation for hyperglycemia above.
- For hypoglycemia (<80 mg/dL): Give IV dextrose bolus (2–3 mL/kg D10W) and recheck blood sugar in 20 minutes.
- Recurrent or refractory hypoglycemia should be treated with additional IV boluses of dextrose or initiation of dextrose infusions (D5W at maintenance rates).

Postoperative Management

- Allow child to take fluids/food postoperatively per surgical protocol.
- Initiate continuous dextrose containing fluids IV (D5 and 1/2NS at maintenance) if child is unable to meet maintenance oral intake.
- Once child is able to tolerate PO intake, family may resume home insulin regimen unless otherwise directed by the diabetes consult service.
- Check blood sugars every 2 hours. May give Novolog insulin correction every 3 to 4 hours as needed for hyperglycemia according to dose guidelines in Section 2.
- Call diabetes consult service for:
  - Ketones
  - Vomiting
  - Persistent low blood sugars (below 80 mg/dL)
  - Persistent high blood sugars requiring more than two corrections with Novolog as described above
  - All patients requiring an overnight hospital admission for surgical indications

At Time of Discharge, Advise Family to:

- Check blood sugar every 2 hours for first 4 hours. After the first 4 hours, family may resume checking blood sugars according to usual routine.
- Give injections to correct for high blood sugar readings using usual correction factor.
- Give injections to cover all meals and snacks using usual insulin: CHO ratio.
- Check for and treat ketones as per usual protocol.

the serum glucose level is recommended for the prevention of hypoglycemia, independent of the glucose-insulin regimen chosen. Postoperative insulin administration is determined by the time of resumption of oral or enteral feeding and by the postoperative blood glucose concentration. The endocrinologist and surgeon should be active partners in the choice of an appropriate insulin regimen because they will be responsible for monitoring glucose homeostasis after the patient leaves the post-anesthesia care unit (PACU). For day surgery patients, contingency planning for insulin management and mechanisms for follow-up and consultation should be clearly defined for members of the care team and family.

Adrenal Insufficiency

Background

Glucocorticoid production by the adrenal glands is regulated by the hypothalamic-pituitary-adrenal (HPA) axis beginning with hypothalamic release of corticotropin-releasing hormone (CRH) that stimulates the pituitary gland to produce adrenocorticotropic hormone (ACTH). The ACTH released by the anterior pituitary stimulates the adrenal cortex to produce cortisol, which then provides negative feedback on CRH and ACTH release to complete the cycle.

Primary adrenal insufficiency is uncommon in children, but secondary deficiency is common after exogenous steroid usage, such as that administered for the treatment of inflammatory (e.g., Crohn disease, asthma) or autoimmune (e.g., lupus, juvenile idiopathic arthritis) disease. HPA suppression is thought to place steroid-dependent children at increased risk for complications in the perioperative period because they may be unable to respond to stress with an appropriate increase in the adrenal secretion of glucocorticoid. Dosages of cortisol or its equivalent that exceed 15 mg/m²/day for more than 2 to 4 weeks will likely produce HPA suppression. A study in children with relatively short-term exposure to prednisolone or dexamethasone (5 and 3 weeks, respectively) for treatment of acute lymphoblastic leukemia showed that recovery of normal adrenal function (in response to ACTH stimulation) had a very wide range, occurring between 2 weeks and 8 months.

Although high dosages, prolonged therapy, and short duration between discontinuance of therapy and the surgical procedure increase the likelihood of HPA suppression, no practical test is available that unequivocally identifies patients who will need intraoperative steroids. Nevertheless, there is a poor correlation between tests that indicate normal HPA function and dose or duration of glucocorticoid therapy or basal cortisol levels. Clinically significant events rarely occur during the perioperative period in patients who were receiving steroid medications for diseases other than adrenal insufficiency even if no perioperative steroids were administered.

Perioperative Steroid Management

Glucocorticoid deficiency is treated with cortisol (hydrocortisone) replacement. The importance of cortisol replacement for patients with known adrenal insufficiency should not be underestimated, although vastly excessive doses are unwarranted. In the nonstressed condition, normal cortisol output is between 6 and 8 mg/m² per day. The normal replacement dose prescribed for nonstressed children is 10 to 15 mg/m²/day; the dose is double the normal production because of factors of bioavailability and half-life.

Over 65 years ago, it was reported that two patients developed irreversible shock perioperatively after glucocorticoid administration was stopped preoperatively. Both patients were found to have adrenal atrophy and hemorrhage at autopsy. These two cases led to suggestions for "stress" steroid coverage in the perioperative period. The need for supraphysiologic doses of steroids in the perioperative period has also been extrapolated from the observed rise in serum cortisol and other endogenous stress hormones in healthy children. The normal adrenal gland responds to physiologic stress (e.g., fever, acute illness, trauma, and surgery) by secreting anywhere from 3 to 10 times the normal production of cortisol. However, it is unclear that the stress response in healthy patients is necessary or beneficial; the theoretical correlation of a diminished cortisol response with clinically adverse outcomes is unproven. Additionally, steroids are known to have deleterious effects that can be especially significant in the perioperative, including immunosuppression, impaired wound healing, surgical site dehiscence, and hyperglycemia.

Although the 2016 Endocrine Society practice guideline recommends hydrocortisone supplementation for 1 to 2 days even for minor surgery, it acknowledges that the regimen "places a higher value on the prevention of underdosage than on reducing potential negative effects of short-term overdosage" as "underdosing of glucocorticoids in an adrenal crisis is potentially hazardous."

As modern anesthetic techniques result in better management of pain, fluids, electrolyte, and volume status, the physiologic stress of surgery has been reduced significantly. Nevertheless, a high index of suspicion should be maintained in all patients at risk for HPA axis suppression. In the case of hypotension or shock that is refractory to fluids or bolus doses of vasopressors (e.g., phenylephrine, ephedrine), steroid administration should be considered.

Importantly, the anesthesia provider must consider the type of glucocorticoid administered, its duration of action, the route of administration, and the timing of doses. The most common doses used for perioperative steroid coverage range from 25 to 100 mg/m² of hydrocortisone hemisuccinate (Solu-Cortef), given intravenously at the induction of anesthesia. If indicated, subsequent IV doses should be given every 6 to 8 hours because of the short half-life of hydrocortisone. The dosing regimen should be commensurate with the degree of stress.

Dexamethasone is up to 30 times as potent as hydrocortisone, and its glucocorticoid effects can last as long as 72 hours. Patients receiving dexamethasone for PONV prophylaxis or to reduce airway swelling or intracranial pressure do not require additional steroids in the perioperative period. In the postoperative period, the steroid dose is tapered to a level commensurate with the residual stress. The physiologic stress of anesthesia and surgery is unlikely to last more than 72 hours. Patient should return to their usual oral preparation as soon as they can tolerate and absorb oral medication.

HPA suppression also can result from modes of steroid administration other than oral, including topical, nasal spray, and inhalers. Although adrenal suppression is rarely symptomatic with these modes of administration, some drugs, especially fluticasone propionate (Flovent) and triamcinolone acetonide (Nasacort), in high chronic doses have been associated with growth failure and adrenal suppression. With surgical stress, patients with adrenal suppression may become symptomatic, as has been reported for other kinds of stress. Numerous cases of acute adrenal crisis have been reported in children receiving inhaled corticosteroids for prolonged periods. Anesthesiologists should maintain a high index of suspicion of adrenal suppression if an asthmatic child on inhaled steroids develops refractory hypotension or hypoglycemia in the perioperative period.

References

1. Jefferies C, Rhodes E, Rachmiel M, et al. ISPAD Clinical Practice Consensus Guidelines 2018: Management of children and adolescents with diabetes requiring surgery [published correction appears in Pediatr Diabetes. 2019 Feb;20(1):137]. *Pediatr Diabetes.* 2018;19(Suppl 27):227–236. https://doi.org/10.1111/pedi.12733.

Suggested Readings

Agiostradu G, Anhalt H, Ball D, et al. Standardizing Clinically Meaningful Outcome Measures Beyond HbA1c for Type 1 Diabetes: A Consensus Report of the American Association of Clinical Endocrinologists, the American Association of Diabetes Educators, the American Diabetes Association, the Endocrine Society, JDRF International, The Leona M and Harry B Helmsley Charitable Trust, the Pediatric Endocrine Society, and the T1D Exchange. *Diabetes Care.* 2017;40(12):1622–1630. https://doi.org/10.2337/dc17-1624.

Coursin DB, Wood KE. Corticosteroid supplementation for adrenal insufficiency. *JAMA.* 2002;287(2):236–240. https://doi.org/10.1001/jama.287.2.236.

Hsu AA, von Elten K, Chan D, et al. Characterization of the cortisol stress response to sedation and anesthesia in children. *J Clin Endocrinol Metab.* 2012;97(10):E1830–E1835. https://doi.org/10.1210/jc.2012-1499.

Ismael H, Horst M, Farooq M, Jordon J, Patton JH, Rubinfeld IS. Adverse effects of preoperative steroid use on surgical outcomes. *Am J Surg.* 2011;201(3):305–309. https://doi.org/10.1016/j.amjsurg.2010.09.018.

Liu MM, Reidy AB, Saatee S, Collard CD. Perioperative Steroid Management: Approaches Based on Current Evidence. *Anesthesiology.* 2017;127(1):166–172. https://doi.org/10.1097/ALN.0000000000001659.

Partridge H, Perkins B, Mathieu S, Nicholls A, Adeniji K. Clinical recommendations in the management of the patient with type 1 diabetes on insulin pump therapy in the perioperative period: a primer for the anaesthetist. *Br J Anaesth.* 2016;116(1):18–26. https://doi.org/10.1093/bja/aev347.

Taylor LK, Auchus RJ, Baskin LS, Miller WL. Cortisol response to operative stress with anesthesia in healthy children. *J Clin Endocrinol Metab.* 2013;98(9):3687–3693. https://doi.org/10.1210/jc.2013-2148.

11

The Premature Infant

FATIMAH HABIB AND RONALD S. LITMAN*

In the last several decades, the incidence of prematurity in the United States has risen to 11.5%.[1] Maternal risk factors for prematurity include absence of prenatal care, low socioeconomic status, tobacco abuse, poor nutrition and genitourinary tract infections, to name only a few. Despite a relative increase in prematurity, perinatal mortality rates have decreased to approximately 6 in every 1000 live births.[2] Late-preterm births, defined as delivery at 34 to 36 weeks' gestation, have significantly increased over the last 15 years. This may partly explain both the rise in the incidence of prematurity and the decrease in perinatal mortality.

Despite improvements, prematurity remains an independent risk factor for increased morbidity and mortality during infancy and childhood. Singleton infants born between 34 and 36 completed weeks' gestation have a three-fold risk for dying in the first year of life compared with term infants. Those born between 32 and 33 completed weeks of gestation have an almost seven-fold risk for dying in the first year of life. The extremely premature infants remain at high risk for chronic morbidity with a rate of 20% to 50%, which contributes heavily to learning and motor disabilities. Prematurity-related disabilities account for about 50% of all childhood disabilities.[1]

Definitions

It is useful to review some common definitions. The **premature infant** is often defined as a viable newborn delivered after the 20th completed week of gestation and before full term, with an arbitrary weight of 500 to 2499 g at birth. The preterm infant is born at any time before the 37th completed week (259 days) of gestation (although most clinicians usually consider infants born any time in the 37th

week to be full term). Preterm can be further subclassified into *late preterm* (34–36 weeks' gestation), *moderate preterm* (32–34 weeks' gestation), *very preterm* (28–32 weeks' gestation), and *extremely preterm* (less than 28 weeks' gestation).[1] **Low birth weight (LBW)** is defined as less than 2500 g at birth. **Very low birth weight (VLBW)** is defined as less than 1500 g at birth. **Extremely low birth weight (ELBW)** is defined as less than 1000 g at birth.

Although the severity of the medical problems described in this chapter is directly correlated with decreasing gestational age, there is a growing recognition that the late preterm (LP) infants[3] have associated risks. LP infants make up 74% of all preterm births and 8% to 9% of total births. The last 6 weeks of gestation are a critical period for neural and respiratory development. LP infants also have an increased risk for the need for resuscitation at birth, feeding difficulty, jaundice, hypoglycemia, temperature instability, apnea and respiratory distress. The mortality rate during infancy is tripled compared with full-term infants. LP infants are more vulnerable to brain injuries and have a tripled risk for developing cerebral palsy, adverse developmental outcomes and academic difficulties up to 7 years of age.

Respiratory Distress Syndrome

Premature infants are born with a deficiency of alveolar type 2 pneumocytes, which are responsible for surfactant production. Surfactant is mainly comprised of phosphatidylcholine, which lowers surface tension inside the alveoli, thus preventing alveolar collapse. Type 2 pneumocytes begin to appear in the fetus by the 22nd week of gestation, and surfactant is primarily produced during the second trimester of pregnancy. Fifty percent of surfactant is produced by the 28th week of gestation, and production is usually complete by 36 weeks.

Surfactant deficiency is associated with a clinical syndrome of pulmonary insufficiency known as *respiratory distress syndrome* (RDS), formerly termed *hyaline membrane*

---

*Many thanks to Dr. Erin Pukenas and Dr. Greg Dodson for contributing to previous versions of this chapter.

disease (HMD). The incidence and severity of RDS is inversely correlated with gestational age; it affects approximately one-half of infants born between 26 to 28 weeks' gestation and 30% of infants born at 30 to 31 weeks' gestation, and is infrequent in infants born after the 35th week of gestation. RDS contributes to a large portion of premature deaths. Approximately 50% of premature infant deaths from the age of 12 hours to 14 days can be attributed in part to RDS. Just over 40% of premature deaths in the first month of life can be attributed to complications of RDS.[4] Conditions that decrease surfactant production and increase the incidence of RDS include perinatal asphyxia, maternal diabetes, multiple pregnancies, cesarean section delivery, precipitous delivery, cold stress and a history of affected siblings. Prenatal factors that increase fetal stress and, therefore, increase surfactant production and lower the risk for RDS include pregnancy-associated hypertension, maternal opiate addiction, prolonged rupture of the membranes and antenatal administration of corticosteroids.

Absence or deficiency of surfactant leads to widespread atelectasis, decreased lung compliance, and loss of functional residual capacity (FRC). This correlates with the clinical manifestations of RDS that usually appear shortly after birth and include tachypnea, nasal flaring, audible grunting, chest wall retractions, and use of accessory muscles of respiration. Severely affected infants with substantial ventilation-to-perfusion mismatch will demonstrate cyanosis and respiratory failure. Blood gas analysis will usually reveal hypoxemia, hypercarbia, and metabolic acidosis. The classic finding on chest radiography[5] in infants with RDS is a bilateral diffuse ground-glass appearance and multiple air bronchograms. On occasion, these radiographic findings may not develop until the second day of life.

Treatment of RDS initially includes supplemental oxygen to achieve a target PaO_2 between 55 and 70 mm Hg. Ideal oxygen targets are still unknown, but an oxygen saturation of 90% to 94% is typically the goal in most institutions. Oxygen therapy is a balance between too much (hyperoxia can lead to increase incidence of retinopathy of prematurity) or not quite enough (hypoxia can lead to increased incidence of necrotizing enterocolitis and higher mortality risk). The optimal first mode of respiratory support for suspected RDS is continuous positive-pressure support, often delivered as nasal CPAP. Ideally, the oxygen should be heated and humidified and the pressures delivered, measured, and controlled. CPAP, between 6 to 9 cm H_2O, with early administration of surfactant is considered optimal management of RDS.[6,7] In prematurely born infants at risk for developing RDS, artificial surfactant is administered into the lungs via an endotracheal tube shortly after delivery. More recently, less invasive means of delivery have made it possible to avoid intubation up front and potentially altogether. A small catheter advanced into the trachea while the child spontaneously ventilates, with CPAP support, is used to deliver surfactant directly into the trachea.

Studies have shown that this less invasive method is just as beneficial as endotracheal administration but may have an indirect benefit considering intubation can potentially be avoided.[8] Nebulized surfactant and pharyngeal deposition of surfactant are even less invasive means of administration which are currently under investigation.[6]

If RDS is suspected at birth, the child is placed initially on CPAP. A high-flow nasal cannula has been shown to be inferior to CPAP because most infants often require escalation to CPAP as a rescue therapy. Any sign of worsening oxygen requirements is indication for artificial surfactant therapy.[6] Early administration of surfactant using a low treatment threshold (Fio_2 <0.45) is preferable to selective surfactant therapy at a higher threshold (Fio_2 >0.45) and results in less pulmonary air leak, chronic lung disease, and decreased need for mechanical ventilation in the first week of life.[7] Instituting mechanical ventilation is indicated if the infant on CPAP cannot maintain an arterial oxygen tension above 50 mm Hg while breathing inspired concentrations of oxygen up to 100%. Additional indications for mechanical ventilation include persistent pH less than 7.2, and central apnea that is unresponsive to pharmacologic therapy.

Because oxygen toxicity and pulmonary barotrauma/volutrauma are thought to be responsible for the development of neonatal chronic lung disease, the goals of mechanical ventilation in the infant with RDS are to achieve relative normoxemia (PaO_2 >50 mm Hg), mild (permissive) hypercapnia ($PaCO_2$ in the range 40–65 mm Hg), and a normal pH (>7.2), depending on the infant's clinical status, while minimizing the concentration of inspired oxygen and the level of artificially maintained lung pressures. A modest amount of positive end-expiratory pressure (PEEP) may be used (3–5 cm H_2O) and ventilatory settings are weaned aggressively as the infant improves.

The majority of infants with RDS who require mechanical ventilation are placed on conventional ventilators that deliver continuous breathing cycles, usually at a rate between 30 and 50 breaths/min. Some studies suggest synchronous intermittent mandatory ventilation may shorten the duration of intubation and decrease oxygen requirements compared with conventional ventilation. Infants who are unresponsive to conventional ventilation may be switched to high frequency jet ventilation (HFJV), which can attain respiratory rates of 150 to 600 breaths/min, or an oscillating type ventilator that can deliver 300 to 1800 breaths/min. The main advantage of these unconventional ventilators is the ability to decrease mean airway pressure and tidal volumes while maintaining the ability to oxygenate and eliminate carbon dioxide.

Some methods used to decrease duration of mechanical ventilation include caffeine therapy and postnatal steroids in the form or systemic or inhaled corticosteroids.[6] Additional doses[9] of surfactant can be administered at regular intervals if respiratory distress persists and may also result in less RDS-related morbidity and mortality. Extremely premature neonates administered surfactant in the delivery room may have improvement in short-term outcomes and milder bronchopulmonary dysplasia (BPD). Some have recommended the prophylactic use of surfactant after resuscitation in extremely premature neonates to further protect the immature lung (<27 weeks' gestation).

Intraoperative Ventilator Management

In infants with RDS, intraoperative ventilator management using the anesthesia machine can be challenging. Attempts to duplicate preoperative settings often result in hypoxemia and/or hypercarbia. This is partly because of differences in ventilatory equipment, anesthetic-related changes in chest wall and lung compliance, and surgical conditions that affect the efficiency of ventilation. The primary goal of intraoperative ventilation in premature infants is avoidance of hypoxemia (PaO_2 <60 mm Hg, or SpO_2 <90%). Secondary goals include avoidance of a high inspired oxygen concentration and high mean airway pressures.

Volume targeted ventilation (VTV), starting at volumes of 5 mL/kg, prevents lung overdistension and ensures less variable tidal volumes. Traditionally, pressure-limited ventilation has been used in neonates because it is protective against higher peak inspiratory pressures (PIP) and complications such as pneumothorax. However, VTV allows for automatic weaning of PIP in real time as compliance improves and compared with pressure limited ventilation, benefits of VTV include less mechanical ventilation time, less incidence of BPD, and fewer air leaks.[6,10] During abdominal or thoracic surgery, where lung and chest wall compliance are changing minute by minute, experienced pediatric anesthesiologists with an "educated hand" will manually ventilate the infant and constantly adjust inspiratory pressures while maintaining adequate volumes, viewing the operative field and "feeling" changes in compliance.

PEEP is often used in infants with RDS to maintain alveolar patency, increase and stabilize FRC, and decrease ventilation-perfusion mismatch. Preoperative levels of PEEP should be maintained intraoperatively. Increasing PEEP may increase PaO_2 but may also increase $PaCO_2$ (secondary to decreased tidal volume) and interfere with venous return, which affects cardiac output in very small infants. In infants with RDS, excess PEEP may also have a deleterious effect on lung compliance. The optimal PEEP is that at which FiO_2 is low with acceptable blood gases and hemodynamic stability.[6,10]

In general, respiratory rates between 30 and 50 breaths/min are adequate for small infants with RDS. Increasing the respiratory rate will increase alveolar ventilation and decrease $PaCO_2$ without affecting PaO_2 if the inspiratory/expiratory ratio remains the same.

Inspiratory-to-expiratory (I/E) ratios in infants with RDS range from 1:1 to 1:3. Increasing the inspiratory component will facilitate opening of atelectatic areas, with a resultant increase in PaO_2. However, increasing the inspiratory time may substantially increase mean airway pressure, with the potential for barotrauma. Furthermore, a shortened expiratory time may cause air trapping and predispose to interstitial emphysema and pneumothorax. Carbon dioxide elimination is not usually affected by changing the I/E ratio.

Outcome of RDS

In most cases, the severity of RDS reaches a peak in 3 to 5 days and is followed by a gradual improvement, provided the infant is not burdened by additional medical problems. In severe cases, ventilatory therapy may be associated with the development of interstitial emphysema, pneumothorax, pulmonary hemorrhage and death. Infants who survive severe RDS are likely to develop neonatal chronic lung disease or bronchopulmonary dysplasia.

Apnea of Prematurity

Apnea is commonly defined as a cessation of breathing for greater than 20 seconds or less if accompanied by bradycardia (heart rate 30 beats/min less than baseline) or hypoxemia (SpO2<90%), cyanosis or pallor.[11] Apnea is extremely common in premature infants, with an incidence that increases with decreasing gestational age. Essentially, all extremely premature infants have apnea of prematurity. Up to 25% of neonates with birth weights of less than 2500 g and up to 84% of infants with birth weights less than 1000 g exhibit some form of apnea. Approximately 50% of infants with birth weights less than 1500 g experience apnea that must be managed pharmacologically or by ventilatory support. Apnea of prematurity usually resolves by the 52nd week after conception. The correlation between apnea and gestational age has implications for both the NICU and postanesthesia care. Generally, all premature infants born less than 35 weeks gestational age will require monitoring in the NICU because of their increased risk for having apneic events, potentially associated with bradycardia. Similarly, because formerly premature infants may develop apnea after stressful events such as general anesthesia, most hospitals and institutions have a policy for admission for cardiorespiratory monitoring of formerly premature infants postanesthesia depending on their gestational age.[11]

Apnea is classified as central (lack of respiratory effort) or obstructive (lack of airflow in the presence of respiratory effort). Most apneic events in prematurely born infants are mixed (some combination of central and obstructive apnea).

Apnea of prematurity is likely caused by neuronal immaturity of the respiratory control center in the brainstem and the peripheral chemoreceptors. Vital organ blood flow decreases significantly[12] during bradycardic events in these infants. However, the association of apnea of prematurity with long-term neurodevelopmental outcomes is not clearly defined. Limited studies indicate that persistent apnea resolving up to or after 36 weeks postmenstrual age may be associated with higher rate of worse neurodevelopmental outcomes; however, it is difficult to distinguish whether the outcomes are caused by apnea or other prematurity-related comorbidities.[11]

Acute episodes of apnea are treated initially with tactile stimulation and simple airway maneuvers to relieve upper airway obstruction (e.g., chin lift or jaw thrust). Bag-mask positive pressure breathing is required if breathing does not resume spontaneously or if hypoxemia continues. Infants with recurrent apneic episodes are placed on prophylactic stimulant therapy consisting of methylxanthines (i.e., caffeine and aminophylline). Nasal CPAP is often used in combination with methylxanthines and is effective in decreasing the severity and number of apneic episodes. It works by maintaining airway patency and decreasing risk for obstruction.[11] Mechanical ventilation is used as a last resort in infants who continue to demonstrate life-threatening apneic events despite pharmacologic therapy. Anemia has been thought to contribute to apnea of prematurity based on a decreased oxygen carrying capacity in anemic infants. Blood transfusions have shown to decrease the number of apneic episodes; however, only short-term effects have been noted, and further studies for long term effects are required.[11,13]

Patent Ductus Arteriosus

A patent ductus arteriosus (PDA) is a common finding in preterm infants with respiratory disease. In normal newborns, the ductus arteriosus closes within the first few days of life and is functionally closed within the first 72 hours of life. This process is initiated by the normal increase in blood–oxygen tension and decreased levels of circulating maternal prostaglandins. The incidence of a PDA in premature infants is inversely related to birth weight and gestational age. Virtually all shunting through a PDA in a preterm infant is left to right, and only in larger infants is persistent pulmonary hypertension with right-to-left shunting across a PDA an issue. In premature infants, a PDA is associated with exacerbation of respiratory distress syndrome, increased oxygen requirements or prolonged need for mechanical ventilation, increased risk for developing bronchopulmonary dysplasia, cardiovascular instability, the development of intraventricular hemorrhage, renal dysfunction and oliguria, necrotizing enterocolitis, cerebral palsy and mortality[14].

A symptomatic PDA may be closed in the early newborn period by pharmacologic therapy using indomethacin,[15] transcatheter occlusion or surgical ligation. Side effects of indomethacin include platelet and renal dysfunction. The American Heart Association recommends[16] that infants with congenital heart disease repaired with prosthetic material or device should receive procedure-associated subacute bacterial endocarditis (SBE) prophylaxis for 6 months after artificial closure.

Assessing hemodynamic significance of a PDA is accomplished by physical exam, echocardiography, and serum biomarkers such as b-type natriuretic peptide (BNP) or N-terminal pro-BNP (pro-BNP). Some physical exam findings for patients with PDA include a classic, coarse systolic murmur heard at the left sternal border, prominent arterial pulses, an increased precordial impulse, decreased diastolic pressure with wide pulse pressure and/or decrease in systolic and diastolic blood pressure. Pulmonary congestion may be seen on chest x-ray. A patient with a hemodynamically significant PDA may have trouble weaning oxygen requirements or weaning from ventilator support. Hemodynamically significant PDA has been associated with lower cerebral oxygen saturation, though the long-term clinical ramifications are unclear. A more comprehensive definition of "hemodynamically significant" PDA needs to be identified.[17]

There is ample evidence to show that routine, early assisted closure of PDA, whether medical or surgical in all preterm infants, does not necessarily improve outcomes in the long term. Whether to selectively assist closure in infants deemed high risk for development of complications is still unclear and requires more study.[17] Knowing that prolonged patency of PDA in premature infants is a major cause of morbidity and mortality, having a way to identify those infants at risk for persistent PDA and associated complications, could potentially facilitate early treatment and prevent future morbidity.[14]

Anemia of Prematurity

Anemia in premature infants is often more severe and protracted than the physiologic anemia of infancy. This "anemia of prematurity" refers to anemia associated with low reticulocyte count and low erythropoietin concentration in preterm infants, usually those born at less than 32 weeks gestational age. It occurs usually in the first month of life[18,19] and is most commonly attributed to decreased production of erythropoietin, decreased erythrocyte production, decreased erythrocyte lifespan, and frequent blood sampling. Its incidence increases with decreasing gestational age. Up to 75% of infants weighing less than 1000 g receive a red cell transfusion at some time during their hospitalization. Anemia of prematurity has been implicated as a cause of apnea of prematurity, poor feeding, inadequate weight gain, persistent tachycardia and unexplained persistent metabolic acidosis. There has been shown to be a correlation between anemia, blood transfusions and necrotizing enterocolitis,[20] retinopathy of prematurity and bronchopulmonary dysplasia.[18]

Treatment options for anemia of prematurity may include transfusion of red cells, recombinant erythropoietin (EPO) and observation. Asymptomatic infants with adequate nutrition and who are not acutely ill may be followed with serial hematocrit measurements. Multiple studies have established premature infants' response to recombinant human EPO after exogenous administration. However, there is no universal agreement regarding its safety and dosing. Additionally the question remains whether EPO therapy will eliminate the need for transfusion completely or decrease the amount of donor exposures.[19]

Blood transfusion is the mainstay for the treatment of anemia of prematurity. Debate still exists regarding the indications for treatment. Triggering hemoglobin levels vary between centers and range between 7 and 12 g/dL, depending on the concurrent illness of the infant. Some centers administer EPO and iron to these infants. Most centers agree that the infant's hemoglobin level should be greater than 10 g/dL before any surgical procedure. In older infants recovering from prematurity, lower hemoglobin levels (7–10 g/dL) are tolerated in the absence of symptoms and a reticulocyte count that demonstrates active production of red blood cells. In general, neonatologists tend to keep infants' hemoglobin levels in direct relationship to their concomitant comorbidities.

Intraventricular Hemorrhage

Intraventricular hemorrhage (IVH) describes a serious condition almost exclusively seen in premature infants that involves spontaneous bleeding into and around the lateral ventricles of the brain. The bleeding originates in the subependymal germinal matrix, an area surrounding the lateral ventricles that contains fragile blood vessels in the premature brain. This fragility is no longer seen in most infants born at term.

The incidence of IVH increases with decreasing birth weight and decreasing gestational age; it occurs in up to 70% of infants with a birth weight less than 750 g, and most cases occur between birth and the third day of life. Additional predisposing factors include trauma, acidosis, anemia, RDS, hypoxic-ischemic injury, seizures, hypocarbia and use of vasopressors. Episodes of acute blood pressure fluctuation accompanied by rapid increases or decreases in cerebral blood flow, cerebral blood volume or cerebral pressure, such as might be observed during endotracheal intubation without administration of a sedative or anesthetic agent, can lead to development of IVH. Rapid infusion of a hyperosmolar solution, such as sodium bicarbonate, has also been shown experimentally to induce IVH in the premature brain. Decreased incidence or severity of IVH has been correlated with administration of antenatal glucocorticoids.[21]

IVH is typically classified into four stages of relative severity, based on ultrasound examination of the brain. Higher grades of bleed correlate with worse clinical symptoms and neurodevelopmental outcome. Grading of IVH is shown in Table 11.1.

TABLE 11.1	Ultrasound-based Grading of Intraventricular Hemorrhage in Neonates and Infants[22]
Grade of IVH	Severity of IVH Based on Ultrasound Examination
I	Bleeding confined to the periventricular germinal matrix
II	Bleeding into the lateral ventricle without ventricular dilatation
III	A substantial amount of bleeding into the lateral ventricle that causes ventricular dilatation
IV	Bleeding that extends into the brain parenchyma

Clinical manifestations of IVH include signs of abrupt neurologic changes in the first several days of life, such as hypotonia, apnea, seizures, loss of the sucking reflex, and a bulging anterior fontanelle. More severe cases manifest as unexplained anemia or hypovolemic shock.

IVH into or beyond the lateral ventricles may result in an obliterative arachnoiditis that causes blockage of cerebral spinal fluid (CSF) resorption and/or blockage of CSF flow at the aqueduct of Sylvius. This leads to a communicating hydrocephalus, which often necessitates ventriculo-peritoneal shunt placement early in life.

Bleeding into the brain parenchyma causes areas of hemorrhagic infarction and leads to the development of periventricular leukomalacia (PVL). PVL, which consists of cavitary cysts in the white matter surrounding the ventricles, is thought to be the single strongest predictor of cerebral palsy later in life. PVL may develop in patients without prior history of IVH or parenchymal hemorrhage.

Retinopathy of Prematurity

Retinopathy of prematurity (ROP), formerly called *retrolental fibroplasia* (RLF), is a disease of the premature infant that is associated with arrest or disruption of neurovascular growth of the immature retina that is characterized by two phases. It is one of the major preventable causes of blindness and occurs globally. ROP occurs when the growth of the retinal vessels is arrested before their full maturation and growth into the periphery of the retina (phase 1). New abnormal vessels proliferate in the area of devascularization (phase 2) at around 33 weeks postmenstrual age and are characterized by their propensity for abnormal growth, hemorrhage, and edema, all which may lead to retinal scarring and loss of vision.[23,24]

Risk factors for development of ROP include low gestational age, low birth weight, prolonged oxygen exposure,[25] mechanical ventilation, low glucose levels, increased exogenous insulin administration, episodes of bacteremia,[26] other neonatal infections such as fungal infections[27] and comorbidities. The precise concentration of inspired oxygen or PaO_2 that results in retinal vessel vasoconstriction is unknown and probably varies between patients. There are even reports of cyanotic infants who have developed ROP.

The incidence of ROP has declined in mildly premature infants because of the recognition of hyperoxia as a major contributing factor. However, the overall incidence of ROP has remained steady because of improved care and survival of extremely premature infants. Early treatment or prevention in at-risk infants includes careful titration of oxygen, though the optimal saturation is still unclear. Most studies agree that an oxygen saturation by pulse oximeter of 90% to 95% is more than adequate.[24] Most infants with mild to moderate disease will attain normal vision without treatment; advanced disease is treated by laser ablation of the avascular retina, intravitreal injection of anti-VEGF antibodies and vitrectomy, or retinal cryotherapy to prevent retinal detachment and vision loss. Long-term follow-up is necessary until adulthood because complications such as recurrence of ROP, refractory errors and retinal detachment can occur later in life.

Does oxygen administered during general anesthesia cause or exacerbate ROP? Although scattered reports implicate oxygen administration during general anesthesia as a contributing factor, this does not support withholding oxygen in fear of causing or exacerbating ROP. Intraoperatively, the oxygen saturation (SpO_2) should be maintained in the 90% to 95% range in extremely premature infants. In the presence of anemia, this saturation should be increased. Hyperoxia has also been shown to be a risk factor in promoting oxidative stress in preterm neonates, thus putting them at risk not only for ROP but also for white matter injury and potentially irreversible adverse neurodevelopmental consequences. Therefore, anesthesiologists should avoid hyperoxia in the perioperative period if possible.[28]

Hypoglycemia

Glucose is a crucial substrate for proper brain growth and development. In utero, glucose is maternally derived by transfer through the placenta. After birth, the newborn infant brain receives glucose by exogenous sources or endogenous gluconeogenesis from glycogen stores. However, glycogen is accumulated in the fetal liver mostly during the third trimester of pregnancy. Therefore, premature infants are at risk for developing hypoglycemia caused by insufficient glycogen storage in the liver, low levels of glycogen synthesis and formation and delay/difficulty in feeding (insufficient intake). The energy needs for neonates is about 3 to 6 times higher (per weight) than adults as a result of a higher metabolism. Not only do they have less glucose, but they actually require more.[28] This risk is also increased in infants with low birth weight, intrauterine growth retardation, infants of diabetic mothers and infants suffering from hypothermia, respiratory distress, polycythemia, or perinatal asphyxia. The recommendation by the Directory of the United States Neonatal Hypoglycemia is that routine glucose screening should occur early in all high-risk newborns.[29]

The definition of hypoglycemia has not been well delineated; however, it can be broken down into categories of severe (<35 mg/dL), moderate (35–47 mg/dL), and mild (47–70 mg/dL). Recent studies show that mild hypoglycemia or short-lived moderate hypoglycemia does not necessarily translate into future neurodevelopmental delays. However, enough evidence exists to prove that untreated hypoglycemia can lead to severe irreversible neurocognitive and neurodevelopmental impairments later in life.[28] Therefore, hypoglycemia should be treated aggressively. Currently, neonatologists advocate treatment of blood glucose levels <50 mg/dL, or more if there are symptoms. Symptoms of hypoglycemia include tremors (or jitteriness), irritability, cyanosis, neonatal convulsions (e.g., eye-rolling, limpness), apnea, high-pitched or weak cry or refusal to eat. Premature newborns that are not expected to receive glucose by enteral feedings are administered 10% dextrose intravenously, with a target glucose infusion rate of 8 mg/kg/min by the second day of life. Symptomatic hypoglycemia is treated with intravenous bolus dosing of 10% dextrose (2–4 mL/kg) until the symptoms resolve and the blood glucose has risen above normal levels. Rebound hypoglycemia commonly occurs; therefore, these infants are placed on a continuous glucose infusion and blood glucose levels are monitored frequently.

Premature or formerly premature infants can easily develop hypoglycemia during the preoperative fasting interval because of immature gluconeogenic pathways or insufficient glycogen stores, as discussed earlier.[28] For this reason, premature infants who present for surgical procedures under general anesthesia will be receiving glucose solutions in the immediate preoperative period. Because the stress response that accompanies the onset of surgery usually results in an elevation of blood glucose (catecholamine surge leading to increased cortisol and glucagon levels and insulin suppression),[28] many pediatric anesthesiologists will reduce the rate of the maintenance glucose infusion by 50% or more at the beginning of the surgical procedure. Subsequent intraoperative glucose measurements are usually performed on an hourly basis and the glucose infusion adjusted accordingly.[28] Symptoms of hypoglycemia will go unnoticed under anesthesia so checking intraoperative glucose frequently is vital. Postoperatively, symptoms of hypoglycemia may be misinterpreted as normal postoperative symptoms; therefore, glucose monitoring should be continued in recovery.

References

1. Glass HC, Costarino AT, Stayer SA, Brett CM, Cladis F, Davis PJ. Outcomes for extremely premature infants. *Anesth Analg.* 2015;120(6):1337–1351. https://doi.org/10.1213/ANE.0000000000000705.
2. Gregory ECW, Drake P, Martin JA. Lack of change in perinatal mortality in the United States, 2014–2016. *NCHS Data Brief.* 2018(316):1–8.
3. Kugelman A, Colin AA. Late preterm infants: near term but still in a critical developmental time period. *Pediatrics.* 2013;132(4):741–751. https://doi.org/10.1542/peds.2013-1131.
4. Patel RM, Kandefer S, Walsh MC, et al. Causes and timing of death in extremely premature infants from 2000 through 2011. *N Engl J Med.* 2015;372(4):331–340. https://doi.org/10.1056/NEJMoa1403489.
5. Chest radiography. https://www.aafp.org/afp/2007/1001/afp20071001p987-f2.jpg. Accessed on October 5, 2021.
6. Sweet DG, Carnielli V, Greisen G, et al. European Consensus Guidelines on the Management of Respiratory Distress Syndrome – 2019 Update. *Neonatology.* 2019;115(4):432–450. https://doi.org/10.1159/000499361.
7. Kandraju H, Murki S, Subramanian S, Gaddam P, Deorari A, Kumar P. Early routine versus late selective surfactant in preterm neonates with respiratory distress syndrome on nasal continuous positive airway pressure: a randomized controlled trial. *Neonatology.* 2013;103(2):148–154. https://doi.org/10.1159/000345198.

8. Aldana-Aguirre JC, Pinto M, Featherstone RM, Kumar M. Less invasive surfactant administration versus intubation for surfactant delivery in preterm infants with respiratory distress syndrome: a systematic review and meta-analysis. *Arch Dis Child Fetal Neonatal Ed.* 2017;102(1):F17–F23. https://doi.org/10.1136/archdischild-2015-310299.

9. Soll R, Ozek E. Multiple versus single doses of exogenous surfactant for the prevention or treatment of neonatal respiratory distress syndrome. *Cochrane Database Syst Rev.* 2009(1):CD000141. https://doi.org/10.1002/14651858.CD000141.pub2. Published 2009 Jan 21.

10. Klingenberg C, Wheeler KI, McCallion N, Morley CJ, Davis PG. Volume-targeted versus pressure-limited ventilation in neonates. *Cochrane Database Syst Rev.* 2017;10(10):CD003666. https://doi.org/10.1002/14651858.CD003666.pub4. Published 2017 Oct 17.

11. Eichenwald EC, Committee on Fetus and Newborn, American Academy of Pediatrics. Apnea of prematurity. *Pediatrics.* 2016;137(1):e20153757. https://doi.org/10.1542/peds.2015-3757.

12. Perlman JM, Volpe JJ. Episodes of apnea and bradycardia in the preterm newborn: impact on cerebral circulation. *Pediatrics.* 1985;76(3):333–338.

13. Zagol K, Lake DE, Vergales B, et al. Anemia, apnea of prematurity, and blood transfusions. *J Pediatr.* 2012;161(3):417–421. e1. https://doi.org/10.1016/j.jpeds.2012.02.044.

14. Mezu-Ndubuisi OJ, Agarwal G, Raghavan A, Pham JT, Ohler KH, Maheshwari A. Patent ductus arteriosus in premature neonates. *Drugs.* 2012;72(7):907–916. https://doi.org/10.2165/11632870-000000000-00000.

15. Fowlie PW, Davis PG, McGuire W. Prophylactic intravenous indomethacin for preventing mortality and morbidity in preterm infants. *Cochrane Database Syst Rev.* 2010;2010(7):CD000174. https://doi.org/10.1002/14651858.CD000174.pub2. Published 2010 Jul 7.

16. Wilson W, Taubert KA, Gewitz M, et al. Prevention of infective endocarditis: guidelines from the American Heart Association: a guideline from the American Heart Association Rheumatic Fever, Endocarditis, and Kawasaki Disease Committee, Council on Cardiovascular Disease in the Young, and the Council on Clinical Cardiology, Council on Cardiovascular Surgery and Anesthesia, and the Quality of Care and Outcomes Research Interdisciplinary Working Group [published correction appears in Circulation. 2007 Oct 9;116(15):e376-7]. *Circulation.* 2007;116(15):1736–1754. https://doi.org/10.1161/CIRCULATIONAHA.106.183095.

17. Benitz WE, Committee on Fetus and Newborn American Academy of Pediatrics Patent ductus arteriosus in preterm infants. *Pediatrics.* 2016;137(1). https://doi.org/10.1542/peds.2015-3730.

18. Colombatti R, Sainati L, Trevisanuto D. Anemia and transfusion in the neonate. *Semin Fetal Neonatal Med.* 2016;21(1):2–9. https://doi.org/10.1016/j.siny.2015.12.001.

19. Juul S. Erythropoietin in anemia of prematurity. *J Matern Fetal Neonatal Med.* 2012;25(Suppl 5):80–84. https://doi.org/10.3109/14767058.2012.716987.

20. Singh R, Shah BL, Frantz 3rd ID. Necrotizing enterocolitis and the role of anemia of prematurity. *Semin Perinatol.* 2012;36(4):277–282. https://doi.org/10.1053/j.semperi.2012.04.008.

21. Ballabh P. Pathogenesis and prevention of intraventricular hemorrhage. *Clin Perinatol.* 2014;41(1):47–67. https://doi.org/10.1016/j.clp.2013.09.007.

22. Parodi A, Govaert P, Horsch S, Bravo MC, Ramenghi LA, eurUS.brain group Cranial ultrasound findings in preterm germinal matrix haemorrhage, sequelae and outcome. *Pediatr Res.* 2020;87(Suppl 1):13–24. https://doi.org/10.1038/s41390-020-0780-2.

23. Hellström A, Smith LE, Dammann O. Retinopathy of prematurity. *Lancet.* 2013;382(9902):1445–1457. https://doi.org/10.1016/S0140-6736(13)60178-6.

24. Cayabyab R, Ramanathan R. Retinopathy of prematurity: therapeutic strategies based on pathophysiology. *Neonatology.* 2016;109(4):369–376. https://doi.org/10.1159/000444901.

25. Lloyd J, Askie L, Smith J, Tarnow-Mordi W. Supplemental oxygen for the treatment of prethreshold retinopathy of prematurity. *Cochrane Database Syst Rev.* 2003;2003(2):CD003482. https://doi.org/10.1002/14651858.CD003482.

26. Tolsma KW, Allred EN, Chen ML, Duker J, Leviton A, Dammann O. Neonatal bacteremia and retinopathy of prematurity: the ELGAN study. *Arch Ophthalmol.* 2011;129(12):1555–1563. https://doi.org/10.1001/archophthalmol.2011.319.

27. Fagerholm R, Vesti E. Retinopathy of prematurity - from recognition of risk factors to treatment recommendations. *Duodecim.* 2017;133(4):337–344.

28. McCann ME, Lee JK, Inder T. Beyond anesthesia toxicity: anesthetic considerations to lessen the risk of neonatal neurological injury. *Anesth Analg.* 2019;129(5):1354–1364. https://doi.org/10.1213/ANE.0000000000004271.

29. Zhou W, Yu J, Wu Y, Zhang H. Hypoglycemia incidence and risk factors assessment in hospitalized neonates. *J Matern Fetal Neonatal Med.* 2015;28(4):422–425. https://doi.org/10.3109/14767058.2014.918599.

12

The Formerly Premature Infant

OLIVIA NELSON, WALLIS T. MUHLY, AND RONALD S. LITMAN

With the advent of antenatal steroids, surfactant therapy, and the overall improvement in care of extremely premature infants, mortality from medical problems of prematurity has decreased. However, as survival rates of premature infants increase, the incidence of chronic medical conditions related to prematurity has also increased. As a consequence, anesthesia providers are exposed to a growing number of infants and children who were born prematurely and have a variety of chronic medical conditions that may influence their response to anesthesia. These patients have a higher risk for complications while sedated[1] or anesthetized,[2] and this risk persists into young adulthood.

Bronchopulmonary Dysplasia

The impact of prematurity on lung development and function will influence the preoperative evaluation of the formerly premature child. The terminology used to describe neonatal respiratory disorders can be confusing so to clarify: any pulmonary disease resulting from a neonatal respiratory disorder is termed chronic lung disease of infancy[3] (CLDI). Causes of CLDI vary based on age. Bronchopulmonary dysplasia (BPD) is the most common form of chronic lung disease, and it is defined as the need for supplemental oxygen for at least 28 days after birth. It is categorized as mild, moderate, or severe, which is determined by the required amount of oxygen or respiratory support at 36 weeks postmenstrual age for infants born before 32 weeks and at 56 days for infants born greater than 32 weeks gestation.[4,5]

A distinction has been made between "old" and "new" BPD.[6] Old BPD occurred in near-term infants during the saccular and late alveolar stages of lung development (see Chapter 1), some of whom had direct lung injury in the form of pneumonia, sepsis, aspiration, or congenital heart or lung malformations. They were treated with prolonged, aggressive mechanical ventilation with high oxygen concentrations and developed a severe form of CLDI with histopathology consistent with diffuse alveolar hyperplasia, wide-spread inflammation, peribronchial smooth muscle hypertrophy and parenchymal fibrosis. In contrast, the histopathology in new BPD does not reveal diffuse inflammatory changes or alveolar hyperplasia. Instead, the histopathology is consistent with an arrest of alveolar development with large simplified alveoli leading to a reduced surface area for gas exchange and fewer alveolar-airway attachments that predispose to small airway collapse.[6] Because the alveoli and pulmonary arterioles grow in parallel, patients with BPD may also have pulmonary hypertension. BPD-related pulmonary hypertension[7] typically has a fixed component related to decreased vascular surface area and a dynamic component because of increased vascular reactivity.

The clinical manifestations of the classic, more severe form of BPD include tachypnea, rales, bronchospasm, and a persistent requirement for supplemental oxygen. Carbon dioxide retention is a prominent finding and is presumably because of increased dead space ventilation. Radiographic abnormalities include hyperinflation, bleb formation, and interstitial densities (Fig. 12.1). Infants with severe BPD may also demonstrate episodes of sudden, severe bronchospasm, and cyanosis after agitation or physical stimulation ("BPD spells"). These are thought to be caused by nearly complete tracheal collapse as a result of underlying tracheomalacia, a complication of prolonged mechanical ventilation. These episodes are treated with sedation or calming of the infant combined with application of continuous positive airway pressure (CPAP) or positive pressure ventilation in the event of unremitting hypoxemia.

The clinical manifestations of the new milder form of BPD are characterized by a more benign clinical course with respect to respiratory support, but the pulmonary pathology in these children should not be underestimated (Fig. 12.2). Formerly premature children still have a higher incidence of wheezing secondary to small airway collapse related to impaired alveolar development and the rate of readmission for respiratory tract infection in the first year of life[8] is higher compared with children born at term. Thus, a concerted effort should be made to reduce exposure to passive smoke inhalation and viral infection in formerly

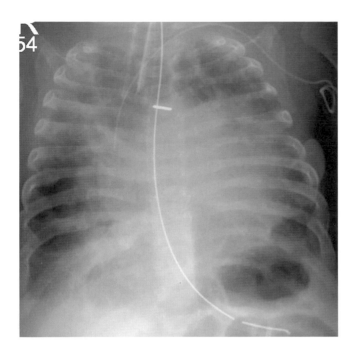

• **Fig 12.1.** Chest radiograph shows areas of hyperinflation and emphysema with adjacent dense areas of atelectasis. This picture is characteristic of old BPD. (From: Bancalari EH, Jain D. Bronchopulmonary dysplasia in the neonate. In: Martin RJ, Fanaroff AA, Walsh MC, eds. *Fanaroff and Martin's Neonatal-Perinatal Medicine: Diseases of the Fetus and Infant*. 11th ed. Philadelphia: Elsevier; 2020 [chapter 69]: 1256–1269.)

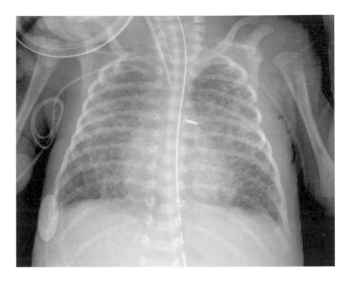

• **Fig. 12.2.** Chest radiograph from an infant with new BPD showing generalized homogenous opacities with an interstitial pattern. (From: Bancalari EH, Jain D. Bronchopulmonary Dysplasia in the Neonate. In: Martin RJ, Fanaroff AA, Walsh MC, eds. *Fanaroff and Martin's Neonatal-Perinatal Medicine: Diseases of the Fetus and Infant*. 11th ed. Philadelphia: Elsevier; 2020 [chapter 69]: 1256–1269.)

premature infants with BPD. The wheezing exhibited by children with BPD is often mistaken for asthma and as a result these children may receive unnecessary steroid or beta-agonist therapy. As noted above, this new form of BPD is not an inflammatory process like asthma and is unlikely to have a significant clinical response to steroid treatment. Additionally, airway obstruction in BPD is only partially reversed with beta-agonist therapy. As the infant with mild BPD grows, there is a comparatively less bronchospastic component than with the more severe form. However, studies of school age children show that pulmonary function tests continue to show obstructive disease[9] despite apparent resolution of symptoms, and one study[10] demonstrated that adults who were born premature had an increased incidence of respiratory symptoms compared with those born full term.

With all forms of BPD, ventilatory management is focused on the minimization of barotrauma or volutrauma and the prevention of atelectasis. Attempts to limit inspired fractional concentration of oxygen will help prevent oxygen toxicity. Debate continues about the ideal ventilatory setting (volume limited or pressure limited) or the use of positive end expiratory pressure (PEEP) in patients with BPD to optimize oxygenation and ventilation while limiting damage to the lung. For ventilatory management in the NICU, it appears that volume targeted ventilation may have lower morbidity and mortality[11] compared with pressure limited

ventilation. Although PEEP maintains functional reserve capacity functional reserve capacity (FRC) and reduces atelectasis, the optimal PEEP level[12] for neonates and formerly premature children is unknown. Ideal tidal volumes with mechanical ventilation remain controversial: some authors argue for 5 to 7 mL/kg while others suggest that lower volumes of 4 to 6 mL/kg might be best.

Anesthetic Management of Infants With BPD

Preoperative assessment of infants with BPD is focused on optimization of their respiratory status, with particular regard for treating underlying bronchoconstriction. Infants with BPD that present for surgery with a concomitant upper respiratory tract infection have a higher risk for an adverse respiratory event during the perioperative period (e.g., laryngospasm, bronchospasm, hypoxia, etc.) and may require prolonged oxygen support postoperatively. Therefore, postponement of elective procedures may be warranted.

Infants with severe BPD who are likely to develop bronchospasm and cyanosis during physical stimulation should receive an anxiolytic premedication. Tracheal intubation should be avoided if possible. Whenever feasible, a laryngeal mask airway (LMA) is preferred. If tracheal intubation is performed, a "deep extubation" may be warranted to avoid bronchospasm. In abdominal procedures, a regional analgesic technique is indicated for adequate postoperative pain control and to avoid chest wall splinting and to preserve the ability to cough without pain. There are insufficient data in

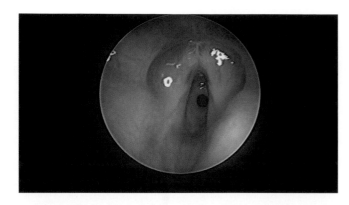

• **Fig 12.3.** Iatrogenic subglottic stenosis after prolonged endotracheal intubation in a neonate. (From: Otteson TD, Wang T. Upper Airway Lesions in the Neonate. In: Martin RJ, Fanaroff AA, Walsh MC, eds. *Fanaroff and Martin's Neonatal-Perinatal Medicine: Diseases of the Fetus and Infant.* 11th ed. Elsevier; 2020 [chapter 68]: 1244–1255.)

infants with BPD with which to predict the incidence of intraoperative or postoperative pulmonary complications.

Laryngeal and Tracheal Injury

Premature infants who required prolonged endotracheal intubation and mechanical ventilation are prone to develop injury to the laryngeal and tracheal tissues, which results in scarring and upper-airway narrowing. Fibrotic narrowing of the airway typically occurs at the level of the cricoid cartilage and is termed subglottic stenosis (SGS) (Fig. 12.3). Historically, the incidence of clinically significant SGS[13] ranged from 0.9% to 8.3% in infants who survived prolonged mechanical ventilation in the neonatal period. However, there is speculation that with improved ventilatory management of the premature neonate the incidence may be declining. An Australian study found that the incidence of severe SGS requiring airway reconstruction[14] approached 0.005%. Regardless of these changes, the anesthesia provider should prepare smaller diameter endotracheal tubes when planning to anesthetize a formerly premature infant, and attention should be paid to any resistance encountered when attempting to pass the tube through the vocal cords or subglottic area. After extubation, these children may develop stridor as a result of further tracheal narrowing from acute subglottic edema. Therefore, the endotracheal tube should permit an air leak below 30 cmH$_2$O to help prevent excessive swelling of the subglottic mucosa.

Tracheal and bronchial injury that occurs during repeated deep suctioning techniques might result in lower airway narrowing and granuloma formation. Tracheobronchomalacia may occur in up to 50% of former premature infants. It is thought to be partially responsible for the tracheal collapse that manifests as wheezing or cyanosis during "BPD spells."

Postoperative Apnea

Former premature infants who are growing and otherwise doing well may demonstrate central apnea[15] after administration of general anesthesia[16] for elective surgical procedures, such as an inguinal herniorrhaphy. These episodes of postoperative apnea may be accompanied by bradycardia and may require bag-mask assisted ventilation to relieve the hypoxemia. The cause of this phenomenon is unknown, but it is probably related to the effects of general anesthetic agents on the immature respiratory control center[17] in the brainstem.

Both retrospective and prospective studies have been performed in an attempt to delineate the types of patients at risk for postoperative apnea. Characteristics of premature infants found in early studies to be more likely to develop postoperative apnea[18] included low gestational age, low postconceptional age (PCA), preoperative apnea of prematurity, anemia (usually defined as a hemoglobin level <10 g/dL), history of pulmonary disease[19] (e.g., BPD). The PCA at which postoperative apnea will not occur is unknown; however, there are no reports of postoperative apnea in infants older than 60 weeks PCA. (These statements are based on older studies that attempted to determine PCA-based risk, but the term "postconceptional age" has been abandoned[20] in favor of the more reliable "postmenstrual age.") The true risk for an individual patient is indeterminate and is likely a continuum based on the infant's gestational and chronologic age, and coexisting medical conditions. Lower rates of apnea in recent studies may reflect the effects of newer, shorter-acting anesthetics or differences in how apnea was measured.

Strategies for Preventing Postoperative Apnea

Recognition of the existence of postoperative apnea prompted a number of investigators to develop anesthetic strategies designed to prevent it in susceptible infants. These strategies have included use of spinal anesthesia, preoperative transfusion, and administration of caffeine in the perioperative period.

In 1984, Chris Abajian, a pediatric anesthesiologist from the University of Vermont popularized spinal anesthesia for small infants. Since publication of that report,[21] numerous additional publications have examined the benefits and risks[22] of spinal or epidural anesthesia in this patient population for lower abdominal or groin procedures. Most reported series confirm that spinal or epidural anesthesia is associated with a lower incidence (but not complete absence) of postoperative apnea,[23] as long as additional systemic sedative agents are avoided. However, a randomized controlled trial[24] in patients undergoing inguinal herniorrhaphy under regional versus general anesthesia found similar rates of overall apnea (0–12 hours), albeit with less early apnea (0–30 min) and less invasive interventions required in the regional anesthesia group. Infants with significant neurologic risk factors or birth at less than 26 weeks of gestation were excluded. Infants at risk for postoperative apnea who receive regional anesthesia with sedation should receive the same postoperative apnea monitoring as that used after administration of general anesthesia. There is currently a debate in the pediatric anesthesia community concerning the appropriate level of postoperative monitoring in infants receiving regional anesthesia without sedative supplementation. Although some centers routinely discharge these infants on the day of surgery, others require overnight monitoring.

At one point in history, there appeared to be an association between anemia and an increased risk for postoperative apnea[25]; thus the argument for preoperative transfusion in the formerly premature infant. However, later studies suggested that the benefit may be small[26] and not significant enough to outweigh the potential risks of transfusion which may include worsening of BPD or necrotizing enterocolitis. Thus, this practice has been largely abandoned.

Perioperative administration of caffeine[27] decreases the incidence of postoperative apnea, bradycardia, and hypoxemia in susceptible infants. Anesthesiologists caring for infants at risk for postoperative apnea should proactively consult with their center's neonatologists and develop a treatment plan for the administration of perioperative caffeine. For NICU patients undergoing surgery, communication between anesthesiologist and neonatologist is crucial. The patient may currently be receiving caffeine and may not require a perioperative dose. Other patients may be going home soon after surgery; thus a perioperative dose of caffeine will complicate discharge planning because of the long half-life of caffeine. In formerly premature infants who present for elective surgery after discharge from the hospital, caffeine is administered on a case-by-case basis, after assessment of the risk factors and discussion with the infant's neonatologist.

References

1. Havidich JE, Beach M, Dierdorf SF, Onega T, Suresh G, Cravero JP. Preterm versus term children: Analysis of sedation/anesthesia adverse events and longitudinal risk. *Pediatrics.* 2016;137(3):e20150463. doi:10.1542/peds.2015-0463.

2. Vlassakova BG, Sinnott SM, Askins N, et al. The Anesthesia perioperative "Call for help"–Experience at a quaternary pediatric medical center: Analysis of 67,564 anesthesia encounters. *Anesth Analg.* 2018;127(1):126–133. doi: 10.1213/ANE.0000000000003353.

3. Allen J, Zwerdling R, Ehrenkranz R, et al. Statement on the care of the child with chronic lung disease of infancy and childhood. *Am J Respir Crit Care Med.* 2003;168(3):356–396. doi: 10.1164/rccm.168.3.356.

4. Jobe AH, Bancalari E. Bronchopulmonary dysplasia. *Am J Respir Crit Care Med.* 2001;163(7):1723–1729. doi: 10.1164/ajrccm.163.7.2011060.

5. Glass HC, Costarino AT, Stayer SA, Brett CM, Cladis F, Davis PJ. Outcomes for extremely premature infants. *Anesth Analg.* 2015;120(6):1337–1351. doi: 10.1213/ANE.0000000000000705.

6. Baraldi E, Filippone M. Chronic lung disease after premature birth. *N Engl J Med.* 2007;357(19):1946–1955. doi: 10.1056/NEJMra067279.

7. Latham GJ, Yung D. Current understanding and perioperative management of pediatric pulmonary hypertension. *Paediatr Anaesth.* 2019;29(5):441–456. doi: 10.1111/pan.13542.

8. Lamarche-Vadel A, Blondel B, Truffer P, et al. Re-hospitalization in infants younger than 29 weeks' gestation in the EPIPAGE cohort. *Acta Paediatr.* 2004;93(10):1340–1345. doi: 10.1080/08035250410032926.

9. Doyle LW, Faber B, Callanan C, Freezer N, Ford GW, Davis NM. Bronchopulmonary dysplasia in very low birth weight subjects and lung function in late adolescence. *Pediatrics.* 2006;118(1):108–113. doi: 10.1542/peds.2005-2522.

10. Narang I, Rosenthal M, Cremonesini D, Silverman M, Bush A. Longitudinal Evaluation of Airway Function 21 Years after Preterm Birth. *Am J Respir Crit Care Med.* 2008;178(1):74–80. doi: 10.1164/rccm.200705-701OC.

11. Wheeler KI, Klingenberg C, Morley CJ, Davis PG. Volume-targeted versus pressure-limited ventilation for preterm infants: a systematic review and meta-analysis. *Neonatology.* 2011;100(3):219–227. doi: 10.1159/000326080.

12. Bamat N, Millar D, Suh S, Kirpalani H. Positive end expiratory pressure for preterm infants requiring conventional mechanical ventilation for respiratory distress syndrome or bronchopulmonary dysplasia. *Cochrane Database Syst Rev.* 2012;1:CD004500. doi: 10.1002/14651858.CD004500.pub2. Published 2012 Jan 18.

13. Walner DL, Loewen MS, Kimura RE. Neonatal subglottic stenosis-incidence and trends. *Laryngoscope.* 2001;111(1):48–51. doi: 10.1097/00005537-200101000-00009.

14. Leung R, Berkowitz RG. Incidence of severe acquired subglottic stenosis in newborns. *Int J Pediatr Otorhinolaryngol.* 2007;71(5):763–768. doi: 10.1016/j.ijporl.2007.01.014.

15. Kurth CD, LeBard SE. Association of postoperative apnea, airway obstruction, and hypoxemia in former premature infants. *Anesthesiology.* 1991;75(1):22–26. doi: 10.1097/00000542-198704000-00006.

16. Kurth CD, Spitzer AR, Broennle AM, Downes JJ. Postoperative apnea in preterm infants. *Anesthesiology.* 1987;66(4):483–488. doi: 10.1097/00000542-199107000-00005.

17. Zhao J, Gonzalez F, Mu D. Apnea of prematurity: from cause to treatment. *Eur J Pediatr.* 2011;170(9):1097–1105. doi: 10.1007/s00431-011-1409-6.

18. Coté CJ, Zaslavsky A, Downes JJ, et al. Postoperative apnea in former preterm infants after inguinal herniorrhaphy. A combined analysis. *Anesthesiology.* 1995;82(4):809–822. doi: 10.1097/00000542-199504000-00002.

19. Massoud M, Kühlmann AYR, van Dijk M, et al. Does the incidence of postoperative complications after inguinal hernia repair justify hospital admission in prematurely and term born infants? *Anesth Analg.* 2019;128(3):525–532. doi: doi.org/10.1213/ANE.0000000000003386.

20. Engle WA. American academy of pediatrics committee on fetus and newborn. Age terminology during the perinatal period. *Pediatrics.* 2004;114(5):1362–1364. doi: doi.org/10.1542/peds.2004-1915.

21. Abajian JC, Mellish RW, Browne AF, Perkins FM, Lambert DH, Mazuzan JE Jr. Spinal anesthesia for surgery in the high-risk infant. *Anesth Analg.* 1984;63(3):359–362.

22. Krane EJ, Haberkern CM, Jacobson LE. Postoperative apnea, bradycardia, and oxygen desaturation in formerly premature infants: prospective comparison of spinal and general anesthesia. *Anesth Analg.* 1995;80(1):7–13. doi: 10.1097/00000539-199501000-00003.

23. William JM, Stoddart PA, Williams SA, Wolf AR. Post-operative recovery after inguinal herniotomy in ex-premature infants: comparison between sevoflurane and spinal anaesthesia. *Br J Anaesth.* 2001;86(3):366–371. doi: 10.1093/bja/86.3.366.

24. Davidson AJ, Morton NS, Arnup SJ, et al. Apnea after awake-regional and general anesthesia in infants: The general anesthesia

compared to spinal anesthesia (GAS) study: comparing apnea and neurodevelopmental outcomes, a randomized controlled trial. *Anesthesiology.* 2015;123(1):38–54. doi: 10.1097/ALN.0000000000000709.

25. Welborn LG, Hannallah RS, Luban NL, Fink R, Ruttimann UE. Anemia and postoperative apnea in former preterm infants. *Anesthesiology.* 1991;74(6):1003–1006. doi: 10.1097/00000542-199106000-00006.

26. Westkamp E, Soditt V, Adrian S, Bohnhorst B, Groneck P, Poets CF. Blood transfusion in anemic infants with apnea of prematurity. *Biol Neonate.* 2002;82(4):228–232. doi: 10.1159/000065891.

27. Welborn LG, Hannallah RS, Fink R, Ruttimann UE, Hicks JM. High-dose caffeine suppresses postoperative apnea in former preterm infants. *Anesthesiology.* 1989;71(3):347–349. doi: 10.1097/00000542-198909000-00005.

Suggested Reading

Lauer R, Vadi M, Mason L. Anaesthetic management of the child with co-existing pulmonary disease. *Br J Anaesth.* 2012;109(suppl 1):i47–i59. doi: doi.org/10.1093/bja/aes392.

13

Preanesthetic Preparation of the Pediatric Patient

GREGORY DODSON, ANASTASIA DIMOPOULOU, THEOKLIS ZAOUTIS, AND RONALD S. LITMAN

The "10 P" Checklist

Cognitive aids, in the form of checklists, are techniques that ensure completeness with multistep processes and aid attention to detail. We devised the 10 P checklist to help anesthesia providers prepare for cases (Table 13.1). This checklist is divided into preoperative, intraoperative, and postoperative considerations, and it will form the basis of the organization for this chapter.

The Patient: History and Physical Exam

The preoperative history should focus on concurrent medical diseases and their treatment, currently administered medications, previous allergic reactions, previous problems with administration of anesthetics, and family history of problems with anesthesia. Anesthetic complications that tend to recur include airway obstruction, postoperative nausea and vomiting, and severity of postoperative pain. If a previous anesthesia record is accessible, it must be thoroughly reviewed. The history of anesthetic problems in the family is focused on detecting susceptibility to malignant hyperthermia or presence of pseudocholinesterase deficiency. Some concurrent medications may influence the anesthetic technique. For example, anticonvulsants tend to shorten the duration of action of the aminosteroidal neuromuscular blockers.

TABLE 13.1	The 10 P Cheklist: What to Discuss With Your Attending Before the Case
Patient	Discuss the patient's history, physical exam, previous anesthetics, and implications of any comorbidities.
Procedure	Discuss the procedure and its considerations for anesthetic management.
Premedication	Discuss the premedication and dose to order.
Preoperative Fasting	Discuss the fasting orders. Healthy children should be encouraged to drink clear liquids up to 2 hours before the scheduled procedure time.
Preoperative labs	Appropriate tests are chosen depending on the medical condition of the patient and the nature of the surgery.
Perioperative monitoring	Additional monitors are obtained if dictated by the medical condition of the patient or the nature of the surgery.
Positioning	Preparations are made to enhance patient safety when using a position other than supine.
Plan	An anesthetic plan for induction, maintenance, and emergence from general anesthesia is formulated based on a combination of the above factors.
Pain control	Plans are formulated for intraoperative and postoperative analgesic requirements. This often includes a regional anesthesia technique.
Postoperative concerns	Considerations are given for possible postoperative concerns and complications on the medical condition of the patient and the nature of the surgery. Plans are made for possible ICU admission and ventilatory management if necessary.

ICU, Intensive care unit.

TABLE 13.2	Maternal Medical Conditions and Their Effects on the Newborn
Maternal Condition	**Effect on Newborn**
Diabetes	Increased incidence of congenital anomalies, hypoglycemia, macrosomia, polycythemia, cardiomyopathy, hypocalcemia, immature lung disease, hypomagnesemia. hyperbilirubinemia
Oligohydramnios	Renal anomalies, fetal distress, growth retardation
Polyhydramnios	Tracheoesophageal fistula
Low alpha-fetaprotein levels	Trisomy 21 (Down syndrome)
Rh sensitization	Hydrops fetalis, or milder forms of hemolytic anemia
Antepartum bleeding	Anemia, hypovolemia
Premature membrane rupture	Neonatal infection, sepsis
Meconium-stained amniotic fluid	Interstitial pneumonitis
Systemic lupus erythematosus (SLE)	Congenital third-degree heart block
Myasthenia gravis	Neonatal myasthenia
Preeclampsia	Neutropenia and thrombocytopenia
Graves disease	Hypothyroidism or hyperthyroidism
Chorioamnionitis	Neonatal infection, sepsis

TABLE 13.3	Maternal Medication Effects on the Newborn
Aspirin and other NSAIDS	Hemorrhage. pulmonary artery hypertension
Opioids	Neonatal depression, or abstinence
Cephalosporins	Hyperbilirubinemia
Sulfonamides	Hyperbilirubinemia
Anticonvulsants	Congenital anomalies
Warfarin (Coumadin)	Congenital anomalies, developmental delay, seizures
Antithyroid medications	Hypothyroidism
Beta-blockers	Neonatal bradycardia, hypoglycemia
Cocaine	Congenital anomalies, placental abruption
Magnesium	Respiratory depression, hypotonia, sensitivity to neuromuscular blockers
Ritodrine	Hypoglycemia
Terbutaline	Hypoglycemia
Alcohol	Fetal alcohol syndrome: dysmorphic facies, growth retardation, developmental delay
Tobacco	Prematurity, IUGR placental abruption and previa
Lithium	Cardiac anomalies
Isotretinoin	Micrognathia, cardiac and CNS anomalies
ACE inhibitors	Hypotension, oliguria

ACE, Angiotensin-converting enzyme; *CNS,* central nervous system; *IUGR,* intrauterine growth retardation.

When anesthetizing a neonate, the preoperative history should also focus on the medical histories of the parents and the course of pregnancy and delivery. Some maternal medical conditions (Table 13.2) and medications administered during pregnancy (Table 13.3) may affect the health of the newborn.

A history of an allergy to a medication is common in children presenting for surgery. All children who require insertion of tympanostomy tubes have been exposed to at least one type of antibiotic. Many of these children report development of a rash after administration of antibiotics with a penicillin, cephalosporin, or sulfa base and have not undergone further diagnostic testing to determine the cause of the rash. The anesthesia practitioner has no accurate way of determining the true allergic status of the child, other than by history, or report from the parent. Studies have consistently shown that history of a drug allergy does not accurately predict positive skin testing. In many cases, more detailed questioning of the parent reveals that the reaction was not allergic in nature. For example, a parent may report that their child is allergic to morphine because it caused the child to experience somnolence or itching.

The focus of the preoperative physical exam is on the cardiovascular system, respiratory system, neurologic function, and other indicators of normal function.

Examination of the cardiovascular system begins with a measurement of vital signs such as heart rate and blood pressure. Normal values for heart rate and blood pressure vary with age, gender, weight, and height. Active and irritable infants will not have accurate vital signs, which are irrelevant in otherwise healthy children. Likewise, auscultation of the heart in a healthy child is so low yield that one could argue that it is unnecessary and will inevitably lead to the presence of the "normal" murmur, inviting further discussion and possible evaluation.

If this occurs, the parents should be queried as to whether or not the murmur had been previously detected, and whether there was any previous cardiac evaluation. If the

TABLE 13.4	Key Elements of the Preanesthetic Physical Exam
Observation	**Implications**
General	
Hypotonia or hypertonia	Neurologic or metabolic disease
Cyanosis	Cardiac disease, sepsis
Pallor	Anemia, poor cardiac output
Cardiovascular	
Abnormal murmur	Congenital heart disease
Abnormal or absent pulses	Coarctation of the aorta, poor cardiac output
Respiratory	
Tachypnea, abnormal lung sounds (e.g, wheezing, rales, rhonchi), use of accessory muscles of respiration, grunting	All are nonspecific findings in a variety of respiratory or cardiac disorders
Head and Neck	
Abnormal craniofacial anatomy (e.g., micrognathia). limited mouth opening or jaw mobility, limited neck mobility	Indicators of possible difficulty with ventilation or intubation

TABLE 13.5	Reasons to Obtain Cardiology Consultation for a Previously Undetected Heart Murmur

History

- Poor exercise tolerance (or feeding intolerance in an infant)
- Patient was supposed to have a cardiology evaluation but it was never done
- Congenital heart disease in immediate family
- Cyanotic episodes

Physical Exam

- Murmur present in diastole
- Systolic murmur grade III or louder
- Absent or abnormal peripheral pulses
- Cyanosis, pallor, or poor capillary refill

murmur has not been previously detected, the anesthesiologist must quickly decide whether or not to continue with the anesthetic or cancel the case pending cardiology consultation to determine the cause of the murmur. Nearly all murmurs in otherwise healthy children can be classified as normal flow murmurs. These are not louder than II/VI, are usually vibratory in nature, and occur in systole over the pulmonary or mitral areas of the chest wall (Table 13.4). Cardiology consultation should be obtained if the characteristics of the murmur are different or if there are other findings relevant to the cardiovascular system on history or physical exam.

Important elements of the respiratory system include the upper and lower airways. Facial structure and mandibular mobility should be examined for clues to a possible difficult ventilation or difficult tracheal intubation. Loose teeth should be suspected in children between 5 and 10 years of age. The anesthesiologist should manually remove an extremely loose tooth after induction of anesthesia as a precaution against its unintentional dislodgement and passage into the bronchial tree. Lung auscultation in healthy children is probably not necessary; however, children with a history of reactive airway disease and those with a concurrent upper respiratory tract infection should be assessed for expiratory wheezing. Room air pulse oximetry should be performed; a value less than 96% should warrant an investigation of respiratory abnormalities. In general, respiratory rates greater than 44 breaths per minute are considered abnormal, except in otherwise healthy neonates and small infants, in whom normal breathing rates can occasionally reach 70 breaths per minute.

Additional elements of the physical exam will be largely dependent on the preexisting medical condition of the child and the nature of the surgery (Table 13.5). For example, a focused neurologic exam is indicated before any neurologic or orthopedic surgery, and in children with neuromuscular diseases.

Discussing Risks of Pediatric Anesthesia

During the preoperative informed consent process, it is helpful to know the modern-day risks for general anesthesia in children. A Mayo clinic study[1] revealed an incidence of cardiac arrest in anesthetized children (for noncardiac surgery) of 2.9 per 10,000, although when attributed only to anesthetic causes, the incidence was 0.65 per 10,000 anesthetics. Very few of these patients were initially healthy before the procedure.

A controversial issue in pediatric anesthesia is the extent to which the anesthesiologist should reveal the risks for anesthesia to the parents. Will this discussion increase or decrease parental (or child) anxiety? Should the anesthesiologist discuss the risk for death? What risks are appropriate to reveal? The answers to these questions are not easily found and may partly depend on the informed consent laws of the state in which one practices. Studies universally demonstrate that anxiety is decreased with more information, even though that information may allude to more harmful risks. For example, in a questionnaire study,[2] most parents whose anesthesiologist mentioned the risk for death indicated they were satisfied to hear about this rare risk. Many parents whose anesthesiologist did not specifically mention the risk for death indicated that it should have been mentioned.

This author's practice is to allude to the potentially harmful, yet rare, risks of anesthesia without increasing anxiety by stressing the overall safety of the procedure. One such dialog to the parents of a healthy child for elective surgery is as follows: "I don't expect any risks or complications. We can never say never, but the risk for a life-threatening complication is extremely rare. Overall the anesthesia is extremely safe, and one of us will always be there." Of course, comorbidities and type of planned procedure increase any risk. For example, the overall risk for respiratory complications is increased in children with obesity.[3] Therefore, the discussion should be appropriately tailored on a case-by-case basis.

Allowing Parents Into the Operating Room

The time of induction of anesthesia represents a frightening time for both patients and parents. Because many parents assert that they possess a right to be with their child during any and all phases of their child's hospitalization, many centers have promoted a culture of parental presence during induction of anesthesia (PPIA). The benefits of this practice are obvious as the child may be less anxious if their parent is soothing them in an unfamiliar location surrounded by strangers.

However, studies have clearly shown that parental presence does not alter the behavioral distress of the child, nor does it alter outcomes such as negative postoperative behaviors. Parental presence is not superior to preoperative sedatives[4] such as midazolam for preoperative anxiety and in certain patients may be associated with increased anxiety[5] when the child is calm and the parent is anxious. Furthermore, many parents are terrified as they observe the placing of a mask over their child's face, watching their child become limp as consciousness is lost, and the occasional episode of upper airway obstruction that may occur. Yet when queried, parents who have been with their child in the OR during induction universally feel that they have done the right thing for their child.

If a decision is made to allow a parent into the OR during induction, the anesthesiologist should fully explain the events that will occur during induction. Three major points should be addressed:

1. There should be an explanation of the nature of the procedure and the possible effects on the child (excitation, limpness, airway obstruction, etc.).
2. The parent must agree to leave immediately at any time when requested by an OR staff member.
3. The parent must agree to leave immediately once the child has lost consciousness. One of the surgical team members or another OR staff member should accompany the parent from the OR to the parents' waiting area.

Some institutions will ask a parent to sign a written agreement to these terms and a waiver of liability should the parent suffer an injury secondary to fainting or other calamity.

Procedure

An important aspect of the preoperative discussion is the procedure. Some procedures require nonroutine anesthetic management. For example, thyroid excision may require intraoperative and postoperative calcium measurements, which necessitates a large IV capable of blood draws. These decisions should be made preoperatively, ideally at the morning huddle with the surgeon.

Premedication

Why is it important to avoid a "Brutane" induction?

The most important outcomes related to preoperative distress in children are postoperative behavioral disorders. These include nightmarish sleep disturbances, feeding difficulties, apathy, withdrawal, increased level of separation anxiety, aggression toward authority, fear of subsequent medical procedures and hospital visits, and regressive behaviors such as bed wetting. Although these disturbances are primarily present within the first two postoperative weeks, in some children they may last longer. Much has been made of this issue in the recent literature, but the concept is not new. In 1953,[6] Eckenhoff demonstrated that postoperative personality changes were associated with younger age and unsatisfactory inductions. However, that study was conducted in an era that we would not recognize.

Today, many different modalities are used in an attempt to decrease fear and anxiety in patients and their families. They include preoperative informational materials that consist of discussions, tours, written literature, videotapes, and even comic books.[7] In some institutions, the Child Life department assumes an active role in development of these programs and coordinates their efforts with anesthesia personnel. In carefully performed and controlled studies, however, these aforementioned interventions do not fare much better than placebo in decreasing the incidence of postoperative behavioral disturbances. Although distraction techniques[8] are often effective for allaying anxious behavior during induction of anesthesia (Fig. 13.1), premedication with an anxiolytic drug such as midazolam is the only proven intervention to decrease these undesirable outcomes.

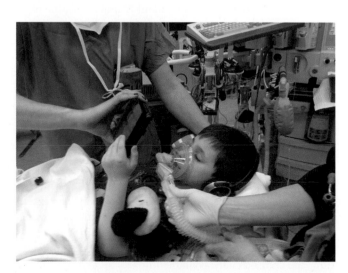

• **Fig 13.1.** Ideal induction. Child watching a movie while using noise cancelling headphones. Photo credit: Ronald S. Litman.

Allaying Parental Anxiety

One of the most important preoperative responsibilities of the pediatric anesthesiologist is to allay anxiety in the parents and other family members. During the preoperative visit the anesthesiologist, while talking to the parents, should initiate contact and communication with the child. It does not matter if the child is too young to understand, or is too premedicated to remember any events. The parents will key in on the anesthesiologist's manner and how they relate to the child. Asking the child about their interests, and performing a simple fist-bump maneuver,[1] will establish confidence and minimize parental anxiety.

Pharmacologic Preparation

Premedication of pediatric patients before induction of anesthesia can accomplish several goals, the primary one being anxiolysis, with a subsequent decrease in the incidence of postoperative negative behaviors. Other indications include preinduction of anesthesia, pain relief, drying of secretions before airway manipulation, vagolysis, and decreasing the risk for pulmonary aspiration of gastric contents. Preoperative sedation may be administered via any route, the most common being oral because the majority of children do not have an existing IV catheter. Rectal premedication is acceptable in toddlers, and in some centers the nasal route is preferred for midazolam. Few centers in the United States administer intramuscular premedication or place IV catheters preoperatively.

There are various options for treatment of preoperative anxiety. None, however, are ideal; each has drawbacks. Principles of pharmacologic treatment of patients dictate that a drug should be administered to target its specific action and not one of its side effects. In other words, anxiety should be treated with an anxiolytic (not an analgesic in the form of a lollipop); pain should be treated with an analgesic; and so on. A benzodiazepine is the best treatment for preoperative anxiety. Options include midazolam, the most commonly administered premedication, and diazepam.

Children above the age of about 9 months will benefit from preoperative anxiolysis because this is about the age of onset of separation anxiety from parents. Yet some studies report that only 25% of children less than 3 years of age are treated for preoperative anxiety.

Midazolam

Oral midazolam is the most common preoperative anxiolytic for children because it possesses most of the properties of the ideal premedication (Table 13.6). The one exception is that it usually leaves an unpleasant aftertaste when administered orally; many children will attempt to spit it out if it is not swallowed rapidly. After oral administration, the commercially available midazolam syrup is rapidly absorbed from the stomach. The absolute bioavailability of midazolam averages 36%, within a variable and large range

TABLE 13.6	Characteristics of the Ideal Premedication

- Effective and reliable anxiolysis and sedation
- Amnesia of preoperative events
- Facilitates induction of anesthesia
- Short latency period to onset of action
- Minimal respiratory and cardiovascular effects
- Easy to administer (for patient and staff)
- Short duration of action
- Lowers intraoperative anesthetic requirements
- Blocks unwanted autonomic (vagal) reflexes
- Prevents excessive airway secretions
- Does not contribute to PONV

PONV, Postoperative nausea and vomiting.

(9%–71%). This large range in bioavailability is consistent with most oral medications administered to children. In a large study, the plasma concentration/time curves of midazolam and its alpha-hydroxy metabolite were highly variable and independent of the age of the child and the dose administered. Approximately 14%[10] of children that receive oral midazolam do not demonstrate effective anxiolysis.

Caution should be observed in children who are receiving erythromycin (or its derivatives) because it can prolong the duration of action of midazolam via cytochrome P-450 inhibition. In children who are currently receiving erythromycin, the midazolam dose should be reduced by at least 50%.

Clinical sedative effects are seen within 5 to 10 minutes of oral midazolam administration and appear to peak 15 to 30 minutes after administration. By 45 minutes, its sedative effects have dissipated in most children. Pharmacodynamic studies indicate that sedation level is directly correlated with plasma concentration of midazolam. However, plasma concentrations of midazolam do not correlate with anxiety scores at the time of induction.

The sedative effect of midazolam is best described as inebriation rather than sleepiness. Therefore, after administration, children should be confined to a bed or a parent's lap and be observed at all times by medical personnel. Important cardiorespiratory side effects are not observed[11] in healthy children but may be seen[12] in children at risk for upper airway obstruction. Dysphoria may occur in some children. Anterograde amnesia is a favorable clinical effect after most doses of oral midazolam and may be responsible for the decrease in postoperative behavioral disturbances.

Most anesthesiologists find that an oral dose of 0.5 to 0.7 mg/kg results in the best clinical efficacy. However, a pharmacodynamic study[13] showed that a dose as low as 0.25 mg/kg results in reliable preoperative anxiolysis. There are no data to indicate the most appropriate maximum dose, but most anesthesiologists use between 10 and 20 mg.

Studies are conflicting, but some evidence indicates that midazolam premedication results in longer times to discharge postoperatively after surgeries of relatively short duration. Nevertheless, its preoperative advantages outweigh this disadvantage.

Nasal administration of midazolam can be accomplished in the form of nose drops or a nasal spray. The required dose (0.2–0.3 mg/kg) is lower than with oral administration and its reliability in producing anxiolysis is excellent. However, its administration is associated with an unpleasant burning of the nasal cavity. Plasma concentrations of midazolam are generally higher after nasal administration compared with the oral route. Respiratory depression has been reported on occasion after nasal administration. For these reasons, pediatric anesthesiologists tend to use the nasal route of administration infrequently.

If a child has a preexisting IV catheter, it should be used to administer midazolam. Pharmacokinetic studies indicate a beta-elimination half-life of less than 2 hours in children. The half-life of both midazolam and its major metabolite tend to increase with advancing age during childhood. The onset of IV midazolam is almost immediate and the peak sedative effect is shortly thereafter. The duration of action varies between 2 and 6 hours, with most of the sedative effect dissipating within 30 minutes of a single dose. A standard dose of IV midazolam is 0.05 mg/kg, which can then be titrated to effect, depending on the clinical situation.

Rectal administration of midazolam in doses of 0.5 to 1.0 mg/kg effectively produces preoperative anxiolysis equivalent to that seen with nasal or oral administration. There is no specific rectal formulation; the IV formulation is most often used and can be diluted with water for injection into the rectal cavity. Children less than 2 years of age are most amenable to this route of administration. The child should be placed prone and the midazolam administered via a lubricated catheter. Once administered, the buttocks should be held closed for several minutes. A small amount of air can also be injected via the catheter to help advance the remaining midazolam solution into the rectal cavity.

Clonidine

Clonidine, an alpha-2 adrenergic agonist, has been tested as an orally administered sedative premedication in children. In doses between 2 and 4 μg/kg, oral clonidine will produce adequate sedation and anxiolysis before induction of general anesthesia. A distinct advantage of clonidine is its ability to decrease intraoperative anesthetic requirements. However, its onset of action is greater than 60 minutes, so it is not be suitable for use in the ambulatory setting. Furthermore, compared with oral midazolam for children undergoing tonsillectomy, clonidine provides less anxiolysis at the time of separation of the child from the caretaker and at induction of anesthesia. An additional disadvantage of clonidine is its ability to blunt the heart rate response to administration of atropine. For these reasons, clonidine is not used routinely as a premedication in children.

Dexmedetomidine

Gaining traction in the hunt for an ideal premedication, dexmedetomidine[14] has grown in popularity because of its increased availability and decreased cost. Dexmedetomidine is a centrally acting selective alpha-2 agonist, which has an anxiolytic and sedative effect. A number of studies have shown improved sedation parental separation, and mask acceptance scores with the added benefit of lower postoperative delirium risk and increased postoperative analgesia compared with midazolam and ketamine. Dexmedetomidine is bioavailable when given orally and rectally but has a slower onset of action than midazolam with these two routes; however, benefit has been shown when given via nebulizer[15] at a dose of 2 ug/kg.

Ketamine

Ketamine can be used as a premedication in children, in both oral and intramuscular forms. At an oral dose of 5 mg/kg, it reliably produces a state of sedation and disassociation within 20 minutes of its administration. Larger doses have been associated with more reliable anxiolysis at the expense of longer postoperative times to awakening and discharge. It may be a useful substitute in children known to exhibit dysphoric reactions to midazolam, or as an additive to midazolam in children who may be in pain, or difficult to calm. Advantages of its use include a low incidence of respiratory depression and a possible decrease in intraoperative anesthetic requirements. It also possesses analgesic and amnestic properties. Disadvantages include increased oral and airway secretions, an increased incidence of postoperative emesis, and an occasional association with adverse postoperative reactions such as delirium, dysphoria, nightmares, and hallucinations. These latter effects have not been observed when ketamine has been used as a premedication. To date, studies have not demonstrated clear advantages of ketamine over midazolam as a premedication in children.

Intramuscular ketamine is used when children are unusually combative and refuse all attempts at medical attention, including refusal to ingest an oral premedication. It is most often used in developmentally delayed adolescents who are unable to understand their circumstances and will not cooperate with IV catheter placement or inhalational induction. To reduce the volume of the amount injected, the concentrated form (100 mg/mL) should be used in a dose of 2 to 6 mg/kg. Larger doses result in greater efficacy at the expense of longer times to emergence from general anesthesia, especially for surgeries of relatively short duration. We prefer a lower dose with the modest goal of obtaining sufficient sedation to facilitate IV catheter insertion or mask induction. Some anesthesiologists will include atropine in the injectate in an attempt to reduce airway secretions.

Zolpidem

Zolpidem,[16] a hypnotic and GABA agonist, is a safe and effective treatment in adults and children for insomnia. Available orally, it has been shown to be as effective as midazolam in achieving sedation for parental separation. Although not used extensively, its utility may lie in children who have previously had adverse reactions when given midazolam as a premedication.

Anticholinergics

In the past, anticholinergic drugs such as atropine and gly-copyrrolate were routinely administered to children in the preoperative period. The major indication was to prevent bradycardia associated with halothane or succinylcholine. An additional indication was to prevent vagal-induced bradycardia during airway manipulation in neonates and small infants. Because halothane and succinylcholine are no longer routinely used in children, anticholinergic premedication is no longer routinely administered. However, many pediatric anesthesiologists may include IV atropine at the beginning of induction of anesthesia when using succinylcholine for full-stomach precautions, or when anesthetizing neonates. The concept that bradycardia will result from too small a dose of atropine (<0.1 mg) in small infants has proven erroneous.[17] One disadvantage to the use of atropine is its ability to cross the blood-brain barrier and cause central anticholinergic effects. These are manifested in infants in the postoperative period as irritability and crying for up to several hours. An additional theoretical disadvantage of atropine is its propensity to lower esophageal pressure within 2 minutes of its administration. This may increase the risk for passive regurgitation of gastric contents into the esophagus.

Perioperative Antimicrobial Prophylaxis

Appropriate use of perioperative antimicrobial prophylaxis (PAP) is essential to attain optimal patient outcomes; inappropriate dose, timing, and drug choice can raise the risk for surgical site infection (SSI). Common principles of PAP are as follows:

- The optimal time for administration of preoperative doses is within 60 minutes before surgical incision to maximize tissue concentration. Some agents, such as fluoroquinolones and vancomycin, require administration over 1 or 2 hours; therefore, the administration should begin within 120 minutes before surgical incision.
- Selection of appropriate antimicrobial agents on the basis of the surgical procedure, the most common pathogens causing SSIs for a specific procedure, the safety profile, the patient's medication allergies, and published recommendations. The agent that is administrated must be safe, inexpensive, and with an antimicrobial spectrum that is appropriate and as narrow as possible.
- Dosage adjustment based on patient body weight. Obesity has been linked to an increased risk for SSI. The pharmacokinetics of drugs may be altered in obese patients, so dosage adjustment based on body weight may be warranted in these patients.
- Intraoperative redosing of prophylactic antimicrobial agents, if the duration of the procedure exceeds two half-lives of the drug or there is excessive blood loss during the procedure.
- Discontinuation of PAP within 24 hours after completion of surgery (48 hours for cardiothoracic surgery). Inappropriately prolonged duration can increase the risk

for *Clostridium difficile* infection and contribute to the development of multidrug resistant organisms.

- In clean and clean-contaminated procedures, do not administer additional prophylactic antimicrobial agent doses after the surgical incision is closed in the operating room, even in the presence of a drain.[18]
- Use of parenteral antimicrobial agents and oral antimicrobials for the reduction of the risk for SSI after colorectal procedures. For most patients, a mechanical bowel preparation combined with oral neomycin sulfate plus oral erythromycin base or with oral neomycin sulfate plus oral metronidazole should be given in addition to intravenous prophylaxis. The oral antimicrobials should be given as three doses over approximately 10 hours the afternoon and evening before the operation and after the mechanical bowel preparation.

Preoperative Preparation of the Patient

- Showering or bathing of patients with an antiseptic agent, such as chlorhexidine, the night before surgery has been shown to reduce bacterial colonization of the skin.
- Hair should not be removed at the operative site unless the presence of hair will interfere with the operation. If hair is removed, remove immediately before the operation, preferably with electric clippers. Do not use razors.

Preoperative Fasting

Traditional fasting times have been based on studies that tracked the rate of gastric emptying of substances that varied by content (Table 13.7). For example, clear liquids are rapidly emptied from the stomach, regardless of age. Children of all age groups who ingest clear fluids 2 hours before induction of anesthesia have a similar gastric volume and pH as those fasted for longer periods. Those studies formed the basis for the maxim that clear liquids are allowable until 2 hours before scheduled surgery. However, even shorter fasting intervals (e.g., 1 hour) are now acceptable on

TABLE 13.7	**CHOP Preoperative Fasting Guidelines**

- Clear liquids until 1 hour before surgery
- Breast milk until 3 hours before surgery
- Formula:
  - Infants <6 months until 4 hours before surgery
  - Infants >6 until 6 hours before surgery
  - Nonhuman milk and solids until 8 hours before surgery

Healthy patients scheduled for surgery after 13:00 h are permitted to eat one of the following before 06:00 h: a single slice of dry toast (no butter, jam, peanut butter, or cream cheese, etc.) or up to 1 cup of dry, plain Cheerios (no milk or yogurt). Having toast or plain Cheerios before 07:00 h may limit flexibility in the event of patient cancellation because anesthesia and surgery cannot in most situations start until 6 hours after eating these foods. To maximize a child's chances of safely moving ahead in the surgical schedule, we recommend no solids after midnight and clear liquids up until 2 hours before surgery.

the basis of the lack of demonstrable harm[19] from doing so, and that actual fasting times are usually significantly longer than anticipated.

Clear liquids generally consist of any fluid that can easily be seen through. Exceptions include cola soda and black coffee, which are allowable. The presence of fat in a liquid will delay gastric emptying, and the presence of pulp in a fruit juice may worsen an aspiration episode. Opinion is mixed on whether or not gelatin (Jell-O) should be considered a clear liquid.

Our current practice is that children should be encouraged to drink clear liquids 1 hour before induction of anesthesia. Advantages to this practice include a decreased risk for hypotension after induction,[20] hypoglycemia at the time of induction of anesthesia, decreased irritability of the child, and increased parental satisfaction.

There is no consensus as to the maximal amount of clear liquids that can be ingested. Some studies have used a certain amount by weight, some have limited the amount to 8 ounces, and others have allowed unlimited amounts. The amount of clear fluids ingested 2 hours before surgery does not seem to influence subsequent gastric volumes. Therefore, an unlimited amount should be allowed within the prescribed time frame.

Breast-fed infants[21] can be allowed to nurse up until 3 hours before surgery. Breast milk contains a large amount of fat and empties slower from the stomach than clear liquids. However, there is some evidence that breast milk has a faster gastric emptying time than some infant formulas. Furthermore, many breast-fed infants will not be able to drink other types of liquids from a bottle. Because pulmonary aspiration is extremely rare in healthy infants, the advantages of allowing a relatively short fasting interval for breast milk probably outweigh the disadvantages.

Infant formula is completely emptied from the stomach within 4 hours in most children. Compared with infants allowed clear liquids[22] up to 2 hours before surgery, infants who ingest formula 4 hours before surgery have similar values for gastric volume and pH. Therefore infants should be allowed to ingest formula up to 4 hours before surgery. Obesity does not adversely affect residual[23] gastric volumes or gastric pH.

There is divided opinion about the most appropriate fasting interval after gum chewing. Although this activity may comfort some adolescents and may encourage gastric emptying, some studies demonstrate increased gastric volumes after gum chewing, and some anesthesiologists fear a dangerous aspiration potential risk if the gum wad is swallowed. Overall, the benefits of preoperative gum chewing[24] up until the time of the administration of premedication most likely outweigh the risks.

Laboratory Testing

Hemoglobin determination is probably the most commonly performed preoperative blood test in children. Each center varies with regard to its requirement for preoperative hemoglobin testing in healthy children. Some children's hospitals mandate routine preoperative hemoglobin testing in infants under a certain age, usually around 2 to 4 months. Unfortunately, there are little or no data to guide current recommendations for obtaining preoperative hemoglobin values in this age range. Emerging technology such as noninvasive cooximeters[25] have been shown to reliably screen children who meet preoperative venipuncture criteria for hemoglobin assessment, thus eliminating the study altogether in patients with near normal values. Additional blood tests, radiographs, and urinalyses are not obtained in healthy pediatric patients before most surgical procedures. These studies are determined solely by the medical condition of the patient and the nature of the surgical procedure.

Collection of a preoperative type-and-screen or type-and-crossmatch to prepare for a potential blood transfusion will depend on the nature of the surgery and the expected blood loss. In general, if a blood sample is sent to the blood bank because of a possible anticipated transfusion, a hemoglobin value should also be obtained. Coagulation studies are not routinely performed except when there is a history of a bleeding disorder in the child or their family. Some surgeons will require these tests before elective tonsillectomy. A recent study suggests that using thromboelastography[26] may be more reliable than the classic coagulation profile to assess coagulation in neonates.

Perioperative Monitoring

The preoperative discussion should include whether nonstandard monitors (e.g., arterial or central line) should be placed. In some cases (e.g., scoliosis repair), these decisions are part of standard practice. In others, they may be influenced by the discussion with the surgeon at the morning huddle.

Positioning

The preoperative discussion should include strategies for nontraditional (e.g., prone) positioning and the additional safety measures that will protect against patient injury, such as padding, soft gel bolster placement, etc.

Plan

This part of the discussion should focus on the anesthetic plan, which mainly includes drug and airway choices (see Chapter 19).

Pain Control

Here the focus of the preoperative discussion centers around choices for postoperative pain control. The main decision is usually whether or not there is a role for regional analgesia (see Chapter 20) and plans for administration of opioids and nonopioid analgesics.

Postoperative Concerns

Lastly, postoperative concerns should be addressed (Chapter 31). Mitigation strategies of possible complications should be considered (e.g., patient with sleep apnea undergoing tonsillectomy).

References

1. Flick RP, Sprung J, Harrison TE, et al. Perioperative cardiac arrests in children between 1988 and 2005 at a tertiary referral center: a study of 92,881 patients. *Anesthesiology*. 2007;106(2):226–414. https://doi.org/10.1097/00000542-200702000-00009.
2. Litman RS, Perkins FM, Dawson SC. Parental knowledge and attitudes toward discussing the risk of death from anesthesia. *Anesth Analg*. 1993;77(2):256–260. https://doi.org/10.1213/00000539-199308000-00008.
3. Tait AR, Voepel-Lewis T, Burke C, Kostrzewa A, Lewis I. Incidence and risk factors for perioperative adverse respiratory events in children who are obese. *Anesthesiology*. 2008;108(3):375–380. https://doi.org/10.1097/ALN.0b013e318164ca9b.
4. Kain ZN, Mayes LC, Wang SM, Caramico LA, Krivutza DM, Hofstadter MB. Parental presence and a sedative premedicant for children undergoing surgery: a hierarchical study. *Anesthesiology*. 2000;92(4):939–946. https://doi.org/10.1097/00000542-200004000-00010.
5. Kain ZN, Caldwell-Andrews AA, Maranets I, Nelson W, Mayes LC. Predicting which child-parent pair will benefit from parental presence during induction of anesthesia: a decision-making approach. *Anesth Analg*. 2006;102(1):81–84. https://doi.org/10.1213/01.ANE.0000181100.27931.A1.
6. Eckenhoff JE. Relationship of anesthesia to postoperative personality changes in children. *AMA Am J Dis Child*. 1953;86(5):587–591. https://doi.org/10.1001/archpedi.1953.02050080600004.
7. Kassai B, Rabilloud M, Dantony E, et al. Introduction of a paediatric anaesthesia comic information leaflet reduced preoperative anxiety in children. *Br J Anaesth*. 2016;117(1):95–102. https://doi.org/10.1093/bja/aew154.
8. Marechal C, Berthiller J, Tosetti S, et al. Children and parental anxiolysis in paediatric ambulatory surgery: a randomized controlled study comparing 0.3 mg kg−1 midazolam to tablet computer based interactive distraction. *Br J Anaesth*. 2017;118(2):247–253. https://doi.org/10.1093/bja/aew436.
9. Fleur N. In The World Of Global Gestures, The Fist Bump Stands Alone. Goats and Soda (website). July 19, 2014. Accessed 20.07.21. https://www.npr.org/sections/goatsandsoda/2014/07/19/331809186/in-the-world-of-global-gestures-the-fist-bump-stands-alone.
10. Kain ZN, MacLaren J, McClain BC, et al. Effects of age and emotionality on the effectiveness of midazolam administered preoperatively to children. *Anesthesiology*. 2007;107(4):545–552. https://doi.org/10.1097/01.anes.0000281895.81168.c3.
11. von Ungern-Sternberg BS, Erb TO, Habre W, Sly PD, Hantos Z. The impact of oral premedication with midazolam on respiratory function in children. *Anesth Analg*. 2009;108(6):1771–1776. https://doi.org/10.1213/ane.0b013e3181a324c3.
12. Litman RS. Airway obstruction after oral midazolam. *Anesthesiology*. 1996;85(5):1217–1218. https://doi.org/10.1097/00000542-199611000-00049.
13. Coté CJ, Cohen IT, Suresh S, et al. A comparison of three doses of a commercially prepared oral midazolam syrup in children. *Anesth Analg*. 2002;94(1):37–43. https://doi.org/10.1097/00000539-200201000-00007.
14. Pasin L, Febres D, Testa V, et al. Dexmedetomidine vs midazolam as preanesthetic medication in children: a meta-analysis of randomized controlled trials. *Pediatr Anaesth*. 2015;25(5):468–476. https://doi.org/10.1111/pan.12587.
15. Abdel-Ghaffar HS, Kamal SM, El Sherif FA, Mohamed SA. Comparison of nebulised dexmedetomidine, ketamine, or midazolam for premedication in preschool children undergoing bone marrow biopsy. *Br J Anaesth*. 2018;121(2):445–452. https://doi.org/10.1016/j.bja.2018.03.039.
16. Hanna AH, Ramsingh D, Sullivan-Lewis W, et al. A comparison of midazolam and zolpidem as oral premedication in children, a prospective randomized double-blinded clinical trial. *Paediatr Anaesth*. 2018;28(12):1109–1115. https://doi.org/10.1111/pan.13501.
17. Eisa L, Passi Y, Lerman J, Raczka M, Heard C. Do small doses of atropine (<0.1 mg) cause bradycardia in young children? *Arch Dis Child*. 2015;100(7):684–688. https://doi.org/10.1136/archdischild-2014-307868.
18. Berríos-Torres SI, Umscheid CA, Bratzler DW, et al. Centers for Disease Control and Prevention Guideline for the Prevention of Surgical Site Infection, 2017 [published correction appears in JAMA Surg. 2017 Aug 1;152(8):803]. *JAMA Surg*. 2017;152(8):784–791. https://doi.org/10.1001/jamasurg.2017.0904.
19. Isserman R, Elliott E, Subramanyam R, et al. Quality improvement project to reduce pediatric clear liquid fasting times prior to anesthesia. *Paediatr Anaesthesia*. 2019;29(7):698–704. https://doi.org/10.1111/pan.13661.
20. Simpao AF, Wu L, Nelson O, et al. Preoperative fluid fasting times and postinduction low blood pressure in children: a retrospective analysis. *Anesthesiology*. 2020;133(3):523–533. https://doi.org/10.1097/ALN.0000000000003343.
21. Litman RS, Wu CL, Quinlivan JK. Gastric volume and pH in infants fed clear liquids and breast milk prior to surgery. *Anesth Analg*. 1994;79(3):482–485. https://doi.org/10.1213/00000539-199409000-00013.
22. Greeley WJ, Cook-Sather SD, Harris KA, Chiavacci R, Gallagher PR, Schreiner MS. A liberalized fasting guideline for formula-fed infants does not increase average gastric fluid volume before elective surgery. *Anesth Analg*. 2003;96(4):965–969. https://doi.org/10.1213/01.ane.0000055807.31411.8b.
23. Cook-Sather SD, Gallagher PR, Kruge LE, et al. Overweight/obesity and gastric fluid characteristics in pediatric day surgery: implications for fasting guidelines and pulmonary aspiration risk. *Anesth Analg*. 2009;109(3):727–736. https://doi.org/10.1213/ane.0b013e3181b085ff.
24. Poulton TJ. Gum chewing during pre-anesthetic fasting. *Paediatr Anaesth*. 2012;22(3):288–296. https://doi.org/10.1111/j.1460-9592.2011.03751.x.
25. Zeng R, Svensen CH, Li H, et al. Can noninvasive hemoglobin measurement reduce the need for preoperative venipuncture in pediatric outpatient surgery? *Paediatr Anaesth*. 2017;27(11):1131–1135. https://doi.org/10.1111/pan.13229.
26. Kettner SC, Pollak A, Zimpfer M, et al. Heparinase-modified thrombelastography in term and preterm neonates. *Anesth Analg*. 2004;98(6):1650–1652. https://doi.org/10.1213/01.ane.0000115149.25496.dd.

Suggested Readings

Bratzler DW, Dellinger EP, Olsen KM, et al. Clinical practice guidelines for antimicrobial prophylaxis in surgery. *Am J Health Syst Pharm*. 2013;70(3):195–283. https://doi.org/10.2146/ajhp120568.

Colletti A. Observe Standard NPO Times for Pediatric Patients Receiving Post-Pyloric Feeds. SPA Newsletter Website. Fall 2019. Accessed 20.07.21. https://www2.pedsanesthesia.org/newsletters/2019fall/procon%20colletti.html.

Elliott L, Isserman RS, Fiadjoe JE. An Argument Against Fasting. SPA Newsletter. Fall 2019. Accessed 20.07.21. https://www2.pedsanesthesia.org/newsletters/2019fall/procon%20elliott.html.

Heikal S, Stuart G. Anxiolytic premedication for children. *BJA Educ*. 2020;20(7):220–225. https://doi.org/10.1016/j.bjae.2020.02.006.

14

Fluid and Blood Administration

DEBORAH SESOK-PIZZINI, GRACE E. LINDER, AND RONALD S. LITMAN

A variety of intravenous fluid and blood products are administered to children in the perioperative period. Indications include preoperative deficit replacement, ongoing maintenance requirements, fluid loss replacement, and treatment of anemia and hypovolemia. This chapter describes the use of these fluid and blood products in pediatric patients in the perioperative period.

Normal Fluid Requirements

Water Requirements

Water maintenance rates in children are based on studies that demonstrated a direct association between metabolic rate and water requirements. In general, water requirements on a per-kilogram basis increase with decreasing size of the child. This is secondary to the higher metabolic rate with decreasing size and the relatively greater evaporative loss from body surfaces in smaller children because of a higher ratio of body surface area to weight. Prematurely born infants have an even greater rate of evaporative loss because of thinner, more permeable, vascularized skin. In general, the amount of evaporative water loss per kilogram is inversely proportional to the gestational age.

In a very influential paper[1] published in 1957, Holliday and Segar developed an easily remembered formula for calculating caloric requirements of the "average" hospitalized child (>2 weeks of age) based on bodyweight. They also demonstrated that the water requirement in milliliters was equal to the total energy expended (i.e., 1000 mL of water is required for every 1000 kcal expended). Thus the formula for caloric requirements can easily be used to calculate daily water requirements using the "4–2–1 rule" (Table 14.1).

Subsequent studies during pediatric surgery demonstrated that intraoperative caloric and fluid requirements are less than those calculated by Holliday and Segar. Nevertheless, for the vast majority of healthy children undergoing surgery, these formulae will consistently prevent perioperative fluid and electrolyte abnormalities, and thus, are still in use today.

Electrolyte Requirements

For each 100 calories metabolized in 24 hours, the average child requires 3 mEq of sodium, 2 mEq of potassium, and 2 mEq of chloride. These recommendations are based on the approximate electrolyte concentration of human breast and cow's milk, and the resulting normal urine osmolality after milk ingestion. In most otherwise healthy hospitalized children, these electrolyte requirements will be met by administering a solution of 0.2% sodium chloride with 20 mEq of added KCl per liter at the normal maintenance rate (Table 14.2).

In the perioperative period, it is necessary to replace surgical losses in addition to providing maintenance fluids and electrolytes. Therefore we commonly use solutions that contain a greater percentage of sodium. This better approximates the fluid that is associated with losses during surgery and avoids hyponatremia that would result from large infusions of a hypotonic fluid, especially in the face of an increase in antidiuretic hormone release caused by the stress of surgery. Lactated Ringer's (LR) solution (or similar) meets these needs for the majority of surgical procedures in children. Normal saline contains 154 mEq/L of sodium and is preferred when replacing large amounts of isotonic fluid because LR is somewhat hypotonic.

Intraoperative Fluid Requirements

Intraoperative fluid administration is required to meet the body's needs for ongoing losses secondary to metabolism and water and electrolyte losses caused by medical and/or surgical conditions. Additional fluid deficits are incurred

TABLE 14.1	Maintenance Fluid Requirements in Children: The "4 2 1 Rule"
Bodyweight (kg)	Maintenance Rate
0–10	4 mL/kg/h
11–20	40 mL+2 mL/kg/h for each kg over 10 kg
21–70	60 mL + l mL/kg/h for each kg over 20 kg

TABLE 14.2	Electrolytes Contained in 1 Liter of Lactated Ringers Solution^	
Electrolyte	**Amount**	
Sodium	130 mEq	
Potassium	4 mEq	
Calcium	3 mEq	
Chloride	109 mEq	
Lactate	28 mEq	

^Not including ions for adjusting pH

during preoperative fasting and intraoperative evaporation and third-spacing.

Replacement of Preoperative Deficit

Normally, children presenting for elective surgical procedures have incurred a fluid deficit during the preoperative fasting interval. Although ingestion of clear liquids is often encouraged up to 1 or 2 hours before the scheduled procedure time, depending on institutional guidelines, many children have fasted for a longer time. Many pediatric anesthesiologists feel that this deficit should be replaced with isotonic fluid to compensate for anesthetic-induced vasodilatation and unexpected intraoperative or postoperative fluid and blood loss. Preoperative fasting deficits are calculated by multiplying the hourly maintenance rate by the number of hours the child fasted. Traditionally, 50% of this deficit is replaced in the first hour of intravenous hydration and 25% in each of the next 2 hours. For relatively short, minor surgeries, a volume of 4 mL/kg of isotonic solution has been suggested as an appropriate replacement volume that covers the preoperative deficit and intraoperative maintenance requirements.

Children presenting for emergency surgery may have increased fluid losses secondary to fever, vomiting, edema, and blood loss. Therefore these children should receive earlier and more aggressive volume replacement, until establishment of normal urine production (1–2 mL/kg/h). Keep in mind that aggressive fluid deficit replacement is associated with a decrease in core body temperature.

Glucose Administration

Because of the normal hyperglycemic response to surgery, healthy infants over about 1 month of age do not require addition of glucose to intraoperative maintenance fluids. Children at risk for intraoperative hypoglycemia include[2] those less than a month of age, weight for age <5th percentile, ASA status ≥III, having a gastric or jejunal tube, poor feeding, and abdominal surgery. These children should have intermittent glucose checks during anesthesia. A 2% dextrose solution[3] appears to provide the best balance between the risk for hypoglycemia and hyperglycemia, which may cause an osmotic diuresis.

Hospitalized neonates, especially those born prematurely, will often be receiving increased amounts of glucose to compensate for limited glycogen reserves. Because most of these patients will demonstrate a hyperglycemic response to the stress of surgery, this author's practice is to initially administer the same solution at half its original rate, check blood glucose values at least hourly, and readjust the rate if necessary. Normal saline or LR solution is then used to replace any deficit or intraoperative isotonic fluid loss.

Children who received clonidine premedication or neuraxial blockade before the surgical incision may not develop the intraoperative hyperglycemic stress response. These patients should receive a maintenance fluid that contains dextrose or should undergo intraoperative blood glucose monitoring at regular intervals.

Replacement of Intraoperative Fluid Losses

In addition to insensible losses and ongoing metabolic needs, fluid is lost intraoperatively as a result of evaporation from exposed tissues, "third-spacing," and surgical blood loss. Third-spacing is the transfer of relatively isotonic fluid from the extracellular volume space to a nonfunctional interstitial compartment, and is triggered by surgical trauma, infection, burns, and other mechanisms of tissue injury. The amount of volume lost to the third space can be estimated based on experience with the particular type of surgery, observation of the surgical field, and the clinical response to volume replacement.

Insensible fluid losses during minor procedures will average less than 3 mL/kg/h. This value will increase based on the location and extent of the surgical injury. For example, a neonate undergoing an exploratory laparotomy for necrotizing enterocolitis and gangrenous bowel may require 50 to 100 mL/kg/h to maintain euvolemia. Most thoracic and neurosurgical procedures require 5 to 10 mL/kg/h.

Intraoperative fluid losses are replaced with an isotonic, nonglucose-containing solution such as LR, NS, or Plasmalyte. When using crystalloid to replace surgical blood loss, three times as much crystalloid solution should be administered as the amount of estimated blood lost. End points of intraoperative volume replacement include an appropriate blood pressure and heart rate, and adequate tissue perfusion as evidenced by a urine output near or above 1 mL/kg/h.

Massive amounts of replacement with each solution carry unique disadvantages. Because of its slightly hypotonic nature, large amounts of administered LR solution are associated with a decreased serum osmolality and development of edema. Large amounts of administered NS are associated with development of dilutional or hyperchloremic acidosis.

Postoperative Intravenous Fluids

In the 1980s it was recognized that some healthy children developed life-threatening hyponatremia after otherwise uncomplicated surgery. Much has been written on this topic with ample warnings about use of hypotonic solutions when not indicated. Unless specifically indicated, hypotonic solutions should not be used for maintenance fluids in children after surgery.

Blood Products

The most commonly administered blood products in the perioperative setting are packed red blood cells (RBCs), fresh frozen plasma (FFP), platelets, and cryoprecipitate. Fresh whole blood[4] may also be used in special circumstances such as children less than 2 years old undergoing complex cardiothoracic surgery and children undergoing craniofacial surgery. For each blood product, a standard 150 to 260-micron blood filter is used for administration.

Pretransfusion Testing

Before a surgical procedure where blood loss is anticipated, a type-and-crossmatch will ensure compatible blood is available for the patient. Once a patient's ABO (Rh) type is confirmed, an antibody screen will detect clinically significant antibodies that are likely to cause hemolysis. In the event that one of these antibodies (e.g., Rh, Duffy, Kell, Kidd) is confirmed, a donor red blood cell unit is prepared that is negative for that particular antigen. RBCs and platelets require specific ABO and Rh compatible blood (Table 14.3). FFP requires ABO type compatible blood (Table 14.4). In situations where a patient does not have a current or previous red blood cell antibody, an electronic or computer crossmatch can be used to detect ABO incompatibility.

Cryoprecipitate and platelets may be given out of type, but platelet transfusions require special precautions for smaller volume patients where hemolysis because of incompatible anti-A or anti-B is more likely. In these cases, blood banks may volume-reduce or wash platelets when ABO type-specific or type-compatible platelets are unavailable or they may identify donors with low-titer anti-A and anti-B antibodies when minor ABO-incompatible platelets must

TABLE 14.3	ABO Blood Group Antigens and Antibodies	
Blood Group	ABO Antigen on RBC	ABO Antibody in Plasma
A	A	Anti-B
B	B	Anti-A
O	None	Anti-A, Anti-B, Anti-AB
AB	A,B	None

TABLE 14.4	Selection of FFP and Platelets by ABO Group	
Recipient ABO	First Choice	Second Choice
A	A	AB
B	B	AB
AB	AB	None
O	O	A, B, AB

be used. Also, platelets should be Rh-type compatible especially for Rh-negative females of childbearing age to prevent anti-D formation. The universal donor for red blood cells is O and the universal donor for plasma is AB. Platelets are considered a plasma product.

Fresh Whole Blood

Fresh whole blood (FWB) is available on a limited basis depending on the blood center. The definition of "freshness" is undetermined, but one study[4] showed that whole blood <48 hours old may provide improved hemostasis and donor limitation for pediatric cardiothoracic patients compared with separate blood components. One recent study[5] examined the use of O low titer anti-A and anti-B uncrossmatched FWB in injured children with hemorrhagic shock. Similar to other blood products, FWB must undergo standard infectious disease testing before administration. FWB may be manufactured as a leuko-reduced product, but if not, CMV-seronegative FWB should be considered for low birth weight premature infants.

Red Blood Cells

Because whole blood is transfused only under special circumstances, RBC concentrates are almost exclusively administered to correct anemia in pediatric surgical patients. In general, there are few differences between children and adults with regard to the indications for perioperative red blood cell (RBC) administration (Table 14.5).

The primary objective of red cell administration is to enhance oxygen delivery to the peripheral circulation. A secondary objective is to maintain the circulating blood

TABLE 14.5	Guidelines for Perioperative Red Blood Cell Transfusion in Children

- Emergency surgical procedure in a child with preoperative anemia (hemoglobin <7 g/dL)
- Hemoglobin <8 g/dL in children with signs and symptoms of anemia, or while on chemotherapy/radiotherapy
- acute blood loss with signs of hypovolemia
- Hemoglobin <10 g/dL in children with pulmonary disease

Based on recommendations from Roseff SD, Luban NL, Manno CS: Guidelines for assessing appropriateness of pediatric transfusion, Transfusion 42:1398-1413, 2002.

volume. Preoperative red cell transfusion before an elective surgical procedure is rarely justified, unless the patient is anemic and symptomatic. Although the incidence of postoperative apnea in premature infants is decreased when the hemoglobin level is >10 g/dL, red cell transfusion is not indicated with mild anemia (7–10 g/dL), provided adequate postoperative monitoring in an intensive care setting is available.

In children without preoperative anemia, intraoperative red cell administration is often based on attainment of the maximum allowable blood loss (MABL) (Table 14.6):

$$MABL = Weight(kg) \times Estimated\ Blood\ Volume(EBV)$$
$$\times (H_o - H_1) / H_{AV}$$

where H_o is the child's original hematocrit, H_1 is the lowest acceptable hematocrit, and HAV is the average hematocrit, $(H_o + H_1)/2$[6].

The lowest acceptable hematocrit, H_1, is determined before the onset of the surgical procedure and is based on the health of the child and the clinical situation. The estimated blood volume is calculated based on the patient's age and size (see Table 14.6).

RBCs should be transfused with an end-point of achieving an improvement of clinical symptoms. Most preparations of red cell concentrates have a hematocrit between 55% and 75%, depending on the storage solution. Washed or plasma-reduced RBCs will have a hematocrit of <80%. On average, 10 mL/kg of packed RBCs will increase the hemoglobin by 2 to 3 g/dL. Most pediatric transfusions range between 10 and 15 mL/kg. Larger volumes may be required during periods of hypovolemic shock, or when acute blood loss is >15% total blood volume.

TABLE 14.6	Estimated Pediatric Blood Volume (EBV)

Age	EBV (mL/kg)
Premature infant	90–100
Full-term newborn	80–90
Infant 3 months to 1 year	70–80
Child >1 year of age	70

There are several types of preservative solutions that will prolong the shelf life of RBCs to 42 days. Each contains a variable amount of adenine, citrate, dextrose, and phosphate. Some contain mannitol. As the duration of blood storage increases, the amount of extracellular potassium increases,[7] the pH decreases, and red cell levels of 2, 3-diphosphoglycerate decrease. Prior concerns for hepatic toxicity with adenine and renal toxicity with mannitol are based on animal studies. The literature is inconclusive for the adverse effects of additive solutions with regard to large volume transfusions in humans, and many hospitals report safe blood transfusions with additive solutions for large volume transfusions including ECMO patients. For most children with simple small volume transfusions (<15 mL/kg), many hospitals are routinely using additive solutions without the need for additional washing. In cases where more massive transfusion is anticipated or rapid transfusion is administered through a central line, fresh RBC concentrates are often used to mitigate the risk for a hyperkalemic reaction. Institutional protocols for "freshness" vary from 5 to 21 days old. Because blood banking procedures differ between institutions, anesthesiologists should be familiar with their hospital's specific storage procedures for children (Table 14.7).

Massive Transfusion

Massive transfusion is defined as the acute administration of one or more blood volumes. Complications of massive transfusion in pediatric patients include dilutional thrombocytopenia,[8] disseminated intravascular coagulation (DIC), hypothermia, metabolic acidosis, hyperkalemia, hyperglycemia, hypocalcemia, and volume overload.

In the emergency transfusion situation, uncrossmatched type O red blood cells may be administered before a completed type-and-crossmatch. Because O red blood cells are a scarce resource, patients may be safely switched back to their own blood type providing there is no evidence of donor antibodies in the patient's plasma or on the patient's red blood cells. A direct antiglobulin test (DAT) will help determine whether antibody is present on the patient's cells.

TABLE 14.7	Storage and Shelf Life of Blood Components

Component	Storage Temperature	Shelf Life
Whole blood	1–6° C	35 days
RBCs	1–6° C	35–42 days
Platelets	20–24° C	5 days
FFP	< −18° C	1 year
Cryoprecipitate	< −18° C	1 year

FFP, Fresh frozen plasma; RBC, red blood cell.

Although type-specific blood is preferred, because of ABO shortages or preference for direct donation with a compatible but not type specific donor, O red blood cells may be used. Also, O red blood cells may be used for neonates with evidence of hemolytic disease of the newborn or with maternal anti-A, anti-B, or anti-A,B antibodies present. Even with residual plasma in anticoagulated blood with preservatives, washing is often not indicated when O red blood cells are used, especially in emergent situations. This is because of the very low residual titer of any anti-A and anti-B in the plasma when red blood cells are stored in additive solutions.

Fresh Frozen Plasma

Fresh frozen plasma (FFP) is administered to correct bleeding secondary to a documented or presumed coagulation factor deficiency. A prothrombin test (PT) or activated partial thromboplastin time (aPTT) may indicate the need for FFP, but often the turnaround time for these tests is inadequate for decision making in the OR. Some hospitals have implemented thromboelastography (TEG) testing[9] as a more rapid point-of-care test to determine coagulopathy in the surgical patient. TEG may be particularly useful for cardiothoracic or liver transplant cases to predict bleeding. In the absence of TEG, the anesthesiologist relies on clinical evidence of bleeding and estimated blood loss as a high probability of a coagulopathy. The most common perioperative cause of coagulation factor deficiency is dilutional, as a result of massive transfusion of crystalloid or RBCs, especially in neonates. FFP is not indicated for volume expansion without coagulation abnormalities. References values for TEG in pediatric patients have been published.[10]

The dose of FFP will depend on the desired correction of coagulation factor activity. In general, the minimum blood activity level of coagulation factors for physiologic hemostatic effects is approximately 25% of the normal level. The appropriate dose of FFP that will raise the level of coagulation factors to 25% can be determined by first calculating the plasma volume:

$$Plasma\ Volume \left(\frac{ml}{kg} \right) = \left[\begin{array}{c} Total\ blood\ volume \left(\frac{ml}{kg} \right) \\ \times (1 - hematocrit) \end{array} \right]$$

Therefore for an average child with a hematocrit of 43%:

$$Plasma\ Volume \left(\frac{ml}{kg} \right) = \left[70 \left(\frac{ml}{kg} \right) \times (1 - 0.43) \right]$$
$$= 40 \left(\frac{ml}{kg} \right)$$

If we assume that the administered FFP contains 100% level of coagulation factors, then the volume administered to achieve 25% activity will be 25% × 40 mL/kg (=10 mL/kg). One unit of FFP contains approximately 200 to 250 mL, so a 20 kg child will require 200 mL (1 unit)

of FFP. Alternatively, a general rule of thumb is that 10 to 15 mL/kg will raise factor levels 15% to 20%.

FFP contains a relatively large amount of citrate, so if administered rapidly (>1 mL/kg/min) it may cause a transient decrease in ionized calcium and decrease in arterial blood pressure.[11] In most children, the hypocalcemia is transient because the citrate is metabolized rapidly. However, children with a limited ability to mobilize calcium (e.g., neonates) or a decreased ability to metabolize citrate (e.g., liver failure) may require exogenous calcium administration. FFP is not subjected to inactivation of infectious pathogens, and thus, may transmit infectious diseases. A solvent detergent-treated plasma product called *Octaplas* is currently approved for replacement of multiple coagulation factors in patients with acquired deficiencies because of liver disease, or who are undergoing cardiac surgery or liver transplantation. Octaplas is manufactured from pooled plasma in a process that inactivates enveloped viruses. It is currently not FDA approved for pediatric use, but postmarketing studies are ongoing.

Platelets

Intraoperative thrombocytopenia is usually dilutional as a result of massive blood transfusion but may result from an underlying illness such as necrotizing enterocolitis, malignancy, or DIC. General indications for the administration of platelets to children include a platelet count $<50\times10^9$/L in a patient undergoing an invasive procedure or minor surgery, or $<100\times10^9$/L in a patient undergoing major surgery. Critically ill premature infants at risk for intracranial hemorrhage should receive platelets when the platelet count is $<100\times10^9$/L, even in the absence of active bleeding. Approximately 5 to 10 mL/kg of platelets from either a random donor or an apheresis unit should result in a rise in platelet count of 30 to 50 x 10^9/L. Patients approaching an adult body weight of 50 kg may only require one unit of apheresis platelets to achieve a therapeutic rise in platelets. Less of an increase in the platelet count will be observed in the presence of sepsis or a consumptive coagulopathy or in patients with previously formed HLA antibodies against HLA Class I antigens present on the platelet surface. If immunologic refractoriness is suspected, communication with the blood bank is needed to confirm HLA antibodies, and assess the need for HLA-matched or crossmatched platelet donors.

Cryoprecipitate

Also sometimes called *cryoprecipitated antihemophilic factor*, cryoprecipitate is a source of fibrinogen, factor VIII, factor XIII, and vWF. When a concentrated source of fibrinogen is required for patients unable to tolerate large volumes of fluid, such as patients in liver failure, cryoprecipitate is the product of choice. Doses of 1 to 2 units/10 kg will increase a child's fibrinogen level to 60 to 100 mg/dL. In infants, a dose of one unit is sufficient for hemostasis. The dose may also be calculated from the difference between the current and desired concentration of fibrinogen using the following calculations:

$$Plasma\ volume = (1 - hematocrit) \times 0.7 \left(\frac{dL}{kg}\right) \times weight(kg)$$

$$Dose(Units) =$$
$$\left[Desired\ fibrinogen\ increment \left(\frac{mg}{dL}\right) \times Plasma\ volume \right]$$

Factor VIII deficiency and von Willebrand disease can be treated with cryoprecipitate but recombinant and virus-inactivated products are preferred. Cryoprecipitate may also be a source for fibrin glue along with bovine thrombin, to achieve rapid topical hemostasis. However, fibrin sealants, composed of virus-inactivated fibrinogen, may be a preferred commercial source because of greater bonding, more rapid preparation time, and a safer virus-inactivated profile.

Leukoreduction

Nearly all blood centers in the United States perform prestorage leukoreduction on all cellular blood components. The goals of leukoreduction are to remove white blood cell (WBC) associated infectious agents (cytomegalovirus) and to protect against human leukocyte antigen (HLA) sensitization. It may also decrease the incidence of febrile nonhemolytic transfusion reactions, and alter the immunomodulation that occurs after transfusion of cellular blood components. Leukoreduction removes approximately 99% of WBCs; fewer than 5×10^6 WBCs should remain in the blood product. Leuko-reduced RBCs and platelets are considered "CMV-safe" and may be used in some hospitals for a substitute for CMV seronegative products.

Irradiation

Gamma irradiation of cellular blood components destroys the proliferative capacity of WBCs and is used to prevent transfusion-associated graft vs. host disease (TAGVHD). TAGVHD occurs when transfused lymphocytes engraft and proliferate in the transfusion recipient's bone marrow, and is fatal in over 95% of patients.

Irradiated blood should be administered to immunocompromised children and those with normal immunity who share an HLA haplotype with the donor (i.e., first- or second-degree relatives), which would enable the donor lymphocytes to engraft without being initially destroyed by the recipient. Determination of irradiation is usually institution-specific with regard to the types of patients that are considered immunocompromised (Table 14.8).

The expiration date of irradiated red blood cells is decreased to 28 days postirradiation, if the available shelf

TABLE 14.8	Criteria for Using Irradiated Blood Products

- Patient with decreased cellular immunity
- Premature infant
- Fetus receiving transfusion in utero
- Bone marrow transplant recipient
- Critically ill child
- Patient receiving chemotherapy that results in severe immune suppression
- Donated blood from a first- or second-degree relative

life was greater than 28 days. This is because of concerns of irradiation effects on erythrocyte membranes accelerating storage abnormalities. When red cell concentrates are irradiated, the potassium level rises rapidly after 3 days of storage, and can reach 7 mEq/L after 2 weeks of storage. Therefore hyperkalemia may occur during rapid and/or massive transfusion of irradiated blood, and when transfusing premature infants or children with renal failure. Some hospitals may even wash irradiated blood after a certain number of days in order to decrease the incidence of hyperkalemic reactions.

Photoinactivation

Pathogen reduction and inactivation methods are available now for platelets (Intercept) and are under investigation for red blood cells (Mirasol). Intercept platelets are manufactured using amotosalen (a psoralen derivative) and ultraviolet light in a manufacturing process that inactivates bacteria, viruses, and parasites. On-going post marketing studies are evaluating the safety of amotosalen-treated platelets in pediatrics, specifically evaluating the frequency of assisted mechanical ventilation required to treat severe pulmonary complications in hematology-oncology patients (PIPER Surveillance Study).

Complications of Blood Product Administration

Complications from blood product administration range from common mild allergic and febrile reactions, to rare fatal hemolytic reactions. Although the general public is usually most concerned about the risk for viral infection from transfusions, the leading causes of transfusion-related mortality include acute hemolysis because of ABO incompatibility (usually a result of human error), bacterial contamination, and transfusion-related acute lung injury (TRALI).

Transfusion Reactions

Transfusion reaction symptoms vary and may include hives, fever, chills, hypertension, hypotension, tachycardia, headache, pain, coughing, renal failure, DIC, shock, or respiratory distress. In general, blood banking standards recommend that transfusions be immediately discontinued for anything other than a mild allergic transfusion reaction of hives only. Once a reaction occurs, the patient's blood should be submitted to the blood bank for a clerical check and evaluation of hemolysis or icterus in the patient's plasma. The blood bank will also seek the presence of RBC antibodies through a Direct Antiglobulin Test (DAT). If these results are positive, further testing may be recommended before a future transfusion.

ABO Incompatibility

Despite all safeguards, human error accounts for an ABO-incompatible transfusion in up to 1 in 12,000 to 38,000 transfusions and causes approximately 1 in 600,000 to 1.5 million deaths per year in the United States. In fact, ABO errors cause more transfusion-related deaths than transmission of HIV from blood products. Infants and children are at particular risk for these types of errors because of special circumstances that may create labeling errors, such as the confusion of maternal and baby (or placental) samples, multiple births, and failure to apply or remove wristbands in children who are too young to identify themselves. Many centers are now requiring two separate sample specimens or a barrier method such as barcoding before releasing type-specific blood. A variety of methods to prevent these human errors are being investigated, including strategies to convert type A or B donor blood into type O blood by altering the molecular structure of the red blood cells. However, universal type-converted blood or artificial blood is not presently available and we must rely on blood bank safety checks and proper patient identification in order to prevent ABO transfusion errors. Patients experiencing an acute hemolytic reaction are at risk for DIC, shock, and acute renal failure.

Bacterial Contamination

Because of the improved detection[12] of viral agents in the blood supply, the risk for infection from bacterial contamination may now exceed that from viral agents. Bacterial infection is most commonly seen after platelet transfusion compared with red blood cells or FFP because of storage at room temperature. Recipients of components containing gram-negative organisms are at highest risk for transfusion-related death. Currently all platelet products are tested for bacteria using a culture method or an FDA-approved sensitive method for bacterial detection. This regulation has helped reduce the incidence of septic reactions and deaths resulting from contaminated platelet products. More recently proposed FDA guidance will require transfusion services to use either platelets manufactured using an FDA-approved pathogen reduction technology (Intercept) or perform a rapid bacterial test, Platelet PGD Test, before transfusion on day 4 and day 5 of platelet shelf life or perform a secondary culture.

Pathogen-Reduction Technologies

Blood product safety has significantly improved in recent years because of enhancements in blood donor screening, infectious disease testing, and blood product manufacturing. Although the residual risk for viral transmission is low, transfusion-transmitted bacterial infection remains a persistent problem.[13] Platelet products are particularly susceptible to bacterial contamination, as they are stored at 22°C. One in every 5000 platelets units is contaminated by bacteria not detected by current screening methods, and approximately 10% of transfusion-related deaths in the United States are attributable to bacterially contaminated platelets.[14, 15]

Pathogen-reduction technologies have been developed to further reduce rates of transfusion-transmitted bacterial sepsis and to mitigate risk for new and emerging infectious diseases. Current pathogen-reduction techniques use either solvent/detergent or photochemical methods to broadly inactivate bacterial, viral, and protozoal agents. Solvent/detergent methods disrupt lipid membranes and are approved for treatment of acellular blood products including plasma (e.g., Octaplas) and coagulation factors. Photochemical technologies prevent replication of nucleic acids, and, unlike solvent/detergent methods, are not cytocidal, allowing for their use in cellular blood products.

The Food and Drug Administration approved the first pathogen-reduced (PR) photochemical platelet product (INTERCEPT, Cerus) in 2014. The INTERCEPT blood system uses amotosalen, a synthetic psoralen, which binds to RNA and DNA and, upon exposure to ultraviolet A light, forms irreversible cross-links, preventing protein synthesis and cell replication (Fig. 14.1). INTERCEPT platelets have been in use in Europe for over a decade, and in countries that have adopted PR platelet inventories, there have been no reported septic transfusion reactions with > 600,000 INTERCEPT platelet transfusions.[15] The Mirasol system (TerumoBCT) uses riboflavin in combination with ultraviolet B-light to induce nucleic acid damage and pathogen reduction. The Mirasol system is currently under investigation in a Phase III clinical trial in the United States, though it is approved for use in both platelet and whole blood products in Europe.

Clinical trial data and meta-analyses in adult patients support that pathogen-reduced platelets demonstrate equal hemostatic efficacy compared with conventional platelets. Transfusion of PR platelets is, however, associated with reduced posttransfusion platelet recovery and survival, leading to increased platelet utilization and decreased intervals between platelet transfusions.[16] There are limited data on the use of PR platelets in pediatric populations. PR platelets are contraindicated for neonatal patients receiving phototherapy with devices that use a peak energy wavelength of less than 425 nm because of the concern for erythema secondary to possible activation of residual psoralen by the UV lights. Several observational studies that included pediatric patients showed similar rates of transfusion reactions between PR and conventional platelets with an acceptable safety profile

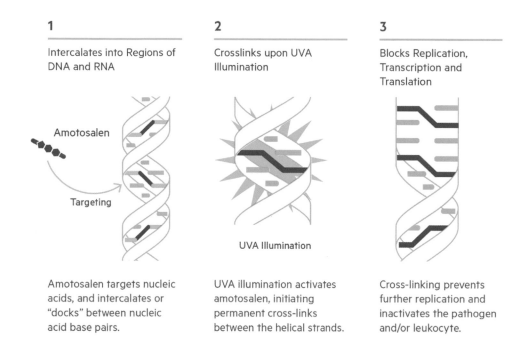

1

Intercalates into Regions of DNA and RNA

Amotosalen

Targeting

Amotosalen targets nucleic acids, and intercalates or "docks" between nucleic acid base pairs.

2

Crosslinks upon UVA Illumination

UVA Illumination

UVA illumination activates amotosalen, initiating permanent cross-links between the helical strands.

3

Blocks Replication, Transcription and Translation

Cross-linking prevents further replication and inactivates the pathogen and/or leukocyte.

• **Fig 14.1.** The INTERCEPT System uses amotosalen—a well-characterized photoactive compound that specifically targets DNA and RNA—and UVA illumination to irreversibly crosslink nucleic acids. In doing so, the INTERCEPT treatment blocks replication of viruses, bacteria, and parasites, rendering them inactive.

in children.[17, 18] A recent study confirmed a small but statistically significant increase in platelet transfusions in pediatric patients receiving PR platelets, however there was no difference in red cell utilization or transfusion reactions between PR and conventional platelets.[19] Though PR technologies show significant promise in reducing transfusion-transmitted infections, additional studies on the use of PR platelets in neonatal and pediatric patients are required.

Transfusion-Related Acute Lung Injury (TRALI)

TRALI is characterized by the development of dyspnea, cyanosis, hypotension, fever, and chills, along with radiologic findings of bilateral pulmonary edema. These findings usually appear within 1 to 6 hours after a blood transfusion, and often progress to hypoxemic respiratory failure with an approximate 6% mortality. The treatment is largely supportive, and may necessitate extracorporeal cardiopulmonary support in severe cases.[20]

TRALI is associated with transfusion of whole blood, packed RBCs, and FFP, with an incidence of one per 5000 to 440,000 unit transfused. TRALI is thought to result from the sequestration of WBCs in the pulmonary microvasculature, which leads to increased vascular permeability and pulmonary edema. It is more likely to occur in children with sepsis or other underlying critical illness. The underlying etiology is likely related to the presence of antibodies against granulocyte or HLA antigens in the donor blood. In the U.S., conversion to an all-male donor plasma supply and/or testing of female multiparous donors for HLA antibodies was implemented to reduce the risk for these reactions.

Circulatory Overload

TRALI is difficult to distinguish from hypervolemia (circulatory overload), with signs and symptoms include shortness of breath, headache, pulmonary edema, congestive heart failure, and hypertension. Once the transfusion is stopped, symptoms typically resolve but the patient may require oxygen and diuretics. To avoid this, transfusions should not exceed 2 to 4 mL/kg/h in a nonemergent situation. Patients with pulmonary or cardiac disease may require slower rates, but all transfusions should be complete within 4 hours.

Transfusion Transmitted Infection

Transfusion transmitted infection remains a serious, albeit less frequent complication from blood transfusion (Table 14.9). Recent adaptation of nucleic acid testing (NAT) has increased the sensitivity of detecting infectious agents in donor blood (e.g., HIV, hepatitis C, West Nile virus) and subsequently decreased the risk for transmission to its lowest value in history. This is because NAT tests for the virus as opposed to previous methods that tested the donor's antibody response to the viral infection. Donor blood is routinely screened for HIV, hepatitis C, hepatitis B, HTLV, syphilis, West Nile virus, Chagas disease, Zika, and babesiosis (endemic areas). Emerging infectious disease testing for Dengue fever are currently under development.

An infection with considerations for neonates and infants is CMV, which resides in the WBCs of many donors

TABLE 14.9	Approximate Risk From Selected Known Transfusion-Transmitted Agents	
Agent	**Risk Per Unit of Blood Transfused**
HIV	1 in 1,467,000
Hepatitis C	1 in 1,149,000
Hepatitis B	1 in 765,000–1,006,000
HTLV-I and HTLV-II	1 in 4,364,000
West Nile Virus	12 cases of transfusion transmission
Chagas disease (Trypanosoma cruzi)	20 cases of transfusion transmission reported in nonendemic areas globally
Babesia species	1 in 18,000
Bacteria, Apheresis Platelets	1 in 107,000

HIV, Human immunodeficiency virus; *HTLV*, human T-lymphotropic virus.

and is transmitted by transfusion of cellular blood components. CMV infection in older, immunocompetent children is associated with a mild illness. However, CMV infection in neonates or immunocompromised children is associated with a severe systemic illness and may be fatal. Therefore providing CMV seronegative blood is critical for these patients. Prestorage leuko-reduced, CMV "safe" blood, is an alternative to providing CMV seronegative blood and is effective in reducing the transmission of CMV. A recent survey by the College of American Pathologists showed that leukoreduction was the primary strategy for mitigating the risk for transfusion transmitted CMV.

References

1. Chesney CR. The maintenance need for water in parenteral fluid therapy, by Malcolm A. Holliday, MD, and William E. Segar, MD, Pediatrics, 1957;19:823–832. *Pediatrics.* 1998;102 (1 Pt 2):229–230.
2. Riegger LQ, Leis AM, Golmirzaie KH, Malviya S. Risk Factors for Intraoperative Hypoglycemia in Children: A Multicenter Retrospective Cohort Study. *Anesth Analg.* 2021;132(4): 1075–1083. https://doi.org/10.1213/ANE.0000000000004979.
3. Nishina K, Mikawa K, Maekawa N, Asano M, Obara H. Effects of exogenous intravenous glucose on plasma glucose and lipid homeostasis in anesthetized infants. *Anesthesiology.* 1995;83(2):258–263. https://doi.org/10.1097/00000542-199508000-00004.
4. Manno CS, Hedberg KW, Kim HC, et al. Comparison of the hemostatic effects of fresh whole blood, stored whole blood, and components after open heart surgery in children. *Blood.* 1991;77(5):930–936.
5. Leeper CM, Yazer MH, Cladis FP, Saladino R, Triulzi DJ, Gaines BA. Use of Uncrossmatched Cold-Stored Whole Blood in Injured Children With Hemorrhagic Shock. *JAMA Pediatr.* 2018;175(5):491–492. https://doi.org/10.1001/jamapediatrics.2017.5238.
6. Gross JB. Estimating allowable blood loss: corrected for dilution. *Anesthesiology.* 1983;58(3):277–280. https://doi.org/10.1097/00000542-198303000-00016.
7. Strauss RG. Red blood cell storage and avoiding hyperkalemia from transfusions to neonates and infants. *Transfusion.* 2010;50(9):1862–1865. https://doi.org/10.1111/j.1537-2995.2010.02789.x.
8. Coté CJ, Liu LM, Szyfelbein SK, Goudsouzian NG, Daniels AL. Changes in serial platelet counts following massive blood transfusion in pediatric patients. *Anesthesiology.* 1985;62(2):197–201. https://doi.org/10.1097/00000542-198502000-00024.
9. Chitlur M, Sorensen B, Rivard GE, et al. Standardization of thromboelastography: a report from the TEG-ROTEM working group. *Haemophilia.* 2011;17(3):532–537. https://doi.org/10.1111/j.1365-2516.2010.02451.x.
10. Chan KL, Summerhayes RG, Ignjatovic V, Horton SB, Monagle PT. Reference values for kaolin-activated thromboelastography in healthy children. *Anesth Analg.* 2007;105(6). https://doi.org/10.1213/01.ane.0000287645.26763.be. 1610-1603.
11. Coté CJ, Drop LJ, Hoaglin DC, Daniels AL, Young ET. Ionized hypocalcemia after fresh frozen plasma administration to thermally injured children: effects of infusion rate, duration, and treatment with calcium chloride. *Anesth Analg.* 1988;67(2):152–160.
12. Busch MP, Kleinman SH, Nemo GJ. Current and emerging infectious risks of blood transfusions. *JAMA.* 2003;289(8): 959–962. https://doi.org/10.1001/jama.289.8.959.
13. Bihl F, Castelli D, Marincola F, Dodd RY, Brander C. Transfusion-transmitted infections. *J Transl Med.* 2007;5:25 https://doi.org/10.1186/1479-5876-5-25. Published 2007 Jun 6.
14. Slonim AD, Joseph JG, Turenne WM, Sharangpani A, Luban NL. Blood transfusions in children: a multi-institutional analysis of practices and complications. *Transfusion.* 2008;48(1):73–80. https://doi.org/10.1111/j.1537-2995.2007.01484.x.
15. Lu W, Fung M. Platelets treated with pathogen reduction technology: current status and future direction. *F1000Res.* 2020;9:F1000 https://doi.org/10.12688/f1000research.20816.1. Faculty Rev-40. Published 2020 Jan 23.
16. Estcourt LJ, Malouf R, Hopewell S, et al. Pathogen-reduced platelets for the prevention of bleeding. *Cochrane Database Syst Rev.* 2017;7(7):CD009072 https://doi.org/10.1002/14651858.CD009072.pub3. Published 2017 Jul 30.
17. Knutson F, Osselaer J, Pierelli L, et al. A prospective, active haemovigilance study with combined cohort analysis of 19, 175 transfusions of platelet components prepared with amotosalen-UVA photochemical treatment. *Vox Sang.* 2015;109:343–352. https://doi.org/10.1111/vox.12287.
18. Snyder E, McCullough J, Slichter SJ, et al. Clinical safety of platelets photochemically treated with amotosalen HCl and ultraviolet A light for pathogen inactivation: the SPRINT trial. *Transfusion.* 2005;45:1864–1875. https://doi.org/10.1111/j.1537-2995.2005.00639.x.
19. Schulz WL, McPadden J, Gehrie EA, et al. Blood Utilization and Transfusion Reactions in Pediatric Patients Transfused with Conventional or Pathogen Reduced Platelets. *J Pediatr.* 2019;209:220–225. https://doi.org/10.1016/j.jpeds.2019.01.046.
20. Nouraei SM, Wallis JP, Bolton D, Hasan A. Management of transfusion-related acute lung injury with extracorporeal cardiopulmonary support in a four-year-old child. *Br J Anaesth.* 2003;91(2):292–294. https://doi.org/10.1093/bja/aeg143.

Suggested Readings

Bailey AG, McNaull PP, Jooste E, Tuchman JB. Perioperative crystalloid and colloid fluid management in children: where are we and how did we get here? *Anesth Analg*. 2010;110(2):375–390. https://doi.org/10.1213/ANE.0b013e3181b6b3b5.

Gibson BE, Todd A, Roberts I, et al. Transfusion guidelines for neonates and older children. *Br J Haematol*. 2004;124(4):433–453. https://doi.org/10.1111/j.1365-2141.2004.04815.xMoritz.Ayus ML JC. Prevention of hospital-acquired hyponatremia: do we have the answers? *Pediatrics*. 2011;128(5):980–983. https://doi.org/10.1542/peds.2011-2015.

Vlaar AP, Juffermans NP. Transfusion-related acute lung injury: a clinical review. *Lancet*. 2013;382(9896):984–994. https://doi.org/10.1016/S0140-6736(12)62197-7.

15

Monitoring

ALLAN F. SIMPAO AND RONALD S. LITMAN

Four monitors are used for virtually every pediatric anesthesia case: pulse oximetry, capnography, electrocardiogram (ECG), and blood pressure measurement. These monitors are components of the Basic Monitoring Standards of the American Society of Anesthesiologists.[1] Temperature monitoring is also performed except in relatively short cases (i.e., <30 minutes duration) where hypothermia or hyperthermia is unlikely, and fluid and blood loss is minimal (e.g., myringotomy and tube insertion). Train-of-four (TOF) nerve monitoring should be used when a neuromuscular blocker is administered. In the following sections, we will review in more detail the use of monitors in pediatric patients.

Pulse Oximetry

Pulse oximetry estimates the oxyhemoglobin saturation by measuring the absorption of two different wavelengths of light, which is dependent on the amount of blood in the tissue and the relative amounts of oxygenated and deoxygenated hemoglobin. The oxygen saturation is then computed by comparing the light absorption ratio to a standard curve of arterial saturations that was determined by experiments on volunteers with arterial blood sampling.

The clinical usefulness of pulse oximetry is to alert the anesthesiologist to impending or actual hypoxemia before the onset of visible cyanosis. However, during rapid decreases in oxygen saturation, the oximetry value usually lags behind the true oxyhemoglobin saturation, such that the recognition of hypoxemia may be delayed. The position of the pulse oximeter probe will affect the rapidity of these changes. Central probe locations (e.g., buccal) will have less of a delay than an upper extremity, which will have less of a delay than a lower extremity. Conversely, the reestablishment of normoxemia may be associated with a persistent low pulse oximetry value for 30 seconds or more.

The precision and accuracy of pulse oximetry measurements in children can be a challenge because of factors such as movement artifact, poor tissue perfusion, low temperature, abnormal hemoglobin, tissue pigmentation, probe site and artificial light. Most oximetry devices have a precision of ±2% when the true oxyhemoglobin saturation is greater than 90%. In the range of oxygen desaturation below 80%, pulse oximetry tends to overestimate the true saturation compared with arterial sampling. The decrement in pulse oximeter precision at lower saturation values differs between manufacturers. Fetal hemoglobin, which is found in neonates and young infants, does not affect the accuracy of the pulse oximeter.

There are no outcome studies that demonstrate a proven benefit from the use of pulse oximetry. However, a single-blinded study[2] (anesthesiologists were not shown the value on the pulse oximeter that was monitored by the investigators) showed that the absence of pulse oximetry resulted in three times as many episodes of hypoxemia (defined as less than 85% saturation) and delayed recognition of hypoxemia compared with having access to the pulse oximeter values. In that study, most of the hypoxemic episodes occurred in children younger than 2 years of age.

Although pulse oximetry is associated with a relatively high rate of false positive alarms (low saturation readings that are not accurate), all alarms must be taken seriously until proven otherwise. When the oximeter displays a low saturation value, the anesthesiologist should immediately turn attention to the adequacy of ventilation by simultaneously evaluating air entry, quality of the capnograph tracing (see below), and the quality of the pulse oximeter signal. Because surgical personnel may unknowingly compress the oximeter probe by leaning on the patient's foot, we prefer to put the oximeter probe on the upper extremity, which can be positioned away from the surgical field. The audible tone on the oximeter should never be turned off or drowned out by loud music, since many anesthesia practitioners listen continuously to the device and respond to a decrease in pitch.

Another use of pulse oximetry is for determination of the heart rate value. The pulse oximeter-derived heart rate can be helpful in certain situations that cause artifact of the electrocardiogram (e.g., electrocautery). Furthermore, concordance between the heart rates on the ECG and the pulse oximeter is one method of verifying that the device is providing accurate saturation information.

The oxygen reserve index (ORi) is a new technology that may prove useful in detecting hypoxemia before it occurs. ORi is a pulse oximeter-based dimensionless index that ranges from 0 to 1 as Pao_2 increases from approximately 80 to 200 mm Hg. A pilot study[3] in 25 healthy children showed ORi detected impending desaturation a median of 31.5 sec before noticeable changes in SpO_2 occurred.

Capnography

Infrared devices that detect exhaled carbon dioxide have been used since the 1970s. They not only measure the $P_{ET}CO_2$ concentration (capnometry), but also display it graphically (capnography). Before 1998, capnography was considered an American Society of Anesthesiologists (ASA) standard monitor for confirming the correct placement and continuous presence of an endotracheal tube. These standards have been since amended and now indicate that capnography should be used to confirm adequate ventilation during the conduct of general anesthesia without an endotracheal tube (e.g., during laryngeal mask airway, face mask, or natural airway anesthesia). Specifically, these guidelines[1] now state:

> "Continual monitoring for the presence of expired carbon dioxide shall be performed unless invalidated by the nature of the patient, procedure, or equipment.... Continual end-tidal carbon dioxide analysis, in use from the time of endotracheal tube/laryngeal mask placement, until extubation/removal or initiating transfer to a postoperative care location, shall be performed using a quantitative method such as capnography, capnometry, or mass spectroscopy."

As in adults, capnography in pediatric patients is used to confirm correct placement of the endotracheal tube and to continuously assess the adequacy of alveolar ventilation. Capnography also provides information about respiratory rate, breathing pattern, airway patency, effectiveness of cardiopulmonary resuscitation, amount of right-to-left intracardiac shunt, change in pulmonary blood flow, and indirectly, the degree of neuromuscular blockade.

The amount of CO_2 in expired gas is a function of the amount produced by the tissues, the alveolar ventilation and the pulmonary blood flow. In pediatric patients, an abnormal increase in $P_{ET}CO_2$ most commonly signifies hypoventilation but may also indicate administration of sodium bicarbonate, release of a tourniquet, abdominal insufflation with CO_2, or increased CO_2 production that occurs with temperature elevation or as an early sign of malignant hyperthermia. Conversely, an abnormally low $P_{ET}CO_2$ may indicate hyperventilation, hypothermia, increased dead space, or a state of low pulmonary perfusion caused by hypotension, venous air embolism, or failure of a systemic to pulmonary artery shunt. An abrupt fall in $P_{ET}CO_2$ can be caused by compression of the trachea and endotracheal tube during intrathoracic surgery or placement of a transesophageal echocardiography probe. Sudden absence of the capnograph tracing can indicate a breathing circuit disconnection, occlusion of the gas sampling line, accidental endotracheal placement of an orogastric tube, or complete loss of cardiac output, while the abnormal presence of inspired CO_2 signifies the presence of a faulty unidirectional valve, exhausted CO_2 absorbent, or when a semiopen circuit is being used, rebreathing secondary to insufficient fresh gas flow. Capnography and capnometry can be used to measure the efficacy of cardiopulmonary resuscitation (i.e., cardiac output generated by chest compressions).

Capnography use in infants and small children[4] (<12 kg) often underestimates the true $P_{ET}CO_2$ value[5] because of the relatively large ratio of dead space to tidal volume. The closer the sampling port is to the endotracheal tube, the more accurate the $P_{ET}CO_2$.

Although mainstream capnography may provide the most accurate $P_{ET}CO_2$ measurement, it adds bulk and dead space to the circuit and may correlate poorly to blood gas values in small infants.[5] Therefore, side-stream capnography is most often employed for pediatric patients. Disadvantages of side-stream capnography in pediatric patients include kinking of the sampling line, slow response time, and with some devices, a relatively large sampling volume. Innovations in capnography ("MICROSTREAM technology,"[6] Covidien, Minneapolis, MN) have enabled a sampling rate as low as 50 mL/min (as opposed to the conventional 150–250 mL/min) without compromising waveform integrity or accuracy of $P_{ET}CO_2$.

Disposable colorimetric CO_2 connectors are commonly used in emergency situations to verify correct endotracheal tube placement.[7] The colorimetric connector changes color from purple to tan to yellow to indicate the presence of carbon dioxide. In one study[8] of pediatric resuscitations, the colorimetric detector was used during cardiopulmonary resuscitation; only patients with a yellow reading had return of spontaneous circulation and survived to ICU admission.

Small infants often lack an alveolar plateau on the capnograph (Fig. 15.1). This can result from a higher respiratory rate, an excessively high sampling flow for the volume of CO_2 produced, excessive dead space in the breathing circuit, or a leak around the endotracheal tube. In most cases, switching the capnograph tubing closer to the patient's airway will reveal a more accurate result (Figs. 15.2 and 15.3).

Electrocardiography

Normal pediatric ECG values differ significantly according to age in the newborn, infants, and children. In pediatric anesthesia, the ECG is most useful for diagnosing intraoperative rate-related arrhythmias, such as bradycardia and supraventricular tachycardia. The ECG

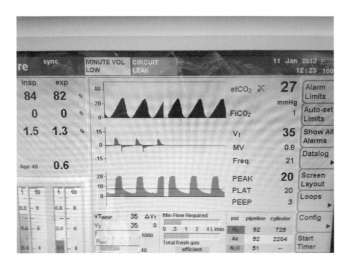

• **Fig 15.1.** Typical capnograph tracing in a small infant. Note the lack of a plateau.

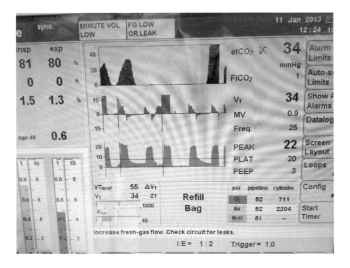

• **Fig 15.2.** The side-stream capnography tubing is switched to a more distal location closer to the patient.

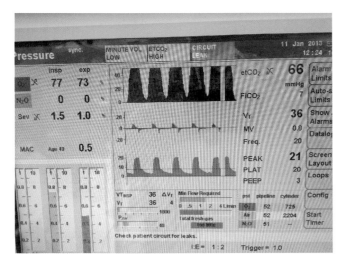

• **Fig 15.3.** When the side-stream capnography tubing is closer to the tracheal tube, the true, higher level of $P_{ET}CO_2$ is revealed. The capnograph appears to have a more pronounced plateau.

is less prone to movement-related artifact than the pulse oximeter. In small infants, hypoxemia-related bradycardia may be apparent on the ECG before the pulse oximeter signaling oxyhemoglobin desaturation. The resolution of hypoxemia is signaled by the transition from bradycardia to normal sinus rhythm, often before the pulse oximeter value recovers. Pediatric patients can have ECG changes that are typical of particular pathologic states, such as prolonged QT, myocardial ischemia (ST changes) and hyperkalemia (peaked T waves).

Blood Pressure Monitoring

The ranges of normal blood pressures[9] in children under anesthesia differ according to age and height. Blood pressure monitoring serves as a surrogate for the monitoring and optimization of adequate cardiac output and is performed most commonly using a noninvasive, automated, oscillometric blood pressure device. Oscillometric measurement of systolic blood pressure and heart rate usually correlates well[10] with the Riva-Rocci mercury column method, but it tends to have poor correlation with the diastolic component in children. In most routine cases, measurement of blood pressure should be performed every 3 to 5 minutes throughout the administration of general anesthesia. In children, the blood pressure cuff is placed most commonly on the upper arm, but it can be placed alternatively on the forearm, thigh, or calf.

The width of the blood pressure cuff[11] should equal 40% of the upper arm circumference (or other extremity portion to which it is applied). Too small a cuff is associated with falsely elevated blood pressure values, and too large a cuff is associated with falsely lowered blood pressure values.

While many characteristics of pediatric arterial blood pressure monitoring (e.g., indications and contraindications, transducer setup) are similar to adults, some differences exist. Usual sites of arterial cannulation in pediatrics include the radial,[12] femoral, and posterior tibial[13] arteries.

Neuromuscular Monitoring

The physiologic changes that occur early in life influence the effects of neuromuscular blockers (NMBs) in children. They include alterations in volume of distribution, development of hepatic and renal elimination processes, accumulation of muscle mass, and the maturation of the neuromuscular junction, which result in age-dependent pharmacokinetic and pharmacodynamic responses to NMB.

Monitoring of NMB should take into consideration physiologic and exogenous factors that influence NMB response, such as site and pattern of stimulation, temperature, and concurrent anesthetic and medication administration. The results of nerve monitoring in preschool aged children must be interpreted with caution, as the relationships between neuromuscular blockade parameters (e.g., train-of-four [TOF] ratio) and respiratory function are variable and not well defined. Care should also be taken when interpreting other sites such as posterior tibial or facial nerve, as these sites may have different sensitivities to NMB. Hypothermia may interfere with NMB monitoring: for each degree below 35°C, the adductor pollicis peak twitch height is reduced by 15%.

Responses to different patterns of stimulation (e.g., tetanic, double-burst, TOF) are age dependent.[14] Tetanic stimulation may be difficult to achieve in infants younger than 12 weeks because of fade and posttetanic exhaustion. Double-burst stimulation is more sensitive than tetanic stimulation and correlates well with TOF ratio. TOF stimulation is the most commonly used pattern and can be used from birth; thus it remains the standard measure of recovery from NMB effect.

Inhaled anesthesia affects the pharmacodynamic response of NMB in children and is age dependent. For example, in infants up to 2 years old, an intubation dose of NMB demonstrated a longer duration of action during inhalation anesthesia compared with older children. In contrast, a total IV anesthetic (e.g., concurrent propofol and remifentanil infusions) does not interfere with the pharmacodynamic effects of NMB in children.

Elucidating the pharmacodynamics of NMB in children remains an ethical and technical challenge because it is unacceptable to study the effects of partial blockade on respiratory function in conscious or sedated children. Studies have varied in type of anesthesia, calibration of NMB monitors, and determination of signal stabilization, making comparison across studies difficult to perform.

Although the recovery of neuromuscular transmission does not necessarily signal a full recovery of muscle function, the use of TOF monitoring in children facilitates the detection of residual blockade when age-dependent differences are taken into consideration.

Precordial or Esophageal Stethoscope

Although not an essential monitor by ASA standards, many pediatric anesthesiologists find that the precordial (or esophageal) stethoscope gives valuable information during all phases of pediatric anesthesia, especially during transport between hospital locations. Continuous auscultation allows the immediate detection of changes in rate and character of heart and breath sounds, and it is often the first warning of a potential problem such as a right main bronchial intubation or wheezing. Subtle changes in heart sounds often correlate with changes in the depth of anesthesia. During ligation of a patent ductus arteriosus (PDA), a precordial stethoscope can help the surgeon identify the correct structure since clamping the ductus will result in a disappearance of the murmur. Portable digital esophageal stethoscope systems[15] have been developed and reported in the literature.

The precordial stethoscope is placed to the left of the sternum in the 3rd or 4th intercostal space. The esophageal stethoscope is placed in the midesophagus in children with an endotracheal tube or laryngeal mask. Placement depth[16] significantly affects the quality of the auscultated sounds. The proper method for accurate placement of the esophageal stethoscope is to listen while simultaneously advancing the device and placing it at the level where the heart and lung sounds are maximal. In small infants, unintentional placement of the esophageal stethoscope into the stomach can occur easily.

Monitoring During Transport

Although much has been written about the safety of critically ill patients during transport[17] between different hospital locations, similar standards or guidelines for the transport of anesthetized patients between different hospital locations do not exist. However, we believe that the same monitoring standards should exist for patients during transport in the perioperative period, regardless of their level of consciousness or type of airway device and regardless of the distance traveled (e.g., operating room to postanesthesia care unit). With the widespread availability of portable monitors, cardiopulmonary status should be continuously assessed during transport using pulse oximetry and/or capnometry/capnography.

References

1. Committee on Standards and Practice Parameters (CSPP). Standards for Basic Anesthetic Monitoring. *American Society of Anesthesiologists.* https://www.asahq.org/standards-and-guidelines/standards-for-basic-anesthetic-monitoring; 12.13.2020 Accessed 21.07.20.
2. Coté CJ, Goldstein EA, Coté MA, Hoaglin DC, Ryan JF. A single-blind study of pulse oximetry in children. *Anesthesiology.* 1988;68(2):184–188.
3. Szmuk P, Steiner JW, Olomu PN, Ploski RP, Sessler DI, Ezri T. Oxygen reserve index: A novel noninvasive measure of oxygen reserve–A pilot study. *Anesthesiology.* 2016;124(4):779–784.
4. Eipe N, Doherty DR. A review of pediatric capnography. *J Clin Monit Comput.* 2010;24(4):261–68.
5. Badgwell JM, McLeod ME, Lerman J, Creighton RE. End-tidal Pco2 measurements sampled at the distal and proximal ends of the endotracheal tube in infants and children. *Anesth Analg.* 1987;66(10):959–964.
6. Capnography Monitoring. *Medtronic.* https://www.medtronic.com/covidien/en-us/products/capnography.html. Accessed 21.07.20.
7. Bhende MS, Thompson AE, Cook R, Saville AL. Validity of a disposable end-tidal CO2 detector in verifying endotracheal tube placement in infants and children. *Ann Emerg Med.* 1992;21(2):142–145.
8. Bhende MS, Thompdon AE. Evaluation of an end-tidal CO2 detector during pediatric cardiopulmonary resuscitation. *Pediatrics.* 1995;95(3):395–399.
9. de Graaff JC, Pasma W, van Buuren S., et al. Reference values for noninvasive blood pressure in children during anesthesia: A multicentered retrospective observational cohort study. *Anesthesiology.* 2016;125:904–913.
10. Friesen RH, Lichtor JL. Indirect measurement of blood pressure in neonates and infants utilizing an automatic noninvasive oscillometric monitor. *Anesth Analg.* 1981;60(10):742–745.
11. Clark JA, Lieh-Lai MW, Sarnaik A, Mattoo TK. Discrepancies between direct and indirect blood pressure measurements using various recommendations for arm cuff selection. *Pediatrics.* 2002;110(5):920–923.

12. Selldén H, Nilsson K, Larsson LE, Ekström-Jodal B. Radial arterial catheters in children and neonates. *Crit Care Med.* 1987;15(12):1106–1109.

13. Kim EH, Lee JH, Song IK, Kim JT, Lee WJ, Kim HS. Posterior tibial artery as an alternative to the radial artery for arterial cannulation site in small children: A randomized controlled study. *Anesthesiology.* 2017;127(3):423–431.

14. Saldien V, Vermeyen KM. Neuromuscular transmission monitoring in children. *Pediatr Anaesth.* 2004;14(4):289–292.

15. Shin JY, Lim SW, Kim YC, Kim SJ, Cha EJ, Lee TS. Portable digital esophageal stethoscope system. *Annu Int Conf IEEE Eng Med Biol Soc 2010.* 2010:1844–1847.

16. Manecke Jr GR, Poppers PJ. Esophageal stethoscope placement depth: its effect on heart and lung sound monitoring during general anesthesia. *Anesth Analg.* 1998;86(6):1276–1279.

17. Fanara B, Manzon C, Barbot O, Desmettre T, Capellier G. Recommendations for the intra-hospital transport of critically ill patients. *Crit Care.* 2010;14(3):R87.

16

Temperature Regulation

JEREMY JONES AND RONALD S. LITMAN

This chapter reviews the importance of thermoregulation and temperature monitoring in anesthetized children. It addresses the significance of keeping children normothermic and will help the trainee understand why pediatric anesthesiologists become apoplectic when faced with the possibility that the small infant they are caring for may become hypothermic. Important updates in this revision include new information and references regarding temperature control in neonates, and early detection of malignant hyperthermia with assiduous temperature monitoring that results in less morbidity and mortality from the disease.

Normal Temperature Physiology in Children

Body temperature is a result of the balance between heat production by the major organs and heat loss to the environment. There is no standard for normal body temperature; individuals exhibit different temperatures, which will be influenced by the time of day, activity, and so forth. Like adults, children's bodies contain different compartments that exist at different temperatures. The core compartment is composed of the major organs and deep body tissues. The peripheral compartment is composed of the extremities. There is a normal temperature gradient between the core and peripheral compartments that is largely maintained by peripheral vasoconstriction. When the administration of general or regional anesthesia causes vasodilation, there is increased mixing of heat between the core and the peripheral compartments. This usually results in an overall decrease in core temperature after induction of general anesthesia.

As a homeotherm, when an infant is placed in a cooler than normal environment, it will consume oxygen and expend caloric energy in an attempt to maintain a normal body temperature. The neutral thermal environment (NTE)[1] is defined as the environmental temperature range that is likely to result in a body temperature with the lowest metabolic heat production, measured as oxygen consumption. The clinical correlate of this is that if a small infant with lung disease has a preexisting defect in transfer of oxygen into the bloodstream and excretion of carbon dioxide, it is more likely to develop cellular hypoxemia during

hypothermia, when the infant is increasing oxygen consumption and metabolic rate to maintain normothermia. Indeed, studies have documented differences in infant survival rates that were influenced by the temperature in the incubator. In one study, an increase in incubator temperature from 85°F to 89°F was associated with a 15% increase in survival.

Generally, the smaller and younger the infant, the higher the environmental temperature required to achieve the NTE. Graphs[2] have been published that indicate the temperature required to maintain infants in the NTE based on weight and gestational age. For example, for newborns weighing between 1 and 3 kg, this temperature can exceed 85°F (29.4°C). When anesthetizing small infants, you should attempt to replicate these conditions in the operating room in the area immediately surrounding the infant. For a naked infant lying supine on an open platform, it is estimated that the abdominal skin temperature should be between 36.5°C and 37°C to approximate the conditions required to be in an NTE.

Within an NTE, the human infant's oxygen consumption is at its lowest, meaning that it is expending minimal amounts of energy to maintain normothermia. If the environmental temperature is lowered slightly, the infant can use compensatory mechanisms (vasoconstriction, brown fat oxidation) to maintain normothermia. However, when the infant's thermal protective mechanisms can no longer sustain normothermia, its core temperature will drop. Eventually, oxygen consumption will also decrease because the temperature regulation center becomes impaired. Just because an infant's temperature is relatively normal does not mean that it is still residing in the NTE. In fact, its thermal protective mechanisms may be very active and on the verge of failing to maintain normothermia. When the infant's body temperature begins to fall, it is an indication that the thermal stress has been so severe that its normal thermal compensatory mechanisms are being overpowered. Furthermore, the presence of either hypoxemia or hypoglycemia impairs the metabolic response to hypothermia, resulting in a more dramatic decrease in body temperature.

The human infant is born with a well-developed temperature regulating system. However, small infants are prone to hypothermia in cold environments and hyperthermia in overly warm environments mainly because of their relatively large surface area-to-volume ratio. The body surface area-to-volume ratio of a tiny premature infant is three to five times higher than an adult's, and the heat loss per unit body mass is about four times that of the adult. Because of less subcutaneous fat (i.e., less insulation), the range of the environmental temperature in which the infant is able to maintain normothermia is limited compared with the adult. For example, in a naked anesthesiologist, the lower limit of this control range is approximately 0°C (32°F) whereas for the full-term infant it is 20 to 23°C (68°F –73.4°F). Therefore, the temperature within the infant's immediate surrounding area in the OR should be maintained at a minimum of approximately 75°F. Because subcutaneous fat is formed mainly in the third trimester of gestation, infants born prematurely are even more at risk for poikilothermic behavior.

Normal Compensation for Hypothermia

When body temperature begins to vary just slightly away (±0.2°C) from the physiologic set point, involuntary compensatory mechanisms will attempt to return the body's temperature back to normal. There are a number of these compensatory mechanisms. Those that are most important in small children and that are most different from adults will be reviewed.

When most of us feel cold, we instinctively seek a warmer location, put on another layer of clothes, increase our muscle activity to generate heat, or cuddle with a loved one. Infants cannot do any of these (although it is often heard from neonatal intensive care unit [NICU] nurses that babies will instinctively find the warmest corner of their isolette).

Older children and adults have the capability to shiver, the high-intensity involuntary rhythmic muscle activity that is probably the most significant means by which adults produce heat. Young children do not have the capability of efficient shivering. Once anesthetized (even without muscle paralysis), efficient shivering is greatly attenuated until the process of awakening.

Nonshivering thermogenesis describes a cold-induced increase in oxygen consumption and heat production that is not inhibited by muscle relaxants. In small infants, nonshivering thermogenesis is probably the most important means of heat production in a cool environment. The thermogenic effector organ—brown fat—is the most significant contributor to nonshivering thermogenesis in the small infant. In the human infant, brown fat accounts for 2% to 6% of total bodyweight and is located in the abdominal cavity surrounding the kidneys and adrenal glands, in the mediastinum, and between the scapulae. As opposed to the more abundant white fat, brown fat cells are rich in mitochondria, contain a dense capillary network, and are richly innervated with sympathetic nerve endings. When norepinephrine release is stimulated by sympathetic activity, triglycerides are hydrolyzed to free fatty acids and glycerol, with heat production resulting from enhanced oxygen consumption and uncoupling of the electron transport chain mediated by the protein thermogenin. Immediately after an infant

is exposed to a cold stimulus the metabolic rate begins to increase, even before core body temperature decreases. Even a mild cold stimulus such as unheated preoxygenation can trigger the onset of an increase in metabolic heat production. In infants exposed to a cold environment, nonshivering thermogenesis is capable of doubling the metabolic rate. However, the decrease in temperature required to initiate nonshivering thermogenesis is unknown. In one study[3] of infants anesthetized with propofol and fentanyl, there was a lack of nonshivering thermogenesis with a temperature drop of 2°C.

Thermoregulatory vasoconstriction occurs in the peripheral compartments in response to cold receptors on the skin. It serves to limit heat loss to the environment. In children undergoing abdominal surgery with isoflurane anesthesia, thermoregulatory vasoconstriction is attenuated by an average of about 2.5°C less than the unanesthetized state. This is similar to the values found in anesthetized adults.

Complications of Hypothermia in Infants

Hypothermia sets into motion a variety of physiologic compensation mechanisms that increase oxygen consumption and may adversely affect normal physiology.[4] Cooling results in release of norepinephrine. This, along with the direct effects of hypothermia, results in widespread vasoconstriction. Peripheral vasoconstriction may restrict oxygen delivery to tissues and cause cellular hypoxia that manifests as a metabolic acidosis. Pulmonary vasoconstriction will increase pulmonary arterial pressures[5] and cause increased susceptibility to right-to-left shunting at the atrial level through a patent foramen ovale and through a patent ductus arteriosus. This will result in additional peripheral tissue hypoxia. NICU patients with hypothermia require more respiratory and cardiac interventions.[6]

Mild hypothermia (34°C–36°C) in healthy infants and children during peripheral procedures probably does not result in adverse effects, and does not influence postoperative recovery indices. Postoperative shivering[7] is uncommon in children. In an audit[8] of 1507 children, 3.5% experienced shivering. Risk factors included use of intravenous induction agents, age older than 6 years, and prolonged duration of surgery. Clonidine has been shown to decrease occurrence of postoperative shivering.

Heat Loss During Anesthesia

After induction of general anesthesia, an initial decrease in core temperature results from the redistribution of heat from the core to the periphery. This is largely caused by a combination of direct vasodilation by the anesthetic agents and an anesthetic-induced inhibition of thermoregulatory vasoconstriction that occurs at a lower than normal core temperature. In children the administration of general anesthesia blunts the ability of the central nervous system to trigger compensatory vasoconstriction by approximately 2.5°C, compared with approximately 0.2°C in the unanesthetized state. This threshold is similar to that of adults. Because infants and small children have a relatively greater proportion of their body mass contained in the core compartment, they may, at least initially, lose proportionately less heat because of redistribution of core heat to the periphery. Their relatively small extremities will not absorb as much heat from the core compared with an adult.

After this initial decrease in core temperature from redistribution, infants will likely continue to lose heat to the environment at a faster pace than older children and adults. This is mainly caused by their relatively large surface area-to-volume ratio, paucity of subcutaneous fat, immature epidermal barrier, and limited capacity for metabolic heat production. In addition, there is a relatively greater contribution to body cooling from unwarmed intravenous solutions and sterile irrigating solutions.

Mechanisms of Heat Loss to the Environment

Radiation is the process by which heat is lost from the child to any colder surrounding structures (e.g., walls in the operation room [OR]) by the transfer of photons and is not influenced by the temperature of the surrounding air. Radiation normally accounts for the greatest percentage of heat lost during anesthesia. During transport of a neonate to and from the operating room, heat lost through radiation can be decreased by use of a double-shelled incubator, or another type of barrier between the infant and the surrounding incubator walls, such as a blanket.

Conduction refers to the direct transfer of heat between contiguous structures. Examples include loss of heat from the child to the operating room table, or the hypothermic effect of infusion of cool intravenous fluids. Because of the relatively larger surface area-to-volume ratio of infants, conduction may influence heat loss more in infants than in older children or adults. Heat lost by conduction is reduced by using a warming mattress beneath the child, increasing the ambient temperature in the operating room, use of a forced warm air blanket on nonsurgical areas of the body, and warming infused intravenous fluids and sterile prep solutions.

Convection is the loss of heat by the movement of air flowing past the surface of the skin. The best way to minimize heat lost through convection is to cover all exposed parts of the child with a sheet or blanket.

Evaporation is the loss of heat by the energy depleted when water dissipates from exposed surfaces of the body, such as the skin, visceral organs, and respiratory epithelium. Evaporative heat loss is minimized by humidification of inspired gases, covering exposed skin surfaces, and using warmed sterile prep solutions.

Prevention and Treatment of Perioperative Hypothermia

Preoperative warming of the extremities is perhaps the most effective method for prevention of the initial decrease in temperature as a result of redistribution. However, this is not practical in most children. Therefore, more effective

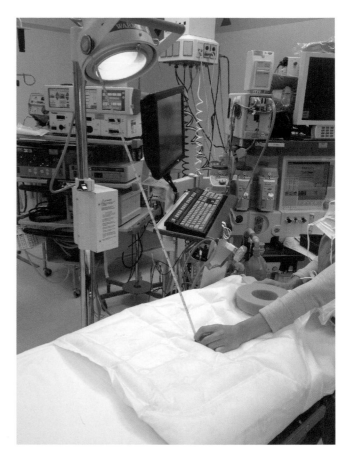

• **Fig 16.1.** Infant radiant warmer. To keep small infants warm during induction, we use a radiant warmer (a.k.a., "French Fry light"). The ruler indicates the minimum safe distance between the light and the infant to prevent burns. Photo credit Ronald S. Litman

means must be used to prevent large decreases in temperature. Every attempt should be made to achieve cutaneous warming by covering all exposed areas with sheets or blankets. This will significantly decrease radiant, convective, and evaporative heat losses. Many institutions use radiant warmers, which are kept over the infant during induction of anesthesia and placement of lines and monitors (Fig. 16.1). These devices may help prevent heat loss via evaporation and conduction of heat to the surrounding cold air.

Airway humidification can prevent evaporation. There are two methods with which to humidify the airway. The simplest is by using a heat and moisture exchanger (HME) to passively trap the patient's own heat and moisture within the airway (Fig. 16.2). The second is the placement of an active humidification device within the anesthesia breathing circuit (Fig. 16.3). This device can both prevent heat loss and add heat to the child's body via the respiratory tract. However, its use is probably not warranted for peripheral surgery of relatively short duration, and we have largely discontinued its use, even in major cases, because it was physically cumbersome to use, and did not seem to make a significant different in temperature outcomes.

Heated water-filled mattresses may be used to prevent conductive heat loss from the infant to the OR table and

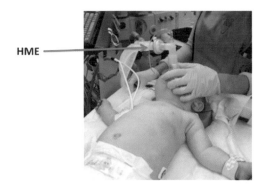

HME

• **Fig 16.2.** Heat and moisture exchanger. All our circuits contain a heat and moisture exchanger (HME) to conserve humidity and heat from the airway and lungs. Photo credit Ronald S. Litman.

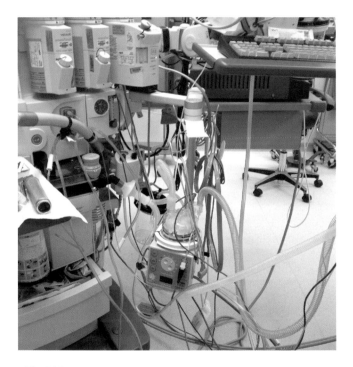

• **Fig 16.3.** Active humidification device within the anesthesia breathing circuit. Photo credit Ronald S. Litman.

to transfer heat to the infant. However, its safe temperature range is narrow: if it is set below 35°C, infants may lose heat to the mattress, and above 38°C there is the possibility of overheating and burns. It is likely most effective in infants weighing less than 10 kg. All infusions, sterile scrubbing, and preparation solutions should also be warmed to prevent conductive heat loss within and around the child's body.

Forced-air warming blankets (e.g., Bair-Hugger, 3 M, St. Paul, MN) prevent heat loss to the environment and may even effectively warm patients via radiant shielding and convection. There is no evidence that forced-air warming devices contribute to surgical site infections. Of all devices, these are one of the most effective and should be used in all cases where hypothermia is possible.

Because infants have relatively low maintenance fluid flow rates, it is difficult to determine whether the warming of intravenous fluids is an effective means of preventing or correcting hypothermia. However, in one study,[9] infants younger than 1 year of age who were hypothermic in the postanesthesia care unit (PACU) had the most efficient rewarming when prewarmed intravenous fluids were administered in addition to a warming blanket.

Lastly, one of the most effective methods for prevention of hypothermia in small children is warming the OR environment. The walls of the OR will become warmed and result in a decrease in loss of radiant heat from the patient. One must be sensitive, however, to the comfort of the surgeons and nurses[10] under the hot operating lights. Therefore, the OR should be maintained warm, but then, once the child is covered with blankets and a forced-air warming blanket, the air temperature can be turned down for comfort after ensuring that the child's core temperature is in the satisfactory range.

In 2020, the results of an important multicenter process improvement protocol for maintenance of perioperative normothermia in NICU patients were published[11]. Process measures to maintain preoperative normothermia (36.5°C –37.5°C) included prewarming the OR, heating the transport isolette during transport to the OR, and minimizing time in preoperative holding area. Intraoperative process measures included continuous temperature monitoring, warming intravenous and irrigation solutions, and actively warming the infant using a combination of a forced-heated air device, chemically heated mattress, warming lights, and covering all exposed skin. Postoperative process measures mainly consisted of transfer back to the NICU in a heated isolette while keeping the infant covered and lying on a chemical heat mattress. This 2-year process resulted in an average decrease in postoperative hypothermia of nearly 50%.

Where Should Temperature Be Measured?

For the purposes of elective general anesthesia cases in low-risk children, axillary temperature measurement is equally as effective as tympanic, nasopharyngeal, or esophageal sites. However, in higher risk populations, or when hypothermia is possible, true representations of core temperature are preferred, such as midesophageal or nasopharyngeal locations. Tympanic membrane temperatures are also reliable but fear of injuring the tympanic membrane dissuades most anesthesiologists from choosing this route. When using distal esophageal temperature monitoring in neonates and small infants during a laparotomy, one must ensure that the tip of the temperature probe has not entered the stomach; falsely elevated readings can result from warming of the stomach if directly exposed to the heat of the overhead lights or warm irrigation solution. Disposable skin temperature devices are generally not considered to be useful in the perioperative environment where diagnosis of temperature alteration is clinically important, but new noninvasive technologies[12] may prove reliable.

Effects of Regional Anesthesia on Intraoperative Temperature Regulation

Regional anesthesia contributes to onset and maintenance of hypothermia because vasodilation of the extremities exaggerates the redistribution of heat from the core component. Furthermore, inhibition of peripheral sympathetic tone may prevent thermoregulatory vasoconstriction and inhibit heat production by utilization of brown fat. However, few studies with modern anesthetic agents in children have been performed to assess the influence of regional anesthesia on intraoperative temperature regulation.

Perioperative Hyperthermia

Intraoperative hyperthermia is often observed during peripheral procedures with minimal heat or fluid loss and when warming maneuvers are being used. Examples include otolarygologic surgeries, dental surgeries, and procedures on the distal limbs. For these types of procedures, it is usually sufficient to use a sheet or light blanket that covers the child's body, and perhaps a warming blanket underneath an infant on the OR table. Use of a forced warm blanket in these situations will usually contribute to hyperthermia.

Although relatively common, postoperative fever (generally thought of as a core body temperature greater than 38°C) in children is a consistent cause of concern. Surgeons worry about wound infections and anesthesiologists worry about postoperative signs of malignant hyperthermia. The fact is, however, that postoperative fever is extremely common in children, and is rarely because of either wound infection or malignant hyperthermia.[13] The precise cause of postoperative fever is unknown, but it is theorized to be a transient adjustment of the body temperature[14] "set-point" as a response to surgical stress. An audit of 150 consecutive pediatric urologic patients revealed that 74% aged younger than 1 year and 28% aged older than 4 years exhibited postoperative fever, none of whom was otherwise clinically ill. Similar incidences have been reported in the pediatric orthopedic, plastic, and tonsillectomy populations. No studies in any particular surgical specialty indicate that postoperative fever alone is a reliable marker of a serious clinical entity.

When asked to evaluate a child with postoperative fever, the anesthesiologist should review the anesthetic and surgical events as a prelude to determining the cause. The child should be evaluated for concomitant upper respiratory tract illness or middle ear infection that may have been present preoperatively. Abnormal lung sounds should prompt investigation of possible lower respiratory tract infection. If the child appears ill, fluid hydration should be continued and the child evaluated for overnight hospital admission.

References

1. Ringer SA. Core concepts: Thermoregulation in the newborn part I: Basic mechanisms. *NeoReviews*. 2013;14(4):e161–e167. doi.org/10.1542/neo.14-4-e161.
2. Sauer PJ, Dane HJ, Visser HK. New standards for neutral thermal environment of healthy very low birthweight infants in week one of life. *Arch Dis Child*. 1984;59(1):18–22. doi.org/10.1136/adc.59.1.18.
3. Plattner O, Semsroth M, Sessler DI, Papousek A, Klasen C, Wagner O. Lack of nonshivering thermogenesis in infants anesthetized with fentanyl and propofol. *Anesthesiology*. 1997;86(4):772–777. doi.org/10.1097/00000542-199704000-00006.
4. Perlman J, Kjaer K. Neonatal and maternal temperature regulation during and after delivery. *Anesth Analg*. 2016;123(1):168–172. doi.org/10.1213/ANE.0000000000001256.
5. Lumb AB, Slinger P. Hypoxic pulmonary vasoconstriction: physiology and anesthetic implications. *Anesthesiology*. 2015;122(4):932–946. doi.org/10.1097/ALN.0000000000000569.
6. Morehouse D, Williams L, Lloyd C, et al. Perioperative hypothermia in NICU infants: its occurrence and impact on infant outcomes. *Adv Neonatal Care*. 2014;14(3):154–164. doi.org/10.1097/ANC.0000000000000045.
7. Kranke P, Eberhart LH, Roewer N, Tramèr MR. Postoperative shivering in children: a review on pharmacologic prevention and treatment. *Paediatr Drugs*. 2003;5(6):373–383. doi.org/10.2165/00128072-200305060-00003.
8. Akin A, Esmaoglu A, Boyaci A. Postoperative shivering in children and causative factors. *Paediatr Anaesth*. 2005;15(12):1089–1093. doi.org/10.1111/j.1460-9592.2005.01646.x.
9. Shen J, Wang Q, Zhang Y, Wang X, Shi P. Combination of warming blanket and prewarmed intravenous infusion is effective for rewarming in infants with postoperative hypothermia in China. *Paediatr Anaesth*. 2015;25(11):1139–1143. doi.org/10.1111/pan.12733.
10. Sultan P, Habib AS, Carvalho B. Ambient operating room temperature: mother, baby or surgeon? *Br J Anaesth*. 2017;119(4):839. doi.org/10.1093/bja/aex307.
11. Brozanski BS, Piazza AJ, Chuo J, et al. STEPP IN: Working together to keep infants warm in the perioperative period. *Pediatrics*. 2020;145(4):e20191121. doi.org/10.1542/peds.2019-1121.
12. Carvalho H, Najafi N, Poelaert J. Intra-operative temperature monitoring with cutaneous zero-heat-flux-thermometry in comparison with oesophageal temperature: A prospective study in the paediatric population. *Paediatr Anaesth*. 2019;29(8):865–871. doi.org/10.1111/pan.13653.
13. Litman RS, Flood CD, Kaplan RF, Kim YL, Tobin JR. Postoperative malignant hyperthermia: an analysis of cases from the North American Malignant Hyperthermia Registry. *Anesthesiology*. 2008;109(5):825–829. doi.org/10.1097/ALN.0b013e31818958e5.
14. Frank SM, Kluger MJ, Kunkel SL. Elevated Thermostatic Setpoint in Postoperative Patients. *Anesthesiology*. 2000;93(6):1426–1431. doi.org/10.1097/00000542-200012000-00014.

17

Routine Airway Management

RONALD S. LITMAN AND MICHAEL R. KING

General anesthesiologists that occasionally anesthetize children should be intimately familiar with the anatomy of the pediatric upper airway. In this chapter, the pertinent features of the pediatric airway and the correct ways to manage the pediatric airway are detailed. Several common and serious complications related to airway management are reviewed. These include laryngospasm, pulmonary aspiration, and negative-pressure (postobstructive) pulmonary edema.

Anatomy of the Pediatric Upper Airway

Unique anatomic airway differences that influence airway management in children include (Fig. 17.1) the following:
- A relatively large occiput in infants, which naturally flexes the neck when in the supine position, causing the infant to assume a natural "sniffing" position.
- A more anterior and cephalad larynx[1] than in the adult, which causes it to be more easily visualized using a straight, rather than a curved laryngoscope (the exact vertebral level is irrelevant).
- A relatively narrow and short epiglottis that is angled into the lumen of the airway, and is often difficult to displace anteriorly during laryngoscopy.
- Smaller size than one might be used to. Small nasal passages are more likely to become obstructed with blood or secretions, and tracheal edema is more likely to increase airway resistance. "Seasoned" anesthesiologists with dwindling eyesight may have trouble with the tiny view of the neonate's larynx through the relatively small view space of a Miller 0 blade.

Dental Development

There are 20 primary ("baby") teeth that are identified by a lettering system[2] that begins with the right upper molar and ends at the right lower molar. Primary teeth erupt starting at about 1 year of age (give or take a few months on either end) and are shed between 6 and 12 years of age. Loose or chipped teeth should be sought for and documented on the anesthetic record. Primary teeth that are very loose should be removed after induction of general anesthesia and before airway instrumentation. To do this, grasp the tooth firmly with gauze and rock it back and forth while pulling or twisting until you oust it from its home. Minor bleeding in the tooth socket abates with firm pressure and, most importantly, all personnel in attendance are expected to contribute to the tooth fairy fund. In adolescents, broken or loose orthodontic hardware should be documented and rubber bands should be removed.

Assessment of the Pediatric Airway

Unlike adults, there are no validated physical characteristics of children (i.e., Mallampati score) that have been definitively associated with the inability to perform mask ventilation or tracheal intubation. Mask ventilation may be difficult for a variety of reasons, including the small size of the neonate, the large tongue of the child with trisomy 21, or the presence of large tonsil and adenoid tissue in toddlers. On the other hand, it is rare that tracheal intubation cannot be accomplished in the prepubertal child unless the child has altered facial or airway anatomy.

Pediatric Airway Management Techniques

Mask Ventilation

In children with normal facial anatomy aged 4 years and older, effective mask ventilation is usually easy to perform. The proper mask ventilation technique for all children is to hold the mask over the mouth and nose with the thumb and forefinger while the middle finger is placed on the bony portion of the mandible. The middle finger lifts the chin to extend the head without externally compressing the anterior neck. The upper part of the mask should rest on the bridge of the nose (Fig. 17.2). Inexperienced practitioners often make the mistake of holding the mask too low, which

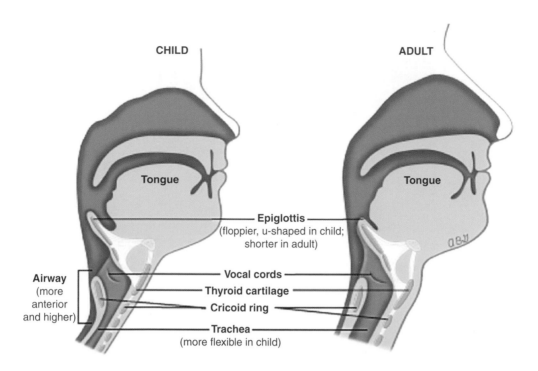

CHILD

ADULT

Tongue

Tongue

Epiglottis
(floppier, u-shaped in child;
shorter in adult)

Vocal cords
Thyroid cartilage
Cricoid ring

Airway
(more
anterior
and higher)

Trachea
(more flexible in child)

• **Fig 17.1.** Anatomic differences between the pediatric and adult upper airway. (Reproduced with permission from Nagler J. Emergency airway management in children: unique pediatric considerations. In: Post TW, ed. UpToDate, Waltham, MA: UpToDate; 2013 Accessed 20.10.10) (Copyright © 2020 UpToDate, Inc. For more information visit www.uptodate.com.)

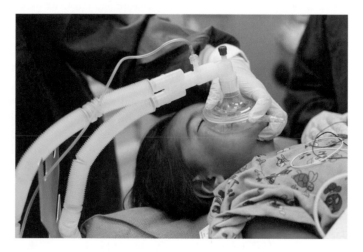

• **Fig 17.2.** Proper position for mask ventilation. (Photograph courtesy Douglas Preuss.)

obstructs the nasal passages. To avoid gastric distention, peak inspiratory pressures should not exceed 15 cmH$_2$O, or less in infants[3] (See Video 17.1).

Airway Obstruction During Mask Ventilation

Difficult mask ventilation during induction of general anesthesia is almost always because of some form of intrinsic airway obstruction. In neonates and small infants, the obstruction is usually caused by soft tissue collapse around the area of the epiglottis. In older children, large tonsils or adenoid tissue is usually responsible. When upper airway obstruction occurs, the practitioner should have in mind a sequential series of corrective maneuvers to relieve the obstruction before more advanced airway instrumentation techniques. The first is chin lift, which stretches and tightens the soft tissue structures along the length of the upper airway and results in an increase in the anteroposterior dimensions of the upper airway (Fig. 17.3). If chin lift is not effective, the next maneuver is jaw thrust (See Video 17.2), which primarily alleviates obstruction caused by the epiglottis protruding posteriorly into the airway. The third maneuver, which is usually done simultaneously with the first two, is application of continuous positive airway pressure (CPAP), which distends all the soft tissues of the pharynx and larynx. Occasionally, when upper airway

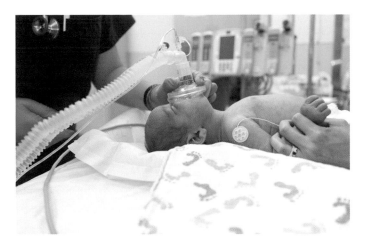

• **Fig 17.3.** Infant mask ventilation. The infant's chin is held in extension with the middle finger of the left hand. (Photograph courtesy Douglas Preuss.)

collapse is severe, as may occur in neonates, it is also necessary to increase peak inflating pressures beyond the recommended 15 cmH$_2$O to distend collapsed airway mucosal surfaces. However, doing so risks gastric insufflation, which may further compromise effective air entry into the lungs. If all of the above maneuvers (which, in aggregate, should not take more than about 30–45 seconds to perform) do not result in an unobstructed upper airway, the next steps include oral or nasal airway insertion, supraglottic airway (SGA) insertion, or tracheal intubation.

Oral Airway Insertion

Insertion of an oral airway establishes airflow by bypassing soft tissue obstruction, or more commonly in preschool-aged children, enlarged tonsils or adenoids. The most commonly used oral airway in pediatric patients is the Guedel type, which contains a central lumen that allows the passage of air and, if needed, a suction catheter. It can be inserted with the aid of a tongue depressor or by initially orienting the distal tip cephalad and then turning it 180 degrees at the posterior aspect of the palate.

Oral airways are sized based on their length (50–80 mm sizes are suitable for most children) or based on an arbitrary scale designated by the manufacturer. The appropriate size is determined by placing the airway adjacent to the child's face to approximate its position in the oral cavity (Fig. 17.4). When appropriately positioned, the distal end of the oral airway should curve along the posterior portion of the tongue, without the proximal end protruding out of the mouth or the distal end extending near the epiglottis. If the chosen size is too small, it can push the tongue against the posterior pharyngeal wall, and if it is too large, it may obstruct the laryngeal inlet.

Nasal Airway Insertion

A nasal airway is a soft flexible tube that can be used to relieve upper airway obstruction and to provide a conduit for delivering oxygen and anesthetic gases. Nasal airways are usually available in sizes 12- to 36-French (French = outer diameter divided by 3 in mm). A "custom" nasal airway can be fashioned by cutting off the appropriate length of an endotracheal tube but this would be less flexible than commercially made nasal airways and cause more trauma to the nasal mucosa.

Before insertion of a nasal airway, the nose should be inspected to assure the absence of significant septal deviation, or other visible causes of narrowing (e.g., polyp) that would interfere with placement of the device. However, nasal patency is not reliably predicted by external visualization. To avoid trauma and bleeding of the delicate nasal mucosa, the nasal airway should be well lubricated and inserted in a posterior caudal direction along the floor of the nasal cavity. A topical vasoconstrictor, such as 0.05% oxymetazoline, can be sprayed into the nasal canal before airway insertion. The proper diameter is determined by approximating the circular diameter of the nasal opening. The proper length of the nasal airway is estimated by measuring the distance from the nares to the tragus of the ear. When appropriately placed, its distal tip should lie at the level of the angle of the mandible between the posterior aspect of the tongue and above the tip of the epiglottis. Some red rubber nasal airways are supplied with a movable ring at the proximal end, with which to adjust the proper length at the tip of the nasal opening.

The most common complication from nasal airway insertion is trauma to the nasal or pharyngeal mucosa that results in bleeding. Adenoidal tissue may be disrupted and bleed into the oropharynx. Occasionally, a friable vessel is encountered in the nasal mucosa and bleeding is brisk. A lesser-known, though not rare, complication is the insertion of the nasal airway device into a false passage behind the posterior wall mucosa of the nasal and oral pharynx. This is not usually accompanied by bleeding, so it may be caused by a patent Thornwaldt[4] bursa. Nasal airways should not be inserted in children with a coagulopathy, neutropenia, or suspicion of a traumatic basilar skull fracture.[1]

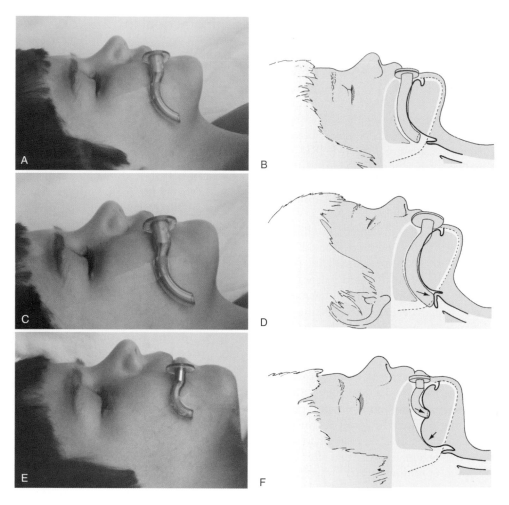

• **Fig 17.4.** The oral airway. The oral airway should curve around the tongue to the angle of the mandible (A, B). A poorly sized oral airway can encroach on the laryngeal inlet (C, D) or obstruction (E, F). (From: Fiadjoe JE, Litman RS, Serber JF. The pediatric airway. In: Coté CJ, Lerman J, Anderson BJ, eds. *A Practice of Anesthesia for Infants and Children*. 6th ed. Philadelphia: Elsevier; 2019: 297–339.e21.)

Supraglottic Airways (SGA)

In the 1990s, the original laryngeal mask airway (LMA) revolutionized airway management and patient safety. It had its shortcomings and improved versions gradually became available. In this section, we discuss the basics about supraglottic airway (SGA) use in children (Table 17.1), using the original LMA as an example because the most has been written about it; but if you want a more detailed discussion, check out the chapters we wrote for the latest editions of Smith or Cote's encyclopedic books on pediatric anesthesia. There, we discuss newer types of SGAs such as the Cobra (Cobra = Engineered Medical Systems, Indianapolis, IN), laryngeal tube, and iGel (iGel = Intersurgical, East Syracuse, NY). Over the years, each of us has developed our favorite SGA for use in children, but there really are no striking clinical differences between them. At The Children's Hospital of Philadelphia (CHOP), we mainly use the Ambu (Ambu = Ambu Inc, Columbia, MD) disposable airways because their preformed shape seems to fit well into the pediatric upper airway without too much displacement or malpositioning.

When the classic LMA was first introduced, it was primarily used as a substitute for the face mask. But over

TABLE 17.1	LMA Sizes for Children	
LMA Size	**Appropriate Weight (kg)**	**Cuff Volume (mL)**
1	<5	2–5
1.5	5–10	3–8
2	10–20	5–10
2.5	20–30	10–15
3	30–50	15–20
4	50–70	25–30

the years, it has also become a substitute for the endotracheal tube in certain procedures such as eye surgery and tonsillectomy (with the flexible LMA). In children with normal airway anatomy, positive-pressure ventilation is easily accomplished through an LMA, but the peak inspiratory pressure should not exceed 15 cmH$_2$O to prevent gastric insufflation. Because of its inability to reliably seal off the trachea, the LMA is not indicated for use in children at increased risk for pulmonary aspiration of gastric contents.

The original models of the LMA were not ideally suited for use in small children. Because of the relatively cephalad location of the pediatric larynx, the LMA (especially sizes 1, 1.5, and 2) was hard to "seat", or position, and commonly became dislodged during surgery. This required either repositioning or replacing with an endotracheal tube. Fiberoptic bronchoscopy and magnetic resonance imaging (MRI) studies demonstrated a high incidence of the epiglottis situated within the aperture of the LMA, despite adequate ventilation. The application of jaw thrust during LMA insertion may prevent downfolding of the epiglottis.

A variety of methods of LMA placement in children have been described. The "Brain" method (named after Archie Brain, the creator of the LMA) consists of pushing the flattened LMA cuff against the hard palate while simultaneously guiding the LMA to slide down into position. Alternatively, it can be inserted with the cuff partially or fully deflated, or inserted with the aperture facing posterior and then turned 180 degrees after passing behind the tongue. There are no advantages to any one method. We usually put some water-based lubricant on the posterior surface of the LMA to decrease the resistance to insertion, and use the Brain method while pulling the jaw anteriorly by grasping behind the lower incisors. In some children, insertion is difficult and causes pharyngeal bleeding. Some children may have a sore throat after LMA placement, but it is not as common as after endotracheal intubation.

During emergence from general anesthesia, the LMA can be removed at any time after suctioning the oropharynx (the child does not need to be deeply anesthetized to prevent laryngospasm, as with "deep" extubation of an endotracheal tube). Removal with the cuff inflated will also facilitate removal of blood or secretions that collect above the cuff. Some providers routinely place an oral airway at the same time as LMA removal.

Endotracheal Intubation

Laryngoscopy

In most children older than about 2 years of age, laryngoscopy is relatively straightforward and technically easy. An unexpected difficult view of the glottis is unusual in children with normal airway anatomy. In neonates and small infants, laryngoscopy can be challenging because of the smaller and more cephalad location of the larynx, and the narrower view through the oropharynx. At CHOP, videolaryngoscopy for infants less than 2 months of age has become mandatory (see A Deeper Dive box, below). The optimal position for laryngoscopy is different than for adults. The relatively large occiput of the small infant naturally flexes the head, while the shoulders lie flat on the table (Fig. 17.5). The anesthesiologist's line of sight should be nearly directly over the child's airway, and the laryngoscope blade is inserted almost perpendicular to the operating room (OR) table to obtain the easiest view of the glottis (Fig. 17.6). This is in contrast to adults, in whom the best glottic view is usually obtained with the laryngoscope blade almost parallel to the OR table.

A variety of pediatric-sized laryngoscope blades are available. A straight blade is most often used to obtain the best glottic view. In infants and small children, the straight blade is usually inserted into the vallecula to tilt the epiglottis anteriorly to view the glottic opening. The infant's small size and anteriorly placed larynx afford the anesthesiologist the opportunity to use the fifth finger of the left hand to push the larynx in a posterior direction to improve the glottic view (Fig. 17.7).

Endotracheal Tubes

Many formulas have been developed to predict the most appropriate size endotracheal tube in children, based on age, weight, or height. All of these formulas have reasonable

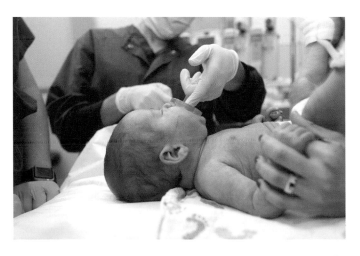

• **Fig 17.5.** The large occiput and neck flexion. The large occiput of the infant provides natural neck flexion. (Photograph courtesy Douglas Preuss.)

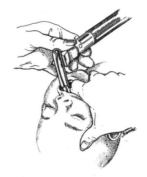
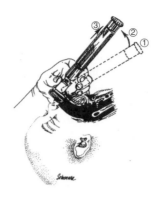

• **Fig 17.6.** The laryngoscope blade is inserted down the center of the tongue and lifts the epiglottis up and out of the way. The final laryngoscope blade angle is more perpendicular to the table in children compared with adults. (From: Lukish JR, Eichelberger MR. Infants and children as accident victims and their emergency management. In: Coran AG, ed. *Pediatric Surgery*. 7th ed. Vol 1. Philadelphia, PA: Saunders; 2012:261–270.)

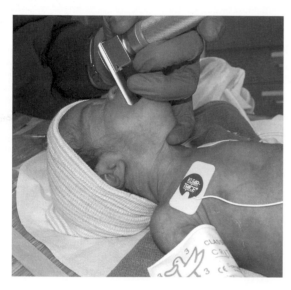

• **Fig 17.7.** Laryngoscopy of an infant. During laryngoscopy of an infant, the 5th finger of the left hand can provide external pressure to improve visualization of the glottis.

TABLE 17.2	Laryngoscope Blade Types and Sizes for Children			
Age	Miller	Wis-Hippel	Macintosh	
Premature neonate	0	—	—	
Term neonate	0–1	—	—	
1–12 months	1	—	—	
1–2 years	1	1.5	2	
2–6 years	2	—	2	
6–12 years	2	—	3	

reliability. The most popular formula for predicting the correct **uncuffed** oral endotracheal tube size is Cole's formula:

$$\frac{16 + Age}{4}$$

A modified Cole's formula can be used to estimate the most appropriate **cuffed** endotracheal tube size.

$$\frac{16 + Age}{5}$$

Once one gains enough experience with pediatric patients, formulas are abandoned in favor of a "mental" chart (Table 17.2). When using a cuffed endotracheal tube (see below), the choice of its size is less important because the cuff can compensate for the selection of too small a tube. On the other hand, manufacturers of endotracheal tubes have a variety of differences[6] with regard to the internal-to-outer-diameter ratios and differences in distal placement of the cuff.

A RAE (Ring-Adair-Elwyn) endotracheal tube is preformed so that the proximal end curves over the chin, and is used for procedures on the mouth or face, where the surgeon sits above the head of the patient. The proximal end of the nasal RAE tube is preformed to rest on the forehead during procedures in the oral cavity or neck. Because a RAE tube is preformed, it is difficult to adjust its length once it is properly placed.

Cuffed versus Uncuffed Tubes

Before the beginning of the 21st century, pediatric anesthesiologists preferred to use uncuffed endotracheal tubes in children up to the prepubertal age group. This practice was based on the notion that the unyielding cricoid ring is functionally the narrowest portion of the upper airway, so a cuff is not necessary to seal off the upper portion of the trachea to provide adequate ventilation and prevent pulmonary aspiration. It was thought that at some uncertain age between 6 and 10 years, the larynx changes shape from conical to cylindrical, and the glottis becomes the narrowest portion; a cuff is then needed to seal off the trachea because the portion of the endotracheal tube that passes the cricoid ring is no longer snug. These hypotheses[7] were based on data obtained from pediatric cadaver specimens, and the clinical observation that an endotracheal tube will often pass easily through the vocal cords, only to meet resistance at the level of the cricoid ring. Furthermore, an uncuffed endotracheal tube will have a relatively smaller external diameter compared with a cuffed endotracheal tube of the same internal diameter. Therefore, a relatively larger-sized internal diameter tube can be inserted comfortably. This will provide relatively less resistance to air-flow, and will facilitate suctioning of secretions.

However, it has now become standard for pediatric anes-thesiologists to use cuffed endotracheal tubes in all children, even neonates. This practice has been the result of the recog-nition that cuffed tubes are not associated with an increased incidence of airway complications,[8] and the dimensions of the pediatric larynx, in fact, do not change their diameter relationships during development.[9] Furthermore, because spontaneous ventilation in intubated children is rare, the increased resistance of the slightly smaller internal diameter tube will not increase work of breathing. Use of a cuffed endotracheal tube will prevent the need to change the tube if it is incorrectly sized, thus sparing the child from an extra laryngoscopic attempt. The very act of changing endotra-cheal tubes while the child is anesthetized increases the risk for laryngeal injury and the concentration of inhaled vapors in the OR environment. Avoidance of a leak around the endotracheal tube will also increase the precision of the val-ues and the waveform pattern of the capnographic tracing.

Additional advantages to using a cuffed tube include the ability to ventilate using higher inflation pressures if necessary, and a theoretical decreased risk for pulmonary aspiration. All of these above-mentioned advantages of cuffed endotracheal tubes have rendered the uncuffed tube nearly obsolete.[10]

The choice of a cuffed tube will influence the incidence of postoperative sore throat.[11] Cuffed tubes with relatively low cuff pressures (below 20 cmH_2O) will result in sore throat incidence of less than 4%, but the use of uncuffed tubes and cuffed tubes with cuff pressures over 20 cmH_2O will significantly increase that incidence.

A newly designed endotracheal tube[12] (Microcuff, Kimberly-Clark) has been developed with the intention of minimizing trauma to the young infant's trachea by prevent-ing mucosal trauma and subsequent inflammation, scarring, and stenosis. It does so by having a thin, low-pressure, high-volume cuff that is more distally placed than normal endo-tracheal tubes, and thus below the vulnerable subglottic area. These types of endotracheal tubes are being used more fre-quently, but there is no proof of definitive benefit over exist-ing endotracheal tubes. This newly designed endotracheal tube is also available in a preformed[13] (i.e., RAE) model.

Confirming Tracheal Location

Methods for confirming tracheal placement include the characteristic rise of the chest wall, absence of gastric

A DEEPER DIVE

The Video Laryngoscopy in Small Infants Trial

The Video Laryngoscopy in Small Infants[14] (VLSI) trial was a multicenter, randomized trial comparing videolaryngoscopy (VL) and direct laryngoscopy (DL) in small infants. Primary outcome measures included first attempt success rates, and secondary outcomes included number of intubation attempts, time to successful orotracheal intubation, frequency of failure to intubate with the randomized device, and frequency of nonsevere and severe complications. Over 500 infants (mean age 5.5 months, Standard Deviation (SD) 3.3) were random-ized (274 in VL group and 278 in DL group). In the VL group, 254 (93%) had first attempt success compared with 244 (88%) of 278 in the DL group ($P = .024$). Severe complications occurred in 4 (2%) infants in the VL group compared with 15 (5%) in the DL group ($P = .009$). There was one esophageal intubation with VL, and seven with DL ($P = .028$).

As a result of this study's findings and accumulating experi-ence with VL in our own departments, we feel strongly that VL will become the standard-of-care method for tracheal intuba-tion in neonates and infants, and possibly older children as well.

inflation, breath sounds in the left axilla, absence of breath sounds over the epigastrium, and a robust capnographic tracing. These are all confirmed simultaneously in the first several seconds after tracheal intubation. When the endotra-cheal tube is placed in the trachea, mist should be observed in the proximal end of the tube during exhalation. In small infants, breath sounds are easily transmitted across the epi-gastrium and chest wall, so auscultation may be less reliable for confirming tracheal placement.

Confirming Proper Endotracheal Tube Dimensions

Diameter

After successful placement of the cuffed endotracheal tube, the cuff should be inflated just to the point at which there is minimal expiratory leak. This is determined by compar-ing the difference between the inspiratory and expiratory tidal volumes displayed on the anesthesia machine. Cuff pressures should be maintained between 10 and 25 cmH_2O to avoid damage to the subglottic mucosa. When the leak pressure is below 10 cmH_2O, the cuff can be slowly inflated to achieve a slightly higher leak pressure. When the pres-sure is above 30 cmH_2O without any cuff inflation, con-sideration should be given to changing the tracheal tube to a smaller size; however, for short surgical procedures, it is unknown whether this tight fit is associated with tracheal injury.

Length

There are several reliable methods for determining the proper length of insertion of the endotracheal tube in chil-dren without resorting to a specific formula.

First, during direct laryngoscopy and insertion of the endotracheal tube through the glottis, the length is noted at which the endotracheal tube has been inserted 2 to 3 cm past the vocal cords. Some endotracheal tube manufacturers place black line markings at the distal end of the tube that are designed to rest at the level of the vocal cords.

Second, for most children with normal airway anatomy, the proper length in centimeters at which to secure the endotracheal tube at the teeth (or gums for infants) is three times the internal diameter of the tube used (in millimeters), assuming that the proper size of endotracheal tube has been chosen.

The last method is to bounce one's fingers along the external trachea in the area of the suprasternal notch while simultaneously feeling the endotracheal tube cuff balloon. If the endotracheal tube is located in the proper position, the cuff will be palpated maximally at the suprasternal notch.

Neck Movement Effects

A number of studies have looked at the effects of different neck movements on the position of the endotracheal tube in the trachea in children. These studies[15] consistently demonstrate the following:
- Neck **flexion** causes the tip of the endotracheal tube to move toward the carina.
- Neck **extension** causes the tip to move away from the carina.
- Lateral **rotation** causes the tip to move away from the carina, although to a lesser extent than occurs during neck extension.
- These findings are similar with both orotracheal and nasotracheal tube placement.

Nasotracheal Intubation

Nasotracheal intubation is safe in children of all ages. Now that we routinely use cuffed tubes, it is probably a good idea to use a half size smaller than the appropriate oral route size. The nasal approach is preferred when an oral tube would interfere with an intraoral surgical procedure. The most common acute complication from nasotracheal intubation is bleeding that results from the tube shearing off nasal or adenoidal friable tissue. This can be decreased by softening the tube by presoaking it in hot water, but we now prefer the red rubber catheter technique.[16] This consists of preinsertion of a lubricated, appropriately sized red rubber catheter through the nasal passage and into the oropharynx (it is initially used as a "sound" in each nasal passage to determine whether one side is more patent than the other). The nonleading flanged end of the rubber tube is attached to the beveled end of the nasotracheal tube to provide a nontraumatic leading edge through the nasopharynx, and then detached when the tracheal tube passes into the oropharynx. Before insertion of the nasotracheal tube, we administer 0.05% oxymetazoline into each nasal passage to further attenuate bleeding.

Nasotracheal tube insertion in children is not technically different than that for adults, except that the unique

TABLE 17.3	Approximate Cuffed Endotracheal Tube Sizes for Full-Term Infants and Children	
Age	Size (Internal Diameter mm)
0–4 months	3.0
4 months–12 months	3.5–4.0
10 months–2 years	4.0
2–3 years	4.5
3–5 years	5.0
6–10 years	5.5
10–14 years	6.0
15–18 years	6.5–7.0

angling of the child's oropharynx usually necessitates the assistance of a Magill forceps to feed the tracheal tube in an anterior direction toward the glottic inlet. Because nasotracheal intubation may result in a transient bacteremia, some centers may choose to administer endocarditis prophylaxis in certain high-risk susceptible children, specifically those described in Table 17.3 of the most recent (2007) iteration of the American Heart Association (AHA) guidelines[17] on prevention of infective endocarditis.

Rapid Sequence Induction

The key components of a rapid sequence induction (RSI) of general anesthesia include preoxygenation, apneic oxygenation after administration of a hypnotic agent and muscle relaxant, and application of cricoid pressure to prevent passive regurgitation of gastric contents into the pharynx. In recent years the standard of care in pediatric anesthesia has been to perform a traditional RSI with the application of "soft" ventilation.[18] This has become the predominant practice because of the increasing recognition that small children desaturate quickly and cannot tolerate brief periods of apnea. In addition, it seems that pulmonary aspiration occurs only rarely in pediatric anesthesia and under unique circumstances (see below). Therefore, cricoid pressure is also decreasingly used.[19] Each of the components of pediatric RSI will be reviewed as they pertain to their usefulness in pediatric patients.

Preoxygenation

Preoxygenation, with the goal of removing nitrogen from the lungs, is performed before RSI to lengthen the duration of apnea before laryngoscopy. In adults, preoxygenation is attained by breathing 100% oxygen for several minutes or asking the patient to take several vital capacity breaths. These maneuvers are not possible in uncooperative children who struggle with face mask application. On the other hand, the relatively smaller ratio of functional residual capacity (FRC) to tidal volume will facilitate a more rapid denitrogenation in children compared with adults. Nevertheless, the optimal length of time for denitrogenation of the pediatric lung has not been determined, although longer preoxygenation times are associated with longer times to desaturation during apnea in children over 2 years of age. A reasonable approach is to administer 100% oxygen for at least 1 minute before rapid sequence induction, or longer until the oxygen saturation increases and stabilizes.

Apneic Oxygenation

Apneic oxygenation is the process by which the lungs continue to take up oxygen in the absence of spontaneous or controlled breathing movements. It occurs by bulk flow of oxygen from an oxygen source (i.e., anesthesia breathing circuit) through a patent upper airway and trachea. Oxygen will continue to flow into the lungs as it is absorbed by the blood passing through the pulmonary vascular bed.

Apneic oxygenation occurs during the phase of RSI that follows preoxygenation and administration of a hypnotic agent plus a neuromuscular blocker. This period is required for the neuromuscular blocker to take effect before performing laryngoscopy. In healthy, nonobese children, oxyhemoglobin desaturation during apnea may not occur for several minutes. In infants and small children, oxyhemoglobin desaturation during apnea will occur rapidly, often within seconds, despite seemingly adequate preoxygenation and denitrogenation. This phenomenon is commonly attributed to the infant's relatively lower FRC while anesthetized, combined with larger oxygen consumption per weight. It is for this reason that, during RSI in infants and small children, positive-pressure ventilation is usually required before endotracheal intubation. When this is performed while cricoid pressure continues, it is termed a "modified" or "controlled" rapid sequence induction.

Cricoid Pressure

Although cricoid pressure reliably occludes the esophagus in infants and children in experimental conditions,[20] its clinical usefulness has never been decidedly demonstrated. In small infants, cricoid pressure may compress the trachea[21] and prevent adequate air entry into the lungs. The pros and cons of cricoid pressure are presented in a 2009 editorial[22] in which the author is critical of its routine use without proven benefit.

Airway Complications

Laryngospasm

Laryngospasm describes a powerful self-protective response of the glottic and supraglottic laryngeal adductor muscles that causes partial or complete airway obstruction during attempts at inspiration (see Video 17.3). Laryngospasm may result from stimulation of a number of anatomic sites, including the nasal mucosa, soft palate, pharynx, epiglottis, larynx, tracheobronchial tree, lung tissue, diaphragm, and abdominal viscera. In anesthetized children, laryngospasm is caused mainly by secretions or blood that contact the laryngeal mucosa in or around the glottic opening. It can also be caused by the laryngeal stimulation that occurs during tracheal extubation in a child who has not fully regained consciousness. Risk factors that increase the likelihood of laryngospasm include an active or recent upper respiratory infection[23] and chronic exposure to secondhand tobacco smoke.[23]

Laryngospasm manifests as partial or complete upper airway obstruction that is not easily relieved by manual airway maneuvers or placement of an oral airway. The distinction between partial and complete upper airway obstruction is important because the treatment of laryngospasm differs between the two conditions. In partial upper airway obstruction, which is diagnosed by the presence of high-pitched inspiratory stridor, a small amount of air entry is possible with the administration of positive-pressure ventilation. This will, in many cases, treat hypoxemia, and allow the passage of anesthetic gases to deepen the level of unconsciousness, thereby alleviating the laryngospasm. Partial laryngospasm can also be alleviated to some extent by applying a jaw thrust maneuver, which stretches the laryngeal structures in an anterior direction and widens the partially obstructed airway. In the absence of hypoxemia, partial upper airway obstruction that does not respond to these conservative measures can be relieved by intravenous administration of a nondepolarizing neuromuscular blocker or propofol, 2 to 4 mg/kg. Hypoxemia is a potent stimulus for the alleviation of laryngospasm, but it should never be relied upon in lieu of pharmacologic therapy because hypoxemia is associated with the development of negative-pressure pulmonary edema (see below) and/or cardiac arrest.[24]

Laryngospasm that causes complete upper airway obstruction usually results in the rapid development of hypoxemia and is not amenable to application of positive airway pressure. When hypoxemia develops, you should immediately give intravenous succinylcholine (as little as 0.1–0.2 mg/kg usually works quickly). If intravascular access has not been established, intramuscular succinylcholine 4 mg/kg should be administered.

A DEEPER DIVE

What is the basis for recommending 4 mg/kg as the intramuscular (IM) dose of succinylcholine that best alleviates laryngospasm? It is based on data[25] showing that 4 mg/kg achieves faster and better relaxation compared with 2 or 3 mg/kg as measured by twitch monitoring. In clinical practice, however, there exists no evidence that the administered dose of IM succinylcholine influences clinical outcomes. We performed a quality review of 248 patients who received IM succinylcholine at our institution over a 17-year period. Doses ranged from 0.5 mg/kg to 7.2 mg/kg, and no correlation with nadir oxygen saturation or need for cardiopulmonary resuscitation was observed (Fig. 17.8).

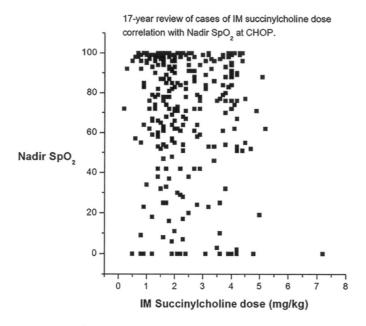

17-year review of cases of IM succinylcholine dose correlation with Nadir SpO$_2$ at CHOP.

• Fig 17.8. Review of airway events requiring intramuscular succinylcholine over a 17-year period at a single institution. The nadir oxygen saturation during events was compared with succinylcholine dose used and did not demonstrate a significant correlation.

Pulmonary Aspiration

Pulmonary aspiration of gastric contents is usually diagnosed when a child demonstrates hypoxemia and respiratory symptoms along with: (1) the direct observation of gastric contents in the pharynx or larynx; or (2) characteristic findings on chest radiography. It is a rare perioperative complication in children, with an estimated incidence ≤0.1% in retrospective studies. Most cases of perioperative pulmonary aspiration in children occur at the time of intubation and, when clinically significant, will cause symptoms within 2 hours. Risk factors for its occurrence include emergency surgery for bowel obstruction or ileus, and lack of sufficient paralysis at the time of laryngoscopy.

In two large retrospective series from 1998[26] and 1999,[27] the majority of children with directly observed pulmonary aspiration of gastric contents were asymptomatic. Symptomatic children developed cough, wheeze, or unexplained hypoxemia with radiologic changes, and some required postoperative mechanical ventilation, but all eventually recovered.

There are no data to indicate the proper preparative pharmacologic regimen for children suspected of being at risk for pulmonary aspiration. A variety of agents theoretically decrease this risk. Metoclopramide is a prokinetic agent, but most studies in children do not show convincing efficacy for its ability to decrease gastric volume or increase gastric pH at the time of induction of general anesthesia. Metoclopramide should not be administered to children with bowel obstruction or ileus. H$_2$ antagonists, such as ranitidine, reduce gastric volume and increase gastric pH in children; however, for optimal efficacy, these agents should be administered at least 2 hours before surgery. Few pediatric anesthesiologists continue to administer prophylactic medications for children at risk for aspiration because there is no known benefit.

Treatment of the child with suspected pulmonary aspiration includes supplemental oxygen and mechanical ventilation as needed for hypoxemia, respiratory distress, or ventilatory failure. Children with mild symptoms such as cough or wheeze should remain in the hospital and monitored appropriately. Asymptomatic children who do not require supplemental oxygen after a witnessed intraoperative aspiration may receive routine postoperative care including discharge home, if appropriate. Chest radiography is indicated only in the presence of respiratory distress or unexplained persistent hypoxemia.

Negative-Pressure (Postobstructive) Pulmonary Edema

Acute pulmonary edema that develops after a brief episode of severe upper airway obstruction is known as negative-pressure (or postobstructive) pulmonary edema. It most often occurs shortly after alleviation of severe laryngospasm, but it can also be observed after upper airway obstruction of any cause. Biting on the endotracheal tube or SGA during emergence can also cause negative-pressure pulmonary edema; thus a bite block should be inserted before emergence, unless the device is removed before the patient regains consciousness.

The exact mechanism of the development of pulmonary edema after upper airway obstruction is unknown; however, the concomitant development of transient hypoxia appears to be an important contributing factor. Most authors speculate that the substantial negative intrathoracic pressure that results when a child attempts to breath against an obstruction results in a dramatic increase in venous return to the right side of the heart. Hypoxemia that accompanies the obstruction leads to sympathetic discharge that promotes systemic vasoconstriction. These two aforementioned processes result in the rapid transudation of fluid and lymph into the alveoli.

The clinical manifestations of negative-pressure pulmonary edema include the rapid development of rales, the appearance of a frothy pink fluid in the endotracheal tube, and a variable degree of hypoxemia. Treatment includes administration of supplemental oxygen, continuous positive airway pressure or positive end-expiratory pressure (if mechanically ventilated), and furosemide. An echocardiogram may be indicated to rule out a cardiogenic cause. In healthy children, symptoms usually resolve within 12 to 24 hours.

References

1. Schwartz DS, Keller MS. Maturational descent of the epiglottis. *Arch Otolaryngol Head Neck Surg.* 1997;123(6):627–628. doi:10.1001/archotol.1997.01900060069012..

2. Eruption Charts. American Dental Association. www.mouth-healthy.org/en/az-topics/e/eruption-charts.

3. Lagarde S, Semjen F, Nouette-Gaulain K, et al. Facemask pressure-controlled ventilation in children: what is the pressure limit? *Anesth Analg.* 2010;110(6):1676–1679. doi:10.1213/ANE.0b013e3181d8a14c.

4. Ghorayeb BY. Tornwaldt's (Thornwaldt's) Bursa / Cyst. Otolaryngology Houston. Updated October 4, 2014. Accessed 21.07.21. http://www.ghorayeb.com/thornwaldtbursa.html.

5. Pandey AK, Sharma AK, Diyora BD, Sayal PP, Ingale HA, Radhakrishnan M. Inadvertent insertion of nasogastric tube into the brain. *J Assoc Physicians India.* 2004;52:322–323.

6. Weiss M, Dullenkopf A, Gysin C, Dillier CM, Gerber AC. Shortcomings of cuffed paediatric tracheal tubes. *Br J Anaesth.* 2004;92(1):78–88. doi:10.1093/bja/aeh023.

7. Eckenhoff JE. Some anatomic considerations of the infant larynx influencing endotracheal anesthesia. *Anesthesiology.* 1951;12(4):401–410. doi:10.1097/00000542-195107000-00001.

8. Khine HH, Corddry DH, Kettrick RG, et al. Comparison of cuffed and uncuffed endotracheal tubes in young children during general anesthesia. *Anesthesiology.* 1997;86(3):627–631. doi:10.1097/00000542-199703000-00015. discussion 27A.

9. Litman RS, Weissend EE, Shibata D, Westesson PL. Developmental changes of laryngeal dimensions in unparalyzed, sedated children. *Anesthesiology.* 2003;98(1):41–45. doi:10.1097/00000542-200301000-00010.

10. Litman RS, Maxwell LG. Cuffed versus uncuffed endotracheal tubes in pediatric anesthesia: the debate should finally end. *Anesthesiology.* 2013;118(3):500–501. doi:10.1097/ALN.0b013e318282cc8f.

11. Calder A, Hegarty M, Erb TO, von Ungern-Sternberg BS. Predictors of postoperative sore throat in intubated children. *Paediatr Anaesth.* 2012;22(3):239–243. doi:10.1111/j.1460-9592.2011.03727.x.

12. Dullenkopf A, Gerber AC, Weiss M. Fit and seal characteristics of a new paediatric tracheal tube with high volume-low pressure polyurethane cuff. *Acta Anaesthesiol Scand.* 2005;49(2):232–237. doi:10.1111/j.1399-6576.2005.00599.x.

13. Weiss M, Dullenkopf A, Böttcher S, et al. Clinical evaluation of cuff and tube tip position in a newly designed paediatric pre-formed oral cuffed tracheal tube. *Br J Anaesth.* 2006;97(5):695–700. doi:10.1093/bja/ael247.

14. Garcia-Marcinkiewicz AG, Kovatsis PG, Hunyady AI, et al. First-attempt success rate of video laryngoscopy in small infants (VISI): a multicentre, randomised controlled trial. *Lancet.* 2020;396(10266):1905–1913. doi:10.1016/S0140-6736(20)32532-0.

15. Weiss M, Knirsch W, Kretschmar O, et al. Tracheal tube-tip displacement in children during head-neck movement-a radiological assessment. *Br J Anaesth.* 2006;96(4):486–491. doi:10.1093/bja/ael014.

16. Watt S, Pickhardt D, Lerman J, Armstrong J, Creighton PR, Feldman L. Telescoping tracheal tubes into catheters minimizes epistaxis during nasotracheal intubation in children. *Anesthesiology.* 2007;106(2):238–242. doi:10.1097/00000542-200702000-00010.

17. Wilson W, Taubert K, Gewitz M, et al. Prevention of Infective Endocarditis: Guidelines From the American Heart Association: A Guideline From the American Heart Association Rheumatic Fever, Endocarditis, and Kawasaki Disease Committee, Council on Cardiovascular Disease in the Young, and the Council on Clinical Cardiology, Council on Cardiovascular Surgery and Anesthesia, and the Quality of Care and Outcomes Research Interdisciplinary Working Group [published correction appears in Circulation. 2007 Oct 9;116(15):e376-7]. *Circulation.* 2007;116(15):1736–1754. doi:10.1161/CIRCULATIONAHA.106.183095.

18. Weiss M, Gerber AC. Rapid sequence induction in children - it's not a matter of time! *Paediatr Anaesth.* 2008;18(2):97–99. doi:10.1111/j.1460-9592.2007.02324.x.

19. Kojima T, Harwayne-Gidansky I, Shenoi AN, et al. Cricoid Pressure During Induction for Tracheal Intubation in Critically Ill Children: A Report From National Emergency Airway Registry for Children. *Pediatr Crit Care Med.* 2018;19(6):528–537. doi:10.1097/PCC.0000000000001531.

20. Trethewy CE, Burrows JM, Clausen D, Doherty SR. Effectiveness of cricoid pressure in preventing gastric aspiration during rapid sequence intubation in the emergency department: study protocol for a randomised controlled trial. *Trials.* 2012;13:17 doi:10.1186/1745-6215-13-17. Published 2012 Feb 16.

21. Walker RW, Ravi R, Haylett K. Effect of cricoid force on airway calibre in children: a bronchoscopic assessment. *Br J Anaesth.* 2010;104(1):71–74. doi:10.1093/bja/aep337.

22. Lerman J. On cricoid pressure: "may the force be with you.". *Anesth Analg.* 2009;109(5):1363–1366. doi:10.1213/ANE.0b013e3181bbc6cf.

23. Schreiner MS, O'Hara I, Markakis DA, Politis GD. Do children who experience laryngospasm have an increased risk of upper respiratory tract infection? *Anesthesiology.* 1996;85(3):475–480. doi:10.1097/00000542-199609000-00005.

24. Bhananker SM, Ramamoorthy C, Geiduschek JM, et al. Anesthesia-related cardiac arrest in children: update from the Pediatric Perioperative Cardiac Arrest Registry. *Anesth Analg.* 2007;105(2):344–350. doi:10.1213/01.ane.0000268712.00756.dd.

25. Liu LM, DeCook TH, Goudsouzian NG, Ryan JF, Liu PL. Dose response to intramuscular succinylcholine in children. *Anesthesiology.* 1981;55(5):599–602. doi:10.1097/00000542-198111000-00027.

26. Borland LM, Sereika SM, Woelfel SK, et al. Pulmonary aspiration in pediatric patients during general anesthesia: incidence

and outcome. *J Clin Anesth*. 1998;10(2):95–102. doi:10.1016/s0952-8180(97)00250-x.

27. Warner MA, Warner ME, Warner DO, Warner LO, Warner EJ. Perioperative pulmonary aspiration in infants and children. *Anesthesiology*. 1999;90(1):66–71. doi:10.1097/00000542-199901000-00011.

Suggested Readings

Engelhardt T, Virag K, Veyckemans F, Habre W. APRICOT Group of the European Society of Anaesthesiology Clinical Trial Network. Airway management in paediatric anaesthesia in Europe-insights from APRICOT (Anaesthesia Practice in Children Observational Trial): a prospective multicentre observational study in 261 hospitals in Europe. *Br J Anaesth*. 2018;121(1):66–75. doi:10.1016/j.bja.2018.04.013.

Cheon EC, Palac HL, Paik KH, et al. Unplanned, Postoperative Intubation in Pediatric Surgical Patients: Development and Validation of a Multivariable Prediction Model. *Anesthesiology*. 2016;125(5):914–928. doi:10.1097/ALN.0000000000001343.

Habre W, Disma N, Virag K, et al. Incidence of severe critical events in paediatric anaesthesia (APRICOT): a prospective multicentre observational study in 261 hospitals in Europe [published correction appears in Lancet Respir Med. 2017 May;5(5):e19] [published correction appears in Lancet Respir Med. 2017 Jun;5(6):e22]. *Lancet Respir Med*. 2017;5(5):412–425. doi:10.1016/S2213-2600(17)30116-9.

Kayashima K, Doi T, Yamasaki R, Imai K. Long-axis Ultrasonic Images of the Pediatric Larynx and Trachea with a Cuffed Endotracheal Tube. *Anesthesiology*. 2017;127(6):1016. doi:10.1097/ALN.0000000000001772.

Lakshmipathy N, Bokesch PM, Cowan DE, Lisman SR, Schmid CH. Environmental tobacco smoke: a risk factor for pediatric laryngospasm. *Anesth Analg*. 1996;82(4):724–727. doi:10.1097/00000539-199604000-00008.

Lorenz LG, Kleine-Brueggeney M, Luepold B, et al. Performance of the pediatric-sized i-gel compared with the Ambu AuraOnce laryngeal mask in anesthetized and ventilated children. *Anesthesiology*. 2011;115(1):102–110. doi:10.1097/ALN.0b013e318219d619.

Mathis MR, Haydar B, Taylor EL, et al. Failure of the Laryngeal Mask Airway Unique™ and Classic™ in the pediatric surgical patient: a study of clinical predictors and outcomes. *Anesthesiology*. 2013;119(6):1284–1295. doi:10.1097/ALN.0000000000000015.

Oberer C, von Ungern-Sternberg BS, Frei FJ, Erb TO. Respiratory reflex responses of the larynx differ between sevoflurane and propofol in pediatric patients. *Anesthesiology*. 2005;103(6):1142–1148. doi:10.1097/00000542-200512000-00007.

Reber A, Wetzel SG, Schnabel K, Bongartz G, Frei FJ. Effect of combined mouth closure and chin lift on upper airway dimensions during routine magnetic resonance imaging in pediatric patients sedated with propofol. *Anesthesiology*. 1999;90(6):1617–1623. doi:10.1097/00000542-199906000-00018.

Shibasaki M, Nakajima Y, Ishii S, Shimizu F, Shime N, Sessler DI. Prediction of pediatric endotracheal tube size by ultrasonography. *Anesthesiology*. 2010;113(4):819–824. doi:10.1097/ALN.0b013e3181ef6757.

Inomata S, Watanabe S, Taguchi M, Okada M. End-tidal Sevoflurane Concentration for Tracheal Intubation and Minimum Alveolar Concentration in Pediatric Patients. *Anesthesiology*. 1994;80(1):93–96. doi:10.1097/00000542-199401000-00016.

Windpassinger M, Plattner O, Gemeiner J, et al. Pharyngeal Oxygen Insufflation During AirTraq Laryngoscopy Slows Arterial Desaturation in Infants and Small Children. *Anesth Analg*. 2016;122(4):1153–1157. doi:10.1213/ANE.0000000000001189.

18

The Difficult Pediatric Airway

ANNERY G GARCIA-MARCINKIEWICZ, JOHN E. FIADJOE, AND RONALD S. LITMAN

In this chapter we review principles of pediatric difficult airway management, with a focus on those entities that cause anatomic or functional airway obstruction above the level of the glottis. We consider causes and treatments of anticipated and unanticipated difficult intubation and difficult ventilation. Finally, we will touch upon updated equipment and techniques for difficult airway management.

The most important aspect of anesthetic management of the difficult airway is having a clear plan and the multiple steps of the back-up plans. It is not enough to have only one or even two back-up plans, but rather three or four, and an exact plan for the worse possible situation: the development of life-threatening hypoxemia. Every anesthesiologist must know precisely the method to alleviate it and save the child's life. This could entail a cricothyrotomy or tracheotomy, which are more technically difficult in small children than in adults.

Proper preparation is essential and will depend on the cause of the expected difficulty. A full explanation of the anesthetic risks and benefits should be discussed with the child's family. An indwelling intravenous catheter is preferred, except when the anesthesiologist feels that provoking or painfully stimulating the child may worsen the upper airway obstruction, as may occur with acute epiglottitis. Another important aspect of pediatric difficult airway management is the presence of adequate help. This could be another experienced anesthesiologist or surgeon or other clinician depending on the clinical circumstances.

The difficult airway is an important cause of cardiac arrest during anesthesia in children. In the first reported pediatric Perioperative Cardiac Arrest (POCA) Registry,[1] respiratory complications accounted for 30 of the 150 reported cardiac arrests, and many of these cases were associated with difficult ventilation or intubation (Table 18.1).

Unlike adults, normal-appearing children rarely present with an unexpected difficult intubation. Therefore in this chapter only the *anticipated* difficult intubation will be reviewed.

Preanesthetic Preparation

The most reliable predictor of a difficult intubation is the patient's history. If a previous anesthetic record is available, it should be reviewed before administering a subsequent anesthetic. Physical examination should focus on anatomic anomalies that involve the head, face, or neck, especially if the child carries the diagnosis of a congenital airway syndrome (Table 18.2).

The anesthesiologist should evaluate the size and mobility of the mandible. The exam should also focus on any anatomic features that cause distortion of the airway or symptoms of airway obstruction (e.g., snoring) when supine. The most likely factor that predicts difficulty with intubation in pediatric patients is a small, malformed, or immobile mandible. Scoring systems that predict the likelihood of a difficult intubation do not exist for children.

The stepwise technical approach to securing tracheal intubation should be well-thought-out before the time of surgery (Fig. 18.1). All necessary airway equipment should be present in the operating room (OR), including the equipment necessary for the second, third, and even fourth options should initial attempts fail. In pediatrics, different sized laryngoscope blades and endotracheal tubes should be within easy reach.

In children with a known difficult intubation, it is preferable to secure venous access while the child is still awake. However, if the child is not amenable, or inspection of the limbs does not show promising possibilities, and if one believes the child will not be difficult to ventilate (based on history or physical exam) then general anesthesia may be induced without prior intravenous (IV) access.

An anticipated difficult intubation can be loosely defined as that which the anesthesiologist feels would be difficult to visualize the airway with standard techniques. In other words, the very nature of the anticipated difficult intubation implies that specialized indirect methods are required for tracheal intubation, and direct laryngoscopy should not be attempted first. With each direct laryngoscopy attempt,

TABLE 18.1 Respiratory Causes of Cardiac Arrest From the POCA[a] Registry

Respiratory Cause	Number of Cardiac Arrests
Laryngospasm	9
Airway obstruction	8
Difficult intubation	4
Inadequate oxygenation	3
Inadvertent extubation	2
Unclear etiology, presumed respiratory	2
Inadequate ventilation	1
Bronchospasm	1
Total	30

(Reproduced with permission from Morray JP, Geiduschek JM, Ramamoorthy C et al. Anesthesia-related cardiac arrest in children: initial findings of the Pediatric Perioperative Cardiac Arrest Registry. Anesthesiology 2000:93:6.)
[a]Perioperative Cardiac Arrest.

TABLE 18.2 Examples of Congenital Airway Syndromes

Syndrome	Clinical Characteristics
Beckwith-Wiedemann	Macroglossia, organomegaly, omphalocele, hypoglycemia
Down (trisomy 21)	Macroglossia
Pierre Robin sequence	Micrognathia, cleft palate, glossoptosis
Treacher Collins	Hypoplasia of the maxilla and mandible, variable eye and ear deformities
Hemifacial microsomia (e.g., Goldenhar) unilateral or bilateral mandibular	Hypoplasia, variable microphthalmia, microtia, macrostomia
Apert	Craniosynostosis, syndactyly
Freeman-Sheldon ("whistling face")	Microstomia, facial anomalies, hand anomalies
Mucopolysaccharidoses	Redundant facial and pharyngeal soft tissue
Klippel-Feil	Cervical vertebral fusion
Crouzon	Craniosynostosis
Stickler	Mandibular hypoplasia, myopia, retinal detachment, joint stiffness
Pfeiffer	Craniosynostosis, polydactyly

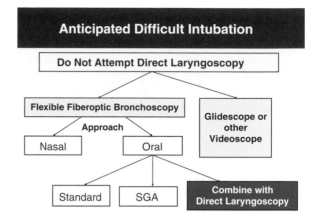

• **Fig 18.1.** Initial approach to the anticipated pediatric difficult intubation.

A DEEPER DIVE

In a multicenter study involving infants and children from the Pediatric Difficult Intubation (PeDI) Registry, the occurrence of a complication was associated with the number of tracheal intubation attempts; the odds of a complication increased 1.5-fold per attempt (Fig. 18.2). Direct laryngoscopy had a very low first-attempt success rate of 3% (16/461) compared with indirect techniques: fiber-optic bronchoscopy 54% (153/284) and video laryngoscopy 55% (101/183). Twenty percent of children had at least one complication, with 2% (15/1018) experiencing cardiac arrest. Temporary hypoxemia was the most common nonsevere complication and occurred in 9% (94/1018) of patients. Overall, complications were associated with multiple intubation attempts (>2), weight less than 10 kg, short thyromental distance, abnormal airway physical examination, and persistent direct laryngoscopy tracheal intubation attempts. Although hypoxemia may be a reversible complication, children have higher oxygen consumption rates than adults and therefore a much faster rate of arterial oxygen desaturation when apneic. When hypoxemia occurs, multiple intubation attempts are more likely, as the intubation attempt is interrupted to ventilate the patient. These nonsevere complications, such as hypoxemia, easily lead to severe complications such as cardiac arrest. Lessons learned from the PeDI Registry include limiting intubation attempts, using indirect techniques initially, and providing passive oxygenation throughout intubation attempts. Passive oxygenation is effective in children, delays the onset of hypoxemia, and provides more time for tracheal intubation.

the severity of airway edema and bleeding will increase and will ultimately decrease the chance of eventual success with more specialized methods.

Techniques

First-line indirect techniques include video laryngoscopy, intubating supraglottic airway (SGA), or the flexible fiberoptic bronchoscope. This choice is influenced by the patient's airway anatomy and is dependent on the experience and personal preference of the anesthesiologist. A

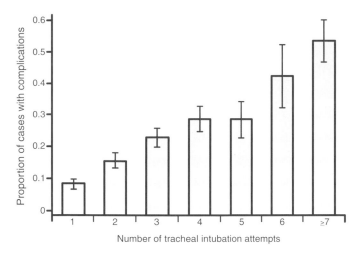

• **Fig 18.2.** The average proportion of cases with complications by the number of required intubation attempts. The odds of a complication increased 1.5-fold per attempt. Each error bar represents mean standard deviation (SD). (From Fiadjoe JE, Nishisaki A, Jagannathan N, et al. Airway management complications in children with difficult tracheal intubation from the Pediatric Difficult Intubation (PeDI) Registry: a prospective cohort analysis. *Lancet Respir Med.* 2016;4(1):37-48.)

detailed explanation of the use of these devices is beyond the scope of this book; however, we will briefly describe the advantages and disadvantages of each technique.

Fiberoptic Bronchoscopy

Flexible fiberoptic bronchoscopy is considered the gold standard technique for managing difficult tracheal intubation in adults and children. In recent years, anesthesiologists have become more adept at manipulating the ultrathin bronchoscope, which may be used inside a 2.5- or 3.0-mm internal diameter endotracheal tube (depending on the manufacturer). In addition, the optical aspects of the equipment have improved to allow better screen resolution. The technique must be practiced on mannikins and normal children before managing the difficult airway (Fig. 18.3).

There are several reasons why bronchoscopy can be more difficult in children compared with adults. First, because of the inherently smaller size of children, smaller bronchoscopes are required. Pediatric bronchoscopes range in size from 2.2- to 4.1-mm diameter. The smallest bronchoscopes lack a working channel; thus there is no conduit for suctioning secretions or blood. Administration of an antisialagogue before beginning the procedure should be considered (not evidence based), and the oropharynx should be suctioned before the bronchoscopic attempt. Oxygen insufflation should not be performed via this port in small children because of the possibility of generating dangerously high intrabronchial pressures and development of a tension pneumothorax.[2]

Second, children have a limited time to oxyhemoglobin desaturation. This is caused by the markedly reduced functional residual capacity (FRC) in anesthetized small children and their relatively high oxygen consumption. Therefore small children require alternate means of oxygenation during intubation attempts. See section below on apneic oxygenation.

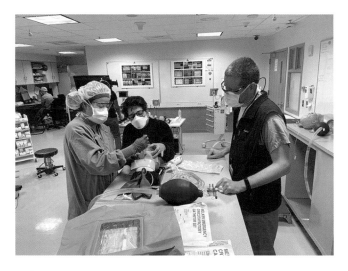

• **Fig 18.3.** Senior pediatric anesthesiologists practice difficult airway techniques on an annual (at least) basis. Photo credit Annery Garcia-Marcinkiewicz.

Third, in smaller children, flexible bronchoscopy performed through an SGA is more difficult than in adults because SGA placement in children is associated with a higher incidence of malpositioning, which leads to an obscured view of the glottic opening. The air-Q intubating laryngeal airway (Salter Labs, Lake Forest, IL, USA) seems to be the optimal choice for an intubation conduit because the lumen of the tube is larger than other types of SGAs, and allows passage of cuffed endotracheal tubes with the pilot balloon.

Finally, the unique anatomic variance of infants and children may influence successful fiberoptic bronchoscopy. If a nasal route is chosen, enlarged adenoidal and tonsillar tissue may obstruct the view and is likely to bleed upon contact. Oxymetazoline can be applied intranasally before insertion of the fiberoptic bronchoscope to minimize bleeding. The relatively more anterior location of the infant glottis may require more extensive anteflexion of the bronchoscope for adequate visualization of the glottic opening.

Video Laryngoscope

In its basic concept, a video or indirect laryngoscope is able to view the larynx using a video camera at the tip of its blade. In the past, pediatric video laryngoscopes were simply smaller adult laryngoscopes. There are now many types of video laryngoscopes manufactured with pediatric-specific designs. One of the simplest ways to classify video laryngoscopes is by whether it is a standard blade or nonstandard blade. Standard (Miller and MacIntosh) blades can be used as direct laryngoscopy, indirect laryngoscopy (completely use the video screen), or as video-assisted direct laryngoscopy. Manipulation of the blade follows the same skills as in direct laryngoscopy. Nonstandard blade video laryngoscopy involves the use of hyperangulated blades such as the traditional GlideScope (Verathon Inc., Parkway Bothell, WA, USA) and the Storz C-MAC D-blade (Karl Storz, Tuttlingen, Germany). Direct laryngoscopy with these blades will not reliably expose the glottic opening; they require different skills. Devices with greater curvature (hyperangulation) of the blade typically provide better visualization of an anterior larynx; however, they also require a more curved trajectory of the endotracheal tube, which increases difficulty. Hyperangulated blades, such as the GlideScope, are advantageous in the management of difficult airways compared with direct laryngoscopy. Having a styletted endotracheal tube that is curved to match the curve of the GlideScope blade will help facilitate manipulation into the field of view and into the glottic opening (Video 18.1).

Tracheal intubation of children with micrognathia or macroglossia is challenging with any video laryngoscope because it is often difficult to manipulate both the laryngoscope and the endotracheal tube within the small pharynx. An alternative option is the use of a combined technique (e.g., a fiberoptic bronchoscope along with a video laryngoscope.) Video screens of each device are placed side by side and at least two operators are required. Benefits of this technique include visualization of the laryngeal inlet with video laryngoscopy, and visual control of the passage of the ETT over the fiberoptic bronchoscope into the trachea.

Intubation via a Supraglottic Airway

Supraglottic airways (SGAs) can be life-saving devices, particularly if difficulty with ventilation is encountered. An appropriately placed SGA allows the patient to continue breathing spontaneously throughout the induction and intubation attempts. However, the SGA poses a particular challenge to insertion of cuffed endotracheal tubes, as the pilot balloon may be larger than the proximal opening of the SGA. Newer designs, such as the air-Q (Salter Labs, Park Forest, IL, USA) allow easier placement of an endotracheal tube. The airway tube of the air-Q is shorter than the classic laryngeal mask airway (LMA), and the opening is wider, thus allowing passage of a cuffed endotracheal tube with less resistance. Nevertheless, fiberoptic bronchoscopy should be used to facilitate the advancement of the endotracheal tube into the trachea via the air-Q device. Table 18.3 summarizes the relationship between the size of LMA and the sizes of endotracheal tubes and fiberoptic scopes that fit.

In addition to fiberoptic bronchoscopy and video laryngoscopy, there exist several additional methods to directly or indirectly visualize the glottis and perform tracheal intubation. These include optical stylets such as the Bonfils (rigid) and Shikani (malleable, firm) types and the lighted stylet (also known as the lightwand). Details of the use of these devices are beyond the scope of this book but can be found in textbooks on advanced pediatric airway management.

Apneic Oxygenation

Oxygenation is the most important principle of airway management in any patient. Infants and small children may develop hypoxemia rapidly during apnea because of

TABLE 18.3 Pediatric-Sized Laryngeal Mask Airways and Compatible Endotracheal Tubes[a]

Inner Diameter of LMA (mm)	Maximum Lubricated Uncuffed ETT Inner Diameter (mm)	Maximum FOB Size[b]	Maximum Lubricated Cuffed ETT Inner Diameter (mm)
1.0	3.5	2.7	3.0
1.5	4.0	3.0	4.0
2.0	5.0	3.5	4.5
2.5	6.0[c]	4.0	5.0
3.0	—	5.0	6.0
4.0	—	5.0	6.0

[a]Based on experiments performed by author. *ETT*, endotracheal tube
[b]As per LMA North America. *FOB*, Fiberoptic bronchoscope.
[c]Largest available uncuffed endotracheal tube available at The Children's Hospital of Philadelphia.

their relatively higher oxygen consumption along with their decreased FRC while anesthetized. If not immediately corrected, this can quickly lead to cardiac arrest, particularly in the pediatric difficult airway. Therefore it is imperative that apneic time be minimized. Some studies have found benefits in providing supplemental oxygenation to children during prolonged tracheal intubation, such as preservation of normoxemia and decrease in the overall rate of desaturation.

Transnasal humidified rapid-insufflation ventilatory exchange (THRIVE) is a technique that provides high-flow humidified oxygen through a nasal trumpet and allows continuous oxygen delivery during the intubation attempt. THRIVE has proven beneficial in adults, prolonging apneic oxygenation time, and enabling unhurried intubation in adults with difficult airways. A randomized trial[3] found THRIVE to be beneficial in infants and children. Children in the THRIVE arm maintained their transcutaneous hemoglobin saturation at least twice as long as the those in the same age range in the control group. Transcutaneous CO_2 increased to a similar extent in both arms. Nasal oxygen during efforts securing a tube (nasal oxygen during efforts securing a tube [NO DESAT]) uses a simple nasal cannula to provide standard low-flow oxygen while tracheal intubation is performed. In adults and children, apneic oxygenation during intubation delays oxyhemoglobin desaturation. There are a variety of other creative ways to provide supplemental oxygenation during intubation attempts (Fig. 18.4A–C)

Etiologies of Difficult Intubation

Pierre Robin Sequence

The Pierre Robin sequence (Fig. 18.5) consists of micrognathia, glossoptosis, and cleft palate. These infants may have an obstructed upper airway from the small anatomic space afforded by their small mandible. The condition is most severe at birth and tends to improve with age. A mandibular advancement procedure is usually performed in the first weeks of life but if airway obstruction is severe and life-threatening at birth, tracheostomy is indicated. Concomitant congenital anomalies may lead to other necessary surgical interventions such as cleft palate repair or placement of tympanostomy tubes. Tracheal intubation in these infants may be extremely difficult or impossible. Mask ventilation in these infants is usually accomplished, especially when aided by placement of an oral airway. SGA placement is often essential for establishing ventilation or to provide a guide for tracheal intubation.

Treacher Collins Syndrome

Treacher–Collins syndrome (TCS) (Fig. 18.6A–B and Video 18.2) consists of hypoplasia of the maxilla and mandible, and variable eye and ear deformities. It results from failure of the first branchial arch to develop between the 3rd

and 5th weeks of gestation. Without repair, these features do not improve with age and their presence can make children difficult or impossible to ventilate or intubate via direct laryngoscopy. Like other severe airway anomalies, the SGA is indispensable for airway management. However, TCS may be associated with restricted mandibular movement; thus oral intubation or SGA insertion may be impossible. Children with TCS associated with limited mouth opening may require awake or sedated nasal fiberoptic intubation.

Hemifacial Microsomia

The most important anomaly in hemifacial microsomia that renders these children difficult to intubate is mandibular hypoplasia. Additional variable clinical features include microphthalmia, microtia, and macrostomia (Fig. 18.7), which result from malformations of the first and second pharyngeal arches. These children are usually easy to mask ventilate, and may often be easily intubated by direct laryngoscopy. Difficult intubation is likely when the unilateral mandibular hypoplasia is severe, or the hypoplasia is bilateral. As with the aforementioned congenital facial anomalies, the SGA is an effective method for ventilating and facilitating intubation in this patient population.

Anticipated Difficult Ventilation From Upper Airway Obstruction

The expected difficult ventilation is one of the most angst-provoking situations in pediatric anesthesia. There is good reason for this: small children with transient or mild upper airway obstruction may rapidly become hypoxemic. How does one know when a child will be difficult to ventilate? The history and physical exam, and possibly some radiologic studies, will almost always indicate the answer to this question. One of the most reliable indicators is previous difficulty with ventilation during a recent anesthetic, assuming there were no clinical changes since that time. Conversely, if the child was easy to ventilate during a recent anesthetic, then one can be reasonably confident that the child will still be easy to ventilate, but we have seen cases where this was not the case. For these reasons, it is imperative to obtain the previous anesthetic record or directly talk to the anesthesiologist who was present. If there were no previous anesthetics, other aspects of the history can indicate ease of ventilation. Was the child previously sedated for a radiologic procedure? If so, were there any ventilation difficulties? How does the child sleep at night? Are there obstructive episodes? Are they related to the position of the child?

On physical exam, signs of clinically important upper airway obstruction include the presence of neck and chest wall retractions, and inspiratory stridor. Intrathoracic airway obstruction is characterized by expiratory stridor or wheezing. The oxyhemoglobin saturation is another indicator of airway patency. A value below 94% on room air is indicative of upper airway obstruction.

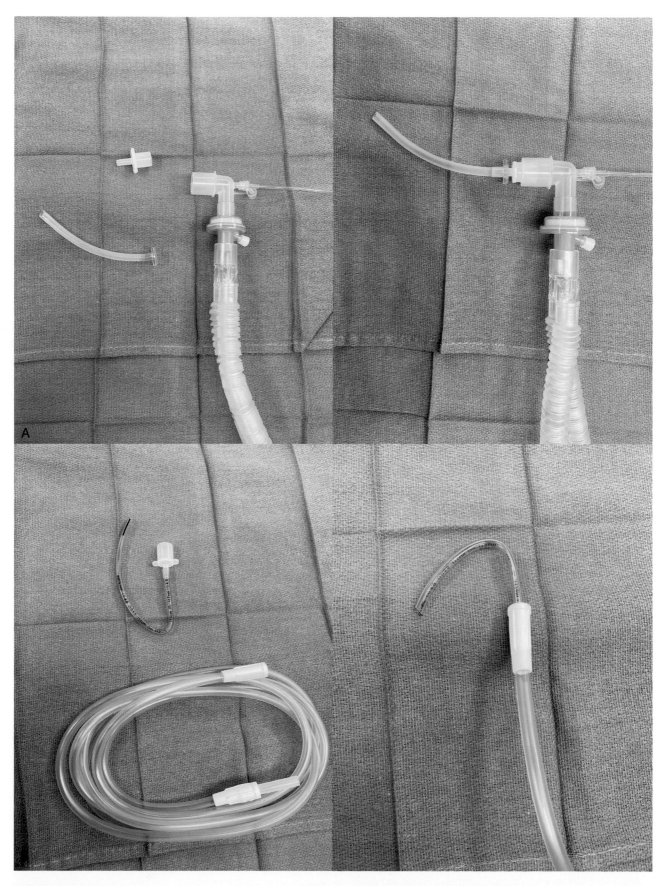

• **Fig 18.4.** Common ways in which supplemental oxygenation can be provided during intubation attempts. (A) A nasal airway or nasal cannula can be attached to the anesthesia circuit via an endotracheal tube adaptor to produce transnasal humidified rapid-insufflation ventilatory exchange (THRIVE). (B) Oral RAE tube attached to oxygen source and placed in side of mouth. (C) Oxygen source connected to air-Q. Flexible bronchoscopy introduced through elbow adaptor.

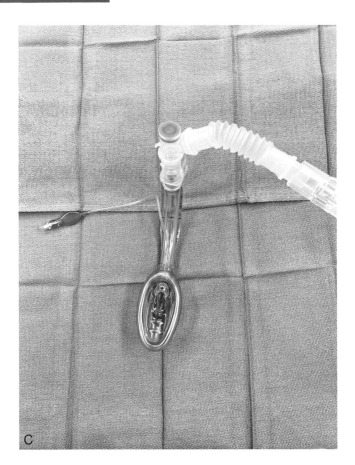

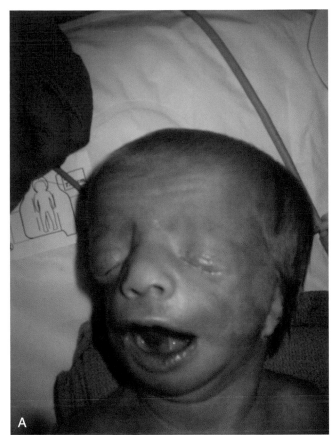

• **Fig 18.4.—cont'd**

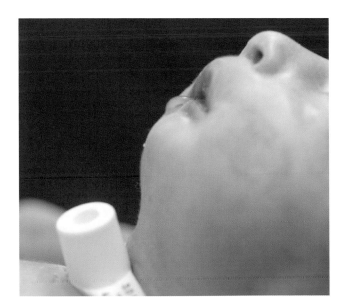

• **Fig 18.5.** Mandibular hypoplasia of Pierre Robin syndrome This infant required a tracheostomy soon after birth to allow optimal oxygenation and ventilation without obstruction because of mandibular hypoplasia. (From Stricker PA, Fiadjoe JE, Lerman J. Plastic and reconstructive surgery. In: Coté CJ, Lerman J, Anderson BJ, eds. *Coté and Lerman's A Practice of Anesthesia for Infants and Children*. 6th ed. Elsevier; 2019: 804-819.e6.)

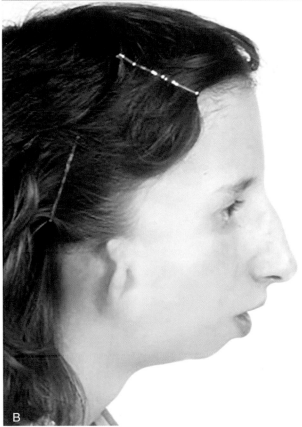

• **Fig 18.6.** Typical facies of Treacher Collins syndrome in a (A) newborn and (B) older child. (From Posnick JC. Treacher Collins syndrome: perspectives in evaluation and treatment. *J Oral Maxillofac Surg*. 1997;55(10):1120-1133. doi:10.1016/s0278-2391(97)90294-9.)

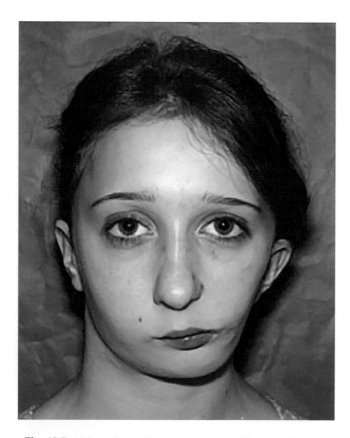

• **Fig 18.7.** Unilateral hemifacial microsomia. (From Wolford LM, Bourland TC, Rodrigues D, Perez DE, Limoeiro E. Successful reconstruction of nongrowing hemifacial microsomia patients with unilateral temporomandibular joint total joint prosthesis and orthognathic surgery. *J Oral Maxillofac Surg.* 2012;70(12):2835-2853.)

Anticipated Difficult Ventilation

MOST IMPORTANT A PRIORI DECISION:
Am I reasonably certain that hypoxia can be avoided by either maintaining spontaneous ventilation **or**

SGA insertion**?**

YES — NO

| ANESTHETIZED INTUBATION | AWAKE OR SEDATED INTUBATION |

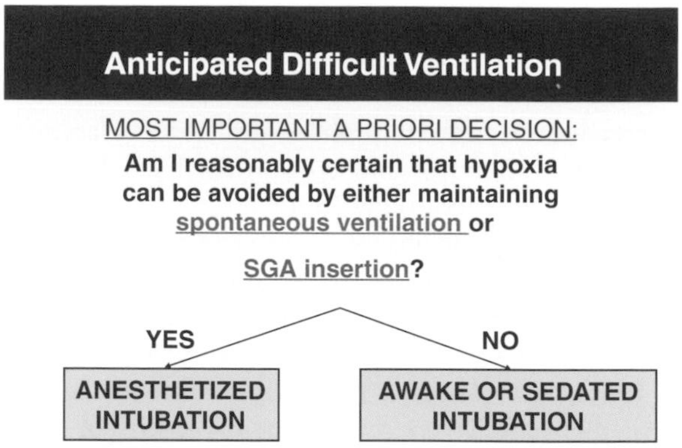

• **Fig 18.8.** Initial thought process for airway management in the child with an anticipated difficult ventilation.

Examination of previous radiologic studies may also help determine the possibility of ventilation difficulty. Important examples include the following:

- Lateral neck radiograph for the "thumb sign" of epiglottitis
- Neck radiograph or computed tomography (CT) for evaluation of the severity of a retropharyngeal abscess
- Neck CT for evaluation of masses encroaching on the upper airway that are not visible externally (e.g., cystic hygroma)
- Neck and chest CT for evaluation of the extent to which an anterior mediastinal mass compresses the trachea (a 50% reduction of the tracheal diameter may indicate critical tracheal compression and the inability to ventilate adequately after induction of general anesthesia)
- Thoracic magnetic resonance imaging (MRI) for diagnosis of a vascular ring, and to evaluate the severity of tracheal compression
- Chest radiograph of a child who has aspirated a foreign body (this may not indicate ease of ventilation but will indicate additional problems that may impact anesthetic management, such as extent of pneumonitis or degree of unilateral hyperinflation)

When approaching the child who may be difficult to ventilate, the first and most important decision is whether or not to proceed with tracheal intubation with the child awake with mild sedation or fully anesthetized (Fig. 18.8). Awake intubations are rarely performed in children because of their inability to cooperate with the procedure. However, if one believes that there exists the possibility of hypoxemia despite SGA placement, then an awake or mildly sedated technique should be performed. Fortunately, this situation is rare in pediatric patients for the very reason that there exist few situations where one feels that SGA insertion would be unsuccessful.

If an awake intubation is planned, it helps to anesthetize the child's upper airway passages with local anesthesia. A local anesthetic solution can be administered by nebulizer, but this is variably effective because of the uncooperative nature of small children. Most anesthesiologists prefer to sedate children using a combination of a benzodiazepine and opioid because the effects can be rapidly reversed. Others prefer small titrations of ketamine (0.25 mg/kg doses) because of its tendency to preserve upper airway patency at concentrations that reliably impair consciousness. The combination of ketamine and dexmedetomidine has also been used to maintain spontaneous ventilation and dexmedetomidine and a benzodiazepine such as midazolam. Propofol, when used judiciously, can also be used effectively when one suspects a reasonable chance of being able to successfully ventilate using positive pressure. Inhalational general anesthetic agents may also be used. Sevoflurane will provide rapid loss of consciousness but has the possibility of rendering the child apneic. A classic and time-honored technique is to maintain spontaneous ventilation while slowly deepening the level of anesthesia (Fig. 18.9). While maintaining spontaneous ventilation, laryngoscopy is performed slowly while progressively applying topical local anesthetic to more distal portions of the pharynx and larynx. If central or obstructive apnea occurs during this procedure, the anesthesiologist must be prepared to either rapidly attempt endotracheal intubation or insert a laryngeal mask to prevent development of hypoxemia.

Infectious Causes of Difficult Ventilation

Three important infections potentially cause life-threatening airway obstruction: retropharyngeal abscess, laryngotracheobronchitis (croup), and epiglottitis. Each has unique clinical characteristics (Table 18.4).

A retropharyngeal abscess is a bacterial infection that occurs behind the oral pharynx anterior to the prevertebral fascia. It is characterized by sore throat, fever, neck stiffness, and odynophagia. It is diagnosed by characteristic findings on a lateral cervical spine radiograph (Fig. 18.10) or CT scan of the neck. If severe, treatment consists of incision

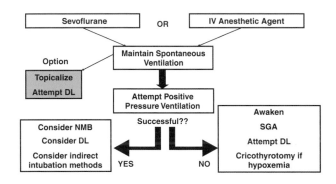

• **Fig 18.9.** Algorithms for managing the child with an anticipated difficult ventilation. DL = direct laryngoscopy; NMB = neuromuscular blockade; SGA = supraglottic airway; IV = intravenous.

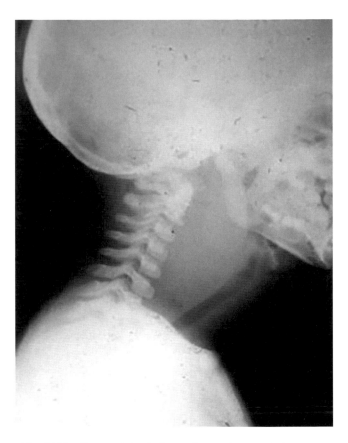

• **Fig 18.10.** Characteristic findings of retropharyngeal abscess on lateral neck radiograph. Photo credit Ronald S. Litman.

TABLE 18.4	Comparison of Infectious Causes of Upper Airway Obstruction		
	Retropharyngeal Abscess	**Laryngotracheobronchitis**	**Epiglottitis**
Age	2–8 years	6 months–3 years	2–5 years
Pathology	Lymphatic drainage or contiguous spread of pharyngeal or oral infections.	Inflammation that affects subglottic tracheal mucosa and entire tracheobronchial tree.	Supraglottitis: severe swelling of epiglottis, arytenoids, and surrounding tissue.
Prominent Clinical Features	Sore throat, fever, neck stiffness, difficulty swallowing, neck swelling, tonsillitis, pharyngitis, cervical lymphadenopathy.	Viral prodrome (upper respiratory tract infection), low-grade fever, barking cough, variable degree of inspiratory stridor, hoarseness; rarely progresses to fatigue and respiratory failure.	High fever, toxic appearing, drooling, throat pain, difficulty swallowing; seated position and leaning forward preferred.
Radiography	Lateral neck radiograph: widening of the retropharyngeal soft tissues; also identified on CT scan.	Anteroposterior neck radiograph: "steeple" sign indicating tracheal mucosal edema.	Lateral neck radiograph: "thumb" sign of swollen epiglottis, prevertebral thickening, hypopharyngeal enlargement on lateral view.
Treatment	Tracheal intubation, incision and drainage, antibiotics.	Cool mist, steroids, nebulized 2.25% racemic epinephrine.	Tracheal intubation until resolved, (usually 2–4 days), antibiotics.

and drainage under general anesthesia with precautions for possible difficult ventilation.

Laryngotracheobronchitis (croup) is a viral-mediated inflammation of the lower portion of the upper airway. It causes edema of the trachea below the glottic level and can be diagnosed on anteroposterior cervical radiography (Fig. 18.11). Treatment consists of cool mist, steroids, and nebulized racemic epinephrine in severe cases. Tracheal intubation is rare except in cases of hypoxemia that do not respond promptly to nebulized epinephrine and oxygen therapy.

Epiglottitis is a bacterial infection that involves all the supraglottic structures (Fig. 18.12). Because the advent of the vaccination against *Hemophilus influenzae* type B, the organism that causes childhood epiglottitis, it is only occasionally seen in children, such as those with incomplete immunizations. Nevertheless, when it occurs, it can cause life-threatening upper airway obstruction. The treatment consists of immediate induction of general anesthesia followed by endotracheal intubation or surgical tracheostomy, followed by a course of antibiotics. Management of epiglottitis begins when the child presents with stridor in the emergency department. Every hospital should have an epiglottitis protocol that consists of immediate consultation with the otolaryngology and anesthesiology services once epiglottitis is suspected in any child.

Tracheal intubation for epiglottitis should be performed in the OR under deep inhalational anesthesia that maintains spontaneous ventilation until it is proven that positive-pressure ventilation is possible. If feasible, nasotracheal intubation should be performed because the child will be intubated for several days, but this depends largely on the preferences of the pediatric ICU. Although direct laryngoscopy may appear to be easy, difficulty may arise because of severe swelling of all the supraglottic structures with obliteration of the glottic opening. Maintenance of spontaneous ventilation may help the anesthesiologist identify the tiny glottic opening by observing bubbles at the site. If the

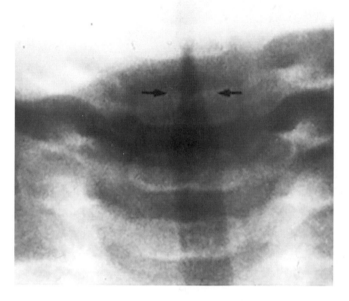

• **Fig 18.11.** Characteristic findings of laryngotracheobronchitis (croup) on anteroposterior cervical radiography. Photo credit Ronald S. Litman.

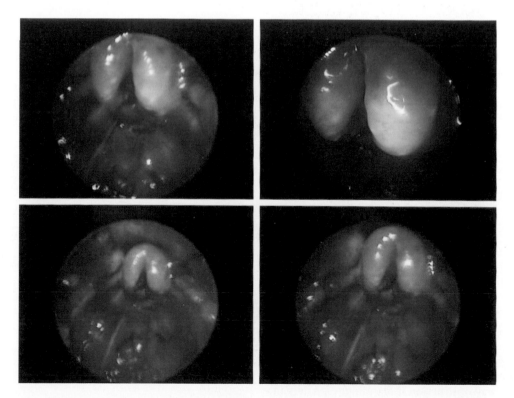

• **Fig 18.12.** Classic swelling of epiglottis and all supraglottic structures.

Every institution should have a protocol that details the steps necessary to treat a patient with suspected epiglottitis:*
1. Every attempt should be made to keep the child calm. A parent should be allowed to comfort the child up to and including during the induction of general anesthesia. No attempt should be made to place the child supine. If the diagnosis of epiglottitis is seriously entertained, radiographs should not be performed.
2. The following departments should be immediately consulted:
   a. Anesthesiology
   b. Otolaryngology
   c. Surgical suite: If OR space is not immediately available, the child should be taken to the intensive care unit (ICU) or recovery room; the child should not be transported until appropriate notifications and preparations are complete.
3. Prepare the child for transport:
   a. Have a gurney available to travel with the patient, but do not lay the child supine.
   b. The child can remain in the parent's arms or lap.
   c. A full O$_2$ tank should accompany the patient and provide supplemental blow-by oxygen.
   d. Have an Ambu bag with appropriately sized face mask.
   e. Have an intubating laryngoscope with appropriately sized and smaller sized endotracheal tubes.
   f. Have portable suction.
   g. Be ready with propofol and succinylcholine.
   h. Transport the child and the parents only when physician experienced in emergency airway management is in attendance. The anesthesiologist attending is always in charge.
4. During the vulnerable period before intubation, handling of the child should be kept to a minimum; no oral examinations and no unnecessary needle sticks. The IV catheter is inserted by the best qualified person.
5. When ready for intubation, the anesthesiologist performs an inhalation induction with a volatile agent, with the otolaryngologist present in the room for possible emergency tracheotomy.
6. After the endotracheal tube is appropriately inserted and ventilation is assured, less urgent procedures such as changing to a nasotracheal tube, blood work, and administration of intravenous antibiotics may be performed. Routine data entry should be dealt with only after the child is safe.
7. After tracheal intubation, the child is transported to the ICU with adequate sedation and possibly paralysis. Restraints may be required to prevent life-threatening self-extubation.
8. If intensive care monitoring and support are not available, the child should be transported with a physician skilled in emergency airway management to an appropriate facility.

*Adapted from Parsons DS, Smith RB, Mair EA, Dlabal LJ. Unique case presentations of acute epiglottic swelling and a protocol for acute airway compromise. *Laryngoscope* 1996;106:1287–1291.

child is apneic an assistant can push on the child's chest, which may also produce bubbles at the glottic opening. Age-appropriate and smaller endotracheal tubes with stylets inserted should be immediately on hand. A supraglottic airway would not be helpful in this situation because it would be situated above the level of the obstruction. If life-threatening hypoxemia occurs before tracheal intubation, an immediate surgical tracheostomy or cricothyrotomy is indicated. The child should remain heavily sedated or paralyzed for transport to the ICU. The endotracheal tube should be secured well to ensure against accidental extubation.

Postoperatively, there are several methods used to determine when the child's trachea can be safely extubated. Some physicians will wait until a leak is heard, which indicates a decrease in the amount of glottic swelling. Others may directly inspect the glottis by direct laryngoscopy or flexible bronchoscopy to assess residual glottic swelling. The child should also be afebrile, an indication that the bacterial infection is adequately treated.

Unanticipated Difficult Ventilation

Unanticipated airway obstruction is alarming, especially in small infants because of the rapidity with which hypoxemia develops. Common causes include passive airway collapse, enlarged tonsils or adenoids, and laryngospasm.

Whatever the cause, the sequence of correctional maneuvers is similar in all cases (Fig. 18.13). The anesthesia provider should first seek to optimally reposition the head and neck while simultaneously checking for appropriate face mask

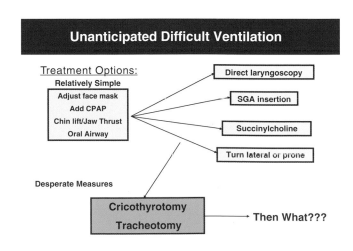

• **Fig 18.13.** Clinical pathway for the unanticipated difficult ventilation.

placement and calling for assistance. A common error in face mask placement in small children is to place the mask too low on the face such that a portion of the nose is obstructed. Chin lift with or without jaw thrust may also alleviate obstruction. Continuous positive airway pressure (CPAP) can be applied to the upper airway by partially closing the pop-off valve. Rapid ventilations are delivered at a high inspiratory pressure until the child's chest is seen to rise, and adequate ventilation is confirmed by capnography and rise in oxyhemoglobin saturation. This technique will effectively relieve upper airway obstruction in many cases caused by passive collapse of the pharynx or adenotonsillar hypertrophy, but will not alleviate complete laryngospasm. The next action to take is to place an oral airway. In cases of airway obstruction caused by enlarged tonsils or adenoids, this will almost always be curative unless there is additional cause for the obstruction.

If these maneuvers fail, and the oxyhemoglobin saturation is still decreasing, the anesthesia provider is faced with a dire situation and must take immediate action. One of three possible actions is appropriate at this point (or any time earlier in this time sequence):

1. Immediately insert an SGA to establish adequate ventilation except when the obstruction is caused by laryngospasm. One would have to be very confident that the obstruction is not being caused by laryngospasm if placing an SGA during a severe hypoxic episode. Appropriately sized SGAs should be immediately available in every anesthetizing location.

2. Immediate tracheal intubation can be performed when one is confident of intubating skills and doubts exist as to the cause of the obstruction. This option is commonly considered in neonates. If laryngospasm is occurring, it is sometimes possible to introduce a styletted endotracheal tube into the glottic opening.

3. Administer succinylcholine. Because laryngospasm is a common cause of unrelenting upper airway obstruction in children, succinylcholine should be administered if conventional methods fail to reverse hypoxemia. It should be administered intravenously if possible, but can also be given intramuscularly (4 mg/kg), with relief of laryngospasm within a minute. One should never withhold succinylcholine during hypoxemia for fear of provoking bradycardia. If the child developed bradycardia as a result of the hypoxemia, the heart rate will increase with the establishment of normoxemia and will not be made worse because of administration of succinylcholine. If laryngospasm occurs but is not associated with hypoxemia, other options for relief include a bolus of propofol (2–3 mg/kg) or administration of a nondepolarizing neuromuscular blocker, such as rocuronium (1.6 mg/kg). These would also be viable options if there were absolute contraindications to succinylcholine (e.g., myopathy, MH susceptibility (MH = malignant hyperthermia).

Desperate Measures

In the rare instance that none of the above measures is successful and the child is becoming dangerously hypoxic, desperate last-chance measures must be performed immediately. These include the following:

Reposition the Patient

If an anterior mediastinal mass is suspected and conventional measures (e.g., rigid bronchoscope) have failed to reestablish ventilation and normoxemia (see Chapter 8), the child should be repositioned to the lateral or prone position. This maneuver may alleviate obstruction of the lower trachea or great vessels surrounding the heart.

Cricothyrotomy

There are several techniques available for creating a surgical airway. A tracheotomy is preferred but may not be rapid enough even if appropriate personnel are available. The most feasible action at this point is usually percutaneous placement of a cricothyrotomy, an opening in the cricothyroid membrane located between the cricoid and thyroid cartilages. Though several commercially made kits are available, the most efficient method is to place a 14- or 16-gauge angiocatheter through the cricothyroid membrane. Once this is properly placed into the child's trachea, one has several options with which to provide oxygenation. Every anesthesiologist should have a plan for oxygenation via cricothyrotomy for every case, every day. One method is to attach a 3.0 endotracheal tube adaptor to the hub of the angiocatheter, which can then be connected to the anesthesia breathing circuit. Another method is to attach the barrel of a 10-mL syringe to the angiocatheter and place a cuffed endotracheal tube within the barrel. Many other successful methods of oxygenation have been described. Of note, there are several challenges with performing cricothyrotomy in infants and children. Cricothyrotomies have a high failure and complication rate, particularly in infants. Known complications from this technique in children include pneumothorax, pneumomediastinum, bleeding into the airway, and misplacement of the angiocatheter through the trachea or into a false lumen within the tracheal wall. In general, cricothyrotomy is not a feasible option in small infants, given their cricothyroid membrane is very soft and small risking laryngeal fracture and severe airway injury.

Tracheotomy

If a qualified surgeon is present, and if it is feasible that a tracheotomy can be rapidly secured, this option may be preferable over cricothyrotomy. However, it cannot be overstated how difficult this technique is in small children.

Extubation of the Difficult Airway

Removal of the breathing tube from a difficult airway patient can provide its own share of challenges. In addition to preexisting factors, such as difficult anatomy, masses, or trauma, there is a chance that the child who has been intubated is developing airway edema that can result in complications after extubation. Precautions to reduce swelling include steroid administration, and elevating the head of the bed for several hours postoperatively. This waiting period also allows additional time for the anesthetic agents to completely wear off.

References

1. Bhananker SM, Ramamoorthy C, Geiduschek JM, et al. Anesthesia-related cardiac arrest in children: update from the Pediatric Perioperative Cardiac Arrest Registry. *Anesth Analg.* 2007;105(2):344–350. https://doi.org/10.1213/01.ane.0000268712.00756.dd.

2. Iannoli ED, Litman RS. Tension pneumothorax during flexible fiberoptic bronchoscopy in a newborn. *Anesth Analg.* 2002;94(3):512–513. https://doi.org/10.1097/00000539-200203000-00007.

3. Humphreys S, Lee-Archer P, Reyne G, Long D, Williams T, Schibler A. Transnasal humidified rapid-insufflation ventilatory exchange (THRIVE) in children: a randomized controlled trial. *Br J Anaesth.* 2017;118(2):232–238. https://doi.org/10.1093/bja/aew401.

Suggested Readings

Cook TM, Woodall N, Frerk C. Fourth National Audit P. major complications of airway management in the UK: results of the Fourth National Audit Project of the Royal College of Anaesthetists and the Difficult Airway Society. *Br J Anaesth.* 2011;106(5):617–631. [Part 1: Anaesthesia] https://doi.org/10.1093/bja/aer058.

Fiadjoe JE, Gurnaney H, Dalesio N, et al. A prospective randomized equivalence trial of the GlideScope Cobalt(R) video laryngoscope to traditional direct laryngoscopy in neonates and infants. *Anesthesiology.* 2012;116(3):622–628. https://doi.org/10.1097/ALN.0b013e318246ea4d.

Fiadjoe JE, Nishisaki A, Jagannathan N, et al. Airway management complications in children with difficult tracheal intubation from the Pediatric Difficult Intubation (PeDI) Registry: a prospective cohort analysis. *Lancet Respir Med.* 2016;4(1):37–48. https://doi.org/10.1016/S2213-2600(15)00508-1.

Garcia-Marcinkiewicz AG, Stricker PA. Craniofacial surgery and specific airway problems. *Paediatr Anaesth.* 2020;30(3):296–303. https://doi.org/10.1111/pan.13790.

Greib N, Stojeba N, Dow WA, Henderson J, Diemunsch PA. A combined rigid videolaryngoscopy-flexible fibrescopy intubation technique under general anesthesia. *Can J Anaesth.* 2007;54(6):492–493. https://doi.org/10.1007/BF03022046.

Isono S, Ishikawa T. Oxygenation, not intubation, does matter. *Anesthesiology.* 2011;114(1):7–9.

Jagannathan N, Kho MF, Kozlowski RJ, Sohn LE, Siddiqui A, Wong DT. Retrospective audit of the air-Q intubating laryngeal airway as a conduit for tracheal intubation in pediatric patients with a difficult airway. *Paediatr Anaesth.* 2011;21(4):422–427. https://doi.org/10.4097/kjae.2016.69.4.390.

Park R, Peyton JM, Fiadjoe JE, et al. The efficacy of GlideScope(R) videolaryngoscopy compared with direct laryngoscopy in children who are difficult to intubate: an analysis from the paediatric difficult intubation registry. *Br J Anaesth.* 2017;119(5):984–992. https://doi.org/10.1093/bja/aex344.

Peyton J, Park R, Staffa SJ, et al. A comparison of videolaryngoscopy using standard blades or non-standard blades in children in the Paediatric Difficult Intubation Registry. *Br J Anaesth.* 2020 https://doi.org/10.1016/j.bja.2020.08.010.

Steiner JW, Sessler DI, Makarova N, et al. Use of deep laryngeal oxygen insufflation during laryngoscopy in children: a randomized clinical trial. *Br J Anaesth.* 2016;117(3):350–357. https://doi.org/10.1093/bja/aew186.

Weiss M, Gerber AC, Schmitz A. Continuous ventilation technique for laryngeal mask airway (LMA) removal after fiberoptic intubation in children. *Paediatr Anaesth.* 2004;14(11):936–940. https://doi.org/10.1111/j.1460-9592.2004.01354.x.

Windpassinger M, Plattner O, Gemeiner J, et al. Pharyngeal oxygen insufflation during Airtraq laryngoscopy slows arterial desaturation in infants and small children. *Anesth Analg.* 2016;122(4):1153–1157. https://doi.org/10.1213/ANE.0000000000001189.

19

Management of General Anesthesia

VANESSA A. OLBRECHT, JI YEON JEMMA KANG, ANASTASIA DIMOPOULLOU, JEFF FELDMAN, JULIA ROSENBLOOM, THEOKLIS ZAOUTIS AND RONALD S. LITMAN

There are many features of the administration of general anesthesia that differ between children and adults. In this chapter, we discuss those differences, with an emphasis on anesthetic medications and ventilation strategies. We also review the importance of racial disparities in pediatric anesthesia, surgical site infection prophylaxis, and the possibility of neurotoxicity of anesthetics to the developing brain.

In the United States, most children that require general anesthesia undergo inhalational induction by face mask with intravenous (IV) catheter placement after loss of consciousness (Fig. 19.1). Most hospitals have taken pride in their "ouch-less" environment, and thus, parents expect that their children will not undergo any painful injections while awake. This strategy is entirely optional, as some children prefer IV insertion while awake instead of the uncomfortable feeling of having a noxious mask over their face.

Not all (healthy) children that are administered sevoflurane require IV access during general anesthesia. Two common examples are myringotomy for ear tube insertion and computed tomography (CT) scan, mainly because they are very brief procedures.

For difficult IV placement in anesthetized children, it has become standard practice to use ultrasound guidance. The use of ultrasound has higher first attempt success rates[1] and

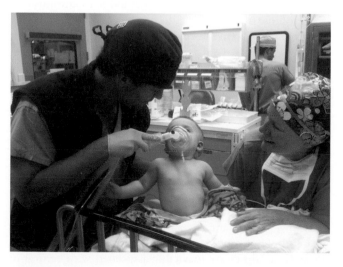

• **Fig 19.1.** Infant mask induction. This beats adults any day!

greater overall success of cannulation than without ultrasound. The short axis out-of-plane technique together with dynamic needle position, where the needle tip is followed as the ultrasound probe is moved proximally, may further increase the success rate of peripheral IV placement in small children.

Sevoflurane

Sevoflurane is the anesthetic agent of choice for inhalational induction of general anesthesia in children because of its relatively low pungency and its lower blood-gas solubility coefficient (0.63) that speeds loss of consciousness.

The minimum alveolar concentration (MAC) of sevoflurane is 3.2% in neonates and infants up to 6 months of age; the MAC of sevoflurane peaks at 3 months of age. In school-aged children, MAC is 2.5%; the concentration that prevents 95% of children from moving in response to a surgical stimulus (ED95) is 2.9%. When 60% nitrous oxide (N_2O) is added to sevoflurane, the MAC is lowered to 2.0%. Summary graphs of MAC according to age have been published.[2]

Induction of general anesthesia with sevoflurane may be accomplished in several different ways. In some cases, the vaporizer is set to the maximal 8% setting from the start. Whether or not this is combined with N_2O, most children will lose consciousness within 5 to 10 breaths.

Most children develop tachycardia during inhalational induction with sevoflurane. Twenty percent of children will develop a nodal rhythm and infants less than 6 months of age may demonstrate lengthening of the QT interval that continues into the postoperative period. These changes, however, do not result in adverse clinical manifestations. Sevoflurane may cause a dose-dependent bradycardia and hypotension in some children, especially those with trisomy 21; pretreatment with IV glycopyrrolate or oral/intramuscular (IM) atropine may be considered in this population.

During the early stages of sevoflurane induction, a peculiar type of agitation may be observed, mainly in teenagers. It consists of muscular rigidity and generalized tonic-clonic or myoclonic movements, and can worry some practitioners that it is the onset of malignant hyperthermia (it is not). It may be caused by electrical seizure activity,[3] especially when concentrations exceed 4.5%. This effect is accentuated with hyperventilation, and is suppressed by N_2O and opioids. These stimulatory effects of the central nervous system are not associated with postoperative sequelae.

Single-Breath Induction Technique

The single-breath induction technique (Video 19.1) will considerably speed the loss of consciousness in older, cooperative children. It is performed by priming the anesthesia circuit and ventilation bag with 70% N_2O and 8% sevoflurane. The distal end of the breathing circuit is sealed off to prevent leakage of sevoflurane into the operating room (OR) environment. The child is instructed to first blow all the air out of their lungs (it is helpful to practice this technique with the child before entering the OR). At the very end of the child's exhalation, the facemask is placed over the child's mouth and nose, and the child is instructed to take "the biggest breath of their life." This technique invariably results in loss of consciousness soon after the vital capacity breath.

Steal Induction

When a child is asleep upon entering the OR, a "steal" induction may be performed. The anesthesia breathing circuit is primed with N_2O and sevoflurane in a similar fashion as that done for the single-breath technique. The child is not touched or moved to the OR table and no monitors are applied. The face mask is moved progressively closer to the child's face without touching it. Once consciousness is lost, the child is moved to the OR table and monitors are applied. Proponents of this technique favor its atraumatic nature and the child's lack of awareness of the OR environment. Opponents of this technique fear that a child could suffer psychological harm if they awaken from a painful procedure without adequate psychological preparation.

Nitrous Oxide

N_2O can be used as an adjunct to inhalational induction because of its ability to reduce the MAC of inhaled agents and to speed the onset of unconsciousness via the second gas effect.[4] It is discontinued when the IV catheter is inserted.

N_2O has been associated with myoclonic movements and even generalized seizures in some unusual cases. Because N_2O decreases the activity of two vitamin B_{12} enzymes, methionine synthetase and thymidylate synthetase, its use has been implicated in the exacerbation of vitamin B_{12} deficiency with development of neurologic symptoms in susceptible patients. Therefore, N_2O should be avoided in children with vitamin B_{12} deficiency or a known homozygous *MTHFR* (methylenetetrahydrofolate reductase gene) mutation. It has also been implicated in causing increased plasma homocysteine concentrations,[5] the clinical significance of which is unknown.

Because N_2O is equally as flammable as oxygen, it should not be used during procedures that carry risk for airway fire, such as a tonsillectomy (especially when using an uncuffed endotracheal tube, which you should not do anyway; see Chapter 22) or laser bronchoscopy, in which the oxygen concentration is lowered as much as possibly safe. Because of these above-mentioned drawbacks of N_2O, its use has markedly decreased in lieu of using higher concentrations of sevoflurane. Also, N_2O will diffuse into the endotracheal tube cuff and may cause tracheal edema from overly high cuff pressures[6] if not monitored.

Propofol

IV induction of general anesthesia is reserved for children with established IV access, those with susceptibility to malignant hyperthermia, and those that require a rapid sequence induction (RSI) technique.

Propofol causes immediate loss of consciousness after administration of 3 to 6 mg/kg. Children require larger induction doses than adults because of a larger volume of distribution. Obese children, however, require less than normal-weight children of the same weight and therefore should receive propofol dosed at ideal bodyweight.[7] Maintenance doses are also larger in children because of greater elimination and clearance. Propofol is particularly well suited for use in asthmatics because it blunts airway responses within its clinical dosing range. Propofol usually causes central apnea when administered as a bolus for induction of general anesthesia. If given in titrated doses, however, apnea can be avoided. The apneic dose of propofol is usually less than the dose required to prevent movement in response to a surgical stimulus. Administration of propofol may cause cardiovascular depression in hypovolemic children or those with a preexisting cardiomyopathy and should therefore be avoided or used with extreme caution.

Propofol injection can cause pain at the injection site. Although different methods have been studied to eliminate this pain, the most reliable method is to administer a small volume of 1% or 2% lidocaine while holding pressure proximal to the vein (i.e., a Bier block technique with your hand). Pressure is held for 5 to 10 seconds to assure that the wall of the vein is anesthetized after which the propofol is administered. This method effectively blunts the pain in most children.

During nonpainful medical procedures that require immobility (e.g., radiologic procedures) propofol can be used in moderate infusion doses (150–250 mcg/kg/min) that preserve spontaneous ventilation. For painful procedures (e.g., bone marrow biopsy, lumbar puncture, burn dressing changes) and surgical procedures that require a total intravenous anesthesia (TIVA) technique (e.g., rigid bronchoscopy, malignant hyperthermia-susceptible patient), greater doses of propofol are required to ensure immobility. These larger doses are inevitably associated with central or obstructive apnea. Alternatively, propofol can be combined with an opioid to decrease the total required propofol dose, but assisted ventilation will almost always be required.

Propofol is manufactured from the lipid components of egg and soy. Although these components may contain trace amounts of the residual protein, there have been no documented allergic reactions. Therefore, our policy has been to administer propofol to children with allergy to soy or egg protein, except in the case of documented anaphylaxis to egg or soy, where we practice more conservatively. Over the course of many years doing this, we are not aware of any allergic reactions.

Ketamine

In some cases, ketamine can be used instead of propofol as an induction and maintenance general anesthetic agent. At clinically useful doses (1–2 mg/kg IV), ketamine usually preserves spontaneous ventilation, upper airway patency, and normal cardiovascular function while providing analgesia and amnesia during painful procedures. Ketamine stimulates the sympathetic nervous system, which may cause undesirable increases in blood pressure, intracranial pressure, and intraocular pressure. However, it is useful for induction of anesthesia in patients in which cardiovascular stability is required, such as in the case of trauma or cardiomyopathy. Ketamine is associated with psychomimetic side effects (e.g., hallucinations, nightmares), increased airway secretions, postoperative nausea and vomiting, and delayed awakening. For these reasons, it has largely been replaced by propofol except for brief sedation for painful procedures and intramuscularly (2–4 mg/kg) as a sedative for uncooperative and/or developmentally delayed children.

Etomidate

Etomidate is mainly used in adults with cardiovascular disease and limited cardiovascular reserve. In these patients, it provides a stable induction with limited cardiovascular perturbation. Like ketamine, it may be useful in the traumatized child who is hypovolemic or in a child with a cardiomyopathy and decreased cardiovascular function. The dose range (0.2–0.3 mg/kg) and side effects (e.g., pain on injection, myoclonus, vomiting) appear to be similar to those in adults, including the risk for delayed adrenal suppression. Because of this risk for adrenal suppression, it is rarely used in pediatrics.

Opioids

Opioids are one component of a balanced anesthesia technique, contribute to postoperative analgesia, and attenuate or prevent postoperative emergence delirium or agitation. The choice of opioid depends on the nature and length of the surgical procedure and the expected duration and intensity of postoperative pain. For example, intranasal or intramuscular fentanyl (1–2 μg/kg) is often administered to children undergoing myringotomy and tube placement.

IV fentanyl is administered for neurosurgical procedures because of the intense analgesia required for scalp incision and placement of skull tongs, and relatively fewer analgesic requirements during the procedure and postoperatively. Morphine or hydromorphone are administered for urologic and abdominal procedures because of the requirement for a relatively longer duration and intensity of postoperative analgesia.

Opioids are commonly included as a component of a TIVA technique for painful surgical procedures. Fentanyl and its congeners (e.g., alfentanil, sufentanil, and remifentanil) are ideally suited for use in TIVA because of their relatively low context sensitive half-time. Remifentanil possesses the most favorable profile as its termination of action is directly related to its metabolism by tissue and nonspecific plasma esterases. Its effects usually dissipate within 5 to 10 minutes of discontinuing the infusion, regardless of the duration of the infusion.

Remifentanil bolus and infusion doses are higher in infants and young children than in adults, reflecting the larger volume of distribution and increased elimination clearance, respectively. Typically, a bolus dose of 1 to 2 μg/kg will be administered over several minutes, followed by an infusion dose of 0.2 to 1 μg/kg/min. This infusion dose is then titrated up or down to achieve the desired analgesic and hemodynamic effects. The use of intraoperative remifentanil has been associated with development of tolerance[8] and increased postoperative pain.

Historically, pediatric anesthesiologists have had concerns about the increased toxicity profile of opioids in the neonatal population because it is possible that opioids (especially the less lipid-soluble drug morphine) are allowed greater access through the blood-brain barrier in neonates and may result in proportionately greater levels in the brain. Furthermore, neonates have been shown to possess increased pharmacodynamic sensitivity, decreased clearance, and a relatively greater depression of CO_2 response curves to opioids compared with older subjects. These maturational changes appear to be most pronounced for morphine in comparison with fentanyl and its analogs. Opioids, like all types of medications administered to neonates, possess substantial interindividual variation in their pharmacokinetic and pharmacodynamic properties; thus, they should be titrated to effect while carefully observing for efficacy and side effects.

Dexmedetomidine

Dexmedetomidine[9] is an α_2-adrenoceptor agonist that is more receptor specific than clonidine. It has been primarily used in pediatric anesthesia to accomplish sedation for medical procedures or postoperative ventilation. Preoperatively, intranasal dexmedetomidine has been used for anxiolysis and sedation before induction of anesthesia. A 2 μg/kg intranasal dose produced faster onset of sedation without significant difference in induction, emergence and recovery compared with 0.5 mg/kg of oral midazolam. Intraoperatively, dexmedetomidine has been used as an adjunct in airway procedures and in both sleep endoscopy and airway imaging. In neurosurgery, it may be used by itself for tumor and epileptic seizure foci resection and mapping. Perioperatively, compared with placebo, dexmedetomidine at a dose of 0.5 to 1 µg/kg can decrease the incidence of emergence delirium by 10-fold. Dexmedetomidine administration is also associated with decreased intraoperative and postoperative opioid use.

Dexmedetomidine administration has been associated with hypotension and bradycardia (up to 30% decrease from baseline). Therefore, it should be avoided in children receiving digoxin, beta blockers, or agents that predispose to bradycardia or hypotension. Administration of an anticholinergic agent after dexmedetomidine has been associated with[10] severe hypertension.

Neuromuscular Blockers

Neuromuscular blockers are often administered to facilitate endotracheal intubation and may be continued intraoperatively to optimize surgical conditions and positive pressure ventilation.

There are developmental physiologic differences that influence the pharmacology of neuromuscular blockers (Table 19.1). During growth in early childhood, the increase in muscle volume increases the number of neuromuscular receptors. Conduction velocity and myelination increase during development and the rate of acetylcholine release progressively increases. Taken together, these are manifested clinically as a greater pharmacodynamic sensitivity to neuromuscular blockers in infants and young children (i.e., neuromuscular blockers are more potent in these age groups). Indeed, unanesthetized newborns demonstrate significant fade when applying 50-Hz tetanic stimulation, which suggests that their acetylcholine supply can be readily exhausted.

In practice, three (or more) times the ED_{95} is administered to assure rapid paralysis and account for pharmacokinetic and pharmacodynamic differences between individual patients. Nondepolarizing neuromuscular blockers are more potent (i.e., longer duration at similar doses) in infants than in children and less potent in children than adults.

Because all neuromuscular blockers are water-soluble and younger children are known to be composed of a relatively

greater volume of body water, the volume of distribution for these drugs is larger in younger children compared with older children and adults. Clinically, this translates to a higher bolus dose required to achieve a given plasma level.

Because neonates and small infants demonstrate enhanced sensitivity to neuromuscular blockers, a lower plasma concentration is required to maintain paralysis so the bolus maintenance dose is the same in a mg/kg basis as it is for adults. Neonates and small infants will also demonstrate a prolonged duration of action because of the larger volume of distribution and the decreased liver function in the newborn period. Because of this latter characteristic, the aminosteroidal relaxants, such as vecuronium and rocuronium, which rely on liver metabolism for their termination of effect, become long-acting agents, often exceeding 60 minutes or more in neonates.

Succinylcholine

Succinylcholine is the fastest acting agent with the shortest duration of action. Despite its many drawbacks in children, it remains the agent of choice for rapid sequence induction and for life-threatening upper airway obstruction, such as laryngospasm. In the latter situation, it can be given IM before establishment of IV access during inhalational induction.

Because succinylcholine is water-soluble, the IV bolus dose required in infants and young children (2 mg/kg) is larger than the dose for older children and adults (1 mg/kg). An intramuscular dose of 4 mg/kg will have an onset of action within a minute, a maximum onset of blockade in 3 to 4 minutes, and duration of action of approximately 20 minutes. In children, its duration of effect is less than in adults because its elimination clearance is more rapid.

There are a number of important side effects and complications of succinylcholine that include vagal-mediated bradycardia, junctional rhythms, or sinus arrest especially after the second dose within a short period of time. Some pediatric anesthesiologists administer an anticholinergic agent before succinylcholine to prevent bradycardia. IV atropine (0.02 mg/kg) and glycopyrrolate (0.01 mg/kg) are equally effective in attenuating succinylcholine-induced bradycardia.

Because of the low overall muscle mass in young children, fasciculations and postoperative muscle pain after administration of succinylcholine are unusual. However, muscle pain, rhabdomyolysis, and myoglobinuria may be observed when repeat doses are given. When these occur after just one dose of succinylcholine, the child should be investigated for an occult myopathy.

Because succinylcholine-induced paralysis causes muscle contraction by simulating the action of acetylcholine, potassium is released from the intracellular space and a transient and clinically insignificant increase in the plasma potassium level normally occurs. However, in patients with muscle atrophy or disorders associated with up-regulation of extrajunctional acetylcholine receptors (e.g., burns), an exaggerated potassium release will occur. The hyperkalemia that develops can lead to arrhythmias, cardiac arrest, and death.

TABLE 19.1	Age-Related Differences in ED_{95} (MG/KG) of Neuromuscular Blockers		
	Infants	Children	Adults
Atracurium	0.24	0.33	0.21
Cisatracurium	0.06	0.06	0.05
Pancuronium	0.065	0.10	0.07
Rocuronium	0.25	0.40	0.35
Vecuronium	0.05	0.08	0.04
Succinylcholine	0.61	0.35	0.29

An important publication[11] in 1997 by Larach et al. alerted the anesthesiology community to a number of cases of succinylcholine-induced life-threatening hyperkalemia in young boys with undiagnosed Duchenne muscular dystrophy. As a result, anesthesiologists generally avoid succinylcholine for routine, elective neuromuscular blockade. But because succinylcholine is still indicated in some situations, all anesthesiologists should be aware that hyperkalemia is manifested as peaked T waves on the electrocardiogram (ECG), which may develop into a wide complex tachycardia, ventricular fibrillation, and asystole. If this occurs, one should not wait to confirm with a blood-potassium level, but should begin immediate treatment with calcium chloride (5–10 mg/kg) or calcium gluconate (50–100 mg/kg) followed by a beta-agonist such as albuterol, insulin and glucose, sodium polystyrene (via orogastric tube), furosemide, and dialysis if clinically indicated.

Succinylcholine-induced hyperkalemia can occur in patients with any type of disease associated with muscle atrophy, especially when progressive (e.g., Duchenne muscular dystrophy) or after an acute muscle injury or burn. Children with cerebral palsy or meningomyelocele demonstrate a normal potassium release after succinylcholine; thus, the use of succinylcholine in these patient groups is not contraindicated.

Along with inhaled anesthetic agents, succinylcholine may trigger malignant hyperthermia (MH) in susceptible patients. When succinylcholine was used routinely, the incidence of MH was estimated to be 1 in 15,000 children. In retrospect, many of these cases were probably rhabdomyolysis-induced hyperkalemia rather than MH, but the possibility of triggering MH is another reason that succinylcholine is no longer used in children electively.

On occasion (1% or more in some studies), masseter muscle rigidity (MMR) may occur after succinylcholine administration. It ranges from a mild difficulty with mouth opening to the complete inability to open the mouth ("jaws of steel"). This may represent a normal response to succinylcholine, especially if underdosed. When severe, or accompanied by generalized rigidity, it can represent an early sign of MH.

If severe MMR occurs, all volatile anesthetics should be discontinued and a nontriggering technique with TIVA administered. Creatine kinase levels should be obtained along with electrolytes and blood gas analysis. The patient should be observed closely for signs and symptoms suggestive of an acute MH crisis. Treatment with dantrolene is not indicated unless there are definitive signs of MH.

Nondepolarizing Neuromuscular Blockers

The nondepolarizing neuromuscular blockers are divided into two major categories based on structure and mode of elimination. The benzylisoquiniliniums (e.g., atracurium, cisatracurium) rely on metabolism by Hofmann degradation and ester hydrolysis by nonspecific plasma esterases for their termination of action. The aminosteroids (e.g., vecuronium, rocuronium) are metabolized in the liver to inactive products that are eliminated by the kidney. A major advantage of the aminosteroids is their efficacy after intramuscular administration.

Atracurium, 0.5 mg/kg, usually produces reliable intubating conditions within 90 seconds after administration. Its duration of action is approximately 30 to 40 minutes but is usually reversible within 20 minutes after administration. Because its metabolism does not rely on hepatic function, its duration of action is predictable, even in neonates. Large doses of atracurium may result in histamine release that is manifested as a macular rash, and rarely, bronchospasm and hypotension.

Cisatracurium is a cis isomer of atracurium and possesses a similar clinical and pharmacokinetic profile except for its increased potency and lack of histamine release. Its onset to maximum block is slower than atracurium. Typically, a dose of 0.15 to 0.2 mg/kg will provide reliable intubating conditions within 2 minutes. Clinical studies in children indicate that administration of cisatracurium is associated with a

A DEEPER DIVE

In Larach's important description of 25 children who had a cardiac arrest within 24 hours of receiving an anesthetic, 20 were previously healthy. The presenting cardiac symptoms included wide complex bradycardia, ventricular tachycardia with hypotension, ventricular fibrillation, and asystole. Hyperkalemia occurred (mean peak serum K^+ 7.4 ± 2.8 mmol/L [median 7.5, range 3.5–14.8]) in 13 of 18 patients in whom potassium level was measured during the cardiac arrest. Eight of the 13 patients with hyperkalemia received both succinylcholine and potent inhaled anesthetics, while one patient received succinylcholine alone, and four received inhaled anesthetics without succinylcholine. Fifteen patients survived, most with eventual return of baseline neurologic function. Of the 13 patients with hyperkalemia, 8 were eventually shown to have an occult myopathy that was previously unknown to the family or anesthesia team. Anesthesiologists should always rule out an occult myopathy in children preoperatively by inquiring about abnormal muscle weakness or delayed (or lost) motor milestones. The failure of a child to walk unassisted by 15 months of age should prompt further evaluation. Clinical features of Duchenne muscular dystrophy include calf muscle hypertrophy, toe walking, and a waddling gait. An elevated creatine kinase level may indicate an occult myopathy.

Based largely on this report, the Food and Drug Administration (FDA) asked the manufacturer to place a **black box warning**[12] in the package insert of succinylcholine. The report and the **black box warning** led to the precipitous decline of elective use of succinylcholine in children.

Succinylcholine Black-Box Warning

"It is recommended that the use of succinylcholine in children should be reserved for emergency intubation or instances where immediate securing of the airway is necessary, e.g., laryngospasm, difficult airway, full stomach, or for intramuscular use when a suitable vein is inaccessible."

slightly longer and less predictable duration of action than atracurium; compared with other agents, cisatracurium is still relatively predictable given its metabolism via Hofmann elimination.

Vecuronium, 0.1 mg/kg, usually provides reliable intubating conditions within 2 minutes. Its duration of action is approximately 40 to 75 minutes but is usually reversible within 30 minutes of administration. School-aged children require relatively more vecuronium to achieve a desired effect and recover faster than infants and adults. Because its termination depends on liver metabolism, the duration of action can be prolonged in neonates and small infants or in patients with hepatic dysfunction. Vecuronium administration is associated with bradycardia when given in combination with fentanyl or one of its analogs. However, vecuronium is not associated with histamine release or bronchospasm.

It is possible to use vecuronium for rapid sequence induction. At a dose of 0.4 mg/kg (four times a typical intubating dose) reliable intubation conditions can be achieved within 1 minute but at the expense of a prolonged duration of action: reversibility may not be possible for more than 90 minutes or shorter with the administration of sugammadex. This large dose can be decreased by also administering an opioid.

Rocuronium has a similar clinical profile as vecuronium and atracurium. Its main advantage is its ability to be given in higher doses (1.2–1.6 mg/kg) to achieve reliable intubating conditions within 1 minute. These higher doses are not associated with the prolonged duration of action seen with vecuronium; reversibility with neostigmine is usually possible within 45 minutes, or much shorter with administration of sugammadex. Therefore, rocuronium is often preferred to succinylcholine for rapid sequence induction in children.

When administered intramuscularly (1.0 mg/kg for infants and 1.8 mg/kg for children), rocuronium provides reliable intubating conditions within 3 minutes at the expense of a prolonged duration of action that may exceed an hour. A deltoid injection provides more reliable plasma levels than a quadriceps injection.

Ventilating Children During General Anesthesia

Pediatric patients undergoing surgery often require mechanical ventilation, especially if intubated. Like most aspects of pediatric care, the tolerance for error is smaller than in adults because small variations can be a significant percentage of the intended therapy. With regard to mechanical ventilation, the most important consideration is that small changes in delivered tidal volume can be a significant percentage of the intended tidal volume. Consequences of unintended variation in tidal volume can be hypoventilation with hypercarbia and atelectasis, or excessive tidal volume with attendant hypocarbia and barotrauma or volutrauma.

On most operating room ventilators, there are both volume and pressure-controlled ventilation modes. With pressure-controlled ventilation, a peak inspiratory pressure is selected (in children with healthy lungs usually between 15 and 18 cmH$_2$O), and the rate is set to achieve the desired carbon dioxide concentration. One should recognize that volume is not guaranteed in pressure mode and will vary with changes in lung compliance. Pressure mode is most useful when changes in lung compliance are not likely although tidal volume monitoring is important. It is useful to set a low tidal volume or minute ventilation alarm close to the desired value so that one will be aware of changes in lung compliance that reduce tidal volume.

Pressure mode has historically been preferred in children because earlier generations of anesthesia ventilators could not deliver small tidal volumes accurately in volume mode. Current approaches to mechanical ventilation emphasize limiting tidal volume to 5 to 7 mL/kg of ideal bodyweight to reduce the potential for ventilator-induced lung injury. Given the desire to control tidal volume, volume controlled (targeted) modes of ventilation make it easier to implement a lung protective ventilation strategy. Modern anesthesia ventilators designed to compensate for the compliance of the breathing circuit are capable of delivering even small tidal volumes accurately. Therefore, volume-controlled ventilation is a very reasonable choice even for small children when using one of these anesthesia ventilators. When using volume-controlled ventilation, a set tidal volume is selected (usually 5–7 mL/kg) and the rate is set to achieve the desired carbon dioxide concentration. Pressure will vary with changes in lung compliance, so it is useful to set an inspiratory pressure limit to prevent excessive pressures because of transient decreases in effective lung compliance like coughing or surgical retraction. Regardless of whether pressure or volume controlled ventilation is used, alterations can be made to the overall ventilation, including changes in the inspiratory to expiratory time ratios and the addition of positive end-expiratory pressure (PEEP) (in healthy children we usually use a PEEP of at least 4–5 cmH$_2$O to prevent loss of FRC) to ensure adequate gas exchange.

It is important to monitor inspiratory pressure, tidal volume and end-tidal CO$_2$ to assess the interaction of the ventilator with the patient. Because arterial blood gas information is not routinely available, assessing oxygenation using SpO$_2$ at an inspiratory oxygen concentration of 25% or less will help guide adjustments to PEEP and tidal volume and the need for recruitment maneuvers. Tidal volumes of 7 mL/kg are adequate for most patients and will result in an end-tidal CO$_2$ measurement that will approximate the arterial CO$_2$ value.

There are different opinions about the value of neuromuscular blockade on ventilatory function during general anesthesia. One study[7] demonstrated a decrease of functional residual capacity (FRC) and ventilation homogeneity after onset of paralysis. In another study of spontaneously breathing children, the performance of a recruitment maneuver to 15 cmH$_2$O resulted in less atelectasis (measured by MRI) than a control group of children that received only CPAP of 5 cmH$_2$O.

A DEEPER DIVE

Equipment Considerations For Mechanical Ventilation Of The Pediatric Patient

An optimal mechanical ventilation strategy requires thoughtful selection of the ventilating parameters (ventilation mode, tidal volume, respiratory rate, I:E ratio, and PEEP) and a mechanical ventilator and breathing circuit to implement the strategy. Not all ventilators are equal however, and the apparatus selected to connect the patient to the ventilator can also impact the outcome. In this "deep dive," we will take a closer look at the features of a modern anesthesia ventilator that facilitate pediatric ventilation and the importance of managing dead space. We will also discuss the pros and cons of using an ICU ventilator in the operating room. If you want to dive even deeper, check out the reference by Feldman entitled "Optimal Ventilation of the Anesthetized Pediatric Patient."

Anesthesia Ventilators

Traditional anesthesia ventilators were not well suited for precise tidal volume delivery so pediatric anesthetists typically selected pressure-controlled ventilation. The compliance of the breathing circuit and the interaction of fresh gas flow with tidal volume were the primary barriers to delivering the desired tidal volume. Because of these factors, there was a significant and unpredictable difference between the volume delivered by the ventilator into the circuit, and the volume delivered to the patient's airway. Modern anesthesia ventilators are capable of compliance and fresh gas flow compensation, overcoming these barriers to precise volume delivery.

If you use an anesthesia ventilator that requires an automated pre-use checkout procedure where the end of the breathing circuit is occluded, you likely have a ventilator with compliance compensation. During this checkout procedure, the ventilator delivers a volume into the circuit to achieve a target pressure. Because the end of the circuit is occluded, no gas actually flows, and the ratio of the volume delivered to the pressure achieved determines the breathing circuit compliance factor in mL/cmH_2O. (Fig. 19.2) Once this compliance factor is known, the ventilator adjusts the volume delivered into the circuit to ensure that the set tidal volume is delivered to the airway. For example, if the circuit compliance is $5\,mL/cmH_2O$, the ventilator adds $100\,mL$ to the set tidal volume at an inspiratory pressure of $20\,cmH_2O$ and the desired volume is delivered to the airway. **It is essential to do the pre-use checkout with the circuit configuration to be used during the procedure.** Expanding the circuit or adding devices after the pre-use checkout will change the circuit compliance altering delivered tidal volume.

Fresh gas flow compensation is intended to eliminate the impact on delivered tidal volume by fresh gas flow. Anesthesia machines approach fresh gas compensation differently but all achieve similar results, namely consistent tidal volume delivery independent of fresh gas flow changes. Not only does tidal volume delivery improve with compliance and fresh gas flow compensation, but tidal volume measurement does as well. To understand the details read the reference by Feldman mentioned previously.

Dead Space: The Ventilation Barrier Hiding in Plain Sight

Dead space in the breathing circuit and lungs is present whenever there is ventilation without gas exchange. Because ventilation requires bidirectional flow, dead space in an anesthesia circuit only exists on the patient side of the wye piece. Devices added to the breathing circuit between the patient and the wye piece add to the dead space. Typical devices include elbows, heat and moisture exchangers, and flexible connectors. Smaller patients are especially sensitive to the increase in dead space and will either experience hypercarbia at a set minute ventilation or require increased minute ventilation to approach a normal level of arterial CO_2. Because arterial CO_2 increases exponentially as dead space increases, it becomes increasingly difficult to control arterial CO_2 (Fig. 19.3). A good rule of thumb is to limit apparatus dead space to less than one-third of the desired tidal volume. This can be especially challenging when caring for patients who weigh less than $5\,kg$ but devices for sampling gas and connecting the breathing circuit to the patient are still required. In that case, the desired tidal volume is about $30\,mL$ and the apparatus dead space is ideally no more than $10\,mL$. **End-tidal CO_2 will be an even less accurate indicator of arterial CO_2 as dead space increases, hiding the impact of dead space on ventilation.** For an even deeper dive, swim over to the references by Pearsall and King.

Do I Need an ICU Ventilator in the Operating Room?

The short answer is that if you are using a modern anesthesia ventilator as described previously, an ICU ventilator is not more capable. Indeed, if the specifications of the anesthesia and ICU ventilators are compared, the differences are not clinically significant for the majority of pediatric patients in the operating room (Fig. 19.4). Furthermore, there are compelling reasons why an anesthesia ventilator is preferable to an ICU ventilator. Most compelling is the ability to transition between mechanical and manual ventilation without the need to disconnect the circuit. The dynamics of surgical procedures often require manual ventilation for lung recruitment and trouble shooting oxygenation problems. ICU ventilators do not provide a manual ventilation capability. Switching from the ICU ventilator circuit to a manual ventilation option compounds the oxygenation problem and risks dislodging the endotracheal tube – not desirable! Anesthesia ventilators also offer the convenience of delivering inhaled anesthetics offering a degree of control over anesthetic depth that is not possible with an intravenous agent.

What Is Successful Mechanical Ventilation?

A successful strategy has three goals:
- The best oxygenation at the least oxygen concentration
- The desired tidal volume with the least inspiratory pressure
- Acceptable CO_2 elimination
  Fortunately, bedside monitors are readily available to monitor how well these goals are achieved.
- **Oxygenation** is readily monitored by reducing the inspired oxygen concentration to approach 21% and observing the oxyhemoglobin saturation by pulse oximetry. Enriched oxygen concentrations will hide oxygenation problems because of V/Q mismatch and provide a false sense of accomplishment.
- **Lung compliance** is also a good indicator of the effectiveness of mechanical ventilation. Strategies that maintain an "open lung" (i.e., prevent atelectasis) will improve lung compliance. Monitor the relationship between pressure and tidal volume either directly or via pressure-volume loops to assess lung compliance.
- **CO_2 elimination** can be assessed by capnography. The gradient between end-tidal and arterial CO_2 is estimated to be 5 to $10\,mm$ Hg which should be reliable if the other indicators of oxygenation and lung compliance are relatively normal.

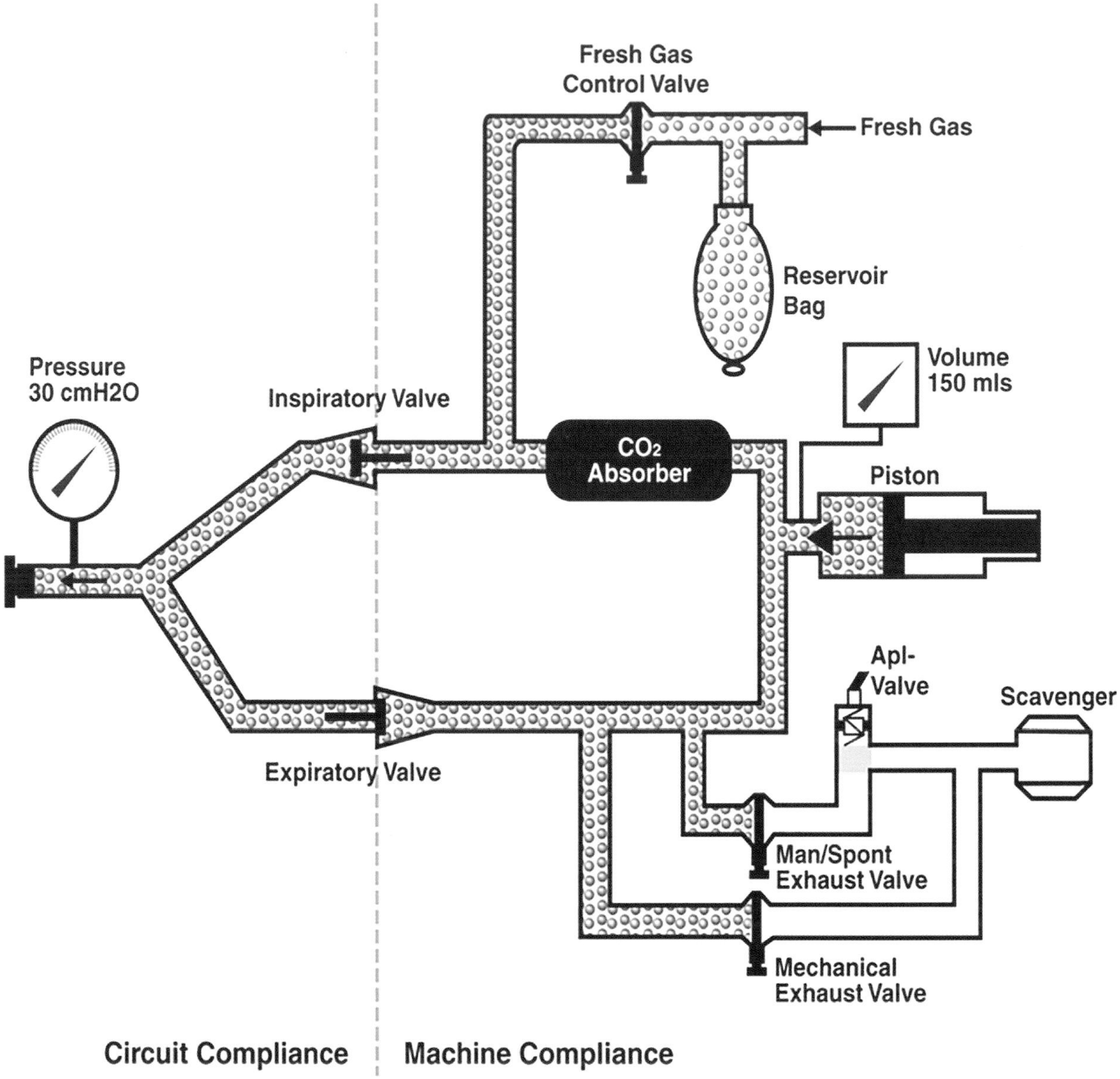

$$\text{System Compliance} = 150 \text{ mls}/30 \text{ cmH}_2\text{O} = 5 \text{ mls/cmH}_2\text{O}$$

• **Fig 19.2.** Example of anesthesia ventilator (piston-type) performing a pre-use checkout to determine the breathing circuit compliance. Ventilator compressed 150 mLs of volume to achieve the target pressure of 30 cmH$_2$O.

Emergence From General Anesthesia

The short duration of action of modern inhaled anesthetic agents makes titration down at the end of the case largely unnecessary. When the surgeon is nearly finished, the anesthesia provider can turn off the vaporizer and in almost all cases, within 5 minutes, the child is actively emerging.

Lest you think the process requires as little skill as we have alluded to, there is the small issue of avoiding postextubation airway obstruction and laryngospasm, which can often ruin your otherwise smooth day in the pediatric operating room. The most reliable method to avoid this annoying (and

dangerous because it can lead to cardiac arrest[13]) complication is to extubate the child's trachea when he or she is sufficiently awake, or sufficiently anesthetized, but never in between.

An "awake" extubation requires good muscular strength, a regular breathing pattern without apneic pauses or breath-holding, and that indefinably high enough level of consciousness that ensures the presence of airway protective mechanisms but also doesn't promote laryngospasm. Let's discuss each of these criteria in more detail.

Before tracheal extubation, each child must have sufficient muscular strength to support upper airway patency. If

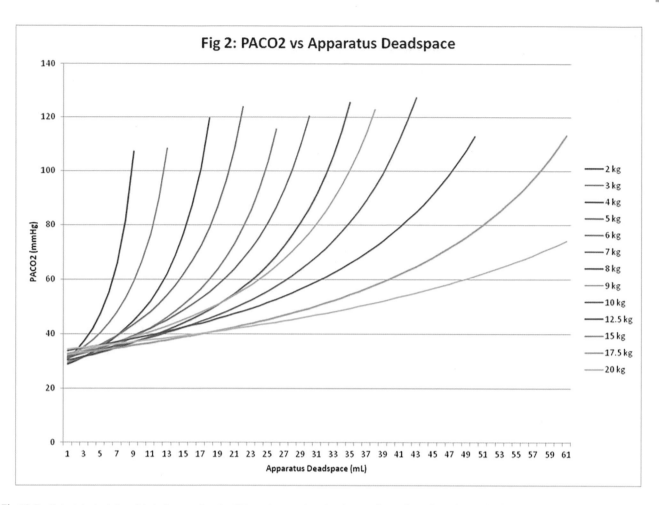

• **Fig 19.3.** Calculated relationship between alveolar CO_2 and apparatus dead space for patients from 2 to 20 kg. Not surprisingly, the impact of dead space is greater as patients get smaller! (From: Pearsall MF, Feldman JM. When does apparatus dead space matter for the pediatric patient?. *Anesth Analg.* 2014;118(4):776–780. doi:10.1213/ANE.0000000000000148.)

Device	Type	Pmax	RR Max	PEEP	Vt min
Babylog	P - ICU	80	150	25	2
Aisys/ Avance	P - Bellows	100	100	30	20
Flow-i	P - Reflectr	80	100	50	20
Apollo	M - Piston	70	100	20	5-20
Perseus	M - Blower	80	100	35	20

• **Fig 19.4.** Comparison of specifications between the Draeger Medical Babylog ICU ventilator and four different anesthesia machine ventilators. Note that reaching the minimum tidal volume of the Babylog requires an additional sensor at the airway. *P*, Pneumatic; *M*, mechanical.

a neuromuscular blocker was administered, a reversal agent should be given, unless the last dose of the paralytic was relatively far in the past and you are convinced of the patient's excellent strength. Many studies have demonstrated a faster recovery from neuromuscular blockade in children compared with adults, but recovery times after administration of reversal agents are probably not age dependent.

Neostigmine is an acetylcholinesterase inhibitor that is used to reverse paralysis from neuromuscular blockade. Because administration of neostigmine can result in

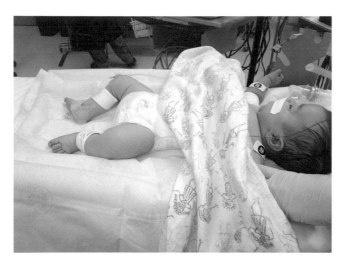

• **Fig 19.5.** During emergence from general anesthesia, hip flexion in an infant will reliably predict sufficient strength for upper airway patency.

bradycardia, glycopyrrolate an anticholinergic agent is routinely coadministered. Other than obvious demonstrations of strength during emergence (e.g., vigorously attempting to remove the endotracheal tube), the ability of the infant or child to flex their hips is an indication of sufficient strength to maintain airway patency independently after removal of the endotracheal tube (Fig. 19.5).

Sugammadex is a noncompetitive antagonist and forms a one-to-one complex with rocuronium and vecuronium. It encapsulates rocuronium in the plasma, reducing its concentration and reverses neuromuscular blockade. Compared with neostigmine,[14] sugammadex has a faster time to reversal; its use has been increasing[15] in the pediatric population.

A typical dose of sugammadex is 2 mg/kg when there are greater than two twitches on train-of-four testing, or 4 mg/kg when there are 1 to 2 posttetanic twitches. A maximum dose of 16 mg/kg can be used for immediate reversal when faced with a "cannot intubate-cannot ventilate scenario" after administration of rocuronium. Mild adverse events[16] include nausea, vomiting, pain, hypotension, and headache. Severe adverse effects observed during preclinical trials include bradycardia and anaphylaxis, although fewer rates of bradycardia have been reported compared with neostigmine. There is also a small chance of recurarization.[17] Unlike neostigmine, sugammadex does not require coadministration with an anticholinergic agent.

After discontinuation of the anesthetic agent and reversal of neuromuscular blockade,[18] children will begin their own spontaneous breathing attempts. These first breaths may appear to be regular, and triggered by the ventilator, but as consciousness increases, these spontaneous breaths will become more irregular with alternating periods of breath holding, and coughing. This temporary phase should not be confused with wakefulness! In fact, during this phase of breath holding and coughing, small infants (especially premature ones with a history of lung disease) will often demonstrate profound decreases in oxygen saturation that are frightening to the entire operating room staff, and prompt

the overhead announcement of "ANESTHESIA NOW" to your location. But as long as the endotracheal tube remains securely in place, air exchange can be maintained by vigorous positive pressure ventilation, which will shortly increase the oxygen saturation. As this occurs, the confident anesthesia provider remains calm and continues to conduct themselves in a manner that leaves no doubt that they are in control of the situation. Indeed, the OR staff's emotions are usually based on the anesthesia provider's reactions to critical situations. During this phase of breath holding, coughing, and oxygen desaturation, the child's lungs should be manually ventilated at a relatively fast rate (>30 breaths per minute) and with a high enough inspiratory pressure to cause observable chest rise. Air entry is confirmed by auscultation and capnographic evidence of CO_2 removal. If the capnograph indicates air exchange, one can be confident that the oxygen saturation will soon begin to rise (the pulse oximeter reading may lag behind). Conversely, if the capnograph does not demonstrate adequate air exchange, the manual ventilation technique must be adjusted to ensure chest rise, (and correct location of the endotracheal tube should be confirmed by auscultation). This may require unusually high inspiratory pressures in small infants with good strength. When the child begins to breathe regularly and maintain normal oxygen saturation without much assistance, the provider can then begin to consider tracheal extubation[19] when signs of wakefulness appear.

Unless the child is pharmacologically weak, the demonstration of wakefulness is the last extubation criterion to appear. Wakefulness will nearly always ensure that the child will assume a regular breathing pattern and adequate airway protective responses. Most children, in the throes of emergence, will not respond to commands to open their eyes or squeeze their fists. Thus the provider is left to infer wakefulness indirectly, by observing spontaneous eye opening, scrunching of the eyebrows, or attempts to cry. Involuntary reflexes such as reaching for the endotracheal tube may not be an indication of wakefulness. In general, always err on the side of leaving the endotracheal tube in too long, for taking it out too soon can certainly ruin your day and you will inevitably end up defending your decision at the monthly quality improvement conference.

Pediatric anesthesiologists often instruct trainees to administer a transient inspiratory hold, up to $30 \text{ cmH}_2\text{O}$ immediately before, and as part of, the last breath before tracheal extubation. The intent of this maneuver is to reverse any existing atelectasis that occurred during the general anesthetic and to restore the FRC. However, controlled studies on the efficacy of this maneuver have not been performed.

Occasionally, in seemingly awake infants, breath holding may develop shortly after tracheal extubation as a result of laryngeal stimulation that occurs during removal of the endotracheal tube. If the infant does not become hypoxemic, we prefer to avoid positive-pressure ventilation but continue to maintain upper airway patency by chin lift and/or jaw thrust. In the majority of cases, the child will resume spontaneous ventilation within a minute and will not develop hypoxemia. In the remainder of children that develop hypoxemia, positive-pressure ventilation is indicated and laryngospasm should be immediately treated with a small dose of IV succinylcholine (0.2–0.3 mg/kg).

Deep Extubation

Occasionally, a situation arises where you think it might be detrimental for the child to regain consciousness and airway reflexes with the endotracheal tube in the trachea. For example, a brittle asthmatic may be at risk for bronchospasm, or perhaps a surgeon may request deep extubation if they are concerned that coughing may disrupt delicate suture placement, for example, in eye surgery. In these cases, the endotracheal tube should be removed from the trachea at a sufficient depth of anesthesia, before the child develops the ability to cough or respond to endotracheal tube movement. Contraindications to "deep extubation" include risk for pulmonary aspiration from gastric contents, or any type of predicted difficulty with mask ventilation or tracheal intubation.

The "deep extubation" technique consists of the following:

- First establish a pattern of regular spontaneous ventilation by gradually lowering the concentration of inhaled agent and, if applicable, reverse the neuromuscular blockade to assure adequate strength. Empty any residual stomach contents with an orogastric tube.
- After establishing a spontaneous, regular breathing pattern, slowly increase the concentration of the inhaled agent to approximately 2 to 3 MAC, within the limits of normal vital signs and maintenance of spontaneous respiratory effort.
- Suction the oropharynx and gently remove the endotracheal tube as you carefully observe for appearance of laryngospasm. Some anesthesiologists prefer to administer lidocaine, up to 1.5 mg/kg, several minutes before deep extubation, to further prevent airway reflexes. Administration of glycopyrrolate to decrease excess secretions may also be considered, but the latency time for this effect is unknown.
- Resume mask ventilation and discontinue the inhaled agent after confirmation that airway reflexes have abated. An oral airway often helps maintain upper airway patency during this phase.

A major consideration when performing a deep extubation is that the child will pass through the lighter stages of anesthesia with an unprotected airway, and often in an area that is not as closely supervised as in the operating room (i.e., postanesthesia care unit [PACU]). Secretions or blood may come in contact with laryngeal structures and precipitate laryngospasm. Therefore, deep extubation should be performed only if the provider has the ability to remain with the child until consciousness is regained, or if the PACU nursing staff possess the experience and training to accommodate the emerging child and promptly recognize upper airway obstruction.

Are Anesthetic Agents Neurotoxic to the Developing Brain?

One of the most important unresolved controversies in modern-day pediatric anesthesia is whether or not the exposure of a young child to anesthetic agents contributes to intellectual or cognitive deficits later in life. Unraveling this mystery has taken center stage for pediatric anesthesiologists since the beginning of the 21st century.

Our current preoccupation with this topic began in 2003 when researchers at the University of Virginia described the appearance of widespread apoptotic neurodegeneration in the brains of 7-day-old rats after exposure to differing combinations of midazolam, nitrous oxide, and isoflurane for 6 hours. More concerning was the correlation of these lesions with persistent memory and learning impairments. Since then, many other animal studies, including some in primate species, have demonstrated similar findings, but the majority of these have used anesthetic exposures greater than typically seen during human exposures.

As a result of these worrisome preclinical studies, an enormous amount of time and money has been spent in academic medical centers throughout the world in an attempt to clarify and elucidate aspects of this potentially catastrophic problem. In 2009, a public-private partnership organization between the FDA and the International Anesthesia Research Society (IARS) was created and named SmartTots (SmartTots.org) whose mission is to organize and fund research that attempts to answer questions, such as:

1. Do these effects occur in humans, or are they confined to animal species?
2. Within what age range is the brain vulnerable to damage from exposure to anesthetic agents?
3. Which anesthetic agents are responsible for brain damage? Is there a dose-related relationship? Are any of these medications relatively safer than any others?
4. What is the duration of exposure that increases the risk for brain damage?
5. Are multiple exposures riskier than a single exposure?
6. Does the nature of the surgical intervention make a difference?
7. What are additional predisposing factors? For example, what role is played by comorbidities that require the child to require surgical intervention in the first place or a patient's socioeconomic status?
8. What is the role of other anesthetic-related physiologic perturbations such as alterations in blood pressure, temperature, glucose, carbon dioxide, prematurity, body temperature, or even head position, to name just a few?
9. What are the specific neurocognitive deficits that are related to anesthetic exposure?
10. Are there any medications that can be administered or substituted in the perioperative period that will mitigate these adverse effects?

Nearly 20 years later, definitive answers to all of these questions are still lacking. At the time of this writing, there have been many single-center database studies that have reported mixed results. Although some showed correlations between anesthetic exposure and learning disabilities later in life, others have demonstrated more reassuring results. In fact, one large long-term study from Sweden demonstrated more of an effect from gender, age at school entry, and level of maternal education, than from exposure to general anesthesia in the first 4 years of life. But on the other hand, an analysis of a Medicaid database from Texas and New York determined that children who experienced a single surgical procedure under the age of 5 years were 37% more likely to be prescribed ADHD medications than unexposed children several years later.

In the face of this current uncertainty, anesthesia providers should follow these commonsense recommendations:

1. Do not perform purely elective surgery or medical procedures that require administration of sedative or general anesthetic agents on children of any age.

   Strictly speaking, there are no purely elective surgeries that we perform in children younger than adolescence. But there are a number of radiologic procedures, especially MRI, that on the surface, appear to have no evidenced-based indication. Young children who are scheduled for MRI with sedation or general anesthesia should be carefully screened with input from the child's pediatrician or neurologist to clarify the true importance for the scan to be performed during early infancy or childhood.

2. Minimize the duration of exposure to general anesthesia in any one procedure.

   We all know instances in which the anesthetic exposure time was unnecessarily prolonged when the attending surgeon is finishing a case in another room, or the medical student is taught how to close a wound, or when an inexperienced anesthesia resident is allowed multiple attempts at intubation or IV insertion. That is not to say that trainees should not learn on children, but these should be closely monitored and of appropriate duration and attempts. Surgical wait times should be minimized by meticulous planning and organization of multiple procedures by different surgeons. Waiting for the surgeon to finish another child's procedure in a nearby operating room (or building!) is never appropriate.

   However, the problem here is that there must be a balance between an anesthetic of prolonged duration and the occurrence of multiple anesthetics of short duration, both of which have been associated with neurocognitive delays in animals. It seems that the best compromise at this time is to limit any anesthetic exposure to under 3 hours duration. Procedures expected to last longer should be proactively discussed between the child's medical, surgical, and anesthetic teams in an attempt to devise a plan for a shorter exposure time.

3. Use regional anesthesia whenever possible.

   There are not many surgical procedures performed in young infants that are not amenable to using local anesthesia to reduce intraoperative anesthetic requirements. When feasible, local anesthesia should be used from the outset of the procedure, not just for the purpose of reducing postoperative pain. In an off-shoot of the GAS study, Dr. Mary Ellen McCann demonstrated that spinal anesthesia for hernia repair resulted in less hypotension compared with general anesthesia.

4. Keep all physiologic parameters well within "normal" ranges.

   Yes, of course we understand that everyone's definition of "normal" may differ, but in general, be conservative with expectations for indices such as the lowest

---

A DEEPER DIVE

Two large multicenter studies have been performed in an attempt to begin to provide answers to some of these questions. Let's take a closer look at those results:

Performed between 2007 and 2013, the **General Anesthesia vs. Spinal Anesthesia (GAS)** study randomized 722 eligible infants less than 60 weeks' postconceptional age throughout the world to receive either general anesthesia with sevoflurane or regional (i.e., spinal or epidural) anesthesia with bupivacaine (without systemic sedation) for inguinal hernia repair. Upon evaluation of neurocognitive function using a variety of tests at 5 years of age, there were no differences between the groups. Published in 2019 in *Lancet,* this is the only prospective and randomized study to address this issue, and provides reassurance that a single exposure to sevoflurane for less than about an hour is not associated with neurocognitive abnormalities 5 years later.

The **Pediatric Anesthesia and NeuroDevelopment Assessment (PANDA)** multicenter study was performed between 2009 and 2015. The researchers administered neurocognitive tests to 105 healthy sibling pairs, between 8 and 15 years of age, with the condition that they were within 36 months of age apart, and only one had been exposed to general anesthesia for inguinal hernia repair before 36 months of age, while the other had not been exposed to general anesthesia before 36 months of age. The results were published in *JAMA* in 2016, and revealed that the sibling pairs did not have demonstrable differences in IQ scores at a mean age of approximately 11 years.

Despite these reassurances, in December, 2016, as a result of the convincing nature of the preclinical evidence and the variable retrospective data results, the FDA issued a "black-box" label warning on all inhalational anesthetics and several anesthetic and sedative agents (e.g., etomidate, ketamine, lorazepam, methohexital, midazolam, pentobarbital, and propofol) stating that repeated or lengthy use of these drugs in children under the age of 3 years or in pregnant women during their third trimester may affect the developing child's brain. The agency further emphasized that regardless of age or maturation, children should not be denied general anesthesia when necessary for essential surgery or painful procedures, as untreated pain and stress is equally detrimental to the developing brain. The label urged health care professionals to balance the benefit of appropriate anesthesia in young children and pregnant women against the potential risks, especially for procedures that may last longer than 3 hours or if multiple procedures are required in children under the age of 3 years.

acceptable intraoperative blood pressure, hemoglobin, glucose level, temperature, and end-tidal CO_2 values.

5. Keep the child's head in a neutral position.

There is evidence that lateral head rotation may diminish blood flow in the jugular veins or carotid arteries. There is no clinical reason why this cannot be accomplished during a surgical procedure that does not involve one side of the head or neck.

Some investigators have begun the search for safer anesthetics or those that may mitigate damage from known neurotoxicants. For example, some preclinical work has been published incorporating dexmedetomidine into the anesthetic regimen, with mixed results on eventual cellular damage from long-term exposure to inhalational agents. Time will tell whether or not pediatric anesthesiologists will routinely include dexmedetomidine in their anesthetic regimen in an attempt to lower the exposure to inhalational agents.

We are left to conclude that there will never be definitive answers that point to the most optimal choices that decrease the risk for anesthetic neurotoxicity in young children, if it indeed exists. To quote Efron et al. in a 2017 editorial, "Sicker children get anesthetics, and sicker children have more developmental issues." Separating causes from associations in this population is a nearly impossible task.

Prevention of Surgical Site Infections

Despite improvements in surgical practices, instrument sterilization methods, and the best efforts of infection prevention practitioners, surgical site infections (SSIs) remain the second most commonly reported health care-associated infection (HAI) in adults and children, representing up to 16% of all infections reported to the National Healthcare Surveillance Safety Network (NHSN) of the Centers for Disease Control and Prevention (CDC). SSIs increase patient morbidity and mortality and health care costs. More specifically, each SSI is associated with approximately 7 to 11 additional postoperative hospital days, while patients with an SSI have a 2 to 11-times higher risk for death compared with operative patients without an SSI. Up to 60% of SSIs have been estimated to be preventable by using evidence-based guidelines.

To reduce the risk for nosocomial SSIs, a systematic but realistic approach must be applied, with awareness that this risk is influenced by the characteristics of the patient, the operation, the health care staff, and the hospital. In theory, reducing the risk is relatively simple and inexpensive, especially compared with the cost of the infections themselves, but in practice it requires commitment at all levels of the health care system. Basic practices for preventing SSI include recommendations where the potential to impact HAI risk clearly outweighs the potential for undesirable effects. These include the following:

- *Skin preparation:* Several antiseptic agents are available for preoperative preparation of skin at the incision site. The iodophors (e.g., povidone-iodine), alcohol-containing products, and chlorhexidine gluconate are the most commonly used agents. Alcohol is highly bactericidal and effective for preoperative skin antisepsis but does not have persistent activity when used alone. Rapid, persistent, and cumulative antisepsis can be achieved by combining alcohol with chlorhexidine gluconate or an iodophor.

- *Surgical attire:* All persons entering the surgical area must wear surgical attire (scrub suits). All head and facial hair, including sideburns and neckline, must be covered (although facial hair is not a recommended practice). Full coverage of the mouth and nose area with a surgical mask is required for everyone entering the operating suite. Sterile gowns must be worn by all personnel participating directly in the operation. Waterproof gowns or aprons should be worn for procedures at high risk for contamination.

- *Operating room asepsis and characteristics:* Adherence to hand hygiene, including nonsurgeon members of the operating team, reduction of unnecessary traffic in operating rooms, and ventilation in the operating room according to published recommendations for proper air handling in the surgical area are essential.

- *Blood glucose control:* Control of serum blood glucose for all surgical patients, including patients without diabetes, will decrease the incidence of SSIs. For patients with diabetes mellitus, reduce glycosylated hemoglobin A1c levels to less than 7% before surgery, if possible. Continue control of blood glucose during the immediate postoperative period—postoperative blood glucose levels should be 180 mg/dL or lower.

- *Perioperative normothermia:* Even mild degrees of hypothermia (<35.5°C) can increase SSI rates. Hypothermia may directly impair neutrophil function or impair it indirectly by triggering subcutaneous vasoconstriction and subsequent tissue hypoxia. In addition, hypothermia may increase blood loss, leading to wound hematomas or need for transfusion, both of which can increase rates of SSI.

- *Tissue oxygenation:* Optimal tissue oxygenation should be attained by administering supplemental oxygen during and immediately after surgical procedures involving mechanical ventilation. Supplemental oxygen is most effective when combined with additional strategies to improve tissue oxygenation, including maintenance of normothermia and appropriate volume replacement.

- *Operative characteristics:* Blood transfusion increases the risk for SSI by decreasing macrophage function. Therefore, reduce the need for blood transfusion to the greatest extent possible. Operative times should be minimized as much as possible without sacrificing surgical technique and aseptic practice.

- *Antibiotic prophylaxis (see also Chapter 13):* Antibiotics should be discontinued within 24 hours after completion of surgery because a prolonged duration can increase the risk for *Clostridium difficile* infection and contribute to the development of multidrug resistant organisms.

A DEEPER DIVE: RACIAL DISPARITIES IN PEDIATRIC ANESTHESIA

- Anesthesia providers should be aware of the research on this topic to provide equitable care so that children are not at increased risk for adverse outcomes from our practices based on their race or ethnicity. Before we examine the research related to pediatric anesthesiology, we must understand the language and definitions of racial and ethnic disparities in health services research. According to the Academy for Health Services Research and Health Policy, health services research examines "how social factors, financing systems, organizational structures and processes, health technologies, and personal behaviors affect access to health care, the quality and cost of health care, and ultimately our health and well-being." Race and ethnicity have definitions that are variable, depending on the researcher or organizing body. For example, the United States Census defines race as "person's self-identification with one or more social groups," and ethnicity as "whether a person is Hispanic or not." The American Sociological Association, by contrast, defines race as "physical differences that groups and cultures consider socially significant while "ethnicity" refers to shared culture such as language, ancestry, practices, and beliefs." Indeed, disparities research may elect to compare white non-Hispanic patients to "minority" children or individualized racial and ethnic groups ("black Americans," "Latinos" "Asian Americans"). In the field of health disparities research, self-identification is considered the "gold standard" for categorization of race and ethnicity. This is because there is significant observer error such that nonwhites are often classified as white. In one dental study, for example, 5% of individuals who self-identified as black and 13.5% as Asian or Pacific Islander were classified as white by their interviewer. Understanding which groups are under study and who defined them will help us to interpret the results of such studies.
- The definition of disparities is likewise dynamic. The Agency for Healthcare Research and Quality (one of twelve agencies within the United States Department of Health and Human Services) states, "healthcare disparity is a difference between population groups in the way they access, experience, and receive healthcare." The IOM's definition differs, "racial or ethnic differences ... that are not because of clinical needs, preferences, and appropriateness of intervention." Understanding and selecting an operating definition of disparities is critical to evaluation of both literature and results.
- To date, eleven studies have been published on racial and ethnic health services disparities in pediatric anesthesia in the United States. All eleven were cohort studies, and ten were based out of a single, tertiary care-institution. In these studies, race and ethnicity were self-reported by patients or parents. The eleven studies were heterogenous: different clinical settings (preoperative, intraoperative, postoperative), populations (definitions of race and ethnicity and ages and surgical cohorts), and outcomes (clinical services). Seven studies focused on disparities in medication administration, two of which also examined management of intraoperative care. Two studies investigated disparities in receipt of blood transfusion; one study looked at anesthesia time; and two studies examined the use of regional anesthesia. The results of these studies are inconclusive. One study suggests that black children less than 5 years of age may be less likely to receive midazolam than white children for elective weekday surgeries, and another study demonstrated no significant difference in the percent of Latino and white children who received midazolam before tonsillectomy and adenoidectomy. Intraoperatively, black children are not less likely to receive intraoperative medications during a laparoscopic appendectomy; Asian, Latino, and Pacific Islander patients may have significantly lower odds of receiving nonopioids; black children may be more likely to receive blood transfusions during spinal surgeries while minority patients may not have an increased or decreased odds of receiving transfusions during cancer surgeries. In the postoperative period, Latino children may receive fewer analgesic medications for tonsillectomy and adenoidectomy and black and minority patients may receive more after tonsillectomy or outpatient surgery, respectively.

References

1. Egan G, Healy D, O'Neill H, Clarke-Moloney M, Grace PA, Walsh SR. Ultrasound guidance for difficult peripheral venous access: systematic review and meta-analysis. *Emerg Med J*. 2013;30(7):521–526. doi: 10.1136/emermed-2012-201652.

2. Nickalls RW, Mapleson WW. Age-related iso-MAC charts for isoflurane, sevoflurane and desflurane in man. *Br J Anaesth*. 2003;91(2):170–174. doi: 10.1093/bja/aeg132.

3. Gilbert S, Sabourdin N., Louvet N, et al. Epileptogenic effect of sevoflurane: determination of the minimal alveolar concentration of sevoflurane associated with major epileptoid signs in children. *Anesthesiology*. 2012;117(6):1253–1261. doi: 10.1097/ALN.0b013e318273e272.

4. Goldman LJ. Anesthetic uptake of sevoflurane and nitrous oxide during an inhaled induction in children. *Anesth Analg*. 2003;96(2):400–406. doi: 10.1097/00000539-200302000-00019.

5. Nagele P, Tallchief D, Blood J, Sharma A, Kharasch ED. Nitrous oxide anesthesia and plasma homocysteine in adolescents. *Anesth Analg*. 2011;113(4):843–848. doi: 10.1213/ANE.0b013e31822402f5.

6. Felten ML, Schmautz E, Delaporte-Cerceau S, Orliaguet GA, Carli PA. Endotracheal tube cuff pressure is unpredictable in children. *Anesth Analg*. 2003;97(6):1612–1616. doi: 10.1213/01.ANE.0000087882.04234.11.

7. von Ungern-Sternberg BS, Hammer J, Schibler A, Frei FJ, Erb TO. Decrease of functional residual capacity and ventilation homogeneity after neuromuscular blockade in anesthetized young infants and preschool children. *Anesthesiology*. 2006;105(4):670–675. doi: 10.1097/00000542-200610000-00010.

8. Yu EH, Tran DH, Lam SW, Irwin MG. Remifentanil tolerance and hyperalgesia: short-term gain, long-term pain? *Anaesthesia*. 2016;71(11):1347–1362. doi: doi.org/10.1111/anae.13602. PMID: 27734470.

9. Mason KP, Lerman J. Review article: Dexmedetomidine in Children: current knowledge and future applications. *Anesth Analg*. 2011;113(5):1129–1142. doi: 10.1213/ANE.0b013e31822b8629.

10. Subramanyam R, Cudilo EM, Hossain MM, et al. To Pretreat or not to pretreat: prophylactic anticholinergic administration before dexmedetomidine in pediatric imaging. *Anesth Analg*. 2015;121(2):479–485. doi: 10.1213/ANE.0000000000000765.

11. Larach MG, Rosenberg H, Gronert GA, Allen GC. Hyperkalemic cardiac arrest during anesthesia in infants and children with occult myopathies. *Clin Pediatr (Phila)*. 1997;36(1):9–16. doi: 10.1177/000992289703600102.

12. Quelicin. (2010). *Succinylcholine Chloride Injection*. Available from: https://www.accessdata.fda.gov/drugsatfda_docs/label/2010/008845s065lbl.pdf

13. Bhananker SM, Ramamoorthy C, Geiduschek JM, et al. Anesthesia-related cardiac arrest in children: update from the Pediatric Perioperative Cardiac Arrest Registry. *Anesth Analg*. 2007;105(2):344–350. doi: 10.1213/01.ane.0000268712.00756.dd.

14. Franz AM, Chiem J, Martin LD, Rampersad S, Phillips J, Grigg EB. Case series of 331 cases of sugammadex compared to neostigmine in patients under 2 years of age. *Paediatr Anaesth*. 2019;29(6):591–596. doi: 10.1111/pan.13643.

15. Nathan N. Emerging kids, emerging questions: sugammadex versus neostigmine in the pediatric population. *Anesth Analg*. 2019;129(4):909. doi: 10.1213/ANE.0000000000004394.

16. Gaver RS, Brenn BR, Gartley A, Donahue BS. Retrospective analysis of the safety and efficacy of sugammadex versus neostigmine for the reversal of neuromuscular blockade in children. *Anesth Analg*. 2019;129(4):1124–1129. doi: 10.1213/ANE.0000000000004207.

17. Carollo D, White WM. Postoperative recurarization in a pediatric Patient after sugammadex reversal of rocuronium-induced neuromuscular blockade: A case report. *A Pract*. 2019;13(6):204–205. doi: 10.1213/XAA.0000000000001023.

18. Murray DJ. Adding science to the decision to extubate children. *Anesthesiology*. 2019;131(4):769–770. doi: 10.1097/ALN.0000000000002921.

19. Templeton TW, Goenaga-Díaz EJ, Downard MG, et al. Assessment of common criteria for awake extubation in infants and young children. *Anesthesiology*. 2019;131(4):801–808. doi: 10.1097/ALN.0000000000002870.

Suggested Readings

Efron D, Vutskits L, Davidson AJ. Can we really suggest that anesthesia might cause attention-deficit/hyperactivity disorder? *Anesthesiology*. 2017;127(2):209–211. doi: 10.1097/ALN.0000000000001736.

Feldman JM. MSE vptimal Ventilation of the anesthetized pediatric patient. *Anesth Analg*. 2015;120(1):165–175. doi: 10.1213/ANE.0000000000000472.

Jevtovic-Todorovic V, Hartman RE, Izumi Y, et al. Early exposure to common anesthetic agents causes widespread neurodegeneration in the developing rat brain and persistent learning deficits. *J Neurosci*. 2003;23(3):876–882. doi: 10.1523/JNEUROSCI.23-03-00876.2003.

McCann ME, de Graaff JC, Dorris L, et al. Neurodevelopmental outcome at 5 years of age after general anaesthesia or awake-regional anaesthesia in infancy (GAS): an international, multicentre, randomised, controlled equivalence trial [published correction appears in Lancet. 2019 Aug 24;394(10199):638]. *Lancet*. 2019;393(10172):664–677. doi: 10.1016/S0140-6736(18)32485-1.

McCann ME, Lee JK, Inder T. Beyond anesthesia toxicity: anesthetic considerations to lessen the risk of neonatal neurological Injury. *Anesth Analg*. 2019;129(5):1354–1364. doi: 10.1213/ANE.0000000000004271.

McCann ME, Withington DE, Arnup SJ, et al. Differences in blood pressure in anfants After general anesthesia compared to awake regional anesthesia (GAS Study-A Prospective Randomized Trial). *Anesth Analg*. 2017;125(3):837–845. doi: 10.1213/ANE.0000000000001870.

Nafiu OO, Chimbira WT, Stewart M, Gibbons K, Porter LK, Reynolds PI. Racial differences in the pain management of children recovering from anesthesia. *Paediatr Anaesth*. 2017;27:760–767. doi: 10.1111/pan.13163..

Olutoye OA, Yu X, Govindan K, et al. The effect of obesity on the ED(95) of propofol for loss of consciousness in children and adolescents. *Anesth Analg*. 2012;115(1):147–153. doi: 10.1213/ANE.0b013e318256858f.

Rosenbloom JM, Mekonnen J, Tron LE, Alvarez K, Alegria M. Racial and ethnic health services disparities in pediatric anesthesia practice: A scoping review. *J Racial Ethn Health Disparities*. 2021;8(2):384–393. doi: 10.1007/s40615-020-00792-w.

Rosenbloom JM, Senthil K, Long AS, et al. A limited evaluation of the association of race and anesthetic medication administration: A single-center experience with appendectomies. *Paediatr Anaesth*. 2017;27(11):1142–1147. doi: 10.1111/pan.13217.

Tobias JD. Current evidence for the use of sugammadex in children [published correction appears in Paediatr Anaesth. 2017 Jul;27(7):781]. *Paediatr Anaesth*. 2017;27(2):118–125. doi: 10.1111/pan.13050.

Zimlichman E, Henderson D, Tamir O, et al. Health care associated infections: a meta-analysis of costs and financial impact on the USA health care system. *JAMA Intern Med*. 2013;173(22):2039–2046. doi: 10.1001/jamainternmed.2013.9763.

20
Regional Anesthesia

ASHA NOOKALA, TARUN BHALLA, ANDREW COSTANDI, RONALD S. LITMAN, AND HARSHAD GURNANEY

Nearly all regional anesthetic blocks in children are performed while they are anesthetized because conscious or sedated children will not cooperate sufficiently to ensure their safety. The main disadvantage of this approach is the theoretical injury of a nerve that would have otherwise been detected in a conscious patient by an immediate reaction of extreme pain or a motor response. However, the worldwide experience[1] of regional blockade in thousands of children has shown the occurrence of nerve damage to be exceedingly rare. This knowledge tips the balance in favor[2] of the benefits of regional anesthesia in the anesthetized and immobile child. Another possible disadvantage of performing a regional technique during general anesthesia is the unreliability of the exact location of block placement. However, peripheral nerve blocks in anesthetized children should now only be performed with the assistance of a nerve stimulator or ultrasound guidance; thus complications as a result of inaccurate block placement are rare.

Central Neuraxial Techniques

Spinal Anesthesia

Spinal anesthesia can be performed in children as an alternative to general anesthesia[5] for lower abdominal, urologic, and lower extremity procedures. The most common use of spinal anesthesia[6] in the pediatric population is for inguinal surgery in the preterm infant at risk for postoperative apnea after general anesthesia, especially in light of recent evidence of the possibility of neurotoxic effects of general

---

A DEEPER DIVE

In 2010, Ecoffrey et al. published[1] the experience of the French-Language Society of Paediatric Anaesthesiologists (ADARPEF) entitled "Epidemiology and Morbidity of Regional Anesthesia in Children." The group collected data from 31,132 regional blocks at 47 institutions, the majority of which were a combination of regional and general anesthesia. The authors found 41 complications, all of which were noted to be minor without long-term sequelae. However, these complication rates were 6 times higher for central (neuraxial) blocks compared with peripheral nerve blocks.

The Pediatric Regional Anesthesia Network (PRAN) was organized in 2006 as a data repository from multiple institutions, with the purpose of determining efficacy and safety of pediatric regional anesthesia techniques. Their first publication[3] in 2012 entitled "A Multi-Institutional Study of the Use and Incidence of Complications of Pediatric Regional Anesthesia" reported 14,917 regional blocks from 2007 to 2010. There were no block-associated deaths or serious complications with sequelae lasting more than 3 months. The majority of complications were associated with continuous catheter blocks compared with single injection blocks. Within the catheter group the majority of complications were reported to be problems with the catheter such as kinking/dislodgement rather than complications of the nervous system.

A subsequent publication[4] by PRAN in 2018 demonstrated similar results in over 100,000 children at 20 US children's hospitals. In this prospective observational study, the risk for a transient neurologic deficit was 2.4:10,000 (95% CI, 1.6–3.6:10,000) and was not different between peripheral and neuraxial blocks. The risk for severe local anesthetic systemic toxicity was 0.76:10,000 (95% CI, 0.3–1.6:10,000); the majority of these cases occurred in infants. The most common adverse events were benign catheter-related failures (4%).

These relatively large prospective observational surveys confirm a low rate of complications associated with pediatric regional anesthesia, without long-term sequelae. Nevertheless, there are extremely rare devastating complications associated with neuraxial blocks in children that all practitioners should be aware of (see Suggested Readings).

TABLE 20.1	**Spinal versus Caudal Epidural Block for the Conscious Infant**	
	Advantages	**Disadvantages**
SPINAL ANESTHESIA	• Lower total dose of local anesthetic (1 mg/kg vs 3–4 mg/kg) • Definite end-point (aspiration of cerebrospinal fluid) • Rapid onset • Dense sensory and motor block	• Limited duration of action (60–90 minutes) • Technically difficult in small infants • Potential for high block with change in position
CAUDAL EPIDURAL	• High rate of success • Longer duration if catheter inserted • Minimal change in level with change in position	• High dose of local anesthetic agents required • Slow onset of action incomplete motor block

anesthesia on the developing brain. Spinal anesthesia is an option when the duration of the surgical procedure is less than 90 minutes. If the procedure is expected to be longer, a combined spinal-epidural or a continuous caudal-epidural anesthesia technique can be considered (Table 20.1). Contraindications to spinal anesthesia include infection at the site, increased intracranial pressure, and clinically significant hypovolemia.

Preoperative considerations before spinal anesthesia include normal fasting guidelines and a stable hemoglobin level. Preoperative application of a topical anesthetic cream over the lumbar spine may decrease pain from the spinal injection. Some pediatric anesthesiologists prefer to obtain IV access before performance of the spinal anesthetic.

Although cardiorespiratory effects are uncommon after spinal block in infants, complications from spinal anesthesia have been reported. Intra- and postoperative apnea, bradycardia, and hypoxemia may occur, necessitating immediate ventilatory assistance and possible atropine administration. A "high spinal" will cause respiratory and neurologic depression with rapid onset of hypoxemia. Therefore vigilance is required during and after the administration of the spinal anesthetic. Hypotension from a spinal anesthetic-induced sympathetic block rarely occurs in children under the age of 5 years. This may be because of the relatively immature sympathetic nervous system in children compared with adults, or because of the relatively smaller intravascular volume in the lower extremities of children such that lower extremity vasodilation does not reduce preload to an appreciable extent. Postdural puncture headache may occur in children. The headache will usually resolve within 3 to 5 days, but in some children, it may last longer.

The choice of intrathecal local anesthetic agent will depend on the expected duration of surgery. A larger dose is required than for adults because of the relatively larger ratio of cerebrospinal fluid (CSF) volume to bodyweight in neonates (6–10 mL/kg) compared with adults (2 mL/kg) and the resulting dilutional effect. Most reports in the literature use 1% tetracaine or 0.5% to 0.75% bupivacaine at doses varying from 0.3 to 1 mg/kg to provide 45 to 90 minutes of effective surgical anesthesia up to the T5–T6 level. To prolong the duration of the spinal block, epinephrine can be added using an "epi wash" which involves drawing up epinephrine (1:1000) into a tuberculin syringe and then ejecting it all out thereby leaving a small amount lining the syringe and the hub of the needle before drawing up the local anesthetic solution.

Spinal anesthesia can be performed in either the sitting or lateral position, depending on the personal preference of the anesthesiologist. Lumbar puncture is performed at the L4 to L5 interspace because the spinal cord in the small infant ends at a more caudad level (L3) than in older children (L1). This landmark can be found parallel to the top of the iliac crest. Using a sterile aseptic technique, a 1.5-inch, 22-gauge spinal needle is most often used and inserted approximately 1 to 2 cm until a light "pop" is felt as the needle penetrates the dura and subarachnoid membrane. When the stylet is removed, free flow of CSF is observed, and the syringe is firmly attached to the hub of the inserted spinal needle (a common cause of a failed spinal block is leakage of the local anesthetic solution during injection). The local anesthetic solution is injected over 5 to 10 seconds. Once the block has been performed, the infant is rapidly placed supine on the operating room table. Precautions should be taken to prevent the infant's legs from being lifted up by operating room (OR) staff, which may result in a high spinal block. When the electrocautery pad is placed on the infant's back, the entire infant should be lifted parallel to the table. The blood pressure cuff should be placed on a numb lower extremity to minimize stimulation of the conscious infant. A few minutes after the spinal block is completed, the anesthesiologist can assess if the infant's legs become limp to assess the success of the spinal block (Fig. 20.1). If the block is not successful, induction of general anesthesia is indicated.

With a successful spinal block, the anesthesiologist is left with a conscious infant who must be kept calm during the surgical procedure because crying or fussing increases intraabdominal pressure, which increases the technical difficulty of inguinal surgery. Most infants will sleep[7] during the procedure or rest quietly if offered a pacifier dipped in glucose water (Fig. 20.2).

What is the course of action when the infant is inconsolable during the surgical procedure? First, the anesthesiologist and surgeon should determine whether the surgical area is properly anesthetized. In some cases of a patchy block, the surgeon can administer local anesthesia into the wound

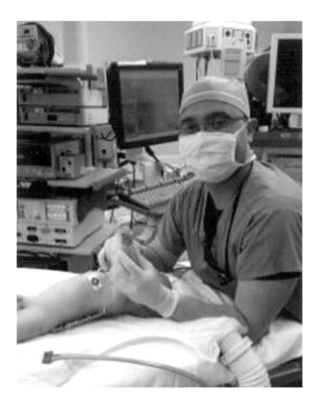

• **Fig 20.1.** Immediately after spinal insertion, the lower extremities should become numb. Andrew is very proud of his working spinal. Photo credit Ronald S. Litman.

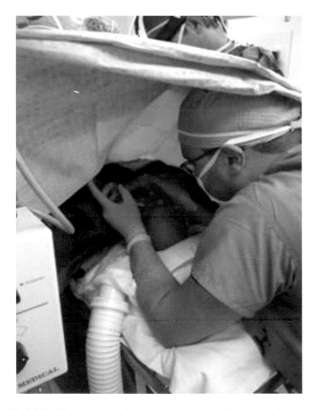

• **Fig 20.2.** The conscious infant must be kept calm when using spinal anesthesia, so Andrew drips glucose water in the infant's mouth while the hernia repair proceeds. Photo credit Ronald S. Litman.

with satisfactory results. However, if doubt remains, induction of general anesthesia is the most prudent action.

Epidural Anesthesia

Epidural anesthesia can be administered in a variety of ways to infants and children. The decision will depend on the nature and duration of the surgical procedure. For ambulatory patients, a single dose of epidural anesthesia is administered, usually via the caudal space. For hospitalized patients, whose pain is expected to be severe for more than a day, insertion of an epidural catheter will provide continuous postoperative analgesia. Ideally, the epidural injection or catheter tip should be located at the level of the surgical incision. In infants, a thoracic level epidural catheter can be threaded cephalad via the caudal space. The use of ultrasound or fluoroscopy[8] can be used to visualize the catheter as it travels from the caudal to the thoracic space to detect coiling of the catheter as it advances cephalad.

The choice of epidural analgesic medications includes a local anesthetic, an opioid, clonidine, or any combination of these. Opioids will usually be used in hospitalized children over 1 year of age who are expected to have severe pain. More specific dosing regimens are discussed in subsequent sections of this chapter and in Chapter 34.

Side effects and complications from epidural analgesia are the same for children as for adults. Common side effects include motor blockade of the lower extremities and urinary retention. Local anesthesia toxicity from accidental intravascular injection is rare and manifests as seizures in an unanesthetized child or cardiac collapse in an anesthetized child. Treatment involves standard resuscitation methods plus the administration of 20% Intralipid emulsion, 1.5 mL/kg. This dose can be repeated as necessary to control cardiac arrhythmias and ideally should be followed by an infusion of 0.25 mL/kg/min titrated to hemodynamic stability. Additional rare complications include epidural hematoma, epidural abscess formation, intraneural trauma causing a residual neurologic deficit, and unintentional dural puncture with spinal blockade. Postdural puncture headache is rarely seen in children less than 8 years of age secondary to the increased volume of CSF and greater CSF turnover. Devastating neurologic complications after seemingly error-free epidural catheter placements have been reported[9] in children.

Caudal-Epidural Anesthesia

The most common neuraxial regional technique in neonates and infants is the caudal epidural block, which is relatively easy to perform once the proper landmarks have been identified. It can be performed before surgery to be used in combination with general anesthesia, performed after surgery to be used for postoperative analgesia, or used instead of general anesthesia for lower abdominal and lower extremity procedures. A caudal epidural block can be performed with the patient in the prone position with the legs tucked under, the lateral position with the hips flexed

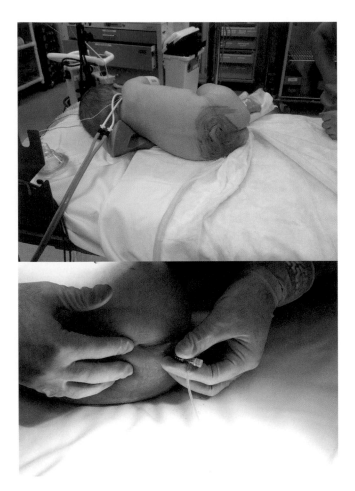

• **Fig 20.3.** (A) Infant prepped and positioned for caudal block. (B) The anesthesia provider's right hand identifies the landmarks while the left hand is used for injection through the sacrococcygeal ligament.

(Fig. 20.3), or even the supine position with the legs lifted up over the head. The important landmarks are the coccyx and the sacral hiatus located between the two sacral cornua. A 22-gauge short-beveled needle is inserted 1 to 2 mm caudad from a point midway between the two cornua. The needle is inserted at a 30- to 45-degree angle to the skin and advanced through the sacrococcygeal ligament. As the needle is advanced through the ligament and into the epidural space, a characteristic loss of resistance is felt. Once the epidural space is entered, care is taken to avoid advancing the needle too far, as the dural sac may extend down as far as S3 or S4 level in small infants (as opposed to S1–S2 in adults), and an unintentional dural puncture may occur. Because ossification of the sacrum is not complete until adulthood, the epidural needle can be accidentally inserted into the sacrum without much resistance. Some anesthesiologists prefer to make a small nick at the skin with an 18-gauge needle to serve as an entranceway for the block needle and to prevent tissue coring.

Before the administration of the local anesthetic solution into the epidural space, the anesthesiologist should attempt to rule out unintentional placement of the catheter or needle into the intravascular or intrathecal space. Initially, the caudal needle is gently aspirated to detect blood or CSF. However, this test is not completely reliable owing to the high compliance of the epidural veins and intrathecal space in children, which collapses easily with even slight negative pressure. A test dose is recommended to help detect intravascular placement of the epidural block. In children, the dose of epinephrine that consistently results in hemodynamic or electrocardiogram (ECG) changes is 0.5 µg/kg. This translates into a test dose of 0.1 mL/kg of a local anesthetic solution that contains epinephrine in a concentration of 1:200,000 (5 µg/mL). Sixty seconds is allowed to elapse to assess for accidental IV or intraosseous injection. Although the efficacy of the test dose has been questioned, especially if administered during the use of inhalational anesthetic agents, its reliability can be increased by observing the change in T-wave amplitude, the heart rate, and the blood pressure response. An increase in T-wave amplitude of greater than 25% over baseline or an increase in heart rate greater than 10 beats/min are indicative of an IV injection of epinephrine. Systolic blood pressure has been described to rise by 15 mm Hg but is less reliable than heart rate or T-wave changes. Changes in any of these parameters indicate an unintentional IV injection and the need to reposition the needle. One caveat to test-dosing in children is that the expected increase in T-wave amplitude in response to IV epinephrine may not occur during a propofol-remifentanil general anesthetic; thus practitioners should rely on the blood pressure response.[10] If no response to the test dose is noted, the remainder of the calculated dose is administered slowly over 1 to 2 minutes while the vital signs are continually monitored for evidence of intravascular injection. The choice of ECG lead does not appear to influence the accuracy of the test dose response.[11]

A caudal epidural block can be achieved using any local anesthetic agent. The concentration and volume of the solution are usually determined by the height and density of the blockade required. The volume of local anesthetic determines the height of the block,[12] which depends on the level of the surgical incision. Volumes of 1.2 to 1.5 mL/kg provide analgesia to the T4 to T6 level. A dose of 1 mL/kg will provide postoperative analgesia for inguinal procedures, while 0.5 to 0.75 mL/kg is sufficient for lower extremity or urogenital procedures. Regardless of the volume used, the concentration is adjusted to ensure that no more than 2.5 mg/kg of bupivacaine or 3 mg/kg of ropivacaine is administered. With bupivacaine, the majority of experience is with the 0.25% solutions. However, effective postoperative analgesia can be achieved using a 0.125% solution, thereby limiting the total dose and decreasing the intensity of the motor block.

Caudal ropivacaine provides a faster onset of analgesia and less motor blockade than bupivacaine. A 0.2% ropivacaine solution provides the best efficacy[13] with the least amount of motor blockade. Although peak plasma concentrations of both bupivacaine and ropivacaine will be achieved 20 to 40 minutes after epidural administration,[14] ropivacaine is absorbed into the systemic circulation more slowly than equivalent doses of bupivacaine. Ropivacaine is less cardiotoxic than bupivacaine at equipotent plasma concentrations and is being increasingly used by pediatric anesthesiologists for regional blockade. Intraoperative bolus doses can be readministered every 1 to 2 hours, or administered as a continuous infusion throughout the procedure (see Table 35.3 in Chapter 35).

Epinephrine can be added to the local anesthetic solution to slightly prolong the duration of action of the sensory block and limit potentially rapid systemic absorption via epidural blood vessels. The addition of clonidine or dexmedetomidine,[15] 1 μg/kg, will enhance the quality and duration of postoperative analgesia when combined with epidural local anesthetics and is now routinely included in the epidural anesthetic solution in many pediatric centers. Concomitant administration of IV dexamethasone has also been shown to prolong the duration[16] of epidural analgesia. The addition of opioids has been found to be beneficial, but must be used with caution and with appropriate postoperative monitoring of the patient's respiratory status.

Thoracic Epidural Analgesia via the Caudal Approach

Segmental anesthesia may be achieved with relatively smaller doses of local anesthetic when the epidural catheter tip is placed in the close vicinity of the spinal segment of the surgical incision. In anesthetized infants, direct thoracic epidural placement may entail the risk for spinal cord trauma and should only be undertaken by those with considerable clinical experience in the technique. Alternatively, in neonates and infants, when thoracic level anesthesia is desired, a catheter can be advanced through the epidural space via the caudal space[17] to the desired level, based on an approximate measurement, or using radiographic or ultrasound guidance. Minor resistance may be encountered, but the catheter should advance relatively easily. If it does not, it is not positioned correctly. Even when it advances easily, there is a high incidence of malpositioning because of coiling of the catheter within the epidural space. Use of a styletted catheter may decrease the incidence of coiling, but may increase the risk for unintentional intravascular and subarachnoid penetration. Once the catheter has been advanced to its expected position, a small amount of nonionic radiographic contrast (Iohexol-Omnipaque 180) is injected while simultaneously obtaining a radiograph or fluoroscopy of the chest and abdomen to identify the level of the epidural catheter and tip and to confirm appropriate placement in the epidural space. Ultrasound can be used in infants younger than 4 to 6 months, and nerve stimulation guidance (Tsui test[18]) is a third way to identify the level of the tip of the catheter.

Direct Lumbar or Thoracic Epidural Analgesia

Direct lumbar or thoracic epidural catheter placement in children differs from that in adults. The first major difference is that the distance from the skin to the epidural space is less in children. In children between 6 months and 10 years of age, the epidural space at the lumbar level will be encountered at a depth of 1 mm per kilogram of weight. The second major difference is that children have a much softer ligamentum flavum than adults. Thus it is more difficult to identify the ligament with certainty during epidural needle placement. An important consequence of these two differences is that unintentional dural puncture is more likely in a child than in an adult. Therefore the epidural space is approached with caution with the loss-of-resistance technique being started just beneath the skin, while advancing the needle slowly until the epidural space is identified. A small skin nick is made at the site before placing the epidural needle so that the pressure required to advance the epidural needle through the skin does not cause the needle to advance too far and puncture the dura. Once the space is identified, an epidural catheter is threaded so that 2 to 4 cm remains in the epidural space. Gentle aspiration for blood or CSF is then performed before the local anesthetic solution is administered. A test dose is given through the catheter using the same diagnostic criteria as described above in the section on caudal block. The initial bolus dose of local anesthesia depends on the level of catheter placement. When the catheter is placed as an adjunct to general anesthesia, 0.25% bupivacaine or 0.2% ropivacaine is used. Suggested starting guidelines for dosing include an initial bolus dose of 0.3 mL/kg (maximum 10 mL) followed by initiation of an epidural infusion of local anesthetic.

Complications of epidural catheter placement and analgesia include dural puncture, nerve root irritation, infection, epidural hematoma, and abscess formation. This technique is contraindicated in children with a coagulopathy (platelet count ≤100,000/mm,[3] an elevated PT (PT = prothrombin time) or elevated PTT (PTT = partial thromboplastin time), or qualitative bleeding dysfunction (e.g., hemophilia or von Willebrands disease). New neurologic deficits and back pain are signs of an epidural hematoma. Placing the epidural below the intercristal line[19] (line connecting the tops of the iliac crests) will avoid direct trauma to the spinal cord.

Neuraxial Opioids

A single administration of a local anesthetic alone may provide up to 8 hours of postoperative analgesia, but in some cases a more prolonged duration of analgesia is required without placing an indwelling catheter. Furthermore, the transient motor blockade that results from administration of local anesthetics is undesirable in some patients. These are indications for administration of an opioid into the spinal or epidural space. Unlike local anesthetics, opioids affect sensory neurons without affecting motor or sympathetic function. When used in combination with local anesthetics, there is an additive effect with an increase in the duration of the regional anesthetic and an improvement in the quality of analgesia while allowing the use of more dilute solutions of local anesthetics. Thus inclusion of opioids may lessen the potential for local anesthetic toxicity and side effects, such as motor blockade.

Intrathecal morphine[20] (3–5 μg/kg per dose) can be used to provide prolonged (usually up to 12 hours) postoperative analgesia. Because of its hydrophilic nature compared with other opioids, morphine tends to stay within the CSF and travel cephalad to the brain. As a result, caudal or lumbar administration may be used to provide analgesia for thoracic procedures. It is best administered before the beginning of the surgical procedure because the onset of action is 20 to 60 minutes.

Opioids can also be administered into the epidural space. Because fentanyl is lipophilic, it is rapidly absorbed into the systemic circulation and is no more advantageous than IV administration. Therefore morphine is most commonly administered epidurally. Dose ranging studies in children have demonstrated that 30 to 50 μg/kg of epidural morphine provides the best balance between sufficient analgesia and lack of respiratory depression.

The most important adverse effect associated with neuraxial opioid administration is respiratory depression. This is particularly true for morphine because significant concentrations persist in the CSF for up to 24 hours after administration. Delayed respiratory depression is associated with the administration of rescue doses of parenteral opioids within about 16 hours after the initial epidural morphine dose. When it becomes necessary to use parenteral opioids in children who have received neuraxial opioids, a mixed agonist-antagonist, such as butorphanol or nalbuphine, may have less effect on respiratory function than a pure agonist, such as morphine. Ongoing monitoring of respiratory function with continuous pulse oximetry is suggested after the administration of neuraxial morphine.

Additional side effects related to neuraxial opioids include pruritus, nausea, vomiting, and urinary retention. Pruritus tends to be more common with intrathecal morphine. Despite being pain-free, pruritis may cause significant distress, requiring treatment with diphenhydramine, nalbuphine, or continuous naloxone infusion, 0.5 to 2 μg/kg/h. The latter can be used to treat pruritus without diminishing the quality of analgesia. The combination of morphine 30 to 50 μg/kg and butorphanol 20 to 30 μg/kg (neuraxial) may decrease the incidence of adverse effects compared with morphine alone.

All patients who receive neuraxial opioids require postoperative respiratory monitoring and are not candidates for home discharge on the day of surgery. In the past, children who had received neuraxial opioids were sent to the intensive care unit (ICU), but with proper training of the nursing staff on a regular postoperative care ward, these children should not require ICU admission. Monitoring should include pulse oximetry when the child is asleep with an evaluation of respiratory rate every 2 hours and sedation scores every 6 hours. With these parameters, changes in respiratory status and increased sedation can be detected early with appropriate intervention. Monitoring should be continued for 16 hours after neuraxial morphine because of the possibility of delayed respiratory depression.

Peripheral Nerve Blocks

Use of peripheral nerve blocks is an effective way to decrease the side effects and complications associated with central blocks. Peripheral nerve catheters can be used in pediatric outpatients.[21] Proper nerve localization is achieved using nerve stimulation, but this has now been replaced (or combined) with ultrasound guidance.[22] Ultrasound guidance enables direct visualization of neurovascular structures, adjacent anatomic structures, needle tip location, and spread of the local anesthetic. In practice, for most blocks, we use both methods simultaneously. If a nerve stimulator is used, avoidance of neuromuscular blocking agents is required. The negative electrode attaches to the insulated needle, the positive electrode attaches to the patient using a standard ECG pad, and the nerve stimulator is set to the low-output setting (0.5–1 mA). The needle is then advanced until a motor response is noted in the desired muscle group of the extremity to be anesthetized. The voltage is turned down to 0.3 to 0.5 mA and a continuing motor response confirms that the needle is in close proximity to the nerve to be anesthetized before injecting the local anesthetic. However, the presence of a continuing motor response below 0.3 mA increases the risk for an intraneural needle tip placement. The use of ultrasound guidance for placement of peripheral nerve blocks provides a visual confirmation of the location of the needle tip relative to the nerve and could decrease the risk for intraneural injections.

Upper Extremity Regional Anesthesia

There are multiple approaches to regional anesthesia of the upper extremity, depending on the specific nerves to be blocked and on the expertise of the practitioner. The axillary block is appropriate for elbow or more distal upper extremity surgery. For this block, the ultrasound probe is placed in the axilla perpendicular to the course of the axillary artery and at the level of the crease formed by the pectoralis major and biceps muscles, to visualize the axillary artery and vein in the short-axis view. The median, ulnar, and radial nerves most likely will surround the artery in a triangular pattern. Using an in-plane approach the needle is advanced and 0.2 to 0.5 mL/kg up to 10 to 20 mL of local anesthetic is injected in a circumferential pattern around the axillary artery producing the characteristic "donut sign." The axillary approach will invariably miss the musculocutaneous nerve; therefore, a separate block can be performed using the same needle insertion site as the axillary block, and injecting part of the local anesthetic solution into the body of the coracobrachialis muscle.

The supraclavicular block is applicable for almost all upper extremity procedures. It is performed with the ultrasound probe placed parallel to the clavicle. A needle is placed in-plane with the local anesthetic deposited around the trunks of the brachial plexus, often referred to as a "cluster of grapes" lateral to the subclavian artery. The infraclavicular block of the brachial plexus is appropriate for humeral shaft, elbow, and distal upper extremity procedures. The ultrasound probe is placed perpendicular under the clavicle and the axillary artery is identified. An appropriately sized needle is placed using an in-plane technique and the local anesthesia is deposited posterior to the axillary artery and spread is observed to the posterior, lateral, and medial cords of the brachial plexus.

Lower Extremity Regional Anesthesia

Femoral Nerve Block

The femoral nerve block provides analgesia for procedures of the anterior portion of the thigh, femoral shaft, and knee. After passing under the inguinal ligament, the femoral nerve divides into an anterior and a posterior branch to supply sensation to the anterior and lower medial portion of the thigh, femur, and knee, as well as sensation to the medial aspect of the leg below the knee down to the foot through the saphenous nerve (terminal branch of the posterior division of the femoral nerve).

To perform this block, a needle is inserted 1 to 2 cm lateral to the femoral artery and 1 to 2 cm below the inguinal ligament. The needle is then advanced at a 45-degree angle in a cephalad direction until a double loss of resistance is felt as the needle passes through the fascia lata and fascia iliaca.

Ultrasound guidance of the femoral block improves the quality and prolongs the duration of analgesia with a lower risk for accidental arterial puncture (Fig. 20.4). Using a linear probe placed along the inguinal crease and below the inguinal ligament, the femoral artery is first identified and confirmed with Doppler. The femoral nerve lies lateral to the artery and appears as a triangular, hyperechoic structure below the fascia iliaca and superficial to the iliopsoas muscle. An in-plane or out-of-plane technique can be used in this block. With the in-plane technique, the needle is inserted from lateral to medial until it penetrates the fascia iliaca. After negative aspiration, 0.2 to 0.3 mL/kg of the local anesthetic is injected until a donut-shaped spread around the femoral nerve is seen.

In the past, dosing for a femoral nerve block typically included up to 1 mL/kg of either 0.2% ropivacaine or 0.25% bupivacaine, but much lower volumes (0.2 mL/kg) are sufficient when ultrasound guidance is used for precise localization of the nerve. Additives such as clonidine[23] have been shown to prolong analgesic duration. Intraneural or intravascular injections are the most likely complications of this block and can be avoided by continuously visualizing the tip of the needle with ultrasound.

Sciatic Nerve Block

The sciatic nerve block is performed for procedures below the knee or posterior thigh. A supplemental block of the saphenous nerve may be required to provide analgesia on the medial side of the ankle. The technique can be performed with the patient in the prone or supine position. With the child in the prone position, the ultrasound probe is placed transversely in the popliteal fossa. The nerve is usually visualized between the biceps and semimembranosus tendons, posterior and lateral to the popliteal artery and popliteal

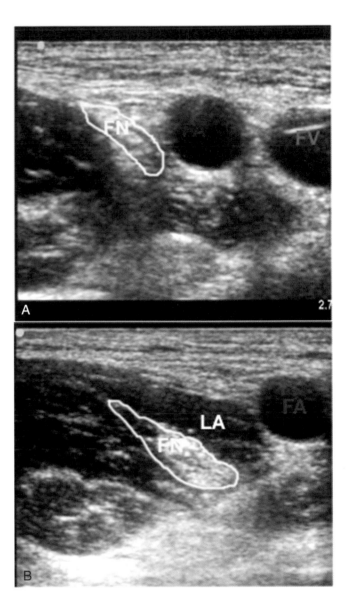

• **Fig 20.4.** (A) The yellow circle identifies the femoral nerve (FN) with ultrasound before administration of local anesthetic. The femoral artery (FA) and femoral vein (FV) are shown for anatomical reference. Photo credit Harshad Gurnaney. (B) Local anesthetic (LA) surrounding the femoral nerve after the block.

vein. After locating the sciatic nerve before it divides, the needle is inserted until the tip is positioned alongside the nerve. After negative aspiration, 0.2 to 0.3 mL/kg of the local anesthetic is then injected until it is seen around the nerve. For patients in the supine position, the foot is supported on a table or small pile of towels. The probe is held on the posterior aspect of the thigh and the needle is inserted on the lateral aspect and directed toward the nerve.

Truncal Analgesia

Ilioinguinal/Iliohypogastric (Hernia) Block

The subcostal nerve (T12), the iliohypogastric nerve (L1), and the ilioinguinal nerve (L1) travel between the internal oblique and transversus abdominis near the iliac crest. These nerves provide innervation to the superficial tissues overlying the inguinal ligament and proximal scrotum. The injection point is 2 cm medial and 2 cm cephalad to the anterior superior iliac spine (ASIS). We perform this block with ultrasound guidance,[24] (Fig. 20.5), which greatly increases the success rate, decreases local anesthetic volume requirements,[25] and decreases the risk for accidentally injuring the bowel or the inferior epigastric vessels. A linear probe is placed on a line connecting the ASIS with the umbilicus, the three muscle layers are identified and the block needle is inserted in or out of plane. Although watching spread of the tissue planes on the ultrasound monitor, 0.2 to 0.5 mL/kg up to 5 to 10 mL local anesthetic is deposited between the internal oblique muscle and the transversus abdominis muscle (Fig. 20.6). Ilioinguinal block is extremely safe except for

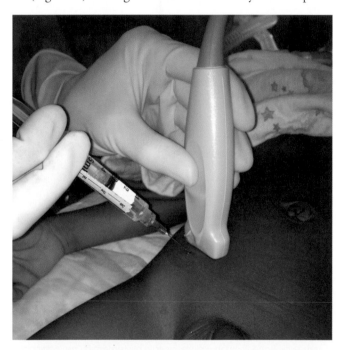

• **Fig 20.5.** Iliohypogastric/ilioinguinal block using ultrasound guidance. Photo credit Tarun Bhalla

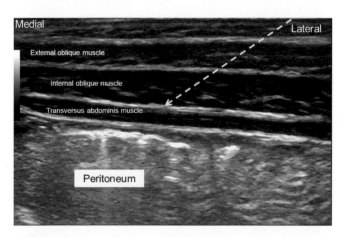

• **Fig 20.6.** Ultrasound view of the abdominal muscle layers during performance of an iliohypogastric/ilioinguinal block. The dotted yellow arrow depicts the location of local anesthetic deposition during this block. Photo credit Tarun Bhalla.

the occasional occurrence of leg weakness because of spread of local anesthetic to the area of the femoral nerve.

Penile Block

A penile block reliably provides anesthesia for procedures involving the distal penis, such as circumcision, or hypospadias repair. The distal end of the penis is innervated by the dorsal penile nerves, which branch off the pudendal nerve (S2–4) at the base of the penis and run along the dorsal side, deep to Buck fascia. These nerves can be anesthetized by injecting local anesthetic solution below the deep fascia at the base of the penis at the 2 and 10 o'clock positions. Alternatively, a penile block can be accomplished by a single midline injection into the subpubic space (Fig. 20.7) This is commonly referred to as a *dorsal penile nerve block* (DPNB). Initially, a "give" is felt as the needle pierces the superficial fascial layer. The needle is further advanced until another more marked give is felt as the needle pierces Buck fascia to enter the subpubic space. After gentle aspiration to rule out an intravascular injection, 3 to 5 mL of 0.25% to 0.5% plain bupivacaine is injected. As this is an end-arterial system, epinephrine is never used in the local anesthetic solution. Complications of DPNB include subcutaneous hematoma at the site of injection (fairly common), and rarely, arterial injection.

Local infiltration of the penis is distinguished from a specific nerve block and is traditionally referred to as a ring block. Between 2 and 3 mL of local anesthetic solution are injected below the deep fascial level at the base of the penis in a circumferential fashion. Practitioners who prefer the ring block to the DPNB cite the inconsistent anatomic location of the dorsal penile nerves and the need for coverage on the ventral side of the penis.

Pharmacology of Local Anesthetics in Children

There are several clinically relevant differences in local anesthetic pharmacology between children and adults. Local anesthetic metabolism is affected by age, especially in the premature infant and neonate where the hepatic, microsomal enzyme system is not fully developed. Protein binding of local anesthetics is decreased owing to the low quantities of albumin and alpha-1-acid glycoprotein produced in the liver during early infancy. This will result in an increased plasma free fraction of the drug, and an increased risk for local anesthetic toxicity. The time it takes for the drug to be absorbed is also a consideration because a rapid rise of the serum concentration is more likely to result in toxicity. Cardiac output and local blood flow of infants is relatively greater than in adults. Therefore systemic absorption of local anesthetics is relatively faster in children, as are peak plasma concentrations. Addition of a vasoconstrictor, such as epinephrine or phenylephrine, can slow the absorption rate and lower the peak serum concentration by 10% to 20%.

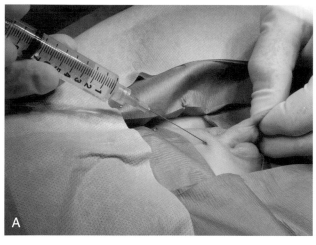
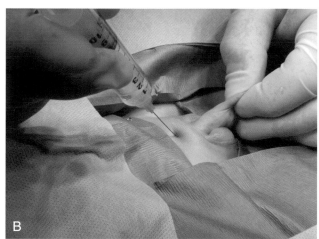

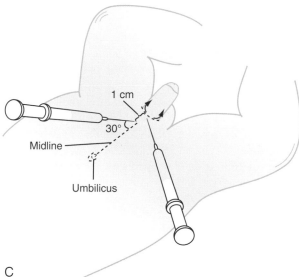

• **Fig 20.7.** Penile block. (A) Dorsal nerve block: a 27- or 25-gauge needle is inserted in the midline, 1 cm above the symphysis pubis at an angle of 30 degrees from the plane of the abdominal wall and directed caudad. (B) After piercing the penile fascia (0.5–1.0 cm) and negative aspiration for blood, 1.0 to 4.0 mL of local anesthetic without epinephrine is injected. (C) Ring block: a 25-gauge needle is inserted at the base of the penis at a 45-degree angle, and a ring of local anesthetic is deposited *(curved arrows)*. This may be done through a single needle placement by redirecting the needle. This block may be used in children in whom a caudal block is contraindicated. (From Suresh S, Polaner DM, Cote CJ. Regional anesthesia, In: Coté CJ, Lerman J, Anderson BJ, eds. *A Practice of Anesthesia for Infants and Children.* 6th ed. Elsevier; 2019:941–987.e9.)

Anatomic differences between children and adults can affect local anesthetic pharmacology. The fat within the epidural space is sparse and loose in infants. Furthermore, the perineural sheath that is located around nerve roots and bundles are more loosely attached to underlying structures in children than in adults. It is for these reasons that injected local anesthetics appear to spread more in children, and cover a greater area of innervation. In addition, the endoneurium is relatively loose in young children and allows rapid exposure of the local anesthetic to the nerve. Thus onset of anesthesia is relatively more rapid than in adults.

With the use of any local anesthetic, regardless of the concentration of the solution, the anesthesiologist must calculate the total milligram dose on a per-kilogram basis to avoid toxic blood levels by administering less than recommended maximum doses (Table 20.2). This is especially important in neonates and small infants. For example, if bupivacaine is used for a caudal anesthetic in a 3 kg baby, the maximum dose that should be used is 1.75 mg/kg or a total of 5.25 mg (70% of 2.5 mg/kg). A 0.25% solution of bupivacaine has 2.5 mg/mL, so a maximum of 2.0 mL of the solution should be used. In general practice, 3 mg/kg of local anesthetic is achieved with either 1.2 mL/kg of 0.25% bupivacaine or 1.5 mL/kg of 0.2% ropivacaine. Even with extreme caution and careful calculation of doses, local anesthetic toxicity can occur. Therefore the practitioner must be familiar with basic resuscitation strategies and the use of Intralipid for rescue from local anesthetic toxicity (Table 20.3).

In summary, these regional block techniques may be used to provide an alternative to general anesthesia, an adjunct to general anesthesia, or to provide postoperative analgesia. Any regional anesthetic technique used in the adult population can theoretically be used in the pediatric-aged patient.

TABLE 20.2 **Maximum Recommended Doses of Local Anesthetics[a,b]**

Maximum Recommended Dose (MG/KG)	
2-Chloroprocaine	20
Tetracaine	1.5
Lidocaine	7
Mepivacaine	7
Bupivacaine	2.5
Ropivacaine	3.5[c]

(From Weinberg GL. Lipid emulsion infusion: resuscitation for local anesthetic and other drug overdose. *Anesthesiology.* 2012 Jul;117(1):180-7. doi: 10.1097/ALN.0b013e31825ad8de. PMID: 22627464; PMCID: PMC4609208.)
[a]Doses should be reduced by at least 30% in infants <3 months of age.
[b]These maximum doses apply to anesthetized children. Doses are reduced in conscious children.
[c]Definitive data are lacking for the maximum dose of ropivacaine.

TABLE 20.3 **Intravenous 20% Lipid Emulsion Dose**

- Bolus 1.5 mL/kg over 1 minute.
- Start an infusion at 0.25 mL/g/min.
- Repeat the bolus for persistent cardiovascular collapse.
- Double the infusion for persistent low BP.
- Continue the infusion for 10 minutes after attainment of cardiovascular stability.

Resource: www.lipidrescue.org accessed 4.29.2022

Given the potential for toxicity, careful calculation of local anesthetic doses (initial bolus dose and continuous infusion) is mandatory.

References

1. Ecoffey C, Lacroix F, Giaufré E, Orliaguet G, Courrèges P, Association des Anesthésistes Réanimateurs Pédiatriques d'Expression Française (ADARPEF) Epidemiology and morbidity of regional anesthesia in children: a follow-up one-year prospective survey of the French-Language Society of Paediatric Anaesthesiologists (ADARPEF). *Paediatr Anaesth.* 2010;20(12):1061–1069. https://doi.org/10.1111/j.1460-9592.2010.03448.x.
2. Bernards CM, Hadzic A, Suresh S, Neal JM. Regional anesthesia in anesthetized or heavily sedated patients. *Reg Anesth Pain Med.* 2008;33(5):449–460. https://doi.org/10.1016/j.rapm.2008.07.529.
3. Polaner DM, Taenzer AH, Walker BJ, et al. Pediatric Regional Anesthesia Network (PRAN): a multi-institutional study of the use and incidence of complications of pediatric regional anesthesia. *Anesth Analg.* 2012;115(6):1353–1364. https://doi.org/10.1213/ANE.0b013e31825d9f4b.
4. Walker BJ, Long JB, Sathyamoorthy M, et al. Complications in Pediatric Regional Anesthesia: An Analysis of More than 100,000 Blocks from the Pediatric Regional Anesthesia Network. *Anesthesiology.* 2018;129(4):721–732. https://doi.org/10.1097/ALN.0000000000002372.
5. Craven PD, Badawi N, Henderson-Smart DJ, O'Brien M. Regional (spinal, epidural, caudal) versus general anaesthesia in preterm infants undergoing inguinal herniorrhaphy in early infancy. *Cochrane Database Syst Rev.* 2003(3):CD003669. https://doi.org/10.1002/14651858.CD003669.
6. Williams RK, Adams DC, Aladjem EV, et al. The Safety and Efficacy of Spinal Anesthesia for Surgery in Infants: The Vermont Infant Spinal Registry. *Anesth Anal.* 2006;102(1):67–71. https://doi.org/10.1213/01.ANE.0000159162.86033.21.
7. Hermanns H, Stevens MF, Werdehausen R, Braun S, Lipfert P, Jetzek-Zader M. Sedation during spinal anaesthesia in infants. *Br J Anaesth.* 2006;97(3):380–384. https://doi.org/10.1093/bja/ael156.
8. Simpao AF, Gálvez JA, Wartman EC, et al. The Migration of Caudally Threaded Thoracic Epidural Catheters in Neonates and Infants. *Anesth Analg.* 2019;129(2):477–481. https://doi.org/10.1213/ANE.0000000000003311.
9. Meyer MJ, Krane EJ, Goldschneider KR, Klein NJ. Case report: neurological complications associated with epidural analgesia in children: a report of 4 cases of ambiguous etiologies. *Anesth Analg.* 2012;115(6):1365–1370. https://doi.org/10.1213/ANE.0b013e31826918b6.
10. Polaner DM, Zuk J, Luong K, Pan Z. Positive intravascular test dose criteria in children during total intravenous anesthesia with propofol and remifentanil are different than during inhaled anesthesia. *Anesth Analg.* 2010;110(1):41–45. https://doi.org/10.1213/ANE.0b013e3181c5f2dc.
11. Ogasawara K, Tanaka M, Nishikawa T. Choice of electrocardiography lead does not affect the usefulness of the T-wave criterion for detecting intravascular injection of an epinephrine test dose in anesthetized children. *Anesth Analg.* 2003;97(2):372–376. https://doi.org/10.1213/01.ANE.0000070230.10328.08.
12. Hong JY, Han SW, Kim WO, Cho JS, Kil HK. A comparison of high volume/low concentration and low volume/high concentration ropivacaine in caudal analgesia for pediatric orchiopexy. *Anesth Analg.* 2009;109(4):1073–1078. https://doi.org/10.1213/ane.0b013e3181b20c52.
13. Khalil S, Lingadevaru H, Bolos M, et al. Caudal regional anesthesia, ropivacaine concentration, postoperative analgesia, and infants. *Anesth Analg.* 2006;102(2):395–399. https://doi.org/10.1213/01.ane.0000194590.82645.4c.
14. Karmakar MK, Aun CS, Wong EL, Wong AS, Chan SK, Yeung CK. Ropivacaine undergoes slower systemic absorption from the caudal epidural space in children than bupivacaine. *Anesth Analg.* 2002;94(2):259–265. https://doi.org/10.1097/00000539-200202000-00006.
15. Tong Y, Ren H, Ding X, Chen Z, Li Q. Analgesic effect and adverse events of dexmedetomidine as additive for pediatric caudal anesthesia: a meta-analysis. *Paediatr Anaesth.* 2014;24(12):1224–1230. https://doi.org/10.1111/pan.12519.
16. Chong MA, Szoke DJ, Berbenetz NM, Lin C. Dexamethasone as an Adjuvant for Caudal Blockade in Pediatric Surgical Patients: A Systematic Review and Meta-analysis. *Anesth Analg.* 2018;127(2):520–528. https://doi.org/10.1213/ANE.0000000000003346.
17. Bösenberg AT, Bland BA, Schulte-Steinberg O, Downing JW. Thoracic epidural anesthesia via caudal route in infants. *Anesthesiology.* 1988;69(2):265–269. https://doi.org/10.1097/00000542-198808000-00020.

18. Tsui BC, Wagner A, Cave D, Kearney R. Thoracic and lumbar epidural analgesia via the caudal approach using electrical stimulation guidance in pediatric patients: a review of 289 patients. *Anesthesiology.* 2004;100(3):683–689. https://doi.org/10.1097/00000542-200403000-00032.

19. Davandra P. Epidural analgesia for children. *Continuing Education in Anaesthesia Critical Care & Pain.* 2006;6(2):63–66. https://doi.org/10.1093/bjaceaccp/mkl001.

20. Ganesh A, Kim A, Casale P, Cucchiaro G. Low-dose intrathecal morphine for postoperative analgesia in children. *Anesth Analg.* 2007;104(2):271–276. https://doi.org/10.1213/01.ane.0000252418.05394.28.

21. Ganesh A, Rose JB, Wells L, et al. Continuous peripheral nerve blockade for inpatient and outpatient postoperative analgesia in children. *Anesth Analg.* 2007;105(5):1234–1242. https://doi.org/10.1213/01.ane.0000284670.17412.b6.

22. Roberts S. Ultrasonographic guidance in pediatric regional anesthesia. Part 2: techniques [published correction appears in Paediatr Anaesth. 2006 Dec;16(12):1305-6]. *Paediatr Anaesth.* 2006;16(11):1112–1124. https://doi.org/10.1111/j.1460-9592.2006.02021.x.

23. Cucchiaro G, Ganesh A. The effects of clonidine on postoperative analgesia after peripheral nerve blockade in children. *Anesth Analg.* 2007;104(3):532–537. https://doi.org/10.1213/01.ane.0000253548.97479.b8.

24. Willschke H, Bösenberg A, Marhofer P, et al. Ultrasonographic-guided ilioinguinal/iliohypogastric nerve block in pediatric anesthesia: what is the optimal volume? *Anesth Analg.* 2006;102(6):1680–1684. https://doi.org/10.1213/01.ane.0000217196.34354.5a.

25. Weintraud M, Lundblad M, Kettner SC, et al. Ultrasound versus landmark-based technique for ilioinguinal-iliohypogastric nerve blockade in children: the implications on plasma levels of ropivacaine. *Anesth Analg.* 2009;108(5):1488–1492. https://doi.org/10.1213/ane.0b013e31819cb1f3.

Suggested Readings

Heydinger G, Tobias J, Veneziano G. Fundamentals and innovations in regional anaesthesia for infants and children. *Anaesthesia.* 2021;76(Suppl 1):74–88. https://doi.org/10.1111/anae.15283.

Kasai T, Yaegashi K, Hirose M, Tanaka Y. Spinal cord injury in a child caused by an accidental dural puncture with a single-shot thoracic epidural needle. *Anesth Analg.* 2003;96(1):65–67. https://doi.org/10.1097/00000539-200301000-00014.

Neal JM, Kopp SL, Pasternak JJ, Lanier WL, Rathmell JP. Anatomy and Pathophysiology of Spinal Cord Injury Associated With Regional Anesthesia and Pain Medicine: 2015 Update. *Reg Anesth Pain Med.* 2015;40(5):506–525. https://doi.org/10.1097/AAP.0000000000000297.

Tsui BC. Innovative approaches to neuraxial blockade in children: the introduction of epidural nerve root stimulation and ultrasound guidance for epidural catheter placement. *Pain Res Manag.* 2006;11(3):173–180. https://doi.org/10.1155/2006/478197.

Walker SM, Yaksh TL. Neuraxial analgesia in neonates and infants: a review of clinical and preclinical strategies for the development of safety and efficacy data. *Anesth Analg.* 2012;115(3):638–662. https://doi.org/10.1213/ANE.0b013e31826253f2.

21

Malignant Hyperthermia

TEEDA PINYAVAT, THIERRY GIRARD, AND RONALD S. LITMAN*

Malignant hyperthermia (MH) is a serious and possibly fatal syndrome of skeletal muscle hypermetabolism and calcium dysregulation that occurs when genetically susceptible individuals are exposed to certain anesthetic "triggering" agents-the potent halogenated inhaled volatile anesthetics and the nondepolarizing neuromuscular blocker succinylcholine.

MH susceptibility is conferred by the inherited or spontaneous (de novo) acquisition of a variant in genetic loci that encode for proteins that are integral for normal functioning of the skeletal muscle excitation-contraction (EC) complex. They include *RYR1*, which encodes for the ryanodine receptor, *CACNA1S*, which encodes for the alpha-1 subunit of the dihydropyridine receptor, and *STAC3*, which has an unknown function in the complex. A current listing of these MH causative variants is located on the European MH Group (EMHG) website.[1]

There are currently two methods to determine MH susceptibility: molecular genetic testing for known MH-causative variants, and an open muscle contracture biopsy. Molecular genetic testing uses an individual's DNA specimen, such as blood or buccal smear. It is noninvasive, and the sample can be sent from anywhere in the world. A positive result (finding the presence of a diagnostic variant) confirms MH susceptibility. A negative result, however, cannot rule out MH susceptibility because of known discordances between contracture testing and molecular genetic results; many families exist in whom a pathogenic variant has not been detected but have been proven MH susceptible either by a convincing clinical event or a positive contracture biopsy. Thus, MH can only be excluded by negative contracture biopsy testing.

A contracture biopsy test requires an open incision (usually from the quadriceps muscle, using either regional anesthesia or trigger-free general anesthesia) for immediate testing to determine the muscle's contractile properties when exposed to halothane and caffeine (Fig. 21.1). Its most important advantage is its high sensitivity (at least 99%); a negative result rules out MH susceptibility. Its main disadvantage is its surgical invasiveness, and limited availability at only several centers throughout the world. In North America the test is called the *caffeine-halothane contracture test* (CHCT) and in European centers it is called the *in-vitro contracture test* (IVCT). The protocols differ slightly, but both have a sensitivity close to 100% and a reasonably high specificity (yielding some possible false positive tests). Because of the size of the muscle required for analysis, children less than about 40 kg weight are usually excluded from testing, but this is biopsy-center dependent.

A person should be tested for susceptibility to MH if they or someone in their family has experienced a clinically suspicious episode of MH during exposure to an anesthetic triggering agent. However, it is very difficult to assess the accuracy of an intraoperative MH diagnosis in the absence of a bedside diagnostic test. When these clinical events are examined carefully, very few are unambiguously attributable to MH. A less common reason for MH susceptibility testing is when a person has experienced exaggerated and unexpected muscle breakdown (i.e., rhabdomyolysis) in response to nonextreme heat exposure or exercise.

The EMHG has published a suggested diagnostic pathway for MH susceptibility testing (Fig. 21.2). Individuals who have experienced a clinically convincing MH event should initially obtain noninvasive molecular genetic testing. This testing, however, is only useful when the analysis demonstrates a known diagnostic MH variant, which confirms MH susceptibility. If a family member has experienced the suspicious MH event, then they should ideally be the first member of the family to undergo testing. In the absence of finding an MH-diagnostic variant, a contracture test is required to exclude or confirm MH susceptibility.

Patients with a positive contracture biopsy without prior molecular genetic investigations should subsequently undergo molecular genetic analysis. If this investigation

*This chapter has been adapted from the more extensive version written by the same authors and will be published in *Smith's Anesthesia for Infants and Children*, 10th Edition (2021). We are grateful to Mary Theroux, who contributed to the original version, and continues to be one of the world's most learned experts on malignant hyperthermia.

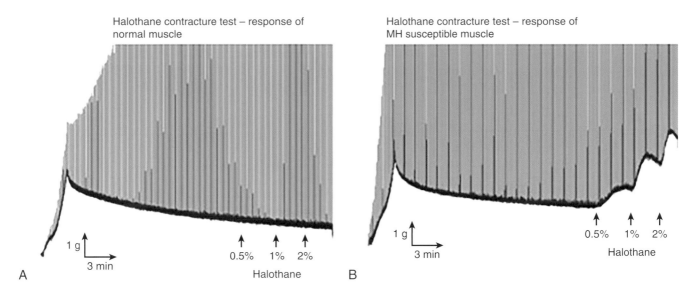

• **Fig 21.1.** Halothane contracture test. The muscle is stimulated electrically throughout the test and the electrically evoked twitches (thin vertical lines) indicate muscle viability. The thick blue line indicates the baseline tension of the muscle. The muscle is initially stretched to its physiologic length (increase in baseline tension) and maintained at this length (decline in baseline tension). Thereafter, any increase in baseline tension is defined as a contracture. (A) In a normal individual as exposure of the muscle to halothane is increased from 0.5 to 2.0%, the baseline tension tends to decrease further. (B) On the other hand, in a susceptible patient a concentration-dependent contracture develops in the presence of halothane. (From: Gupta PK, Hopkins PM. Diagnosis and management of malignant hyperthermia. *BJA Educ.* 2017:17(7):249–254.)

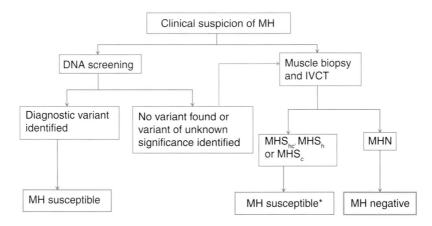

• **Fig 21.2.** EMHG suggested diagnostic pathway for MH susceptibility testing. (From: Hopkins PM, Rüffert H, Snoeck MM, et al. European Malignant Hyperthermia Group guidelines for investigation of malignant hyperthermia susceptibility. *Br J Anaesth,* 2015;115(4):531-539.)

reveals a pathogenic variant for MH, then other members of the family can be tested for that variant at less expense.

The most frequent reason for investigating an individual's MH susceptibility is the suspicion of MH susceptibility in a blood relative, either by a convincing clinical event or diagnostic testing. How closely related should this "proband" be to warrant testing or avoidance of MH triggering agents? Although a classic mendelian inheritance of MH is an over-simplification, the autosomal dominant mode of inheritance is helpful to estimate the risk for MH susceptibility. Each offspring of an MH susceptible parent has a 50% risk to be MH susceptible. With every generation, the risk for MH susceptibility decreases by 50%. Therefore, the next generation (grandchildren) each have a risk for 25% and so on. Using a conservatively high prevalence of MH variants of approximately 1 in 1500 in the general population,

it would take approximately 10 generations to decrease the calculated familial risk to be similar to that of the general population. As this example illustrates, any familial history within 10 generations (essentially everyone) should be cause for suspicion of MH susceptibility and should prompt the use of a nontriggering general anesthetic and referral for susceptibility testing. If ever possible, the family member with the highest risk for MH susceptibility should be tested for MH to rule out, or confirm, the risk for MH in subsequent generations.

Prevalence, Incidence, and Penetrance

The *prevalence* of MH susceptibility is defined as the percentage of people with an MH-causative variant, almost always on the *RYR1* gene. It varies by geographic region throughout the world, and is currently estimated to be as high as 1 in 1500 in some areas.

The *incidence* of MH is defined as the percentage of MH crises that occur during all anesthetic administrations (with triggering agents). Some authors have estimated this incidence to be about 1 in 50,000 to 100,00 cases, but these estimates are unreliable for several reasons. First, it is difficult to know the total number of anesthetics administered with MH-triggering agents (i.e., the denominator). Second, it is difficult to know the total number of true MH cases. Few acute presentations of MH present with unmistakable classic signs. The remainder are a mix of true MH events and other physiologic perturbations that manifest with similar signs as MH. A definitive diagnosis relies on testing after the episode and can be difficult to obtain. In addition, reporting of MH events to a national registry is not comprehensive.

The *penetrance* of MH is defined as the percentage of time that MH occurs when known MH-susceptible individuals are administered MH triggering agents. This has been reported to range from 5% to over 40% and is influenced by different individual and environmental conditions. Approximately one-half of patients who develop acute MH have had one or two previous uneventful exposures to triggering agents. The North American MH Registry (NAMHR) includes a case of a genetically confirmed MH susceptible patient who developed fatal MH on what may have been their 31st exposure to an MH-triggering agent!

Triggering Agents

Nearly all MH reactions are associated with the administration of one of the potent inhalational agents (i.e., halothane, isoflurane, sevoflurane, or desflurane) in a dose dependent manner (the minimum dose is unknown), with or without concomitant administration of succinylcholine. The concomitant use of succinylcholine is associated with a worse clinical presentation of MH. The decrease in use of halothane and succinylcholine in the 1990s is thought to account for an apparent shift in clinical presentation of MH to later in the course of a patient's anesthetic.

Although rare, there appear to be MH cases initiated with succinylcholine alone. The clinical signs of these MH events tend to occur within 10 minutes of succinylcholine administration and are more likely to be associated with masseter muscle rigidity than reactions triggered by the potent inhalational anesthetic gases. Besides the inhalational anesthetic gases and succinylcholine, no other medications or substances, in any class, are causally associated with the occurrence of MH.

Clinical Presentations

MH most often presents as a constellation of physiologic signs indicative of uncontrolled hypermetabolism during the administration of general anesthetic triggering agents (Table 21.1 from Smith's chapter). This includes unexplainable **hypercarbia** that is resistant to increases in minute ventilation, **sinus tachycardia**, and **metabolic acidosis**.

Spontaneously breathing patients will develop **tachypnea** to counteract the respiratory and metabolic acidosis. However, the onset of MH may manifest in a variety of clinical presentations. For example, in some patients the first signs of MH are abnormally prolonged **skeletal muscle contractures**, either generalized throughout the body or confined only to the masseter muscle soon after the administration of succinylcholine. In other patients, the first sign of MH is an **arrhythmia** caused by hyperkalemia from acute **rhabdomyolysis**. These arrhythmias are variable and are thought to depend on the absolute level and rate of rise of serum potassium and the degree of acidosis and sympathetic stimulation. They range from seemingly benign premature ventricular contractions (PVCs) or changes in the electrocardiogram (e.g., peaked T waves, broadened and decreased amplitude of the P wave, widened QRS) to sudden heart block, ventricular tachycardia, ventricular fibrillation, or asystole. **Hyperthermia** may occur any time in the clinical course of MH, from the initial onset to the later stages. It may be indolent, rising slowly without attracting much attention, or accelerated, rising more than one degree Celsius every few minutes in its initial stages. Lack of temperature monitoring and failure to detect hyperthermia has been associated[3] with increased morbidity and death caused by MH. Therefore, core temperature monitoring (e.g. distal esophagus, nasopharynx, tympanic membrane, pulmonary artery, bladder) should be used in all general anesthetics expected to last longer than 30 minutes, or less when perturbations in body temperature are expected because of unique patient or surgical characteristics.

When MH causes **rhabdomyolysis**, serum CK may rise rapidly (>10,000 U/L) within the first several hours, and myoglobinuria may occur, causing the urine to appear tea-colored. Some patients will continue to have increases in CK (>100,000 U/L) within a few days, despite adequate treatment with dantrolene. The speed and extent of the skeletal muscle destruction will determine the relative level of hyperkalemia and its deleterious effects on the heart.

The clinical manifestations of MH have occurred at any time during the administration of triggering anesthetic agents, from induction to emergence.

A common misunderstanding about the presentation of MH is that it may be delayed, even many hours into the postoperative period. This does not seem to be true. In a published analysis of 528 cases of suspected MH reported to the NAMHR, 10 occurred after discontinuation of volatile anesthetic agents. In none of these 10 cases did the first signs of MH appear more than 40 minutes after discontinuation of the volatile anesthetics. Many clinicians worry that acute MH may begin in the postoperative period with hyperthermia as the presenting sign. Based on our experience with calls to the MHAUS hotline, postoperative hyperthermia (i.e., T >39°C) without additional signs of MH is relatively common, but is not associated with an eventual diagnosis of MH.

Signs of MH may differ between adults and children of different age groups. In a review of pediatric MH

TABLE 21.1	Clinical Characteristics of Acute MH

Hypercarbia

- Unexpected and unexplainable increase in $P_{ET}CO_2$ that is resistant to increasing minute ventilation
- Usually one of the first signs of acute MH
- Tachypnea or breathing over the ventilator in a spontaneously breathing patient
- Results in respiratory acidosis
- One of the first signs of MH to abate with successful treatment with dantrolene
- According to the Clinical Grading Score (CGS),[2] a diagnosis of acute MH is consistent with:
  - $P_{ET}CO_2 > 55$ mm Hg with appropriately controlled ventilation
  - Arterial $P_ACO_2 > 60$ mm Hg with appropriately controlled ventilation
  - $P_{ET}CO_2 > 60$ mm Hg with spontaneous ventilation
  - Arterial $P_ACO_2 > 65$ mm Hg with spontaneous ventilation
- Before ascribing to MH, rule out causes of hypoventilation

Sinus Tachycardia

- Usually develops early in the acute MH event and is often one of the presenting signs
- Probably represents a response to the increase in skeletal muscle metabolism, acidosis, sympathetic stimulation, or all combined
- Is not specific for MH but used in combination with additional supporting evidence

Metabolic Acidosis

- Venous or arterial blood sample acceptable
- An arterial base excess more negative than −8 mEq/L or a pH < 7.25 have shown be consistent with acute MH[1]

Muscle Rigidity

- Presenting sign, along with hypercarbia and tachycardia, in some cases of acute MH
- Unusually prolonged and severe ("jaws of steel") masseter muscle rigidity (MMR) after administration of succinylcholine has been associated with the onset of MH
- Generalized rigidity as sustained muscle contractures may also occur early in some patients with MH; however, may be difficult to differentiate the often severe myoclonus that occurs with administration of sevoflurane or propofol
- Skeletal muscle contractures in the presence of neuromuscular blockade should be considered pathognomonic for MH
- Serum creatine kinase (CK) will begin to rise soon after the MH event and may not peak for several days, despite appropriate treatment
- Urine may appear tea-colored from presence of myoglobin

Hyperkalemia

- May occur any time during an MH event
- May cause life-threatening or fatal cardiac arrhythmias such as ventricular tachycardia or fibrillation, or cardiac arrest

Hyperthermia

- May occur early or later in the course of an acute MH event
- May rise as high as 1°C every few minutes
- Severe hyperthermia (> 41°C) associated with development of disseminated intravascular coagulation (DIC)
- Is not indicative of MH when isolated in the postoperative period without other signs of MH

Rhabdomyolysis

- MH consistent with an elevated CK >20,000 U/L after anesthetic that included succinylcholine
- Elevated CK >10,000 U/L after anesthetic without succinylcholine

P_ACO_2, Partial pressure of arterial CO_2; $P_{ET}CO_2$, partial pressure of end-tidal CO_2.

cases from the NAMHR, children less than 2 years of age were less likely to demonstrate classic signs of MH, such as sinus tachycardia, hypercarbia, rapid temperature elevation, and muscle rigidity, and had lower peak serum potassium and CK levels. Infants, however, were more likely to develop skin mottling and had higher peak lactic acid levels.

Episodic RYR1-Related Crises (ERRC)

On rare occasions, MH susceptible individuals may spontaneously develop a life-threatening and sometimes fatal condition that is characterized by muscle rigidity, rhabdomyolysis, and severe hyperthermia in the absence of known anesthetic triggering agents. We have termed these events as *episodic RYR1-related crises* (ERRC). Some of these individuals who have had repeated episodes are able to abort the process by ingestion of oral dantrolene when they begin to experience certain symptoms such as muscle weakness or rigidity, or increasing body temperature, while others have died after sudden presentation of severe muscle rigidity accompanied by accelerated hyperthermia and hyperkalemia.

Clinical Diagnosis of MH

There is currently no bedside diagnostic test to determine whether a patient is experiencing an MH event. Therefore diagnosis of an acute MH crisis depends on clinical suspicion based on the recognition of key clinical features occurring more or less in a temporal pattern after excluding other feasible causes. Two of the most common reasons to suspect MH are unexplainable hypercarbia and hyperthermia. Hypercarbia is almost always associated with hypoventilation from a number of causes; but when these have been ruled out by confirming the adequacy of ventilation, MH should be considered, especially when the hypercarbia is resistant to increases in minute ventilation. When hypercarbia persists and is associated with generalized muscle rigidity (especially if the patient has been administered a nondepolarizing neuromuscular blocker), MH should be strongly suspected and treatment with dantrolene should begin. Unexpected intraoperative hyperthermia is most often associated with iatrogenic overwarming, but when associated with hypercarbia with or without muscle rigidity or other signs of MH, it should prompt the initiation of treatment and measures to reduce core temperature below 38.5°C. When one is unsure of the cause of the hypercarbia or hyperthermia, a blood gas (arterial or venous) may be helpful in determining the extent of metabolic acidosis. A normal blood gas, in most cases, will be sufficient to rule out MH. The ultimate final diagnosis, in most cases, has relied on a retrospective review of the patient's clinical characteristics at the time of the event combined with contracture biopsy and/or genetic test results obtained after the clinical event has resolved.

Treatment

Improving survival from MH is highly dependent on early recognition and prompt initiation of treatment. As soon as the diagnosis is considered reasonable, (i.e., the patient has more than one sign (from Table 21.1) that cannot be explained by an alternative diagnosis) triggering agents should be immediately discontinued and an "MH emergency" declared. There are various treatment components to an MH emergency (Table 21.2). The most important initial steps are to discontinue and clear the triggering agent(s), summon all available personnel to assist, administer dantrolene, and treat symptomatic hyperkalemia, acidosis, and hyperthermia.

Intravenous (IV) dantrolene, 2.5 mg/kg, should be administered as an initial bolus, and additional boluses should be administered every 5 to 10 minutes until reversal of MH signs (e.g., alleviation of muscle rigidity, lowering of $P_{ET}CO_2$, decreasing temperature, etc.).

There are currently two types of dantrolene formulations available for clinical use. The original formulation, dantrolene sodium, is a lyophilized powder that uses the additives mannitol and sodium hydroxide to increase solubility. Each vial contains 20 mg of dantrolene and 3 gm mannitol, and requires 60 mL of sterile water to reconstitute. This formulation is relatively difficult to solubilize before IV administration, often requiring warming and considerable mixing.

The newer formulation, dantrolene sodium suspension (DSS, trade name Ryanodex), contains dantrolene in nanocrystalline particles. These very small particles do not need to be solubilized, but rather form a "nanosuspension" in only 5 mL sterile water that allows a much higher available dantrolene concentration (250 mg/mL) that does not require prolonged mixing or warming. Most importantly, it can be mixed and administered by a single individual. This may be especially advantageous in an ambulatory setting. DSS contains less mannitol (125 mg per vial). Although it makes intuitive sense that the DSS preparation would result in faster treatment of MH, leading to better outcomes, this is impossible to prove in the setting of a clinical trial. The DSS preparation is currently more expensive than the older generic versions, and has slightly shorter shelf life (30 months) compared with older generic versions (36 months).

Dantrolene's effect on lowering $P_{ET}CO_2$ and improving other manifestations of the MH process should be apparent within several minutes of its administration. If multiple doses have been administered (>10 mg/kg) without apparent effect, the diagnosis of MH should be questioned and alternative diagnoses considered.

Complications of dantrolene administration are dose-related and include venous phlebitis and thrombosis at the administration site, and skeletal muscle weakness that may prevent weaning from mechanical ventilation. Because of its alkaline pH of 9.5, it can cause skin necrosis if extravasated. Therefore, dantrolene should always be given through the largest intravenous line available (or preferably a central line) and free flow should be ensured before it is administered. DSS is more alkaline than conventional dantrolene (pH 10.3) and thus, requires heightened vigilance during administration.

Active cooling is sometimes necessary during an MH crisis. Most patients with acute MH that are treated promptly with dantrolene will not develop dangerous levels of hyperthermia and will not require active cooling. If core temperature is above 39°C, surface cooling with cold water blankets and ice packs should be considered first, followed by an infusion of 20 mL/kg of refrigerated IV fluid. Invasive cooling (i.e., peritoneal or bladder irrigation) is rarely necessary. To avoid overcooling and subsequent hypothermia, active

TABLE 21.2	Emergency Treatment for An Acute MH Event[a]

- Discontinue volatile agents and succinylcholine; begin intravenous anesthetic agents if indicated; hyperventilate with 100% oxygen at high flows; intubate trachea if not already; if available, insert charcoal filters into inspiratory and expiratory limbs of anesthesia circuit.
- Call for help and MH cart (if necessary, call MHAUS hotline (1-800-644-9737 in US, 1-209-417-3722 outside the U.S.) for advice on treatment; if free-standing ambulatory surgery center, call 911 for transport to closest full-service medical center.
- Notify surgeon to complete the procedure as soon as feasible.
- Administer IV dantrolene 2.5 mg/kg rapidly through largest bore IV available; repeat as frequently as needed until the patient responds with a decrease in $P_{ET}CO_2$ and muscle rigidity. Large doses (>10 mg/kg) may be required for muscular patients with persistent contractures or rigidity.
  - DANTRIUM/REVONTO: Each 20 mg vial should be mixed with warmed 60 mL sterile water and shaken until clear.
  - RYANODEX: Each 250 mg vial should be mixed with 5 mL sterile water and shaken to form an orange-colored, opaque suspension.
- Large doses (>10 mg/kg) without symptom resolution should prompt consideration of alternative diagnoses.
- Obtain blood gas (venous or arterial) to determine degree of metabolic acidosis. Consider administration of sodium bicarbonate, 1 to 2 mEq/kg dose, for base excess more negative than -8 (maximum dose 50 mEq).
- Cool the patient if core temperature is >39°C or less if rapidly rising. Stop cooling when the temperature has decreased to <38°C.
- Treat hyperkalemia (K > 5.9 or less with ECG changes) with:
  - Calcium chloride 10 to 20 mg/kg (0.1–0.2 mL/kg 10% solution), maximum dose 2 g (20 mL) or calcium gluconate 60 to 100 mg/kg IV (0.6–1 mL/kg of 10% solution), maximum 3 g (30 mL) per dose
  - Sodium bicarbonate, 1 to 2 mEq/kg IV (maximum dose 50 mEq)
- Glucose/insulin
  - For pediatric patients: 0.1 units/kg regular insulin IV and 0.5 grams/kg dextrose
  - For adult patients: 10 units regular insulin IV and 50 mL 50% dextrose
- For refractory hyperkalemia, consider albuterol (or other beta-agonist), kayexalate, dialysis, or ECMO if patient is in cardiac arrest.
- Treat dysrhythmias with standard medication but avoid calcium channel blockers with concomitant dantrolene administration.
- Diurese to >1 mL/kg/hr urine output.
- If CK or K[+] rise, assume myoglobinuria and give bicarbonate infusion of 1 mEq/kg/hr, to alkalinize urine.
- Monitor: core temperature, urine output with bladder catheter, and consider arterial and/or central venous monitoring if warranted by the clinical severity of the patient.
- Follow: HR, core temperature, $P_{ET}CO_2$, minute ventilation, blood gases, K[+], CK, urine myoglobin and coagulation studies as warranted by the clinical severity of the patient.
- When stable, transfer to PACU or ICU for at least 24 hours. Key indicators of stability include:
  - $P_{ET}CO_2$ declining or normal
  - Heart rate stable or decreasing with no signs of ominous dysrhythmias
  - Hyperthermia resolved
  - Muscular rigidity resolved

[a]Adapted from Malignant Hyperthermia Association of the U.S., https://www.mhaus.org/healthcare-professionals/managing-a-crisis/

cooling measures should be discontinued when core temperature has decreased to 38°C.

After initial treatment and stabilization of the acute MH event, 1 mg/kg dantrolene should be administered every 6 hours for at least 24 hours. Dantrolene can then be discontinued when there is no evidence of metabolic acidosis, hyperthermia, muscle rigidity, or increasing CK.

Anesthetizing the Known or Suspected MH-Susceptible Patient

Known or suspected (i.e., before definitive testing) MH susceptible patients can safely receive general anesthesia with a nontriggering anesthetic technique. This technique uses any type of local or general anesthetic (or sedative) agent other than the known triggering agents. This necessitates placement of an intravenous catheter before administration of general anesthesia. In children, this can be facilitated with prior administration of an oral sedative (e.g., midazolam),

topical application of a local anesthetic cream, and inhalation of nitrous oxide during IV cannulation.

Because modern anesthesia machines are variable in the times taken to minimize residual anesthetic levels (possibly up to 100 minutes[4]), the placement of charcoal filters (Fig. 21.3; Vapor-Clean, Dynasthetics, Salt Lake City, UT, USA) on the inspiratory and expiratory sides of the circuit are recommended to reduce the flush time to about 90 seconds. It is also advisable to completely remove the vaporizers from the anesthesia machine or alternatively, place a wide piece of tape over them to act as a reminder that they should not be used (Fig. 21.4).

Although the use of nontriggering anesthetic agents in MH-susceptible individuals is considered safe, one should not proceed without a full supply of dantrolene immediately available, and there should be continuous vigilance for signs of MH. After an uneventful nontriggering anesthetic in these patients, they may be discharged to home or a hospital ward using standard discharge criteria.

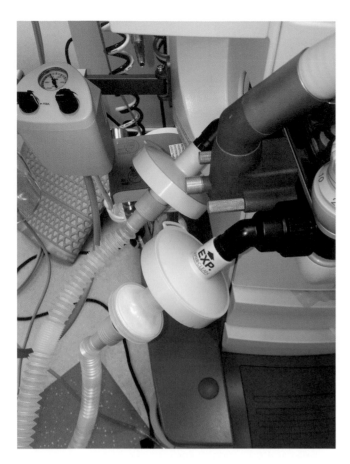

• Fig 21.3. Charcoal filters attached to proximal ends of inspiratory and expiratory limbs of the anesthesia breathing circuit.

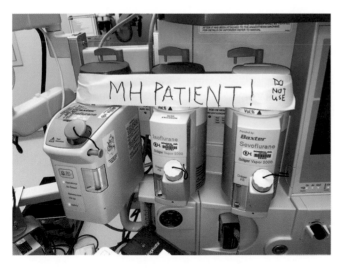

• Fig 21.4. Taped reminder across vaporizers that patient is MH susceptible.

Non-MH Rhabdomyolysis in Children With Myopathies

Although not directly related to MH, there is an important complication from volatile anesthetic agents and succinylcholine that, in the past, was thought to represent MH susceptibility. In 1997 based on reports to the MH hotline, a group of MH specialists published[5] the details of 25 presumed healthy children who developed cardiac arrest soon after receiving succinylcholine. Hyperkalemia was detected in 13 of 18 children who had potassium measurements performed, and 10 children died from the arrest. Upon further analysis, 12 children were diagnosed with a previously unrecognized myopathy (most had Duchenne muscular dystrophy). As a result of this report and others, the Food and Drug Administration issued a black box warning for succinylcholine, and anesthesiologists curtailed their use of succinylcholine for elective neuromuscular blockade in children. Life-threatening hyperkalemia and rhabdomyolysis have also been reported after exposure of children with Duchenne or Becker muscular dystrophy to volatile anesthetics used without succinylcholine. These serious complications of exposure to MH triggering agents are apparently caused by their direct action on atrophic muscles that have upregulation of extrajunctional acetylcholine receptors. Therapy should focus on rapid reversal of hyperkalemia (i.e., calcium, bicarbonate, etc.). Although some of these signs are consistent with acute MH, there is no association with the hypermetabolic response seen during acute MH.

Malignant Hyperthermia Association of the United States

Founded in 1981, the Malignant Hyperthermia Association of the United States (MHAUS) is a nonprofit patient advocacy organization composed of physicians, scientists, and MH-susceptible patients and their families. Its mission is to promote the optimum care and scientific understanding of MH and related disorders. One of the most important services provided by MHAUS is the availability of a telephone hotline (800-MH-HYPER) continuously staffed by physicians with substantial expertise in managing patients with MH.

References

1. The European Malignant Hyperthermia (MH) Group. (2019). http://www.emhg.org. Accessed 21.7.30.
2. Larach MG, Localio AR, Allen GC, et al. A clinical grading scale to predict malignant hyperthermia susceptibility. *Anesthesiology.* 1994;80(4):771–779. doi:10.1097/00000542-199404000-00008.
3. Larach MG, Brandom BW, Allen GC, Gronert GA, Lehman EB. Malignant hyperthermia deaths related to inadequate temperature monitoring, 2007-2012: a report from the North American malignant hyperthermia registry of the malignant hyperthermia association of the United States. *Anesth Analg.* 2014;119(6):1359–1366. doi:10.1213/ANE.0000000000000421.
4. Kim TW, Nemergut ME. Preparation of modern anesthesia workstations for malignant hyperthermia-susceptible patients: a review of past and present practice. *Anesthesiology.* 2011;114(1):205–212. doi:10.1097/ALN.0b013e3181ee2cb7.

5. Larach MG, Rosenberg H, Gronert GA, Allen GC. Hyperkalemic cardiac arrest during anesthesia in infants and children with occult myopathies. *Clin Pediatr (Phila)*. 1997;36(1):9–16. doi:10.1177/000992289703600102.

Suggested Readings

Davis P, Cladis F, eds. *Smith's Anesthesia for Infants and Children*. 10th ed. Philadelphia: Elsevier; 2021.

Dowling JJ, Riazi S, Litman RS. Episodic RYR1-related crisis: part of the evolving spectrum of RYR1-related myopathies and malignant hyperthermia-like illnesses. *A Pract*. 2021;19;15(1):e01377 doi:10.1213/XAA.0000000000001377. Published 21.1.19.

Gupta PK, Hopkins PM. Diagnosis and management of malignant hyperthermia. *BJA Educ*. 2017;17(7):249–254. doi:10.1093/bjaed/mkw079.

Shafer SL, Dexter F, Brull SJ. Deadly heat: economics of continuous temperature monitoring during general anesthesia. *Anesth Analg*. 2014;119(6):1235–1237. doi:10.1213/ANE.0000000000000487.

22

ENT Surgery

WILLIAM RYAN, RONALD S. LITMAN, AND KAREN B. ZUR

Anesthesia for ENT surgery is one of the most challenging because of the frequency of airway obstruction in infants and small children and requisite sharing of the airway that is often at a distance from the anesthesiologist. The trainee must learn a variety of airway management techniques that are appropriate for each type of procedure and the different types of airway instruments used by otolaryngologists.

Ear Surgery

Myringotomy and Tube Placement

Otitis media is a viral or bacterial infection that develops within a transudate in the middle ear space. The fluid accumulation results from eustachian tube dysfunction or adenoid hypertrophy and inflammation. These children present with fever and upper respiratory tract infections that do not abate until the ear fluid is drained. Myringotomy and tube placement consist of the insertion of tiny ventilating tubes through the tympanic membrane to drain fluid from the middle ear and prevent future fluid collections (Fig. 22.1). It is the most common surgical procedure requiring general anesthesia in children.

The major focus of the preoperative assessment is to ensure that the child does not have any lower airway symptoms that indicate acute reactive airway disease or pneumonia, and that the child is no worse than their usual baseline state of health.

The standard anesthesia technique for myringotomy and tube placement consists of an inhaled induction with sevoflurane, with or without nitrous oxide (N_2O). Premedication with a short-acting anxiolytic (e.g., oral midazolam) is institution-dependent. Once the child has reached a depth of general anesthesia sufficient to prevent response to a painful stimulus, the anesthesia provider turns the child's head to the side while maintaining mask anesthesia, and the tubes are placed by the surgeon using a microscope (Fig. 22.2). Intravenous (IV) access is not necessary unless the child has a comorbidity that necessitates administration of IV fluids or medications. Each ear tube insertion typically lasts no more than 5 minutes. Many children will manifest

upper-airway obstruction when the head is turned. This usually resolves with application of continuous positive airway pressure (CPAP) or placement of an oral airway (Fig. 22.3). Laryngospasm may occur if the depth of anesthesia is insufficient. Central or obstructive apnea may occur and is treated with positive-pressure ventilation. An oral airway may also be helpful postoperatively to prevent upper-airway obstruction in the recovery phase.

Significant postoperative pain may occur in some children immediately after the procedure and can occasionally last a few hours. Thus, prophylactic analgesia is indicated. Choices include acetaminophen, ibuprofen, or (rarely) oxycodone. *Intranasal*[1] or intramuscular fentanyl 1 to 2 µg/kg, administered while the child is anesthetized, provides adequate postoperative analgesia and decreases agitation during emergence from general anesthesia without prolonging discharge times. Some anesthesiologists administer intranasal or *intramuscular*[2] ketorolac intraoperatively. In a large retrospective study,[3] combination intramuscular fentanyl and ketorolac was strongly associated with superior postanesthesia care unit (PACU) analgesia, reduced oxycodone rescue, and absence of clinically significant increases in recovery time or emesis incidence, compared with either medication alone. Healthy children may be safely discharged within an hour of completing the procedure.

Tympanomastoidectomy

Indications for a tympanomastoidectomy include chronic otitis media or the presence of a cholesteatoma. A cholesteatoma is a benign cyst made of squamous epithelia. It may present as a continuum of chronic otitis media and can cause damage to the middle ear ossicles leading to hearing loss. Cholesteatomas may be congenital (primary) or acquired (secondary). Secondary causes include tympanic membrane perforation or prior surgery.

A traditional tympanomastoidectomy is performed through an incision behind the ear to expose the mastoid, ear canal, and tympanic membrane or through the ear canal with endoscopic assistance. The ear canal is occasionally widened, and a portion of the mastoid bone is removed to

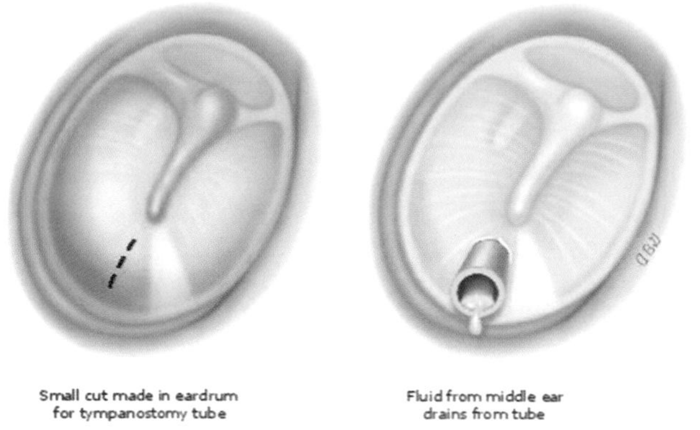

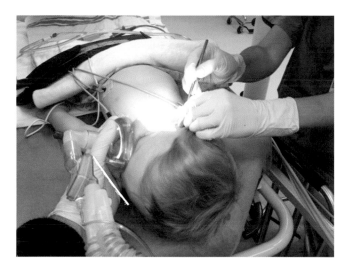

• Fig 22.1. Myringotomy and tube placement. (Reproduced with permission from Klein JO, Pelton S. Patient information: Ear infections (otitis media) in children (Beyond the Basics). In: Basow DS, ed. *UpToDate*, Waltham, MA. Copyright 2013. For more information see www.uptodate.com.)

allow access to the area of pathology. The eardrum is reconstructed, and the cholesteatoma is removed. The procedure is performed in the supine position with the child's head turned away from the side of the surgery. The operating room (OR) table is turned 90 to 180 degrees away from the anesthesia machine (Fig. 22.4). Therefore, you will need to anticipate the requirement of a breathing circuit with sufficient length. During the procedure, the head and neck are completely covered with drapes that will impede access to the airway. There is minimal blood loss or third-space fluid losses. The surgeon may use facial nerve monitoring, which precludes the use of a neuromuscular blocker. A temporary urinary catheter should be considered for procedures greater than 4 hours duration. Hyperthermia is possible if a warming blanket is used. The main postoperative concern is nausea and vomiting, so multimodal antiemetic prophylaxis should be administered. Postoperatively, children may be discharged home if they are well hydrated and do not have severe pain. The infiltration of local anesthesia at the incision site, and administration of oral or rectal acetaminophen will aid in postoperative analgesia. The extubation

• Fig 22.2. Myringotomy and tube insertion. During myringotomy and tube placement, face mask anesthesia is maintained with the child's head rotated laterally. It takes practice keeping the surgical field still, and maintaining upper-airway patency. Courtesy of Ronald S. Litman.

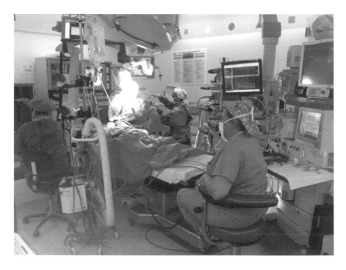

• Fig 22.4. Tympanomastoidectomy position. The OR table is turned 180 degrees away from the anesthetist for ear cases. Courtesy of Ronald S. Litman.

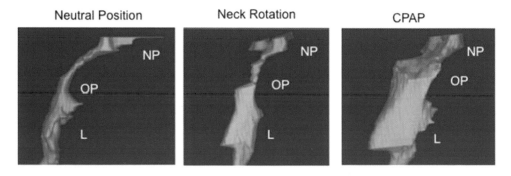

• Fig 22.3. Upper-airway obstruction during lateral neck rotation. 3D reconstructed MRI images of a child's airway (gray-colored) with head in neutral position (left), lateral rotation (center), and lateral rotation with 10 cmH$_2$O CPAP applied. Note significant obstruction of oropharynx (OP) when rotated that widens dramatically with CPAP. *NP*, nasopharynx, *L*, larynx. Courtesy of Ronald S. Litman.

plan should be discussed with the surgeon, who may prefer a deep extubation technique to eliminate coughing, which has been known to cause graft displacement.

Tympanoplasty

A tympanoplasty is a repair of a perforated eardrum, usually with a temporalis fascia graft. It may also involve reconstruction of the bones of the middle ear. A postauricular approach is most often used; however, many otolaryngologists have been now performing this procedure with endoscopic assistance in a transcanal approach. All anesthetic implications and techniques are the same as those for tympanomastoidectomy.

Nasal Surgery

Nasal Cautery

Nasal cautery is performed in children who have chronic epistaxis secondary to friable blood vessels along the anterior portion of the nasal septum. The procedure consists of brief electrocauterization and typically lasts no more than 10 to 15 minutes. Some anesthesiologists may choose to provide mask anesthesia while intermittently removing the mask for the surgeon to cauterize the vessels. Supraglottic mask anesthesia or endotracheal tube placement are reasonable options, especially if the child is expected to bleed into the back of the pharynx. Postoperative analgesia is minimal and usually treated with acetaminophen or ibuprofen.

Nasal Fracture Reduction

Displaced nasal fractures are common in children, usually from falls or sports injuries. The fracture should be reduced within 14 days of the injury, after the initial period of swelling but before healing begins. Closed reduction consists of the manipulation of the nasal bones externally with the assistance of instruments through the nasal openings. Bleeding is typical, though not enough to be clinically important. However, there is a significant amount of blood that enters the nasopharynx. For this reason, most pediatric anesthesiologists will choose laryngeal mask airway (LMA) placement or endotracheal intubation for airway management and will thoroughly suction the pharynx before removal. The surgeon may choose to place a throat pack to minimize the chance of aspirating blood. Postoperative pain in the recovery room may require opioid analgesia, however home-based opioid use is not typically needed. Because postoperative nausea and vomiting are common, a prophylactic multimodal antiemetic approach is indicated.

Juvenile Nasopharyngeal Angiofibroma Resection

A juvenile nasopharyngeal angiofibroma (JNA) is a benign vascular tumor of the posterior nasopharynx that can spread into contiguous structures. Adolescent boys are most often affected and present with chronic nasal obstruction or painless, typically unilateral nasal bleeding that is not associated with trauma. The management of JNA is difficult because the lesion receives abundant vascular blood supply. Most patients will undergo preoperative embolization to limit intraoperative bleeding, which may be severe. An endoscopic nasal approach is then used for complete resection. Preoperative assessment includes a complete blood count, coagulation studies, and a type-and-crossmatch. After induction of general anesthesia and tracheal intubation (usually with a Ring-Adair-Elwyn [RAE] tube), two large-bore IV catheters are inserted for volume replacement and possible blood transfusion. An arterial line is often placed, depending on the extent of the procedure. A temporary urinary catheter should be placed because the duration of the surgery is often many hours. At the end of the procedure the nasal cavity is frequently packed. Depending on the extent of the surgical resection these children may remain intubated at the end of the procedure and mechanically ventilated in the intensive care unit (ICU) until their vital signs and fluid status have stabilized.

Upper Airway Surgery

Laryngomalacia and Supraglottoplasty

Laryngomalacia is the most common cause of chronic extrathoracic airway obstruction in infants. The typical endoscopic findings are of a curled epiglottis and floppy arytenoids with foreshortened aryepiglottic folds that cause the arytenoids to prolapse toward the glottic opening during inspiration, resulting in inspiratory stridor. The symptoms worsen in the first several months of life. The stridor is usually more prominent when the infant is lying supine, crying, or feeding. In most cases, the stridor is loudest between 4 to 8 months of age and resolves during the first year of life. However, some cases may cause chronic hypoxemia and may interfere with normal feeding and subsequent growth. These cases may require surgical intervention, which includes rigid bronchoscopy to rule out synchronous airway lesions and a supraglottoplasty. The purpose of the supraglottoplasty is to trim portions of the supraglottis that obstruct the airway (this is variable in different infants). Most commonly, the aryepiglottic folds need to be lysed and the cuneiform cartilages of the arytenoids may also need to be trimmed. Various instruments may be used including cold steel, CO_2 laser, or shaver. During induction of general anesthesia, infants with laryngomalacia will demonstrate airway obstruction that is not relieved by placement of an oral airway device. Deepening the anesthetic will often relieve the obstruction because of progressive weakening of the diaphragm and decreasing the strength of inspiration. However, during upper-airway obstruction, speed of inhaled induction is slowed. Positive-pressure ventilation is usually easily accomplished in these infants, especially after the onset of neuromuscular blockade. Topical lidocaine is often used to mitigate the risk for laryngospasm during bronchoscopy and supraglottoplasty. When the CO_2 laser is used in the airway, standard laser safety precautions will apply.

Obstructive Sleep Apnea and Tonsillectomy

There are two common reasons why children have their tonsils removed: recurrent infection and obstructive sleep apnea (OSA, or "sleep disordered breathing"). OSA is the result of adenotonsillar hypertrophy, often combined with an abnormally small retropharyngeal space, and altered neuromuscular control of upper-airway patency during sleep. It mainly occurs in children between the ages of 2 and 6 years (although infants and older children may also have it), and is especially prevalent in children with obesity, trisomy 21, neuromuscular disease, and craniofacial abnormalities. The clinical manifestations include partial or complete upper-airway obstruction during sleep, restless sleep, enuresis, morning headaches, behavioral disturbances, and daytime somnolence. Severe cases of untreated long-standing OSA can result in chronic hypoxemia, polycythemia, cor pulmonale, growth delays, behavioral problems, and learning difficulties.

Diagnosis of OSA in children is mainly by clinical characteristics, but an overnight sleep study using polysomnography (PSG) may be performed to confirm the diagnosis and is recommended[4] in children with comorbidities, such as obesity, trisomy 21, craniofacial abnormalities, neuromuscular disorders, sickle cell disease, or mucopolysaccharidoses. OSA is measured by the apnea-hypopnea index (AHI), which is the average number of apnea or hypopnea events per hour. OSA can be categorized as[5] as mild, moderate, or severe (Table 22.1). The most common therapy for pediatric OSA is adenotonsillectomy, which alleviates symptoms in most children.

Preoperatively, some pediatric anesthesiologists reduce the dose of the preoperative sedative in children with OSA, for fear of causing life-threatening upper-airway obstruction if the child is waiting in an unmonitored environment. During induction of general anesthesia, virtually all children with untreated OSA will exhibit partial or complete upper-airway obstruction. Insertion of an oral airway device after loss of consciousness will bypass the obstruction and allow easy bag-mask ventilation. In the immediate postoperative period after adenotonsillectomy, the incidence of airway obstruction is higher in children with OSA compared with those who undergo adenotonsillectomy for recurrent infections. Therefore, children with significant OSA should be monitored closely after the procedure, and those chosen on a case-by-case basis should be kept as an inpatient overnight. Even some time after adenotonsillectomy has been performed, a predisposition toward upper-airway obstruction during sleep or sedation may persist throughout childhood. Children with OSA are more likely to develop adult-type OSA.

Tonsillectomies in otherwise healthy children are performed as outpatient surgery unless the child has OSA and meets one of the criteria for overnight admission[4] (Table 22.2).

Unless there is a history of a bleeding disorder in the child or the family, tonsillectomy patients do not require preoperative lab studies.

The goals of anesthetic management for tonsillectomy are a motionless patient during the procedure, a rapid and smooth emergence, postoperative pain relief, and control of postoperative nausea and vomiting. After induction of anesthesia, a cuffed oral RAE endotracheal tube is inserted to accommodate the mouth-opening device used by the surgeon. The cuff should be inflated to prevent oxygen from entering the surgical field, where it may fuel a fire if electrocautery is being used. Even with cuffed tubes, our routine practice is to keep the inspired oxygen concentration below 30% (without N_2O) to minimize the risk for airway fire. Some pediatric anesthesiologists use a flexible LMA for airway management during tonsillectomy. Some anesthesiologists administer a neuromuscular blocker. Tracheal intubation, however, can be accomplished using deep sevoflurane anesthesia with propofol supplementation. Maintenance of anesthesia usually consists of an inhaled agent, or continuous infusion of propofol, or both. Propofol maintenance is associated with less postoperative nausea and vomiting. IV acetaminophen is now available to contribute to the analgesic regimen, although some centers may place restrictions on its use because of the cost.

Once the endotracheal tube or LMA is appropriately secured, the table is turned 90 degrees. A booster roll may

TABLE 22.1	Categories of Pediatric Obstructive Sleep Apnea	
Type	Apnea-Hypopnea Index (Events Per Hour)	SpO$_2$ < 90% During Total Sleep Time
Mild	1–5	2%–5%
Moderate	5–10	5%–10%
Severe	>10	>20%

TABLE 22.2 Tonsillectomy Admission Criteria

Age <3–4 years

Moderate to severe OSA

Coexisting disease (e.g.,):

- Sickle-cell anemia or other blood disorder
- Trisomy 21
- Obesity
- Bleeding disorder
- Other significant preexisting comorbidities

be placed underneath the shoulders of the patient, and the head is placed in extension. Care must be taken in patients with trisomy 21 because of the possibility of atlanto-axial subluxation (see Chapter 9). When the surgeon inserts the mouth gag, the child's mouth is maximally opened. During this process the endotracheal tube may be pulled out of the trachea or critically compressed. Therefore, you should ensure that ventilatory parameters remain the same as before the gag was placed. In addition, because of the surgeon's viewpoint from above the head of the child, he or she may not notice that certain portions of the lips and tongue have become pinched by the gag. You should carefully observe this process to ensure that injury does not occur.

Adjuvant medications include an opioid for pain and either a 5-HT$_3$ antagonist or dexamethasone[6] (or both) to help prevent postoperative nausea and vomiting. Young children with recurrent hypoxemia because of OSA have reduced opioid requirements[7]; thus titration is essential to avoid respiratory depression. Dexamethasone decreases the incidence of postoperative nausea and vomiting, is associated with improved postoperative fluid intake, and lessens the severity of postoperative pain.

During tonsillectomy, there are several anesthetic concerns. Blood loss varies and may be significant but is difficult to measure. However, it is rarely severe enough to warrant transfusion. Fluids should consist of an isotonic solution to replace the preoperative deficit, blood loss, and minimal insensible losses. Hypotonic fluids should never be used intraoperatively or postoperatively as profound hyponatremia with seizures and cerebral edema may occur. Some surgeons prefer to infiltrate the tonsillar fossae with a local anesthetic to decrease postoperative pain. Others, however, feel that this practice results in a higher incidence of postoperative bleeding and has been associated with brainstem trauma.[8] For this reason, this is no longer an accepted practice during tonsillectomies. At the end of the procedure, the surgeon may pass a soft catheter to suction gastric contents. However, blood is rarely recovered, and there is no evidence that this practice influences the incidence of postoperative nausea and vomiting.

Once the surgeon has completed the procedure, the table is turned back and an oral airway or soft bite block is inserted into the mouth to prevent the child from biting down and compressing the endotracheal tube during emergence. The nasal passages are gently suctioned for secretions and excess blood. The catheter should go no farther than the anterior nasal cavity to avoid irritating the raw adenoid bed in the nasopharynx. Similarly, oral suctioning should be gentle and limited to the anterior midline of the oral cavity so that the tonsillar fossae are avoided. Bright, red blood that is continually suctioned during emergence should prompt an exploration of the area before the child awakens.

There are two schools of thought with regard to the safest and most appropriate method for emergence and tracheal extubation after tonsillectomy: wide-awake versus deeply anesthetized. The major advantage of a wide-awake extubation is the patient's conscious ability to maintain airway patency immediately after the procedure. The main purported disadvantage is an increased tendency for bleeding secondary to coughing and gagging during emergence, which may lead to bleeding at the surgical site. The main advantage of a deep extubation is the avoidance of bleeding during emergence, and the facilitation of throughput in a busy surgical suite. Disadvantages include possible respiratory depression and failure to maintain airway patency, and laryngospasm during the semiconscious phase of emergence as a result of secretions or blood in the larynx.

After an awake tracheal extubation, the child is carefully observed for several minutes to ensure airway patency and the ability to maintain spontaneous ventilation without hypoxemia. The child should be kept in the operating room until he or she demonstrates the ability to maintain a patent airway without jaw thrust or chin lift. Occasionally, an oral airway may be left in place during transport to the postoperative care unit. The classic "tonsil position" with the child lying on one side and with the head lower than the body will facilitate upper-airway patency and draining of secretions from the mouth (Fig. 22.5).

Patients at high risk for airway complications (i.e., OSA, craniofacial abnormalities) should be extubated wide-awake. Coughing during emergence can be minimized by administering a moderate dose of intraoperative morphine (0.05–0.1 mg/kg) and/or dexmedetomidine (0.5 mcg/kg). Using this awake extubation technique, bleeding during emergence and postoperative laryngospasm are infrequent.

Other centers, however, are equally adamant about the efficacy and safety of the deep extubation technique. This technique requires a relatively greater use of inhaled agent and less opioid, to facilitate adequate airway patency after tracheal extubation. If deep extubation is routinely used, the institution must develop a culture within the postoperative

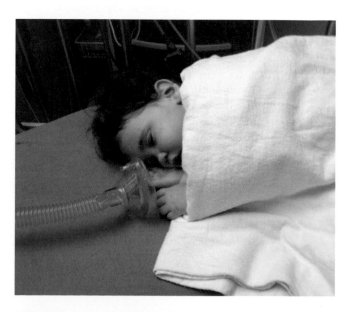

• **Fig 22.5.** Lateral position recovery. Tonsillectomy patients can be recovered in the lateral position, which will optimize upper-airway patency. Courtesy of Ronald S. Litman.

recovery site that facilitates expedient treatment of transient airway obstruction and laryngospasm.

An additional practice model in some institutions consists of the patient being moved to the PACU immediately after completion of the surgical procedure. The child is then allowed to fully emerge from general anesthesia under the watchful care of the PACU staff (which may or may not consist of additional anesthesia personnel). Tracheal extubation is performed when the child is fully awake.

The most important postoperative concern after tonsillectomy is upper-airway obstruction. The precise cause is unknown and may be related to airway edema, residual effects of general anesthesia or opioids, the child's predisposition to upper-airway obstruction, or a combination of these. It occurs more often in children less than 3 years of age, and in children with preexisting sleep apnea. It most often manifests within the first 30 minutes postoperatively. Delayed upper-airway obstruction is uncommon, but when it occurs is usually related to opioid use. Initial treatment consists of optimal placement of the head and neck in a position that is most consistent with airway patency (lateral positioning may be helpful), cool mist in oxygen, and administration of corticosteroids if not already given. If these measures fail to relieve continuing hypoxemia (SpO_2 <90%), placement of a soft lubricated nasopharyngeal airway is indicated (Fig. 22.6). Most children with distress secondary to upper-airway obstruction will allow placement of this device without much of a struggle. If a nasopharyngeal airway is necessary, the child should be admitted to a postoperative hospital unit with close nursing supervision (e.g., intensive care unit). To enhance oxygenation after placement of a nasopharyngeal airway, it can be connected to a ventilation device to administer CPAP (Fig. 22.7). Should the child remain hypoxemic despite placement of a nasopharyngeal airway, tracheal intubation is then indicated, with a trial of extubation at a later time.

Additional postoperative concerns after tonsillectomy are pain relief and postoperative nausea/vomiting (PONV). Opioids should be titrated to achieve sufficient analgesia while avoiding respiratory depression and upper-airway obstruction. Many children will alternate between crying in pain and falling asleep and becoming hypoxemic. This is a continual challenge for the PACU staff. Outpatients with moderate pain may be given oxycodone or equivalent oral analgesic before leaving the facility. There is a growing consensus that administration of ketorolac may be beneficial in this patient population because of its ability to decrease postoperative opioid use, and decrease PONV, sedation, and respiratory depression. But the risk for postoperative bleeding with ketorolac is still not fully understood. Selective COX-2 inhibitors like parecoxib[9] and celecoxib reduce postoperative pain but further studies are warranted. In our practice, celecoxib is now routinely used twice daily on day of surgery and continued for 10 days with significant decreases in postoperative opioid use. Intraoperative IV[10] or rectal administration of acetaminophen[11] may also be helpful. A double-blind, randomized, controlled study[12] found that high-dose dexmedetomidine (2–4 mcg/kg) decreases opioid requirements, and prolongs the opioid-free interval after tonsillectomy, but prolongs length of stay in the PACU compared with fentanyl (1–2 mcg/kg).

Without antiemetic prophylaxis, PONV occurs in up to 75% of children after tonsillectomy. Vomiting can result in exacerbation of bleeding from the tonsillectomy site, dehydration, and inability to take oral analgesics at home. Prophylactic administration of a serotonin antagonist and/ or dexamethasone[13] will decrease the incidence of emesis to less than 20%. One study found that a dose of dexamethasone of 0.0625 mg/kg was equal to higher doses; however, another study[14] demonstrated that higher doses of dexamethasone reduce pain until the second postoperative day. Treatment of ongoing emesis includes maintenance of IV fluids and continuous observation for hypovolemia and anemia. Additional doses of a 5-HT$_3$ antagonist may be administered, but are generally less effective for treating nausea alone. Metoclopramide is usually ineffective in this setting. Most centers will employ one of a number of other antiemetics for refractory vomiting. Children with ongoing nausea or vomiting should have their IV access maintained to provide continuous hydration. If vomiting is continuous and severe, hospital admission is warranted for continuation of IV hydration, analgesics, and antiemetics. The majority of children will no longer manifest nausea and vomiting by

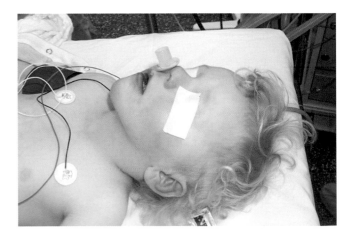

• **Fig 22.7.** Posttonsillectomy airway obstruction can be treated with a soft nasopharyngeal airway attached to an endotracheal tube adapter to attach to a Mapleson circuit to provide CPAP. Courtesy of Ronald S. Litman.

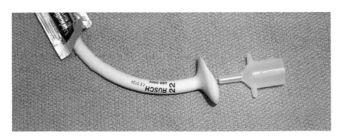

• **Fig 22.6.** An endotracheal tube adapter can be fit into the proximal end of a soft nasopharyngeal airway to facilitate oxygen and CPAP administration. Courtesy of Ronald S. Litman.

the next day. Continued presence of blood in the vomitus should initiate examination for a primary bleed.

Delayed postoperative complaints after tonsillectomy include otalgia, fever, uvular swelling, and temporary velopharyngeal insufficiency that produces a hypernasal voice. In children with significant preoperative obstruction, there is a rare possibility of postobstructive pulmonary edema. If awake hypoxemia is noted in the postoperative period, consider obtaining a chest radiograph to rule out this entity. Postdischarge vomiting can be treated with the oral disintegrating form[15] of ondansetron.

Bleeding Tonsil

Bleeding after tonsillectomy can be severe and life-threatening. *Primary* bleeding occurs in the first 24 hours and is a direct result of residual operative bleeding. *Secondary* bleeding typically occurs 5 to 12 days postoperatively as a result of scab dislodgment. These cases are usually considered surgical emergencies. It is difficult to estimate the actual blood loss because most of it is swallowed, and some children present with bloody emesis. Physical exam should focus on detection of hypovolemia or anemia by checking for signs of dehydration, pallor, tachycardia, and orthostatic changes. Preoperatively, IV access is obtained, and blood samples are sent for a CBC and coagulation studies. An additional blood sample should be retained for possible type-and-crossmatch if the hemoglobin level is low. Aggressive fluid hydration with an isotonic solution is geared toward normalization of vital signs.

The anesthesiologist should review the anesthetic record from the original surgery to determine the presence of problems or issues that would influence the subsequent anesthetic technique (e.g., difficult ventilation or intubation). Small doses of IV midazolam may be titrated shortly before surgery under the direct supervision of an anesthesia provider. The OR should be prepared with a double-suction set-up, several different sized styletted, cuffed, oral RAE endotracheal tubes, and an extra laryngoscope (preferably including a videoscope).

Rapid sequence induction of anesthesia and tracheal intubation is indicated using propofol (ketamine or etomidate if significant hypovolemia is suspected), and succinylcholine or a nondepolarizing neuromuscular blocker. Succinylcholine is usually used because the case almost never lasts more than about 10 minutes, but high-dose rocuronium or vecuronium may be used with sugammadex reversal. If hypovolemia is suspected, a lower dose of propofol should be used to avoid hypotension upon induction of general anesthesia. Alternatively, it can be combined with ketamine, or ketamine can be used alone. Occasionally, the pharynx is filled with blood during direct laryngoscopy, impeding adequate visualization of the laryngeal inlet. These are tense moments; the ENT surgeon should be present in the OR during induction, and the most qualified anesthesiologist available should be managing the airway. Once the airway is secured by tracheal intubation with a cuffed endotracheal tube, the stomach can be suctioned. This should be done by the ENT surgeon under direct vision. Intraoperative anesthetic considerations are the same as for a routine tonsillectomy with the exception of more vigilant attention to blood loss and fluid replacement. Tracheal extubation should occur with the child fully awake because of the possibility of residual blood in the stomach. Postoperative concerns are the same as after routine tonsillectomy and include pain and emesis.

Adenoidectomy

Adenoidectomy is indicated in young children with chronic nasal obstruction, chronic sinusitis, sleep disturbance, or middle ear infections caused by recurrent adenoiditis or eustachian tube obstruction. Chronic upper respiratory illnesses are common, and often do not abate until after the adenoids have been removed. Perioperative anesthetic considerations are essentially the same as for tonsillectomy, except for less postoperative pain, and less chance for postoperative upper-airway obstruction or bleeding. Morphine is often limited to 0.05 mg/kg intraoperatively, and then titrated to achieve analgesia in the PACU. A shorter acting opioid such as fentanyl may also be used.

Peritonsillar Abscess Incision and Drainage

A peritonsillar abscess (PTA) results when bacterial tonsillitis spreads to the tonsillar fossae and soft palate. PTA most commonly presents as unilateral throat soreness, fever, pooling of saliva, dysphagia, and trismus from pterygoid muscle spasm. Patients may be dehydrated from the fever and the inability to drink. Preoperative considerations include administration of IV antibiotics, isotonic fluids, and occasionally, a magnetic resonance imaging (MRI) or computed tomography (CT) scan of the neck to estimate the spread of the infection and severity of airway obstruction. An airway evaluation is often difficult because of the presence of trismus. Preoperative sedatives are avoided if airway obstruction is evident.

Induction of anesthesia will depend on the likelihood of a difficult intubation. If the anesthesiologist suspects a potential difficult ventilation or intubation, spontaneous ventilation should be maintained during induction of anesthesia until it is known that positive-pressure ventilation is successful. If a difficult airway is not suspected, a rapid sequence induction and tracheal intubation are indicated. The trismus will abate upon administration of a general anesthetic and paralytic. The abscess may rupture during direct laryngoscopy, so be prepared with a double-suction set-up, various sized styletted, cuffed, oral RAE endotracheal tubes, and an extra working laryngoscope. Visualization of the glottic opening may be difficult secondary to altered pharyngeal anatomy. The intraoperative anesthetic implications are the same as for a tonsillectomy. Tracheal extubation should take place when the child is fully awake to optimize upper-airway patency. However, postextubation airway obstruction may occur from residual pharyngeal swelling.

Esophageal Foreign Body

In the course of placing objects in their mouths, toddlers will occasionally swallow these objects, which may become trapped in the esophagus. Most commonly, a coin becomes lodged in the proximal esophagus and must then be removed under general anesthesia. Removal using sedation in a non-operating room environment with an unprotected airway is never appropriate. Severe pain and/or airway obstruction are the only reasons this procedure becomes an emergency. Otherwise, the child should be admitted, made NPO, and IV access obtained with administration of maintenance fluids. A radiograph should be obtained just before surgical removal to confirm that the coin has not already passed into the stomach. In the preoperative holding area, IV midazolam may be titrated to effect. Induction and maintenance of anesthesia is routine, with tracheal intubation, and the expectation that this procedure will last no more than 5 to 10 minutes. Therefore, neuromuscular blockade is accomplished with succinylcholine, or intubation is facilitated with a combination of sevoflurane, propofol, and/or remifentanil. If the anesthesiologist suspects a residual full stomach, then rapid sequence induction should be performed. The OR table is turned 90 degrees away from the anesthesiologist and the surgeon uses a rigid esophagoscope to remove the object. The child can be discharged to home after the procedure as long as there was not residual esophageal damage that would require further hospital observation.

Button Battery Ingestion

The number of emergency room visits and fatal outcomes stemming from button battery ingestions has risen in recent years. These ingestions can rapidly result in life-threatening complications. Button batteries vary in voltage and size, but the most common button battery is 3 volts and about the size of a nickel. More than 90% of serious outcomes in children reported between 2000 to 2009 occurred with lithium batteries that were larger than 20 mm, and the younger age group is more likely to suffer devastating consequences[16] because the higher chance of such batteries lodging in the esophagus. The negative electrode produces hydroxide, resulting in an increase in tissue pH and esophageal tissue necrosis within 15 minutes of mucosal contact. Clinically significant tissue damage can occur within 2 hours of battery impaction, which is why such an injury should be managed as a major trauma. Children typically present with nonspecific symptoms such as fever, cough, irritability, and vomiting, and a delay in diagnosis may occur when the ingestion is unwitnessed. Radiographs are used for witnessed or suspected ingestions so that a tailored treatment plan can be made. Esophageal perforation can occur within 24 hours. Other possible complications include long term scarring, tracheoesophageal fistula, esophageal stricture formation, vocal cord paralysis, and parenchymal hemorrhage. The National Battery Ingestion Hotline (1-800-498-8666) at the National Capital Poison Center in Washington, D.C.,

provides information and guidance to both the public and clinicians regarding battery ingestions. Ingestion of honey, sucralfate or local irrigation with acetic acid (in the operating room) have been shown to limit damage after button battery ingestion. These substances may decrease mucosal contact by coating the battery and decreasing the pH of the surrounding tissue. Battery removal in children is considered a life-threatening surgical emergency that requires general anesthesia. A rapid sequence induction may be appropriate. The anesthesia induction agents should be chosen based on the hemodynamic stability of the patient. Each hospital facility should develop a plan for rapid deployment to the operating room in cases of suspected button battery ingestion, including a direct transfer from the helipad to the operating theater.

Dental and Oral Surgical Procedures

The most common dental procedures requiring general anesthesia in children consist of extractions and restorations of teeth. Children are scheduled for this procedure with general anesthesia because of a previous failure using sedative techniques, or if the child has developmental delay or other behavioral or medical problems. Many of these children have preexisting comorbidities that need to be investigated before the day of the procedure. Premedication with an anxiolytic is usually indicated. Uncooperative adolescents with developmental delay may refuse oral premedication and require intramuscular administration of ketamine.

An inhaled induction with sevoflurane is usually performed. Neuromuscular blockade is optional. After the child loses consciousness, a head wrap is snugly applied to the head to use as a secure attachment for the endotracheal tube. A nasotracheal intubation is performed using a nasal RAE tube, aided by a Magill forceps (Fig. 22.8). The table

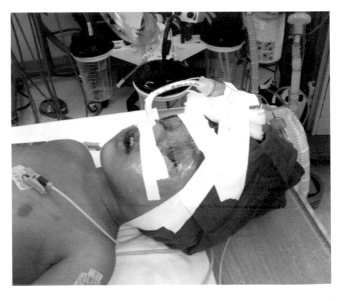

• **Fig 22.8.** A nasal RAE tube is secured to a head wrap to prevent dislodgment during oral surgery. Courtesy of Ronald S. Litman.

may be turned 90 degrees away from the anesthesiologist. Fluid requirements are minimal. Hyperthermia is possible during long procedures; a warming blanket is usually not necessary. Unintentional breathing circuit disconnections or obstructions of the capnograph line are possible hazards. The dentist or oral surgeon will usually infiltrate a moderate amount of local anesthesia. Administration of acetaminophen and/or ketorolac may help alleviate postoperative residual soreness. Titrated doses of an opioid may also be helpful.

Frenulectomy

A frenulectomy (also known as a *frenotomy*) entails incising the frenulum, a midline fibrous band below the tongue. It is indicated for ankyloglossia, a condition of restricted tongue movement because of congenital overgrowth of the frenulum, which can lead to swallowing or speech issues. It may be performed by a dissection technique and sutures, or using laser, or both. Airway management varies depending on the preference of the surgeon and anesthesiologist. Spontaneous ventilation via mask anesthesia or nasopharyngeal airway can be easily accomplished. Others will feel more comfortable with placement of a supraglottic airway (SGA) or endotracheal tube, because of the possibility of bleeding into the back of the pharynx. Postoperative pain is mild to moderate and can be controlled by small doses of opioids and/or ketorolac. The surgeon should use local anesthesia infiltration.

Laryngeal Surgery

Subglottic Stenosis

Subglottic stenosis is an abnormal narrowing of the region below the level of the vocal cords at the level of the cricoid cartilage. It may be present at birth or, more commonly, acquired secondary to chronic inflammation and scarring from the presence of an endotracheal tube. Congenital subglottic stenosis is more common in children with multiple congenital anomalies and children with trisomy 21.

Acquired subglottic stenosis is most often seen in children who require intubations longer than 1 week or children who have had greater than three intubations. The presence of an endotracheal tube causes inflammation and scarring, particularly at the level of the cricoid ring, and a restrictive scar is formed. The clinical manifestations include inspiratory or biphasic stridor during crying or at the time of an upper respiratory tract infection, during which subglottic narrowing increases secondary to edema.

Subglottic stenosis is diagnosed using rigid bronchoscopy under general anesthesia. Positive-pressure ventilation via bag and mask can be difficult when the narrowing is severe. An additional anesthetic implication is the need for an endotracheal tube that is smaller than predicted for age. During the procedure, the risk for laryngospasm is reduced by administration of topical/atomized lidocaine spray

(usually by the surgeon). Severe cases may require treatment with endoscopic dilation procedures, laryngotracheal reconstruction, or placement of a tracheostomy.

Tracheomalacia

Tracheomalacia is a softening of the tracheal cartilage, which then becomes susceptible to collapse when the intraluminal tracheal pressure is less than the extraluminal tracheal pressure. Thus, airway collapse can occur during forceful coughing or exhalation. Congenital tracheomalacia occurs in infants with a tracheoesophageal fistula and some genetic disorders such as trisomy 21 and the mucopolysaccharidoses. Acquired tracheomalacia occurs in children who required long-term mechanical ventilation during early infancy, and in children with tracheal compression lesions such as a vascular ring.

Clinical manifestations of tracheomalacia include noisy breathing (typically described as washing machine sounds), "barky" cough, wheezing, and respiratory distress. These symptoms are often exacerbated during an upper respiratory infection (URI). Many children with tracheomalacia are initially thought to be asthmatic until properly diagnosed. Some may have associated dysphagia from extrinsic vascular compression of the esophagus. Rigid bronchoscopy is required for a definitive diagnosis.

Anesthetic implications for children with tracheomalacia are similar to those for laryngomalacia. Positive-pressure ventilation, especially after administration of a neuromuscular blocker, will open the softened trachea and establish adequate ventilation. Coughing and partial upper-airway obstruction will exacerbate tracheal collapse and rapidly lead to hypoxemia. This is particularly difficult to manage during emergence from general anesthesia and after tracheal extubation. Children with severe tracheomalacia may require a "deep extubation" to avoid these complications.

Microlaryngoscopy and Bronchoscopy

Microlaryngoscopy and flexible or rigid bronchoscopy are used as part of a diagnostic work-up in the evaluation of stridor (e.g., subglottic stenosis, tracheal stenosis), as a therapeutic tool for the treatment of airway lesions (e.g., laryngomalacia, papillomas, cysts), and for the removal of foreign bodies from the upper or lower airways.

A variety of medical conditions may cause airway abnormalities that require diagnostic or therapeutic intervention. As an example, children born prematurely are especially prone to develop subglottic stenosis, and are frequently evaluated for chronic stridor, or inability to be successfully weaned from mechanical ventilation. The one common theme among children presenting for microlaryngoscopy and bronchoscopy is an obstructed upper or lower airway that may worsen with the loss of pharyngeal muscle tone that accompanies induction of general anesthesia. The preoperative history should consist of a thorough review of previous anesthetics and optimization of comorbid conditions.

Physical exam is focused on upper-airway anatomy and the severity of existing airway obstruction. There are no specific requirements for preoperative laboratory testing. Radiographic studies of the head and neck region should be reviewed to assess the potential for airway obstruction during induction of general anesthesia.

Preoperative anxiolysis is tailored to the age and medical condition of the patient. Sedative medications may exacerbate existing airway obstruction and lead to life-threatening hypoxemia. IV atropine or glycopyrrolate may be considered to dry airway secretions, prevent vagal-induced bradycardia, and attenuate cholinergic-mediated bronchoconstriction during airway manipulation. Preoperative communication with the surgeon will facilitate a precise understanding of the procedural components and will enable the anesthesia provider to develop a plan for airway management and the subsequent anesthetic technique.

Flexible Bronchoscopy

Flexible bronchoscopy allows for dynamic assessment of the upper airway during spontaneous respiration and for an evaluation of the peripheral tracheobronchial tree. It is particularly helpful for the evaluation of tracheomalacia, bronchial lesions, and to perform bronchoalveolar lavage.

Flexible bronchoscopy is performed soon after the patient loses consciousness so that spontaneous respiration is maintained. It is commonly performed through a device attached to the anesthesia mask to allow concomitant inhalation of oxygen and inhaled anesthetic during the procedure. Flexible bronchoscopy is initially performed with the head of the OR table facing the anesthesiologist, so that mask ventilation can be optimally continued throughout the procedure.

Rigid Bronchoscopy

A rigid bronchoscope is a stainless-steel hollow tube that is used for diagnostic and therapeutic procedures within the airway below the glottis. The distal end is blunt with several ventilation ports/holes along its side, and the proximal end contains a ventilation side-port that attaches to the standard anesthesia breathing circuit by a 15 mm adaptor (Fig. 22.9). A thinner telescope (Hopkins rod) with an optical eyepiece is placed coaxially within the rigid bronchoscope and allows for magnified and illuminated visualization of the airway (primarily below the glottis) while retaining the ability to provide adequate ventilation. When the telescope is removed, instruments can be passed through the bronchoscope to retrieve foreign bodies, resect masses, and so forth, while maintaining oxygenation and some ventilation (Fig. 22.10). The rigid bronchoscope is particularly suited for difficult airway management because of its ability to bypass laryngeal and tracheal lesions that compress the airway and contribute to difficult ventilation or intubation. It may be lifesaving in the case of a mediastinal mass that is compressing the bronchial tree below the carina.

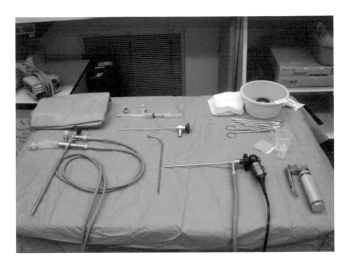

• **Fig 22.9.** Bronchoscopy table set-up contains a variety of instruments to examine the lower airways. Courtesy of Karen Zur.

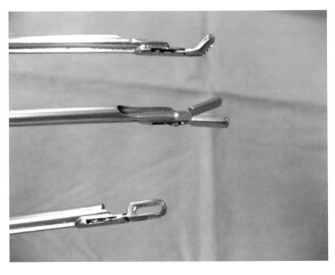

• **Fig 22.10.** The ENT surgeon can choose from a variety of graspers to remove a bronchial foreign body. Courtesy of Karen Zur.

There are a variety of sizes and lengths of rigid pediatric bronchoscopes that are chosen on the basis of the age and size of the child. The bronchoscope size is chosen to give the surgeon the best possible view while causing the least amount of trauma to the glottis and subglottic tissues. The time taken to perform bronchoscopy should be as short as possible to decrease the risk for obstructive edema secondary to vocal cord and subglottic trauma. In some cases, the surgeon may choose to examine the glottis and the subglottis with the telescope alone to minimize trauma to this region. In this case simultaneous ventilation is not possible; preoxygenation will increase the duration of apnea before hypoxemia intervenes. Such airway inspections may also be performed using suspension laryngoscopy with insufflation of oxygen and sevoflurane while maintaining spontaneous ventilation.

Various successful methods have been reported for anesthetizing children for bronchoscopy. Anesthetic induction can be accomplished using inhaled sevoflurane or IV propofol. After loss of consciousness, and before airway manipulation, IV and topical lidocaine can be administered to prevent the occurrence of protective airway reflexes such as gag and laryngospasm. Topical lidocaine within the lower airway may precipitate reflex bronchoconstriction unless preceded by IV lidocaine. Small doses of an opioid can be carefully titrated to maintain spontaneous ventilation, which is maintained during flexible bronchoscopy to evaluate the dynamic function of the airway. Spontaneous ventilation should always be maintained with a potentially difficult ventilation or intubation. Neuromuscular blockers are administered only after positive-pressure ventilation has proved successful.

The anesthetic plan for rigid bronchoscopy will be largely determined by the *a priori* choice of spontaneous or positive-pressure ventilation during the bronchoscopy. This choice is influenced by the personal preferences of the anesthesiologist and surgeon, who must agree on an acceptable technique before administration of anesthesia. There are times, however, when this decision will be made during the case, depending on the surgeon's findings and the patient's clinical condition. With either ventilatory method, these procedures entail a large percentage of time that the child's airway is open (i.e., exposed to the atmosphere when the surgeon removes the optical eyepiece or removes the bronchoscope). There are various ways to administer general anesthesia. For some, a total intravenous anesthesia (TIVA) technique is preferred to decrease OR pollution from inhaled agents and provides an uninterrupted source of general anesthesia to the patient. Others will use suspension laryngoscopy and insufflation of sevoflurane in oxygen through a port in the distal end of the laryngoscope.

There are advantages and disadvantages of both spontaneous and controlled ventilation methods during rigid bronchoscopy. If spontaneous ventilation is maintained, continuous ventilation is occurring, despite interruptions in the anesthesia breathing circuit. For some obstructive lesions, negative-pressure breathing may provide better oxygenation and ventilation. Disadvantages of spontaneous ventilation include the requirement to maintain a sufficient depth of anesthesia to obliterate airway reflexes and prevent patient movement during instrumentation, yet maintain sufficient ventilatory function and hemodynamic stability. Thus, topical anesthesia to the airway is an important component of this technique.

A controlled ventilation technique, which may or may not consist of the administration of a neuromuscular blocker, relies on intermittent positive-pressure breaths between apneic periods when the surgeon instruments the airway. Its advantages include the ability to provide optimal oxygenation and ventilation during the breathing phase, and assurance of lack of patient movement to airway manipulation. An obvious disadvantage is that during periods of apnea, even with preoxygenation, there is a limited time before oxyhemoglobin desaturation will occur, and the child will require additional positive-pressure breaths. Another significant disadvantage is the lack of assurance that positive-pressure ventilation will be successful with an obstructive lesion within the airway, as is sometimes seen with laryngeal papillomatosis (Fig. 22.11). In the case of a foreign body lodged within the bronchial tree (Fig. 22.12), a theoretical disadvantage of positive-pressure is the unintentional movement of the object further distally. This can worsen airway exchange or create a ball-valve effect with hemodynamic consequences secondary to lung compression of vascular structures. This complication is rare. Alternatively, for some procedures and only in select patients, specialized techniques of ventilation such as supraglottic jet ventilation may be used.

Once the child is adequately anesthetized, and just before performing rigid bronchoscopy, the OR table is turned 90 degrees away from the anesthesiologist, while

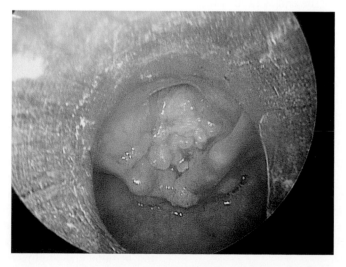

• **Fig 22.11.** Laryngeal papillomatosis obstructing the laryngeal inlet. (From Subramaniam R. Acute upper airway obstruction in children and adults. *Trends Anaesth. Crit. Care.* 2011;1(2):67-73. doi: https://doi.org/10.1016/j.tacc.2011.01.010.)

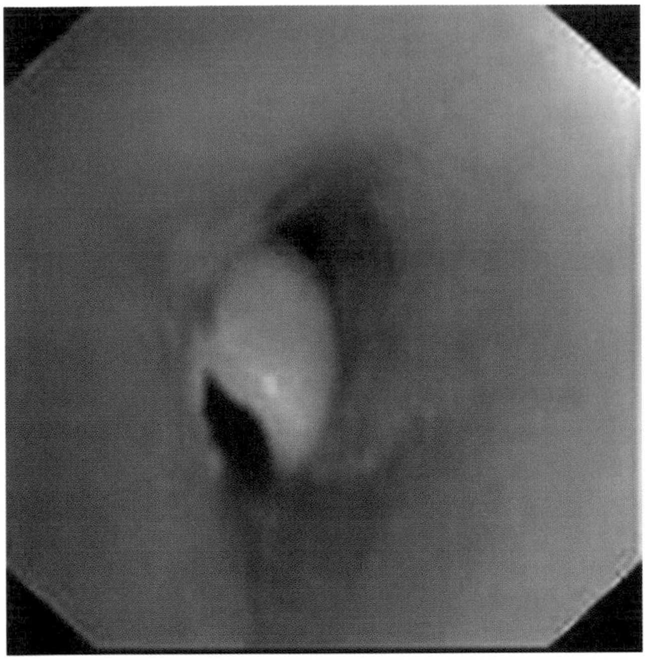

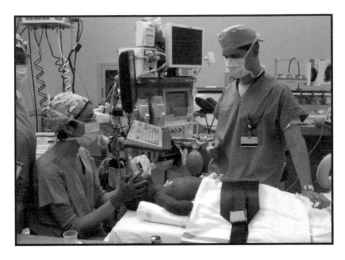

• **Fig 22.13.** For rigid bronchoscopy, the OR table is turned 90 degrees and the airway is shared and managed by the ENT surgeon. Courtesy of Karen Zur.

• **Fig 22.12.** A foreign body with surrounding mucosal inflammation in the left main bronchus. (From: Cakir E, Ersu RH, Uyan ZS, et al. Flexible bronchoscopy as a valuable tool in the evaluation of persistent wheezing in children. *Int. J. Pediatr. Otorhinolaryngol.* 2009;73(12): 1666-1668. doi: https://doi.org/10.1016/j.ijporl.2009.08.016.)

mask ventilation is continued from a side position or by an assistant at the head of the table until the surgeon is optimally prepared to instrument the airway (Fig. 22.13). The goal of the entire process should be a smooth, coordinated, sharing of the child's airway with a combination of optimal oxygenation, ventilation, and surgical exposure.

Suspension Microlaryngoscopy

Suspension microlaryngoscopy is used mainly for procedures of the upper airway and vocal folds, and may or may not include use of the CO_2 laser. The child's head is fixed in a constant position that provides an optimal view of the larynx. An endotracheal tube can be held in place by the suspension laryngoscope, or the surgery can be performed with an apneic technique to provide access to the larynx and airway. If a laser procedure is involved, several types of commercial laser-safe endotracheal tubes are available. Removing the endotracheal tube during the laser treatments will optimize visualization for the surgeon and remove a possible source of an airway fire. Oxygenation and ventilation during microlaryngoscopy procedures are then provided by one of two methods: (1) intermittent endotracheal tube placement between apneic treatments; or (2) spontaneous ventilation by insufflating continuous 100% oxygen through the side-port of the suspension laryngoscopy, via a cut endotracheal tube (ETT) that is inserted in the lateral oral cavity or via a nasal cannula.

If suspension microlaryngoscopy is used in combination with the CO_2 laser, all usual laser precautions should

be strictly followed. The child's eyes should be covered with wet saline gauze, and all skin surfaces are completely covered with sheets or drapes. If a cuffed endotracheal tube is used, the cuff should be filled with water or saline. Some anesthesiologists inject methylene blue into the saline that goes into the cuff to better detect any breakage by the laser. Oxygen concentrations should be as low as possible and N_2O should be avoided to minimize combustibility. A prearranged algorithm should be in place to treat an airway fire. We recommend the four Es of airway fire treatment:

1. Extract (remove the endotracheal tube)
2. Eliminate (turn off the oxygen source)
3. Extinguish (saline flush the airway)
4. Evaluate (rigid bronchoscopy to evaluate the airway)

Bronchial Foreign Body

A variety of different types of edible and inedible foreign bodies commonly become lodged in the distal bronchial tree in children. Toddlers are most affected because of their underdeveloped ability to coordinate breathing and swallowing of small food items such as peanuts. Bronchial foreign bodies are likely to cause distal airway obstruction with development of emphysema, atelectasis, and pneumonia (Fig. 22.12). Children may present with a respiratory illness that runs the gamut from tachypnea and fever to respiratory failure and hypoxemia. A bronchial foreign body is suspected when a toddler presents with the sudden onset of respiratory distress that usually begins with a choking episode. The aspiration event may or may not be observed, and often the type of foreign body is unknown. Confirmation of the diagnosis consists of radiologic demonstration of the foreign body if it is radiopaque and a high level of suspicion. If it is not apparent on radiograph, there may be unilateral emphysema from a ball-valve effect of the distal obstruction. An aspirated peanut will exacerbate the condition by causing a lipoid pneumonitis. Radiographic findings will vary depending on the location and type of aspirated foreign body, and performing decubitus films may help decipher the presence of trapped air suggestive of an inhaled foreign body. Regardless of radiographic findings, if an aspiration event is suspected, bronchoscopy is indicated.

This procedure is usually considered a surgical emergency. Preoperative assessment should be focused on determining respiratory function, administration of antibiotics, and bronchodilator therapy if bronchospasm is present. An IV catheter should be inserted. Midazolam can be titrated to achieve anxiolysis in the preoperative holding area under direct supervision of the anesthesiologist. Induction and maintenance of general anesthesia is the same as described above for rigid bronchoscopy, with a choice between spontaneous or controlled ventilation. Even with publication[17] of large series of patients, insufficient evidence exists to determine the optimal ventilation strategy in these cases.

Neck Surgery

Thyroglossal Duct Cyst

A thyroglossal duct cyst is a congenital mass in the midline of the neck. It is believed to be a remnant of the connection between the foramen cecum of the tongue and the thyroid gland in fetal life (Fig. 22.14). During childhood it can become infected and enlarged, and usually requires excision. These children are usually otherwise healthy. The standard surgical treatment involves removing the cyst along with the midportion of the hyoid bone, termed a *Sistrunk procedure*. Preoperative assessment, induction, and maintenance of general anesthesia are no different from usual care. The anesthesiologist may wish to place a towel wrap around the head with which to secure the endotracheal tube over the forehead. The child is positioned with the neck extended for a transverse midline incision. The anesthesiologist may

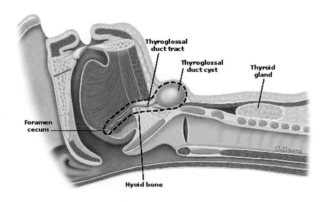

• **Fig 22.14.** Excision of thyroglossal duct cyst and tract. (Reproduced with permission from: Randolph GW, Kamani DV. Thyroglossal duct cysts and ectopic thyroid. In: Basow DS, ed. *UpToDate*, Waltham, MA, 2013. Copyright © 2013 UpToDate, Inc. For more information visit *www.uptodate.com*.)

be asked to depress the base of the tongue to move the cyst to facilitate surgical identification. Surgical risks include unintentional trauma to vascular or airway structures in the neck. Postoperative concerns include hematoma formation with subsequent airway compression.

Branchial Cleft Cyst

Branchial cleft cysts are found on the side of the neck and develop from a failure of involution of one of the branchial clefts during embryonic development. These children are otherwise healthy; perioperative and postoperative anesthetic implications are the same as for the thyroglossal duct cyst.

Neck Mass Biopsy and Excision

When unclassified neck masses in children do not respond to conventional antibiotic therapy, an excisional biopsy is indicated to rule out malignancy or unusual infection. However, when a lymphoma is suspected, there may be an occult anterior mediastinal mass that carries the potential for life-threatening airway obstruction after induction of general anesthesia. Symptoms of an anterior mediastinal mass include coughing or dyspnea in the supine position that is relieved when the child assumes a sitting or prone position. If these symptoms are present, a diagnostic chest radiograph is indicated (see also Chapter 8).

Cystic Hygroma

A cystic hygroma (i.e., lymphangioma) is a malformation of lymphatic vessels in and around the neck. It is associated with Turner syndrome, trisomy 21, trisomy 18 (Edwards syndrome), and Noonan syndrome, although many otherwise healthy children are also affected. Cystic hygromas are often found at birth or in infancy and tend to enlarge during early childhood. The main indication for surgically addressing these congenital lesions is because of functional impact from the mass effect or its location. The occasional child will present for reduction and/or tracheostomy because of respiratory distress from airway compression (Fig. 22.15). Cystic hygromas tend to grow inward and compress the airway. The preoperative assessment should include MRI to delineate spread and evaluate airway patency. A hemoglobin level and type-and-screen should be obtained if an extensive dissection and excision is planned, or if the mass is located near vascular structures of the neck. Induction and maintenance of anesthesia is practitioner dependent and will vary with the severity of the mass and the degree of airway obstruction. Principles of difficult airway management will apply if upper-airway obstruction is suspected. Intraoperative concerns include blood loss, fluid management, hypothermia if the dissection is extensive, and the possibility of nerve monitoring. A temporary urinary catheter should be placed if the procedure is expected to last more than about 4 hours.

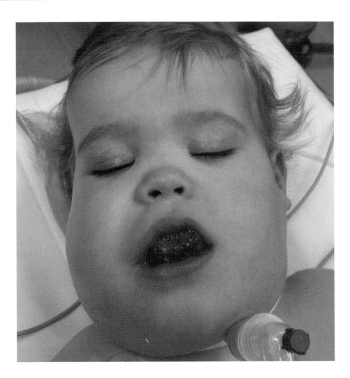

• **Fig 22.15.** Large cystic hygroma requiring tracheostomy in infancy. Courtesy of Ronald S. Litman

Tracheostomy

The term given to creating a hole in the trachea is a matter of debate, with the names *tracheotomy* and *tracheostomy* used interchangeably. In general, tracheotomy is the temporary surgical cutting of the trachea through the anterior neck tissues, whereas tracheostomy entails a more permanent opening into the trachea and placement of the tracheostomy tube.

Over the last decade, there has been a decrease in the number of pediatric tracheostomies[18] being performed, largely because of improvements in airway management by pediatric anesthesiologists and intensive care physicians. However, with an increase in the length of survival of children with complex medical problems and extreme prematurity, a new population of patients requiring tracheostomy is emerging. Several studies have shown that once a tracheostomy is placed, the duration that it is left in place has increased over time because of the increased number of chronically ventilated children. A recent trend shows that the procedure is being performed in younger children, with a peak incidence in patients less than 12 months of age.

The three most common *indications*[19] for a tracheostomy in children are (1) prolonged mechanical ventilation, (2) upper-airway obstruction, and (3) pulmonary toilet. Within each category there are congenital, traumatic, metabolic, infectious, and neoplastic conditions that require tracheostomy. Although the underlying medical conditions may be numerous, the most common diagnoses in pediatric tracheostomy patients are bronchopulmonary dysplasia and neurologic disorders.

The majority of tracheostomies are elective or semielective. The decision to perform an elective tracheostomy is complex and depends on several factors, including the child's underlying medical condition, the severity of airway obstruction, and the difficulty and duration of intubation. In general, a child who is chronically ventilated is initially managed with an endotracheal tube, with the timing of conversion to a tracheostomy dependent on the patient's age and the family and medical team decisions that are specific to each child. Neonates may tolerate endotracheal tube intubation for several months with potentially less laryngeal injury owing to a more pliable airway. On the other hand, in older children and adolescents the laryngeal cartilage is firmer, requiring a tracheostomy to be performed after 2 to 3 weeks of tracheal intubation.

The ideal tracheostomy tube should be made of a material that causes minimal tissue reactivity, can be easily cleaned and maintained, and is available in a variety of sizes and lengths. The tube needs to be rigid enough to prevent kinking or collapse, yet soft enough to be comfortable for the patient. Modern tracheostomy tubes have a 15 mm male connector for the attachment of standard respiratory equipment. The ideal tube also contains an inner cannula that may be removed and cleaned although most pediatric tubes do not have inner cannulas.

Tracheostomy tubes for small children may contain a cuff, if ventilation is required and a leak is present. Cuffed tubes are also used for positive-pressure ventilation and to protect the lower airways from aspiration of secretions. Cuffs can be filled with air or sterile water depending on the tube design. It is preferable to avoid placing a cuffed tracheostomy tube to minimize the chances of tracheal injury. In larger children and adolescents, cuffed adult tracheostomy tubes may be used. In selecting the appropriate tracheostomy tube, both the diameter and length should be considered. The external diameter determines the size of the tube that may be inserted, whereas the inner diameter determines the actual airway size. The diameter of the tube should be large enough to allow adequate air exchange, easy suctioning, and clearance of secretions. If the indication for tracheostomy is assisted ventilation, the size of the tube should be adjusted to prevent excessive air leak. Predictors of the appropriate tube size include the child's age and the size of a preexisting endotracheal tube. Too large a tube will compromise the capillary flow in the tracheal wall, which may result in mucosal ulceration and development of fibrous stenosis. Overinflation of a cuffed tracheostomy tube for a prolonged period may produce similar injuries and may also lead to a dilation of the trachea. These complications may be avoided by selecting the proper sized tracheostomy tube and adjusting the cuff pressure to less than 20 cmH$_2$O. The choice of the tube size is also influenced by visualizing the size of the tracheal lumen.

The length of the tracheostomy tube is important, especially in neonates and infants. A tube that is too short may result in accidental decannulation or the development of a false passage. If a tube is too long, the tip may abrade the carina or rest in the right main bronchus leading to coughing, ventilatory issues and discomfort, and granulation at the carina. With knowledge of the desired and appropriate length of the tracheostomy tube, customized tubes can be ordered with relative ease. Extralong custom-made tubes may be helpful in unusual situations, such as tracheomalacia, post tracheoesophageal fistula (TEF) repair or tracheal stenosis, to span the involved area.

Unless airway obstruction is immediately life-threatening, pediatric tracheostomy procedures should be performed in the operating suite. This creates a well-controlled environment for the child and the personnel performing the procedure. The operating suite provides optimal illumination, proper positioning of the child, and expert nursing care. In addition, a full range of laryngoscopes and bronchoscopes are available to control the airway if necessary.

In children with an indwelling endotracheal tube, the choice of induction and maintenance of general anesthesia is unimportant. However, if the tracheostomy is being performed for acute airway obstruction, principles of difficult airway management will apply (see Chapter 18). Before performing the procedure, the surgeon and anesthesiologist should discuss the method of choice for obtaining and securing the airway. All alternatives should be discussed in the event that the child cannot be intubated successfully. It is preferred to perform the tracheostomy with the child intubated under general anesthesia with paralysis. In certain situations of severe upper-airway obstruction, it may be necessary to perform the tracheostomy with mild sedation and infiltration of local anesthesia, although this situation should be avoided if possible. An SGA is also possible in selected patients.

The tracheostomy is performed supine with the child's neck extended using a shoulder roll. The child should be breathing 100% oxygen in anticipation of a temporary interruption of ventilation, but if electric cautery is being used near the airway, the oxygen level should be as low as possible to minimize the chance of an airway fire. Lidocaine with epinephrine is infiltrated into the subcutaneous tissue one to two fingerbreadths above the sternal notch. A horizontal skin incision is then made at the same site. A vertical midline dissection is performed to expose the tracheal rings. Traction sutures are placed in a paramedian position at the level of the third tracheal ring, to rapidly open the airway should accidental decannulation occur before the tract is established. The trachea is incised vertically in the midline to expose the underlying endotracheal tube. While directly observing the endotracheal tube, the anesthesiologist gradually pulls it back to just above the incision as the surgeon inserts the tracheostomy tube (there is a large air leak during this portion of the procedure). The anesthesia breathing circuit is then connected to the tracheostomy tube; correct placement is confirmed by listening for bilateral breath sounds and observing a normal capnographic tracing. Before these final confirmations, the endotracheal tube should never be completely withdrawn out of the trachea. Flexible tracheobronchoscopy is then performed to identify the distal position of the tracheostomy tube. Proper adjustment or possible replacement of the tracheostomy tube with a different size is done at this stage. The previously placed endotracheal tube is removed just before leaving the operating room or after arrival in the ICU. A postoperative chest radiograph is obtained to further confirm tube position and rule out pneumothorax.

Postoperatively, humidified air by collar or ventilator is provided to prevent excessive dryness and thickening of tracheal secretions. The surgeon performs the first tracheostomy tube change on the fifth to seventh postoperative day after a well-formed tract has been established. The traction sutures are also removed at this time.

Anesthesiologists should be aware of the various complications related to pediatric tracheostomy. Bleeding can occur from superficial tissues, thyroid vessels, or vascular anomalies such as a high-riding innominate artery, and can obstruct the surgeon's view of the opened trachea. Air entry into the subcutaneous tissues may cause a pneumomediastinum, pneumothorax, subcutaneous emphysema, or any combination of those. Anatomic injury to the neurovascular structures in the neck, including the recurrent laryngeal nerve, can also occur. During placement, the tracheostomy tube can be unintentionally placed into a false lumen adjacent to the trachea, or into the esophagus. For these reasons, the endotracheal tube should never be fully removed before final confirmation that the tracheostomy tube is functional.

References

1. Galinkin JL, Fazi LM, Cuy RM, et al. Use of intranasal fentanyl in children undergoing myringotomy and tube placement during halothane and sevoflurane anesthesia. *Anesthesiology*. 2000;93(6):1378–1383. https://doi.org/10.1097/00000542-200012000-00006.

2. Pappas AL, Fluder EM, Creech S, Hotaling A, Park A. Postoperative analgesia in children undergoing myringotomy and placement equalization tubes in ambulatory surgery. *Anesth Analg*. 2003;96(6):1621–1624. https://doi.org/10.1213/01.ane.0000064206.51296.1d.

3. Stricker PA, Muhly WT, Jantzen EC, et al. Intramuscular Fentanyl and Ketorolac Associated with Superior Pain Control After Pediatric Bilateral Myringotomy and Tube Placement Surgery: A Retrospective Cohort Study. *Anesth Analg*. 2017;124(1):245–253. https://doi.org/10.1213/ANE.0000000000001722.

4. Roland PS, Rosenfeld RM, Brooks LJ, et al. Clinical practice guideline: Polysomnography for sleep-disordered breathing prior to tonsillectomy in children. *Otolaryngol Head Neck Surg*. 2011;145(1 Suppl):S1–S15. https://doi.org/10.1177/0194599811409837.

5. Katz ES, Mitchell RB, D'Ambrosio CM. Obstructive sleep apnea in infants. *Am J Respir Crit Care Med*. 2012;185(8):805–816. https://doi.org/10.1164/rccm.201108-1455CI.

6. Steward DL, Grisel J, Meinzen-Derr J. Steroids for improving recovery following tonsillectomy in children. *Cochrane Database Syst Rev*. 2011;2011(8):CD003997 https://doi.org/10.1002/14651858.CD003997.pub2. Published 2011 Aug 10.

7. Brown KA, Laferrière A, Moss IR. Recurrent hypoxemia in young children with obstructive sleep apnea is associated with reduced opioid requirement for analgesia. *Anesthesiology*. 2004;100(4):806–810. https://doi.org/10.1097/00000542-200404000-00009.

8. Murphy C. Two local girls in critical care following tonsillectomies. *Weny News*. March 7th 2019 Accessed October 22, 2020. https://www.weny.com/story/40089529/two-local-girls-in-critical-care-following-tonsillectomies.

9. Li X, Zhou M, Xia Q, Li J. Parecoxib sodium reduces the need for opioids after tonsillectomy in children: a double-blind placebo-controlled randomized clinical trial. *Can J Anaesth*. 2016;63(3):268–274. https://doi.org/10.1007/s12630-015-0560-3.

10. Alhashemi JA, Daghistani MF. Effects of intraoperative i.v. acetaminophen vs i.m. meperidine on post-tonsillectomy pain in children. *Br J Anaesth*. 2006;96(6):790–795. https://doi.org/10.1093/bja/ael084.

11. Capici F, Ingelmo PM, Davidson A, et al. Randomized controlled trial of duration of analgesia following intravenous or rectal acetaminophen after adenotonsillectomy in children. *Br J Anaesth*. 2008;100(2):251–255. https://doi.org/10.1093/bja/aem377.

12. Pestieau SR, Quezado ZM, Johnson YJ, et al. High-dose dexmedetomidine increases the opioid-free interval and decreases opioid requirement after tonsillectomy in children. *Can J Anaesth*. 2011;58(6):540–550. https://doi.org/10.1007/s12630-011-9493-7.

13. Bolton CM, Myles PS, Nolan T, Sterne JA. Prophylaxis of postoperative vomiting in children undergoing tonsillectomy: a systematic review and meta-analysis. *Br J Anaesth*. 2006;97(5):593–604. https://doi.org/10.1093/bja/ael256.

14. Hermans V, De Pooter F, De Groote F, De Hert S, Van der Linden P. Effect of dexamethasone on nausea, vomiting, and pain in paediatric tonsillectomy. *Br J Anaesth*. 2012;109(3):427–431. https://doi.org/10.1093/bja/aes249.

15. Davis PJ, Fertal KM, Boretsky KR, et al. The effects of oral ondansetron disintegrating tablets for prevention of at-home emesis in pediatric patients after ear-nose-throat surgery. *Anesth Analg*. 2008;106(4):1117–1121. https://doi.org/10.1213/ane.0b013e318167cc3a.

16. Litovitz T, Whitaker N, Clark L, White NC, Marsolek M. Emerging battery-ingestion hazard: clinical implications. *Pediatrics*. 2010;125(6):1168–1177. https://doi.org/10.1542/peds.2009-3037.

17. Fidkowski CW, Zheng H, Firth PG. The anesthetic considerations of tracheobronchial foreign bodies in children: a literature review of 12,979 cases. *Anesth Analg*. 2010;111(4):1016–1025. https://doi.org/10.1213/ANE.0b013e3181ef3e9c.

18. Coté CJ, Hartnick CJ. Pediatric transtracheal and cricothyrotomy airway devices for emergency use: which are appropriate for infants and children. *Paediatr Anaesth*. 2009;19(Suppl 1):66–76. https://doi.org/10.1111/j.1460-9592.2009.02996.x.

19. Wetmore RF, Marsh RR, Thompson ME, Tom LW. Pediatric tracheostomy: a changing procedure? *Ann Otol Rhinol Laryngol*. 1999;108(7 Pt 1):695–699. https://doi.org/10.1177/000348949910800714.

Suggested Readings

Okonkwo I, Cochrane L, Fernandez E. Perioperative management of a child with a tracheostomy. *BJA Educ*. 2020;20(1):18–25. https://doi.org/10.1016/j.bjae.2019.09.007.

23

General Surgery

VANESSA A. OLBRECHT, JI YEON JEMMA KANG, AND RONALD S. LITMAN

In this chapter, we review principles of anesthetic management of some common and unique surgical procedures that are within the purview of the general pediatric surgeon. The first section contains a discussion of concerns for intraabdominal procedures, especially in neonates and small infants. The second section reviews the unique aspects of some common surgical conditions of the abdomen that are of interest to pediatric anesthesiologists and describes the key anesthetic implications for each of these conditions. Anesthetic considerations for indwelling vascular access placement (e.g., port placement or Broviac catheters) are also covered.

General Considerations

Intraabdominal procedures in children run the gamut from simple hernia repairs in healthy children to complex bowel resections (e.g., necrotizing enterocolitis) in extremely ill, premature infants. Preoperative assessment allows the anesthesiologist the opportunity to explore underlying comorbidities and the need for preoperative preparation, including volume resuscitation. Many abdominal diseases will present with vomiting and diarrhea and will be accompanied by sequestration of fluid within the abdominal cavity and electrolyte abnormalities. Therefore, estimation of volume status is crucial and preoperative volume resuscitation is often required.

The preoperative physical exam is focused on determination of cardiorespiratory vital signs and evaluation of the child's upper airway. Indicators of hypovolemia include lethargy, weight loss, tachycardia, dry mucous membranes, cold mottled skin, poor peripheral capillary refill, and a sunken fontanel in the young infant. More advanced findings include metabolic acidosis, oliguria, and hypotension.

Abdominal distention may result from bowel edema, accumulation of fluid or air in the bowel, and pneumoperitoneum if intestinal perforation has occurred. It can cause elevation of the diaphragm which leads to a decrease in the patient's functional residual capacity (FRC); in a small infant, this decrease in FRC can lead to atelectasis, alveolar collapse, and ultimately hypoxemia and respiratory failure. Small infants with acute abdominal processes require a full set of preoperative laboratory studies, including a complete blood count with platelets, a comprehensive metabolic panel, and coagulation studies. Although a type and screen may be appropriate in most cases, a type-and-crossmatch should be obtained if there is a possibility of blood loss requiring red cell transfusion. When bowel ischemia is likely, such as with necrotizing enterocolitis, arterial or venous blood gas analysis is indicated to determine the severity of the underlying metabolic acidosis. Premedication should be administered to treat existing pain or anxiety. There is no proven benefit to the administration of medications that aim to prevent pulmonary aspiration of gastric contents and reduce gastric acidity. In fact, metoclopramide, a prokinetic agent, should not be administered if there is the possibility of an intestinal obstruction. Children with suspected bowel obstruction should receive gastric decompression with an indwelling nasogastric tube (orogastric in small infants) before induction of general anesthesia.

Intraoperatively, the major anesthetic considerations include management of hypovolemia, acidosis, and hypothermia. Standard monitors are usually sufficient, but the disease process and any underlying patient morbidity should determine the need for more invasive monitoring such as direct arterial measurement or central venous access. Measures to ensure normothermia include core temperature monitoring (esophageal or rectal), warming of the operation room (OR), humidification of the breathing circuit, use of an intravenous fluid warming device, and use of a forced air or water heating blanket underneath and around the child. Overhead radiant heaters can be used for neonates and small infants during induction of anesthesia and placement of monitors. During a laparotomy in a small infant, beware of advancing the esophageal catheter into the stomach where it will reflect the warmer temperature from the OR lights. An indwelling urinary catheter is indicated if the procedure will last more than about 4 hours or if large intraoperative fluid fluctuations are anticipated.

When a large surface area of bowel is exposed, insensible losses are deceptively high (at least 10 mL/kg/h) and will warrant liberal fluid administration. Hypovolemia can result from unanticipated bleeding, or third space loss from bowel exposure or edema. Neonates with large abdominal defects such as gastroschisis or omphalocele often require more than 50 mL/kg of isotonic fluid over the duration of the procedure. To allow for adequate volume resuscitation, many pediatric anesthesiologists will insert two peripheral intravenous catheters. Isotonic crystalloid solutions are appropriate for most volume resuscitations. The occasional child may require inotropic therapy with dopamine or epinephrine if hypotension persists despite seemingly adequate volume resuscitation, especially when there is an intraabdominal process associated with sepsis.

Infants and children presenting for urgent abdominal surgery are considered to have a full stomach and thus are at increased risk for pulmonary aspiration of gastric contents during induction of general anesthesia. Decreased gastric emptying in these patients may be caused by the pathologic abdominal process or from anticholinergic medications, such as opioids. Children undergoing elective abdominal procedures that are minor and not associated with pathologic processes that interfere with normal gastric emptying can be managed with normal fasting guidelines.

The indwelling nasogastric tube should be suctioned immediately before induction of general anesthesia. It can be removed to facilitate airway management and replaced after insertion of the endotracheal tube.

In most children, rapid sequence induction and intubation (RSI) is similar to that for adults: preoxygenation and administration of a rapid-acting hypnotic agent along with a rapid-acting neuromuscular blocker. The benefit of cricoid pressure to prevent regurgitation and aspiration of gastric contents remains controversial and is still debated.

It is important to remember to maximally maintain upper airway patency while waiting for relaxation to occur; despite the avoidance of manual ventilation, oxygenation can still occur via bulk flow of oxygen from the anesthesia circuit as long as the upper airway is kept open by neck extension and chin lift.

Classic application of RSI is sometimes not possible in certain children. Preoxygenation may not be feasible in the struggling child who refuses mask placement, and apneic oxygenation may be unsuccessful (i.e., result in oxyhemoglobin desaturation) in infants because of their vanishingly small FRC and high oxygen consumption. Furthermore, because the use of succinylcholine may be hazardous in children with undiagnosed myopathies, it is often replaced with rocuronium, which has a longer onset of action, except in very high doses. For all these aforementioned reasons, many pediatric anesthesiologists prefer a modified RSI that consists of "gentle"[1] positive pressure ventilation breaths (i.e., relatively low inspired pressures to cause modest chest rise) before endotracheal intubation. Awake intubations are rarely, if ever, performed on neonates, except during episodes of severe cardiorespiratory instability or suspected difficult airway.

The anesthesia maintenance technique during an abdominal procedure depends on the severity of the child's illness. For procedures that are not expected to require postoperative mechanical ventilation, a balanced technique of an inhaled agent and an opioid is appropriate. When postoperative mechanical ventilation is expected, an opioid-based

technique (while still including sufficient inhaled agent to ensure unconsciousness) is preferred because it can be continued into the postoperative period to decrease the child's overall stress response and provide ongoing analgesia and sedation. In the absence of hypovolemia, small infants and neonates tend to remain hemodynamically stable after relatively large amounts of opioids. Nitrous oxide should probably be avoided even in superficial abdominal wall procedures (e.g., simple hernia repair) because its use is associated with bowel distention.

Regional analgesia via the lumbar or caudal epidural route may be useful for intraoperative and postoperative pain relief when the child is hemodynamically stable and does not demonstrate evidence of bacteremia or sepsis.

Neonates that undergo major abdominal surgery often benefit from postoperative mechanical ventilation. This practice allows liberal titration of opioids and a decreased stress response without the risk for apnea during this phase of large fluid requirements and intravascular fluid shifts secondary to intestinal "third spacing." Muscle relaxation will also assist with ventilation during this "third spacing" stage. The postoperative plan should be proactively discussed with the neonatologists, surgeon, and pediatricians who will be managing the patient in the postoperative period.

A variety of pediatric abdominal procedures are now being performed laparoscopically. This includes appendectomy, pyloromyotomy, hernia repair, Nissen fundoplication, and bowel resection, just to name a few. The most important consideration in the management of patients undergoing laparoscopy is the close monitoring of intraabdominal pressure (IAP) during abdominal insufflation. In older children, the laparoscopic methods and anesthetic implications are the same as for adults. In younger children and infants, increases in IAP may result in cardiopulmonary compromise. In several studies of small children, an IAP less than 12 mm Hg appears to be safe whereas an IAP above 12 mm Hg has been associated with hypotension, bradycardia, and difficulty with ventilation secondary to a loss of FRC and a decrease in lung compliance. In children with cyanotic congenital heart disease, an IAP greater than 6 mm Hg may cause increased pulmonary vascular resistance (PVR) that results in right-to-left shunting.

Despite the small size of vulnerable vessels, carbon dioxide embolism[2] may cause hemodynamic compromise during laparoscopy in infants. Although rare, neonates may be susceptible to this particular complication because of damage or insufflation of a residual patent umbilical vein.

Congenital Diaphragmatic Hernia

A congenital diaphragmatic hernia (CDH) consists of a defect in the diaphragm that allows the abdominal contents to enter and remain within the thoracic cavity during fetal life. It occurs in approximately 1 in 3000[3] live births, is usually accompanied by polyhydramnios, and is often detected by prenatal ultrasound. The most critical consequence of this anomaly is the prevention of normal prenatal lung

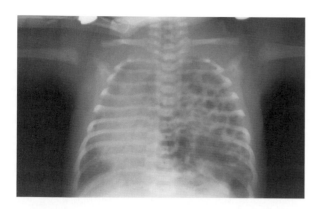

• **Fig 23.1.** Left-sided diaphragmatic hernia in a 1-day-old term infant. Note the bowel gas in the left thorax that displaces the heart and compresses the right lung. The left lung is hypoplastic because it is not allowed to grow normally during fetal development. (From: Crowley, MA, Neonatal Respiratory Disorders, In: *Fanaroff and Martin's Neonatal-Perinatal Medicine.* 11th ed. Philadelphia: Elsevier; [chapter 66]; pages 1203-1230.).

growth. It leads to pulmonary hypoplasia, decreased cross-sectional area of the pulmonary vasculature, and changes in surfactant production and availability. Severe cases may lead to left ventricular hypoplasia.

There are three identified variations of CDH. The most common is the left-sided, posterior defect through the foramen of Bochdalek (Fig. 23.1). This breech of diaphragmatic integrity allows herniation of both small and large bowel and solid organs. Less commonly, CDH occurs through a right-sided or anterior defect through the foramen of Morgagni. These are not usually associated with severe pulmonary hypoplasia, but rather are signs of intestinal obstruction because only a small part of the liver and large bowel become herniated into the thoracic cavity. The least common form of CDH occurs as a hiatal hernia (<2%).

The manifestations of severe CDH are apparent immediately after birth as respiratory distress; they are also often detected before birth via prenatal ultrasound. Newborns with CDH will demonstrate chest wall retractions, tachypnea, cyanosis, absence of breath sounds on the affected side, and the classically appearing scaphoid abdomen that indicates a lack of intestines within the abdominal cavity. Bowel sounds may be heard in the chest. Diagnosis is confirmed by a "baby-gram" radiograph, which demonstrates bowel in the thoracic cavity and a gasless abdominal cavity (Fig. 23.1). Approximately 25% of affected infants have associated cardiac anomalies. Depending on the location of the hernia, the mediastinum may shift and cause cardiac compromise. Although most of these patients are diagnosed at birth, up to 10% of affected patients with mild CDH may remain undiagnosed until later in childhood or even into adulthood.

Pulmonary hypoplasia and hypoxemia are associated with persistent pulmonary hypertension and failure to transition normally from fetal to adult circulatory function. Elevated right-sided heart pressures cause right-to-left shunting through the ductus arteriosus. Persistent hypoxemia, hypercarbia, and acidosis also contribute to keeping the ductus open. Right-to-left shunting can also occur through a patent foramen ovale or ventricular septal defect, if present. This vicious cycle can only be broken by the establishment of normoxemia and normal lung function. Concomitant congenital heart disease contributes to this process and reduces overall survival.

Once diagnosed, management consists of immediate tracheal intubation and institution of mechanical ventilation. Bag-and-mask positive pressure ventilation should be minimized in an effort to reduce gastric distention because the stomach or small intestine may be contained within the thoracic cavity. A naso- or orogastric tube should be immediately inserted to decompress the upper digestive tract. A chest radiograph will confirm the diagnosis and rule out a pneumothorax on the contralateral side.

In the past, infants with CDH were brought immediately to surgery to remove the abdominal contents from the thoracic cavity and allow lung reexpansion and growth. However, this practice was not associated with good results because the affected lung is hypoplastic, not atelectatic. Currently, corrective surgery is performed on a semielective basis within the first few weeks of life when the infant has achieved optimal medical stabilization.

The initial successful management of pulmonary hypertension is the key to survival. In the immediate newborn period, the goal of ventilatory management is to provide oxygenation and ventilation without triggering a pulmonary vasospasm crisis. That goal is a PaO_2 greater than 50 mm Hg, with the acceptance of a lower oxygen saturation and hypercapnia while trying to maintain a pH greater than 7.2. Permissive hypercapnia ($PaCO_2$ of 40–60 mm Hg) has been shown to greatly improve survival. Permitting higher $PaCO_2$ has allowed for less volume and pressure to be used for ventilation, thus, minimizing barotrauma and volutrauma. Inotropic support may be needed to maintain perfusion, and inhaled nitric oxide and milrinone may be utilized to reduce afterload, both of which may improve pulmonary blood flow. The inability to reduce the PCO_2 or reduce the alveolar-to-arterial oxygen gradient to less than 500 mm Hg despite maximal ventilatory techniques (e.g., using the oscillator or jet ventilator) is associated with a poor outcome and is an indication for institution of extracorporeal membrane oxygenation (ECMO). Other signs that indicate the need for ECMO include preductal oxygen saturations less than 85%, peak inspiratory pressures greater than 25 cmH_2O, hypotension resistant to pressors, and inadequate perfusion based on urine output and increasing lactate. Although pulmonary vasodilator therapy with inhaled nitric oxide may help stabilize a patient, it does not reduce mortality or the need for ECMO. CDH surgery consists of an abdominal incision and reduction of the herniated viscera. Repair is planned once the pulmonary system has stabilized. This stabilization is marked by an adequate urine output, normotension, an adequate preductal oxygen saturation, and a pulmonary artery pressure less than systemic arterial pressure. The diaphragmatic defect is closed by primary repair or by using a synthetic patch. In most cases, a chest tube is placed on the affected side, and some surgeons will also insert a contralateral chest tube to protect against pneumothorax from aggressive ventilator therapy. Unexplained intraoperative decreases in lung compliance, hypoxemia, or hypotension are suggestive of a contralateral pneumothorax and should warrant immediate chest tube placement. The surgery can be performed in the operating room after medical stabilization, or in the neonatal intensive care unit (NICU) while the patient remains on ECMO.

Ventilatory management during CDH repair consists of a balance between avoiding barotrauma (particularly in the unaffected normal lung) and decreasing hypoxemia, hypercarbia, and acidosis, all of which increase PVR. Simultaneous pulse oximetry at preductal (right upper extremity) and postductal (lower extremity) sites allow early detection of right-to-left shunting from pulmonary hypertension. Right radial artery cannulation will allow continuous blood pressure measurement and assessment of preductal oxygenation. Additional anesthetic priorities during CDH repair include adequate volume expansion, especially when high ventilatory pressures are required, and use of a high-dose opioid technique to minimize elevations in PVR. It is important to administer adequate intravenous fluids to ensure adequate preload, but care must be taken to avoid pulmonary edema. Mechanical ventilation is continued in the postoperative period in all but the most minor defects.

Biliary Atresia

Biliary atresia occurs in about 1 in 15,000 live births. It is thought to occur as a result of inflammation of the bile ducts leading to obliteration of the extrahepatic biliary tract. The result is that bile cannot be emptied properly from the liver. It manifests as direct hyperbilirubinemia within the first several weeks of life and, if left untreated, can lead to cirrhosis. Infants with biliary atresia require a surgical anastomosis between the duodenum and an intrahepatic biliary duct known as a Kasai procedure.[4] Repair must be done in the first 60 days[5] of life to optimize clinical outcomes. Anesthetic concerns are primarily those of decreased hepatic function and its sequelae, such as clotting factor deficiency, hypoalbuminemia, increased abdominal girth/ascites, and avoidance of medications that are metabolized in the liver. In the absence of a coagulopathy, epidural analgesia is preferred for postoperative pain relief. Long-term postoperative complications after the Kasai procedure include recurrent ascending cholangitis and chronic cirrhosis. Many of these children will ultimately require liver transplantation.

Hirschsprung's Disease

Hirschsprung's disease (congenital aganglionic megacolon) describes a condition of the absence of parasympathetic ganglion cells in the lower colon, leading to a functional obstruction of the large bowel. It is the most common cause of large bowel obstruction in the newborn and typically presents in the first few days of life as abdominal distention

and a failure to pass meconium. The diagnosis should be considered in any neonate that has not passed meconium by 48 hours of life or in any older infant with a history of chronic constipation. On rare occasions, these children may become very ill with toxic megacolon, peritonitis, and colonic perforation. Because of the association with cardiac anomalies (2%–5%) and trisomy 21 (5%–15%), a cardiac work-up may be necessary before operative intervention.

Treatment consists of removal of the nonfunctional part of the colon and reanastomosis to the rectum; a diversion colostomy may or may not be required. In many centers, the intraabdominal resection is accomplished using a laparoscopic approach before the perineal repair.

During the perineal repair, the infant is positioned at the end of the OR table in the lithotomy position. The anesthesiologist should anticipate this relocation and prepare the lengths of the monitoring wires, breathing circuit, and IV tubing accordingly. Maintaining normothermia in the infant may be challenging, so core temperature monitoring is essential with warming of the OR, warming of intravenous fluids, and/or a forced air heating blanket as necessary.

Imperforate Anus

Imperforate anus (anal atresia) is diagnosed shortly after birth on physical exam or after an evaluation for failure of the infant to pass meconium in the first days of life; prenatal ultrasounds are often normal. This anomaly ranges in severity from a mild stenosis with a thin obstructive band that is punctured at the bedside to a more severe atresia that is associated with other anomalies. Although the defect usually appears superficial, it can be associated with underlying pelvic neuromuscular abnormalities. Anal atresia is a component of the VATER syndrome: **V**ertebral anomalies, **A**nal atresia, **T**racheo-**E**sophageal fistula, and **R**enal/genitourinary malformations. The updated acronym, VACTERL, includes **C**ardiac and **L**imb anomalies.

Infants may undergo primary repair in the neonatal period or undergo a staged repair involving a colostomy. Repair of some type is urgent if the child is unable to pass stool. Repair is less urgent in female infants with a rectovaginal fistula that allows passage of meconium. Ultimately, the corrective procedure, a posterior sagittal anorectoplasty (Pena procedure or PSARP), is performed during the first year of life. Unique anesthetic concerns include the delineation of coexisting anomalies and assessment of fluid and electrolyte imbalance. Management of life-threatening comorbidities takes priority over repair. The procedure usually begins in the prone position and is completed in the supine or lithotomy position. Even after correction, these children may suffer from urinary and/or fecal incontinence.

Indwelling Intravenous Access

One of the most commonly performed surgical procedures in children is the intraoperative placement of an indwelling venous catheter such as a Broviac, Hickman, or subcutaneous port. The catheter is usually inserted into one of the central veins of the neck and a portion of it is tunneled underneath the skin for improved stability and to decrease the risk for infection at the site of insertion. Children with chronic diseases will require placement of indwelling venous access for long-term parenteral nutrition, administration of antibiotics, or administration of chemotherapy or other types of chronically administered medications.

Preoperative evaluation of the patient should consist of a thorough review of the patient's underlying comorbidities. Preoperative midazolam can be administered by the oral or intravenous route. There are no unique considerations for induction and maintenance of general anesthesia. The procedure is performed with the child in the Trendelenburg position (to maximize vein size and minimize the risk for venous air embolism), with the head hyperextended and turned to the opposite side of the line insertion. Therefore, after draping of the patient, airway access is limited, and for this reason, we prefer endotracheal intubation for the procedure. Some pediatric anesthesiologists are comfortable with a supraglottic airway.

General anesthesia is also utilized during removal of the tunneled catheter when its use is no longer necessary. The catheter may be used to administer intravenous induction agents at the start of the procedure but should not be removed before establishing adequate peripheral venous access. Significant blood loss can occasionally occur from a tear in the vein that contained the tunneled catheter and a venous air embolism is possible. Endotracheal intubation is not required for this procedure as it often takes less than 10 minutes to perform and surgical draping is minimal.

Inguinal Hernia

Inguinal hernia repair is one of the most commonly performed surgical procedures in children. A unilateral hernia is usually diagnosed on routine physical exam in healthy school aged children. Bilateral hernias occur more commonly in premature infants and because of the potential risk for incarceration, will usually be repaired before the child is discharged from the hospital. Therefore, these children will present with all of the usual medical problems associated with prematurity.

There are many ways to anesthetize children for hernia repairs. Different factors are taken into consideration when deciding on an anesthetic technique, including the health of the child, preference of the surgeon, and the skills of the anesthesia provider. Older children with uncomplicated unilateral hernias can receive maintenance of general anesthesia by facemask or supraglottic airway with inhaled agents. When laparoscopic examination of the contralateral side is performed, endotracheal intubation and neuromuscular blockade may be indicated, depending on the surgeon's preference for abdominal wall relaxation and desired degree of intraabdominal insufflation.

Pain relief for inguinal hernia repair consists primarily of regional analgesia. Caudal analgesia with dilute local anesthesia is often used for bilateral repair, and a peripheral nerve block is used for unilateral repair. However, in ambulatory children in whom a caudal block may cause lower extremity weakness, bilateral peripheral nerve blocks are often performed. Analgesia should be supplemented with a small dose of intravenous opioid and nonopioid analgesics, including acetaminophen and ketorolac.

The anesthetic technique for bilateral hernia repair for the small infant is different from that of the older child. The hernias can consist of large bulging sacs (in the male) and can present a surgical challenge. For these cases, we prefer general anesthesia with neuromuscular blockade and endotracheal intubation. In some cases of extreme prematurity and small size (e.g., less than 3 kg), when the infant is scheduled to return to the intensive care unit, we may choose to maintain endotracheal intubation into the postoperative period while the infant fully recovers. Caudal analgesia is often performed for postoperative pain relief. The use of spinal anesthesia without sedatives[6] is an option in these cases, especially in former preterm infants that may be at risk for development of postoperative apnea. There is a reduction in the risk for postoperative apnea when preoperative sedatives are not used compared with general anesthesia. Infants without a history of apnea in the preoperative period have also shown a reduced risk for postoperative apnea when spinal anesthesia was used compared with general anesthesia. However, the risk of anesthetic failure is higher with spinals compared with general anesthesia.

Intussusception

Intussusception is the telescoping of a portion of bowel (usually the distal ileum) into an adjacent portion of the bowel with subsequent swelling and intestinal obstruction. Occasionally, this obstruction may be severe enough to cause intestinal ischemia and perforation. The classic description is the patient that presents with the triad of vomiting, abdominal pain, and rectal bleeding ("currant jelly" stool). Although the cause of intussusception is generally unknown, it may be associated with a polyp or enlarged intestinal lymph nodes (Peyer's patches). It usually occurs in infants and toddlers (ages 2 months to 5 years). In severe or protracted cases, bowel ischemia and sepsis may develop, and these patients may have severe dehydration and electrolyte imbalances. The diagnosis is confirmed radiographically, via ultrasound or plain film. In younger children up to age 3 years, intussusception can usually be treated by a nonsurgical reduction using a barium or air enema. In older children and those who fail nonoperative reduction, exploratory laparoscopy and manual reduction is required, using general anesthesia with RSI. The primary anesthetic concerns for this procedure consist of fluid resuscitation, correction of electrolyte abnormalities, maintenance of normothermia, and provision of postoperative analgesia.

Malrotation and Midgut Volvulus

Malrotation is defined as an abnormal twisting of the intestine as it migrates back into the fetal abdominal cavity from its embryonic extraabdominal location during the latter part of the first trimester at approximately 10 weeks gestation. When this twisting compromises the blood supply of the intestine (superior mesenteric artery), the condition is known as a volvulus (Fig. 23.2). Malrotation with resulting midgut volvulus is one of the only true pediatric surgical emergencies. Infants who develop volvulus from malrotation usually become symptomatic sometime in the first 2 months of life, although mild cases can remain asymptomatic for years. Symptoms include bilious vomiting or signs of intestinal perforation and ischemia if the volvulus has progressed. These infants can be quite ill and may present with a sepsis-like picture; the condition can be fulminant and fatal if left untreated. Severely ill children may require fluid and blood resuscitation and endotracheal intubation in the preoperative period. Preoperatively, a naso- or orogastric tube is placed to decompress the stomach and antibiotics are initiated to prevent infection. Children with malrotation may have additional congenital anomalies that should be investigated before surgery if time permits.

The treatment of volvulus consists of urgent exploratory laparotomy and a surgical reduction known as a Ladd's procedure. Ischemic bowel is resected at the time of surgery. Viable bowel is untwisted along the mesentery and fixed in a nonrotated position to restore proper blood flow. After

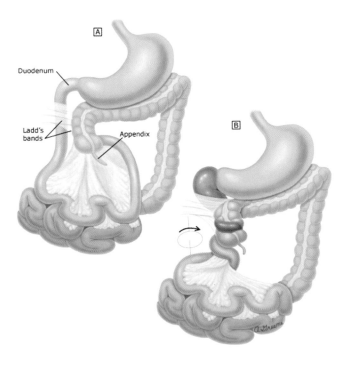

• **Fig 23.2.** Intestinal malrotation, with (right) and without (left) midgut volvulus. (Reproduced with permission from: Brandt ML. (2020). *UpToDate*. In: Post TW, ed. *UpToDate*. Waltham, MA. Copyright © 2020 UpToDate, Inc. For more information visit www.uptodate.com. Accessed 20.9.22.).

the repair, most children are awakened in the operating room and require only routine postoperative care. However, depending on the severity of the child's condition, postoperative mechanical ventilation may be warranted, especially if a "second-look" procedure is planned to assess bowel viability in 24 to 48 hours.

Meckel Diverticulum

A Meckel diverticulum is the most common congenital anomaly of the small intestine. It is a persistence of the omphalomesenteric duct after fetal life that presents as painless rectal bleeding sometime in the first few years of life. Definitive treatment is surgical resection by exploratory laparoscopy. Clinically significant anemia is uncommon. There are no significant anesthetic considerations except for postoperative pain relief if a laparotomy is required.

Necrotizing Enterocolitis

Necrotizing enterocolitis (NEC) is a multifactorial disorder that affects 6–10% of prematurely born infants weighing under 1500 g and carries a mortality of 50% or more. It is the most common gastrointestinal emergency in neonates. NEC is typically a disorder of the premature infant although it can be seen in full term infants with or without underlying systemic disease. Risk factors include prematurity, administration of hypertonic enteral feedings, decreased bowel perfusion, and infection with enteric organisms. Intestinal damage ranges from superficial mucosal injury to full thickness wall necrosis with bowel perforation. NEC initially presents as abdominal distention, vomiting, increased gastric residuals, feeding intolerance, diarrhea, and bloody stools, and can progress rapidly to severe intestinal ischemia, sepsis, shock, and even death. The infant may develop cardiovascular instability, respiratory failure, temperature instability, metabolic acidosis, thrombocytopenia, and disseminated intravascular coagulation (DIC). Although most neonates develop this condition in the first few days of life, it can still occur in the first few weeks of life. Infants who survive an episode of NEC are more likely to suffer from neurodevelopmental morbidity.

Pathologic findings vary from patient to patient. In mild cases, there may be superficial mucosal injury, and severe cases may have bowel ischemia, perforation, and severe peritonitis. Bowel ischemia causes damage to the intestinal mucosa, which allows bowel gas to penetrate the submucosal region and enter the mesenteric veins and portal venous system. Diagnosis is usually made on the basis of an abdominal radiograph that reveals pneumatosis intestinalis (air bubbles within the intestinal wall), dilated loops of bowel, and/or free air within the abdominal cavity or portal venous system.

Prompt diagnosis of NEC is crucial, and treatment varies from medical therapy to surgical exploration[7] depending on the severity of the illness. Mild cases of NEC can be managed conservatively with medical therapy, including gastrointestinal rest, parenteral feeding, and gastric decompression with a large-bore, multiorifice catheter such as a Replogle tube. In addition, these infants require antibiotics and volume resuscitation with isotonic fluids, and, sometimes, blood products. These patients may require placement of a central venous catheter and an arterial line and may require tracheal intubation with mechanical ventilation. In severe illness, in which necrotic or perforated bowel is suspected or in a patient that continues to worsen despite medical therapy, an exploratory laparotomy is performed to examine the bowel in its entirety. An important clinical sign that may indicate the need for surgical intervention is erythema of the abdominal wall. Absolute indication for surgery is pneumoperitoneum secondary to intestinal perforation. Other infants that have identified risk factors may undergo early surgical management to prevent further intestinal necrosis and eventual perforation. Clinical signs include abdominal wall erythema, a palpable abdominal mass, and hypotension. Metabolically, these at-risk infants may show thrombocytopenia, metabolic acidosis, and hyponatremia. Radiographic findings include profound pneumatosis of the bowel, portal venous gas, and pneumoperitoneum. The current trend in management of NEC has been the optimization of medical management with the avoidance of surgery as much as possible; as such, fewer babies are being brought to the OR for surgical management.

When patients are brought to the OR, anesthetic considerations for infants with NEC undergoing abdominal exploration include management of acidosis, hypovolemia, anemia, electrolyte imbalance, and coagulopathy, as well as support of cardiovascular function. An arterial line is recommended to monitor blood pressure closely and to facilitate frequent collection of blood samples. Central venous cannulation will facilitate volume replacement and allow trending of volume status via the central venous pressure (CVP). Inotropic support with epinephrine or dopamine may be necessary to support cardiovascular function. The procedure itself is associated with large amounts of fluid shifts and possible blood loss. The anesthesia provider should be prepared to resuscitate the infant with isotonic fluid (normal saline or Lactated Ringer's solution) and blood products as needed. A type-and-crossmatch is imperative. Postoperatively, these infants remain intubated, sedated, and mechanically ventilated while supportive therapy continues. Recovery and survival are dependent on the extent of bowel ischemia and the severity of the underlying disease. Lower birth weight infants have poorer outcomes.

In a severely ill and unstable patient that develops pneumoperitoneum but that is unlikely to tolerate surgical intervention, a peritoneal drain may be inserted under local anesthesia. Of note, these patients may have respiratory compromise from abdominal distension. Peritoneal drainage rapidly decompresses the abdomen and by removing toxic effluents, healing may improve. However, by not removing necrotic bowel, the patient may also continue to exhibit a cytokine and inflammatory response resulting in a worsening clinical status. Currently, more patients undergo peritoneal drainage as more of a stabilizing measure with subsequent laparotomy rather than as definitive treatment. Ongoing investigation is being done to determine the benefit of this technique compared with early surgical intervention.

Omphalocele and Gastroschisis

Although each of these anomalies represents a distinct anatomic defect, omphalocele and gastroschisis are discussed together because their anesthetic considerations are very similar. Each is a congenital defect that allows a portion of the intestinal viscera to remain outside of the abdominal cavity and requires surgical repair in the newborn period. Large defects are managed with a staged approach if primary closure is not possible. These defects are relatively common, occurring in approximately 1 in 2,000 births. An omphalocele occurs when the visceral organs fail to migrate from the yolk sac back into the abdomen early in gestation and the umbilical ring remains open; the defect is a central lesion and occurs at the insertion of the umbilicus. Gastroschisis is thought to result from an occlusion of the omphalomesenteric artery during early development. As a result, the abdominal viscera herniate through a rent in the abdominal wall, usually to the right of the umbilicus. Omphalocele is more likely than gastroschisis to be associated with additional congenital defects. These occur in 25% to 50% of cases and include chromosome anomalies and cardiac defects. Omphalocele may be a component of the Beckwith–Wiedemann syndrome, which consists of hypertrophy of multiple organs. This syndrome is particularly relevant to the anesthesiologist as enlargement of the tongue may compromise the upper airway and be associated with difficult intubation. Pancreatic enlargement causes hyperinsulinism, which results in hypoglycemia that needs to be monitored intraoperatively.

Infants with gastroschisis are usually born at full term without additional isolated defects. The major pathophysiological difference between the two is that, in omphalocele, the intestinal contents remain covered with the peritoneal membrane (Fig. 23.3), which protects the intestinal mucosa from the irritative effects of amniotic fluid as well as excessive evaporative fluid and temperature loss after delivery. Infants with gastroschisis lack this natural protective covering, and thus, are more prone to dehydration, hypoglycemia, hypothermia, third-space fluid accumulation, electrolyte imbalance, acidosis, bleeding, and sepsis.

Management of omphalocele and gastroschisis begins immediately after birth. The extruded abdominal contents are covered with warm saline dressings and are encased in a sterile plastic bag or wrap (silo) to decrease fluid and temperature loss and discourage infection. A naso- or orogastric tube is placed for gastric decompression, normovolemia is maintained with intravenous hydration, and associated comorbidities are addressed before surgical repair. Antibiotics may be necessary if intestinal abnormalities are suspected.

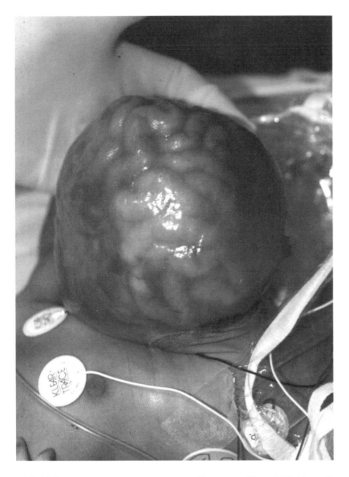

• **Fig 23.3.** Omphalocele before surgery (Courtesy of Ronald S. Litman).

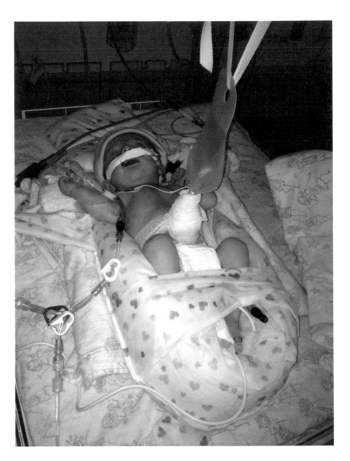

• **Fig 23.4.** Omphalocele silo. Large omphaloceles are treated with a silo and progressive constriction until primary repair (Courtesy of Ronald S. Litman).

Considerations for induction of general anesthesia are similar to those for any newborn infant with a presumed increased risk for a "full stomach" secondary to intestinal obstruction. A modified RSI is usually performed using gentle breaths. Some pediatric anesthesiologists will prefer to temporarily remove the nasogastric tube during induction to facilitate airway management.

Achieving a primary repair is the goal of surgery as failure to replace all of the intestinal contents back into the abdominal cavity increases postoperative morbidity. However, in many cases where the abdominal cavity is too restrictive or when there is not enough skin to close the underlying defect, a partial replacement is performed, and the remaining external viscera is encased in a synthetic silo mesh (Fig. 23.4), allowing for complete repair to occur as a staged procedure. There are several intraoperative adverse physiologic derangements that may occur when the surgeon attempts to place a large volume of abdominal contents back into a small, restrictive abdominal cavity. Cephalad displacement of the diaphragm because of the increase in abdominal contents may significantly decrease FRC and tidal volume, which can lead to difficult ventilation, development of atelectasis, and hypoxemia. During the repair, the anesthetist may need to use manual ventilation to maintain adequate tidal volumes in response to rapid changes in lung compliance.

The presence of hypoxemia despite maximal ventilation may preclude completion of a primary repair.

In addition to its impact on intrathoracic pressure, increased intraabdominal pressure may result in an abdominal compartment syndrome. When this occurs, venous compression leads to a decrease in preload and hypotension and lower limb venous congestion. High intraabdominal pressures may lead to renal artery compression resulting in oliguria and decreased perfusion to the lower extremities. Bowel ischemia may also result secondary to decreased perfusion. Adequate volume and blood replacement and full neuromuscular blockade must be maintained throughout the procedure to optimize the chances for successful primary closure.

All infants, except those with the most trivial repairs, remain mechanically ventilated in the postoperative period. Abdominal compartment syndrome and respiratory compromise may continue postoperatively; therefore, muscle relaxation and adequate sedation are essential for optimal management.

Pyloric Stenosis

Pyloric stenosis describes an abnormality that occurs within the first several weeks of life in which a hypertrophied pylorus obstructs the passage of food from the stomach to the small intestine. With an incidence of up to 1 in 300 live births, it represents one of the most common procedures requiring general anesthesia within the first weeks of life. Clinical manifestations include projectile nonbilious vomiting after feeds, and when severe or protracted, dehydration and failure to thrive. The diagnosis is confirmed by characteristic findings on physical exam (palpation of the hypertrophied pylorus), or ultrasound examination. Chronic emesis causes loss of hydrochloric acid from the stomach, which leads to a hypochloremic, hypokalemic metabolic alkalosis.

Once the condition is diagnosed, these children should be hospitalized and given intravenous rehydration therapy and correction of electrolyte abnormalities. An orogastric or nasogastric tube is inserted, and all feedings are stopped. Rehydration consists of normal saline for reestablishment of normovolemia (some infants may require in excess of 50 mL/kg), and maintenance fluids consisting of D5 ½ NS with potassium chloride added. Pyloric stenosis is a medical and not a surgical emergency.[8] Perioperative morbidity and mortality are associated with surgical correction before normalization of fluid and electrolyte derangements.[9] Serum potassium should be in the normal range, serum chloride should be >100 mEq/L, and correction of the alkalosis to a serum bicarbonate <30 mEq/L are generally indicated before surgery. The kidney will retain chloride as a result of volume contraction. A urine chloride >20 mEq/L suggests that volume status has been adequately restored.

Before induction of general anesthesia, the infant's nasogastric tube should be suctioned and removed, and a large-bore suction catheter (e.g., 14-French) is inserted orally into the stomach and suctioned while tilting the infant in all directions to evacuate any remaining gastric contents. This procedure will completely empty the stomach in nearly all infants. A common anesthetic induction technique is a modified RSI technique[10] that consists of preoxygenation, followed by administration of propofol, succinylcholine or 1.2 to 1.6 mg/kg dose of rocuronium. Gentle (low pressure) positive-pressure ventilation (peak inflating pressure of 10–12 cmH$_2$O) is provided by mask, with an inhalational anesthetic turned fairly high (i.e., sevoflurane at 5%–7%) for a minute or so before endotracheal intubation. Sometimes, cricoid pressure is applied, although correct placement in neonates may be difficult and may also interfere with mask ventilation and airway visualization. A true rapid sequence technique without ventilation is not used because oxyhemoglobin desaturation will usually occur before intubation, and the incidence of pulmonary aspiration is exceedingly low. Awake intubations are no longer performed on children with pyloric stenosis. The use of inhalation induction after gastric suctioning in an infant with intravenous access has been described to be safe, but because of the risk for gastric aspiration more studies need to be established to see if it is equally as safe as a modified RSI. Maintenance of general anesthesia can consist of any inhaled agent; however, sevoflurane or desflurane are preferred because of their ability to be rapidly eliminated. There is no difference in the risk for postoperative apnea between sevoflurane and desflurane, but

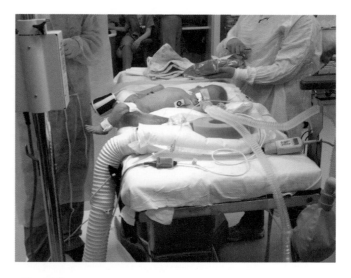

• **Fig 23.5. Pyloromyotomy positioning.** Sideways positioning on the OR table for laparoscopic pyloromyotomy. **(Courtesy of Ronald S. Litman).**

recovery times are slightly shorter with desflurane. Surgical correction consists of a laparoscopic pyloromyotomy in which the pylorus is partially split lengthwise to loosen the constriction (Fig. 23.5). After the myotomy, the surgeon will often request insufflation of the stomach with air via an orogastric tube to test the integrity of the pyloric mucosa. Fluid and blood losses are minimal. The surgeon administers local anesthesia into the skin and subcutaneous tissues. Opioids are avoided in this patient population because of increased risk for opioid-mediated respiratory depression and postoperative apnea that may be magnified because of the effects of metabolic alkalosis on the central control of ventilation. One dose of intravenous or rectal acetaminophen is administered while local anesthetic infiltration in surgical incisions is often performed. If high dose rocuronium is used, reversal can be accomplished using sugammadex.

Regional anesthesia such as spinal, thoracic epidural and caudal anesthesia as the primary anesthetic or as an adjuvant technique to general anesthesia have been described.

References

1. Weiss M, Gerber AC. Rapid sequence induction in children – it's not a matter of time! *Paediatr Anaesth.* 2008;18(2):97–99. doi: 10.1111/j.1460-9592.2007.02324.x.
2. Kudsi OY, Jones SA, Brenn BR. Carbon dioxide embolism in a 3-week-old neonate during laparoscopic pyloromyotomy: a case report. *J Pediatr Surg.* 2009;44(4):842–845. doi:10.1016/j.jpedsurg.2008.11.045.
3. Dingeldein M. Congenital diaphragmatic hernia: management & outcomes. *Adv Pediatr.* 2018;65(1):241–247. doi:10.1016/j.yapd.2018.05.001.
4. Cincinnati Children's. (2020). *Biliary Atresia.* Cincinnati Children's [Last updated 2020]. https://www.cincinnatichildrens.org/health/b/biliary. Accessed 21.7.30.
5. Hopkins CM, Yazigi N, Nylund CM. Incidence of biliary atresia and timing of hepatoportoenterostomy in the United States. *J Pediatr.* 2017;187:253–257. doi:10.1016/j.jpeds.2017.05.006.

6. Jones LJ, Craven PD, Lakkundi A, Foster JP, Badawi N. Regional (spinal, epidural, caudal) versus general anaesthesia in preterm infants undergoing inguinal herniorrhaphy in early infancy. *Cochrane Database Syst Rev.* 2015;2015(6):CD003669. doi:10.1002/14651858.CD003669.pub2. Published 2015 Jun 9.

7. Thakkar HS, Lakhoo K. The surgical management of necrotising enterocolitis (NEC). *Early Hum Dev.* 2016;97:25–28. doi:10.1016/j.earlhumdev.2016.03.002.

8. Kamata M, Cartabuke RS, Tobias JD. Perioperative care of infants with pyloric stenosis. *Paediatr Anaesth.* 2015;25(12):1193–1206. doi:10.1111/pan.12792.

9. Gilbertson LE, Fiedorek CS, Fiedorek MC, Lam H, Austin TM. Adequacy of preoperative resuscitation in laparoscopic pyloromyotomy and anesthetic emergence. *Anesth Analg.* 2020;131(2):570–578. doi:10.1213/ANE.0000000000004446.

10. Park RS, Rattana-Arpa S, Peyton JM, et al. Risk of Hypoxemia by induction technique among infants and neonates undergoing pyloromyotomy. *Anesth Analg.* 2021;132(2):367–373. doi:10.1213/ANE.0000000000004344.

Suggested Reading

Kovler ML, Jelin EB. Fetal intervention for congenital diaphragmatic hernia. *Semin Pediatr Surg.* 2019;28(4):150818. doi:10.1053/j.sempedsurg.2019.07.001.

24
Thoracic Surgery

SAMUEL HUNTER AND LYNNE G. MAXWELL*

Anesthetic care for pediatric thoracic surgery covers a wide range of ages, concomitant disease processes, and surgical pathology. The clinical scenario ranges from an elective, outpatient procedure on an otherwise healthy patient to an emergent procedure in a neonate with a severe underlying illness or associated congenital heart disease. The surgical pathology may have limited physiologic impact on the patient; or, as in the case of an anterior mediastinal mass, a cystic adenomatoid malformation, or a tracheoesophageal fistula, it may result in significant patient compromise. Newer surgical techniques such as thoracoscopy have additional anesthetic implications.

Preoperative Considerations

There exists a spectrum of diseases for which thoracic surgery is required. For example, a child undergoing a thoracotomy and resection of a pulmonary nodule may have no other associated conditions or may have associated pulmonary parenchymal disease that affects the anesthetic management. As is true for all anesthetics, the preoperative history and physical exam should identify acute problems, underlying medical conditions, and previously undiagnosed problems that may affect perioperative management. Preoperative laboratory evaluation depends more on the clinical status of the patient than the procedure itself. Blood loss is usually minimal during most thoracic procedures, but because of the proximity to the great vessels and the risk for unintentional damage to these structures, blood should be immediately available in the operating room (OR). If the surgery is elective, a type-and-crossmatch should be performed in the preoperative period so that crossmatched blood is available at the start of surgery. If the case is an emergency, a blood sample for type-and-crossmatch can be obtained after the induction of anesthesia and the placement of intravascular catheters, provided the blood bank can expedite processing of the specimen and provision of blood products. In surgical procedures with an elevated risk for significant hemorrhage, incision should be delayed until blood is readily available. Other preoperative studies, such as pulmonary function tests (PFTs), an electrocardiogram (ECG), or echocardiogram are not routinely indicated; rather, they are obtained on the basis of the patient's medical history and the indication for the surgical procedure.

In patients with compromised respiratory function, preoperative PFTs may assist in estimating the potential risk for intraoperative or postoperative respiratory complications and aid in ensuring that preoperative therapies, such as antibiotics for pulmonary infections or bronchodilators in patients with reactive airway disease, have been optimized. Preoperative PFTs will also help categorize the type of respiratory disease (obstructive or restrictive) and document the response to bronchodilator therapy. Children with significant respiratory impairment (i.e., PFTs <50% predicted for age) may benefit from noninvasive ventilation after tracheal extubation.

Cognitively normal children older than 6 years are usually able to cooperate with pulmonary function testing. However, there are limited data regarding the utility of PFTs in pediatric patients in guiding anesthetic management and postoperative care decisions. Preoperative PFT results that predict poor outcomes in adults after lung resection (such as VO_2 max <10 mL/kg/min, DLCO <40%, and preoperative FEV_1 <60%) cannot necessarily be applied to pediatric patients because there is generally less comorbidity in children, such as associated cardiac disease, compared with adults. It can be expected that most children will experience small decreases in PFTs after thoracotomy. Preoperative PFTs may not identify all patients at risk for postthoracotomy complications, but they can identify some high-risk patients, which can direct preoperative teaching and optimization of respiratory function. All children undergoing thoracotomy, if old enough, should receive preoperative teaching regarding the use of incentive spirometry and high-flow nebulization therapy.

Systemic disease processes are less frequently encountered in children than adults presenting for thoracic surgery. In oncology patients, however, there may be concerns such as previous chemotherapy or the presence of an anterior mediastinal mass. When evaluating the pediatric oncology patient, careful attention should be directed toward his or her disease process and previous chemotherapeutic regimen and the impact these may have on end organ functioning. One class of chemotherapeutic agents of particular interest to the anesthesiologist are anthracyclines such as doxorubicin, because of their association with congestive heart failure.

In the otherwise healthy patient without signs of airway compromise, several options are available for preoperative anxiolysis. Midazolam, the most commonly administered pediatric premedication, is given orally (0.5 mg/kg up to 10–15 mg) 15 to 20 minutes before anesthetic induction. Additional agents that may be included as part of the premedication process include the following:

- High-flow nebulization of albuterol and an anticholinergic agent such as ipratropium in children with reactive airway disease.
- Corticosteroids for patients with airway reactivity or those having airway procedures that may result in postoperative airway edema.
- Antisialagogue such as glycopyrrolate to decrease secretions and blunt cholinergic-mediated airway reactivity. These drugs may be particularly useful if ketamine is employed due to ketamine's sialagogue effect.

Anesthetic Techniques

Anesthetic induction for thoracic surgery in children can include inhalation with sevoflurane in N_2O and oxygen (with discontinuation of N_2O after loss of consciousness), or an intravenous (IV) anesthetic agent. For patients with obstructive airway lesions (tracheal compression from subglottic stenosis or vascular rings), sevoflurane can be administered with a mixture of oxygen and helium. Because helium is less dense than nitrogen, it decreases resistance in areas of turbulent airflow. After loss of consciousness IV access is secured. Once adequate bag-mask ventilation has been demonstrated, either technique can be followed by the administration of a nondepolarizing neuromuscular blocking agent to facilitate tracheal intubation and provide ongoing neuromuscular blockade during the surgical procedure. Potential contraindications to this method include the presence of an anterior mediastinal mass compressing the distal trachea, or a tracheoesophageal fistula (TEF) where the endotracheal tube tip position should be confirmed below the fistula before the administration of a neuromuscular blocking agent.

Endotracheal intubation then follows, with placement of additional venous access if required and arterial monitoring (when indicated) before the start of the procedure. Because thoracic surgical procedures are frequently performed in the lateral decubitus position, access to the extremities to obtain additional venous sites may be limited once the procedure begins. In patients with normal cardiovascular function, the monitoring of central venous or arterial pressure may offer little additional information to improve or influence anesthetic care. Central venous access is generally reserved for cases in which adequate peripheral IV access is unavailable. If central venous access is necessary, ultrasound-guided internal jugular or subclavian vein cannulation on the side of the procedure is recommended. This avoids the possibility of bilateral pneumothoraces (the surgical pneumothorax

induced on the side of the thoracotomy and the unintentional pneumothorax as a complication of the venous access procedure). The need for placement of invasive hemodynamic monitoring of arterial blood pressure is guided by the clinical status of the child and the specific surgical procedure and the need for postoperative blood pressure monitoring or blood gas sampling requirements. As many of these procedures use one-lung ventilation (OLV), arterial access may be useful to allow intermittent sampling of blood gases. End-tidal CO_2 monitoring may be inaccurate during thoracic procedures because of alterations in dead space and shunt fraction, especially during OLV. Transcutaneous carbon dioxide monitoring may be considered if continuous monitoring of carbon dioxide is indicated.

One-Lung Ventilation Techniques

Thoracic procedures often require lung deflation and minimal movement on the operative side while ventilating the nonoperative lung. Even during thoracoscopy, where insufflation of CO_2 gas may help collapse the operative lung, OLV should be considered if the surgeon requires additional exposure. In the pediatric patient, there are several options for attaining unilateral lung isolation (Table 24.1).

Double-Lumen Endotracheal Tube

A double-lumen endotracheal tube (DLT) is the most common method for attaining lung separation in adult patients. However, the smallest commercially available DLT is size 26-French (Fr), which precludes its placement in children weighing less than about 30 to 35 kg or younger than 8 to 10 years of age. Advantages of DLT over other techniques includes (1) rapid and easy separation of the lungs, (2) access to both lungs to facilitate suctioning, (3) ability to rapidly switch to two-lung ventilation if needed, and (4) ability to administer continuous positive airway pressure (CPAP) or oxygen insufflation to the operative lung, when necessary.

Left-sided DLTs are used almost exclusively as they are relatively easy to insert into the appropriate position and their use eliminates the possibility of obstruction of the right upper lobe bronchus given its short distance from the carina. After placement into the trachea and a 90-degree counterclockwise rotation, the DLT is advanced until resistance is encountered, and the tracheal and bronchial cuffs

TABLE 24.1	Techniques of One-Lung Ventilation in Children

- Double-lumen endotracheal tube (DLT)
- Univent tube (Fuji Systems, Tokyo, Japan)
- Selective unilateral bronchial intubation
- Bronchial blocker
- Fogarty embolectomy catheter
- Arndt endo bronchial blocker (Cook Critical Care, Bloomington, IN, USA)
- Pulmonary artery catheter
- Atrial septostomy catheter

are inflated. Inflation of the bronchial cuff with 1 to 2 mL of air before advancement may help guide the DLT into the correct position, which is verified by auscultation after alternate clamping of tracheal and bronchial lumens and direct visualization using flexible bronchoscopy. When selecting a bronchoscope size, consideration should be given to the fact that the DLT's bronchial lumen is at least 0.2-mm smaller than the tracheal lumen. When using the 26 to 28 Fr-sized DLTs, a neonatal bronchoscope (outer diameter 2.5–2.7 mm) is needed given the small internal diameter of its two lumens.

If lung isolation has not been achieved after insertion, a DLT may be in four possible incorrect locations, one of which is in the esophagus. The remaining three incorrect possibilities are (1) if the tube has not been advanced far enough, both tracheal and bronchial lumens will be in the trachea; (2) if the tube has been advanced too far, both tracheal and bronchial lumens will be in the left main bronchus; (3) and if the tube was unintentionally advanced into the right main bronchus, the bronchial (and possibly the tracheal) lumen will be located in the right main bronchus.

The correct position will have the tracheal lumen opening into the trachea above the carina and the bronchial lumen opening in the proximal left main bronchus. Confirmation should be performed after initial tube placement by end-tidal carbon dioxide ($ETCO_2$) detection, auscultation, and bronchoscopy. After turning the child to the lateral decubitus position, correct DLT positioning should be reconfirmed using repeat auscultation and flexible bronchoscopy.

If postoperative mechanical ventilation is required, consideration should be given to exchanging the DLT to a single-lumen endotracheal tube to prevent airway complications because of the large size of the DLT.

Univent Endotracheal Tube

The Univent tube (Fuji Systems Corporation, Tokyo, Japan) is a single-lumen endotracheal tube with a moveable bronchial blocker built into its sidewall. The bronchial blocker has a central channel, which can be used for the insufflation of oxygen if needed to treat intraoperative hypoxemia during OLV. After the Univent tube is placed into the trachea, the bronchial blocker is advanced into the main bronchus of the operative lung under direct vision using flexible bronchoscopy. The bronchial blocker is angled and therefore may be easily directed to either main bronchus by twisting the proximal shaft. Advantages of the Univent tube include ease of placement, the ability to easily change from OLV to two-lung ventilation (by deflating the bronchial cuff), and (unlike the standard DLT) the ability to pull the bronchial blocker back into its channel and to leave the Univent tube in place for postoperative ventilation.

Univent tubes are available with internal diameters of 3.5 (uncuffed), 4.5, 6.0, 6.5, 7.0, 7.5, 8.0, 8.5, and 9.0 mm (Table 24.2). The outer diameter is larger than that of a conventional endotracheal tube of the same internal diameter. As a point of reference, the outer diameter of the smallest

TABLE 24.2 Inner and Outer Diameters of Standard and Pediatric Univent Endotracheal Tubes

Inner Diameter	Outer Diameter of Standard Tube	Maximum Outer Diameter of Univent
3.5 mm	4.9 mm	8.0 mm[a]
4.5 mm	6.2 mm	9.0 mm[b]
6.0 mm	8.2 mm	11.5 mm[c]

[a]Corresponds to a 6.0 mm internal diameter standard endotracheal tube.
[b]Corresponds to a 6.5 mm internal diameter standard endotracheal tube.
[c]Corresponds to a 8.5 mm internal diameter standard endotracheal tube.

3.5 mm Univent tube is equivalent to that of a standard 5.5 mm cuffed endotracheal tube. The internal diameters of the 3.5 and 4.5 mm Univent tubes limit the passage of a standard pediatric bronchoscope with an outside diameter ≥3.5 mm, thereby requiring an ultrathin pediatric bronchoscope to visualize the bronchial blocker. The external diameters of even the smallest of the Univent tubes is such that they are not feasible for patients less than about 6 to 8 years of age.

Selective Endobronchial Intubation

In infants and young children whose small size precludes placement of a DLT or Univent, there are two additional options for OLV: selective endobronchial intubation with a standard endotracheal tube, or placement of a separate bronchial blocker. The major disadvantage of selective endobronchial intubation is that it is not possible to quickly change from OLV to two-lung ventilation because it requires repositioning of the endotracheal tube from the bronchus into the trachea. Furthermore, movement of the tracheal tube in a small infant in the lateral position under the surgical drapes during a thoracotomy risks hazardous complications such as accidental tracheal extubation. Unintentional movement of the endotracheal tube, which may be associated with surgical manipulation, may dislodge the tube tip from the bronchus into the trachea or the other bronchus. Our practice is to achieve standard endotracheal tube placement in the midportion of the trachea and note the depth of insertion at the gum. The tube is then advanced into the bronchus and the position at the gum is again noted. This allows for a measure of the depth of insertion when manipulating the tube during the surgical procedure. Remember that changes in head and neck position (flexion, extension, rotation) can alter the position of the tip of the tube even if the position at the gum is unchanged and secure.

Right-sided endobronchial intubation is easily accomplished blindly because of the anatomic orientation of the right main bronchus at a less acute angle to the vertical tracheal axis, although these angles tend to be similar in children younger than 3 years of age. A cuffed endotracheal tube is recommended as it facilitates total isolation of the lung, which will help prevent spread of an infectious process or blood from the operative lung to the ventilated nonoperative lung. The cuffed endotracheal tube size chosen for endobronchial intubation of either side should be one-half to one size smaller than usual, based on the patient's age. This is suggested because the cuff adds to the outer diameter of the tube, and the diameter of the bronchus is smaller than the trachea. When selecting an appropriate size for the endotracheal tube, consideration should be given to the fact that the left mainstem bronchus is approximately 0.5 mm smaller than the right mainstem bronchus, which may necessitate a smaller tube size depending on the lung to be isolated.

Blind placement into the left main bronchus is not as straightforward as for the right main bronchus. The usual orientation of the distal bevel of the tube should be reversed (using a stylet) so that the concave segment becomes convex, ensuring that the tip of the stylet does not extend beyond the tip of the tube. When this is done, the angle of the bevel will face the patient's right side with the Murphy eye along the left lateral wall of the trachea. Once the endotracheal tube is positioned in the midportion of the trachea, the stylet is removed and the tube advanced. Other maneuvers suggested to aid the successful left main bronchus placement include elevating the right shoulder, turning the head to the right side, or by applying firm pressure to the right side of the thorax. The authors' preference, and perhaps the easiest technique, is to use bronchoscopic guidance by placement of the flexible bronchoscope through the endotracheal tube and into the left main bronchus, followed by advancement of the tube over the bronchoscope. Fluoroscopic guidance[1] in the supine position with confirmation in the lateral position is a reliable, effective, and more expeditious technique than bronchoscopy for endobronchial endotracheal tube placement in infants. Some practitioners prefer the use of a Magill (no Murphy eye) or Microcuff tube (more distally located balloon cuff, no Murphy eye) to minimize the chance of gas leaking into the operative lung, especially when the main bronchus is short.

Bronchial Blockers

When a DLT or a Univent tube cannot be used because of the patient's size or technical difficulty, a bronchial blocker should be considered. Several different devices can be used as bronchial blockers, including a Fogarty embolectomy catheter and the Arndt[2] (Cook Critical Care, Bloomington, IN, USA) endobronchial blocker. The latter are available in three sizes (5, 7, and 9 Fr) allowing their effective use in the majority of patients. Fogarty embolectomy catheters (2–4 Fr) may be necessary in neonates. Atrioseptostomy and pulmonary artery catheters have also been used, but they have no advantage over the others and are more expensive. All these devices have a balloon at the distal end that when inflated will occlude the bronchus of the operative lung. Those devices with a central channel provide the advantage of allowing suctioning and application of low flow oxygen and CPAP to the operative lung. Because of the small size

of the channel, suctioning will not clear the lung of secretions but it is used to deflate the operative lung and improve surgical visualization. Without the central channel, air or gas cannot exit from the lung once the balloon is inflated; therefore the lung may not completely deflate and may obscure surgical visualization. In these cases, the lung can be manually compressed by the surgeon during a brief period of apnea and the balloon then inflated before the provision of positive-pressure ventilation.

The bronchial blocker can be placed either alongside (extraluminal) or through (coaxial) a standard endotracheal tube. When placed through the tube, there will be a decrease in the internal cross-sectional area, thereby increasing the resistance to airflow. The degree to which this occurs depends on the outer diameter of the bronchial blocker and the inner diameter of the endotracheal tube. When placed inside the endotracheal tube, the blocker may be secured easily as it exits the proximal end of the tube. This can be accomplished using a T-piece bronchoscopic airway adaptor with a self-sealing diaphragm. Other commercially available options include the Arndt adaptor (Cook Critical Care, Bloomington, IN, USA), which has a port for the bronchoscope, one for the anesthesia circuit, and an occlusive port through which the bronchial blocker can be placed. The latter can be twisted to tighten down and hold the bronchial blocker in place. An additional option is to make a small hole in the wall of the proximal endotracheal tube; the bronchial blocker is then passed from the outside to the inside of the tube. The bronchial blocker can then be positioned and secured in place by taping it to the outside of the endotracheal tube, but subsequent manipulation may be more difficult.

The bronchial blocker can be positioned in the main bronchus of the operative side blindly, using fluoroscopic guidance, or most easily and safely under direct vision using flexible bronchoscopy. If bronchoscopy is used, and if the bronchial blocker is passed into the lumen of the endotracheal tube, then the bronchoscope and bronchial blocker must be small enough so both can pass through the endotracheal tube. The ease with which these instruments can be passed through the tube is greatly enhanced by prior application of a silicone spray. The proper fit of these instruments should be checked before induction of anesthesia. Given the external diameter of the bronchial blocker and the neonatal bronchoscope (OD 2.2 mm), a size 4.5 mm or greater tracheal tube is required.

The Arndt bronchial blocker has an inflatable cuff and a central lumen, through which a wire with a looped end can be passed. The bronchial blocker is passed through a specialized adaptor that is placed at the proximal end of the endotracheal tube. This adaptor contains four ports. The bronchial blocker is passed through the appropriate port and placed at the entrance of the endotracheal tube. The bronchoscope is passed through the port and then through the wire loop at the end of the bronchial blocker. The bronchoscope and bronchial blocker are passed under direct vision as a single unit into the main bronchus of the operative side. The wire loop is loosened, and the bronchoscope is withdrawn into the trachea to directly visualize inflation of the blocker balloon. When correct placement has been confirmed, the wire loop is removed from the central channel of the blocker. Once the wire guide is removed from the channel, it cannot be replaced. The Arndt blocker is currently available in three sizes, with the 9-Fr recommended for endotracheal tubes of internal diameter ≥8.0 mm, the 7-Fr for 6.5 to 7.5 mm tubes, and the 5-Fr for 4.5 to 6.0 mm tubes. When the 5-Fr blocker is placed in an endotracheal tube smaller than 6.0 mm, or a 7-Fr placed in an endotracheal tube smaller than 7.0 mm, airway pressures will be increased by 3 to 5 cmH$_2$O.

If a child requires an endotracheal tube smaller than 4.5 mm, it may be necessary to place the bronchial blocker alongside the endotracheal tube if the bronchoscope and bronchial blocker will not fit through its lumen. In such cases, the bronchial blocker can be placed directly into the bronchus on the operative side using direct laryngoscopy, through a rigid bronchoscope or under fluoroscopy. Alternatively, the bronchus on the operative side can be intubated; the bronchial blocker passed through the endotracheal tube, which is then withdrawn completely and the trachea reintubated, so that the bronchial blocker lies on the outside of the endotracheal tube. The authors' preference is to perform direct laryngoscopy, place the bronchial blocker through the glottic opening and into the tracheal lumen followed by tracheal intubation with the endotracheal tube. A flexible bronchoscope is then placed through the endotracheal tube and the bronchial blocker advanced into the bronchus of the operative lung under direct vision.

Regardless of which catheter or placement technique is chosen, there remains a risk for displacement of the bronchial blocker during the surgical procedure or with repositioning of the patient. If this occurs, the bronchial blocker may occlude the tracheal lumen just beyond the endotracheal tube, resulting in inadequate ventilation. Continuous auscultation of breath sounds using a precordial stethoscope on the nonoperative side and monitoring of inflating pressures, respiratory compliance, and P$_{ET}$CO$_2$ should help identify this problem rapidly. Clinical experience suggests that inflating the balloon of the bronchial blocker with saline as opposed to air may limit movement and dislodgment during surgical manipulation. Additionally, with any change in the patient's position, correct placement of the bronchial blocker should be confirmed using flexible bronchoscopy or fluoroscopy. If the patient's respiratory status deteriorates rapidly during the surgical procedure with physiologic compromise, the balloon of the blocker should be deflated and consideration given to rapidly removing the bronchial blocker.

Anesthetic Management During One-Lung Ventilation

After separation of the lungs using one of the techniques described above, general anesthesia is maintained with a combination of IV and inhaled anesthetic agents. Hypoxic pulmonary vasoconstriction (HPV) maintains oxygenation during OLV by restricting pulmonary blood flow to the unventilated lung. In this setting, the administration of a nonspecific vasodilator (e.g., terbutaline, albuterol, isoproterenol, dobutamine, nicardipine, nitroglycerin, sodium nitroprusside, and inhaled anesthetic agents) may impair HPV and decrease oxygenation. The effects of isoflurane, sevoflurane, and desflurane on oxygenation during OLV are similar. Regardless of which inhaled agent is chosen, its expired concentration should be limited to 0.5 to 1.0 MAC to limit the effect on HPV.

With normal preoperative respiratory function, 100% oxygen may not be required to maintain adequate arterial oxygen saturation during OLV. Therefore the fraction of inspired oxygen can be decreased as needed by utilization of an air-oxygen mixture; the addition of air may have the added benefit of less postoperative atelectasis. Anesthesia is supplemented as needed with IV agents such as fentanyl or remifentanil, ketamine, benzodiazepines, propofol, and dexmedetomidine, none of which affect HPV. Ketamine preserves HPV, whereas propofol potentiates pulmonary vasoconstriction during hypoxia.

During OLV, ventilation should be maintained with tidal volumes of 4 to 8 mL/kg and a judicious amount of PEEP (4–6). Lung protective ventilation, which uses PEEP and avoids excessive tidal volumes (≥10 cc/kg), has been shown to reduce pulmonary complications in adults and children undergoing thoracic surgery. Respiratory rate may be adjusted as needed to maintain normocarbia. Pressure-limited ventilation can be used to deliver the same tidal volume with a lower peak inflating pressure compared with volume-limited ventilation. Hypocarbia should be avoided as it may interfere with HPV. The use of OLV may precipitate hypoxemia in children with preexisting lung disease or an alteration of pulmonary function. Treatment of this may require the intermittent provision of two-lung ventilation or a modification of OLV such as oxygen insufflation or application of CPAP to the operative lung. If adequate oxygenation cannot be maintained during OLV using 100% oxygen to the nonoperative side, CPAP of 4 to 5 cmH$_2$O can be applied to the operative lung provided that a DLT, Univent, or bronchial blocker with a central channel has been used. Although this will improve oxygenation, it may also distend the operative lung to some degree and impair surgical visualization. If the above measures fail, it may be necessary to provide intermittent two-lung ventilation. A final option in management of acute severe hypoxemia is for the surgeon to clamp the nonventilated pulmonary artery to reduce shunt fraction.

Anesthetic Management for Thoracoscopy

The reports of successes in the adult population combined with ongoing refinements in technique and the availability of smaller sized equipment have led to the use of thoracoscopy in infants and children. Initially used to biopsy intrathoracic neoplasms, thoracoscopy has now been used in more involved surgical procedures including the treatment of empyema, pleurodesis, and anterior spinal fusion in older children and resection of congenital lung masses, ligation of a patent ductus arteriosus, and TEF ligation and esophageal repair in infants. Various anesthetic techniques have been described in the adult population for thoracoscopy, including local anesthetic infiltration and regional anesthetic techniques; however, in the pediatric population, general anesthesia is required.

The anesthetic technique for thoracoscopy in children is straightforward. After the induction of general anesthesia, OLV is established using one of the techniques previously described. The patient is then positioned in either the supine or lateral decubitus position. After repositioning, the efficacy of OLV is again demonstrated and the endotracheal tube or bronchial blocker repositioned as needed.

There are a number of possible complications related to the thoracoscopic technique. Even more so than with laparoscopy, the rapid absorption of CO_2 from the pleural surfaces necessitates an increase in minute ventilation to avoid hypercarbia. The hemidiaphragm on the operative side, which has been isolated by the technique of OLV, will move cephalad, so trocar entry below the third or fourth intercostal space may result in hepatic or splenic injury. The artificial pneumothorax may decrease blood pressure and cardiac output by altering preload and/or afterload. In addition, inadvertent gas embolism may occur with the use of CO_2 insufflation. CO_2 embolism can occur from direct injection through vascular puncture during insufflation or from the entry of the gas, which is under pressure in the hemithorax, into an internal vessel that has been damaged during the procedure. The physiologic effects and clinical manifestations of gas embolism are dependent on the type and volume of embolized gas, the rate of injection, and the patient's baseline cardiovascular function. The dead space of the equipment should be flushed with a large volume of CO_2 before placement in the patient to avoid insufflation of air, which has more hemodynamic consequences than CO_2 if embolized.

Treatment of gas embolism begins with the immediate cessation of insufflation or release of the artificial pneumothorax. Because CO_2 is rapidly absorbed from the bloodstream, the cardiovascular changes usually reverse rapidly. Additional treatment, determined by the severity of the cardiovascular changes, includes the administration of fluids to increase preload and inotropic agents to augment cardiac contractility. With severe cardiovascular compromise, placement of the patient in the head-down, left lateral decubitus position (Durant maneuver) may displace the gas out of the right ventricular outflow tract into the apical portion of the right ventricle and restore cardiovascular function. Aspiration from a central venous catheter should be attempted if one is present.

At the completion of the procedure, the pneumothorax is evacuated and two-lung ventilation is reinstituted. Several large-volume breaths are delivered to ensure reexpansion of the lung on the operative side. In most cases, residual neuromuscular blockade is reversed and the patient's trachea is extubated.

Postoperative analgesia may be enhanced through the use of local anesthetic techniques. Administration of local anesthesia by the surgeon to the incision site or intercostal nerves under direct visualization is both timely and effective. Neuraxial analgesia in the form of an epidural or paravertebral technique may be employed assuming the absence of any contraindications and may be particularly useful in improving pulmonary outcomes after open thoracotomy. Newer fascial plane nerve block and catheter techniques such as serratus plane[3] blocks and erector spinae blocks[4] may also be of utility in improving postoperative pain control and decreasing opioid consumption.

Neonatal Thoracic Surgery

Thoracic surgery in neonates is primarily performed to correct congenital lung anomalies. These include congenital cystic adenomatoid malformation (CCAM), congenital lobar emphysema (CLE), pulmonary sequestration, and tracheoesophageal fistula (TEF) with or without esophageal atresia. All except pulmonary sequestration have an association with additional congenital anomalies, including congenital heart disease. TEF is often found as part of the VATER (or VACTERL) syndrome. VATER and VACTERL syndrome denote a constellation of abnormalities with the following structures. V = Vertebra; A = Anus (atresia); T = Trachea; E = Esophagus; R = Renal (Kidneys); VACTERL as above plus C = Cardiac, L = Limb. These associations necessitate a thorough preoperative evaluation to identify associated congenital anomalies, including echocardiography to rule out congenital heart disease.

When anesthetizing infants with congenital lung lesions, one of the most important preoperative determinations is whether or not positive-pressure ventilation will cause cardiopulmonary deterioration. This could occur in a lesion that contains a bronchial connection to a segment of lung with abnormal parenchyma, such as CLE. In this condition, positive-pressure ventilation results in progressive distention of the abnormal lobe with compression of normal lung because of a ball-valve effect, leading to hypoxemia. Mediastinal shift may torque the great vessels, causing decreased cardiac output and leading to cardiac arrest. If it is not known whether the lesion connects to a bronchus, spontaneous ventilation is indicated until one-lung ventilation of the contralateral lung is achieved or until the chest is opened. Maintenance of spontaneous ventilation can be achieved by carefully titrating a combination of IV and inhaled induction agents, and endotracheal intubation can be performed without muscle relaxation. A rostrally advanced caudal catheter or thoracic epidural catheter can be used to provide analgesia and aid in the preservation of spontaneous ventilation.

If the application of positive pressure is not of concern, routine IV induction of general anesthesia followed by administration of a neuromuscular blocking agent may be performed. Maintenance of general anesthesia is provided by a combination of an inhaled agent and an opioid or regional anesthetic technique. Nitrous oxide is avoided because of the risk for increasing the size of an air-filled mass.

Postoperative analgesia after neonatal thoracic surgery is best accomplished using an epidural catheter that has been advanced to the thoracic level via the caudal space. Infants who remain on mechanical ventilation can receive a continuous opioid infusion.

Congenital Cystic Adenomatoid Malformation

A CCAM is a cystic, solid, or mixed intrapulmonary mass that may communicate with the normal tracheobronchial tree (Fig. 24.1). A CCAM may grow large in utero, causing cardiac compression, decreased cardiac output with hydrops fetalis, and even fetal demise. Fetal surgery or ex-utero intrapartum treatment (EXIT) procedure is now available in some centers for such lesions. More commonly, a CCAM is detected by prenatal ultrasound or magnetic resonance study, does not compromise the fetus, and is surgically excised in the neonatal period or the first 2 months of life. CCAM may be associated with a mediastinal shift and respiratory distress, which necessitates emergent resection. Most cases, however, are asymptomatic and resection is performed as an elective procedure.

There are few unique anesthetic considerations[5] for CCAM resection. Because most are of the solid variety, positive-pressure ventilation can be accomplished without cardiopulmonary compromise. When open thoracotomy is performed, the CCAM is usually "delivered" out of the chest for resection. Therefore one-lung ventilation is not usually required, but this decision should be made in consultation with the surgeon before the case. Some surgeons have started to perform thoracoscopic resection of CCAM, in which case OLV is desirable.

Congenital Lobar Emphysema

CLE consists of an abnormally emphysematous lobe that communicates with the bronchial tree. It occurs, in order of frequency, in the left upper, right middle, or left lower lobes of the lung. Unless the lesion is large or has been expanded by bag-mask ventilation at birth, the infant is usually asymptomatic initially but may develop wheezing or respiratory distress soon after birth. In the presence of a bronchial connection and abnormal inelastic parenchyma within the lesion, positive-pressure ventilation may lead to rapid expansion because of a ball-valve effect, with compromise of subsequent ventilation and/or cardiac output. Preservation of spontaneous ventilation or minimizing the inflating pressure before establishment of one-lung ventilation will help prevent this complication. If cardiopulmonary deterioration occurs, immediate thoracotomy with delivery of the lobe from the thoracic cavity may be lifesaving.

Reinstitution of two-lung ventilation will be necessary before closure of the chest wall to ensure the absence of an air leak at the site of the bronchial resection and suture ligature. At the completion of the surgical procedure, the infant's trachea should be extubated to avoid the development of an air leak at the bronchial suture/staple line as a result of positive-pressure ventilation. Continuation of thoracic epidural analgesia via caudal catheter into the postoperative period will help maintain spontaneous ventilation and minimize or avoid opioid administration.

Pulmonary Sequestration

A pulmonary sequestration is a portion of nonfunctioning lung tissue that does not contain a bronchial connection. Its blood supply is derived from anomalous vessels (usually bronchial or aortic) with azygos venous drainage, sometimes below the diaphragm. Pulmonary sequestrations may be intralobar (within the pleura of a lobe) or extralobar (within its own pleura). Both types occur mainly in the lower lobes. Intralobar sequestration may be confused with a CCAM, which may also have aberrant subdiaphragmatic venous drainage. Although frequently diagnosed in utero, these lesions are usually asymptomatic at birth, unless the lesion is large and compressing normal lung, or the lesion's blood supply is large and results in high-output cardiac failure. More often, however, these lesions remain asymptomatic until they become infected and present as a pneumonia that is resistant to conservative therapy. MRI imaging or angiography may be required to delineate the blood supply and drainage of the lesion before surgery. Because a pulmonary

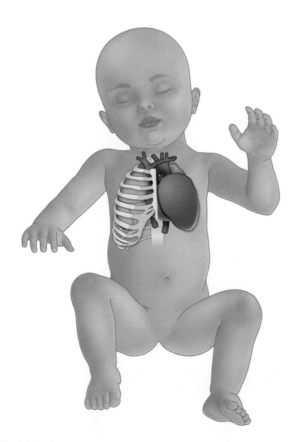

• **Fig 24.1.** Cystic adenomatoid malformation. Illustration by Rob Fedirko. (*Illustration by Rob Fedirko.*).

sequestration has no bronchial connection, there is no risk for overexpansion of the lesion during positive-pressure ventilation, but one-lung ventilation is usually required to allow the surgeon to carefully identify and ligate the arterial supply and venous draining vessels. The presence of aberrant blood flow through the lesion in the operative lung may increase shunt fraction during one-lung ventilation until vascular isolation is obtained.

Tracheoesophageal Fistula

TEF with or without esophageal atresia occurs in approximately 1 in 3000 births and can exist in five different forms (the sixth is isolated esophageal stenosis without a TEF) (Fig. 24.2). Esophageal atresia with a distal TEF (type C) is the most common form (85%). The fistula is usually located slightly above the carina but may also be found as a "trifurcation" at the carina. Any type of esophageal atresia with or without a TEF is usually diagnosed immediately after birth by the inability to pass an orogastric tube into the stomach. Infants with a TEF are distinguished from those with isolated esophageal atresia by the presence of a gastric air bubble on a radiograph. Because TEF is a component of the VATER or VACTERL syndrome, additional congenital abnormalities may be present, including congenital heart disease. Thus an echocardiogram is indicated in the early newborn period and an abdominal ultrasound to detect renal abnormalities. Before surgery, these infants are maintained in a head-up position with a suction tube draining the esophageal pouch, to minimize the possibility of aspiration of gastric and nasopharyngeal contents.

TEF is usually repaired within the first several days of life. A thoracotomy incision is performed on the side opposite the aortic arch (because the vast majority of these children have a left-sided arch, a right thoracotomy is usually performed). The first and most important part of the procedure is ligation of the TEF. The second portion of the procedure involves repair of the esophageal atresia. In most cases, the proximal and distal segments of the esophagus are joined using a primary anastomosis. However, occasionally the two ends are too far apart for primary reanastomosis, and need to be connected at a later date after growth has occurred. At that time either the length of the upper pouch has been increased using a weighted tube or esophageal traction via the Foker technique[6] or, in rare cases, interposition of a section of the infant's colon may be necessary to achieve esophageal continuity. In premature infants smaller than 1800 grams, esophageal atresia repair may be deferred until the infant grows larger because of technical difficulties in these small infants and nutritional deficiencies that may impair proper healing. In these cases, a gastrostomy tube will be placed after the fistula is ligated and the thoracotomy is closed.

An important consideration during induction of general anesthesia for TEF repair is the avoidance of positive-pressure ventilation. Some of this airflow may exit the trachea through the fistula and cause gastric distention, impairing subsequent ventilation and leading to the reflux of gastric contents through the fistula and into the lungs. Cases of massive gastric distention resulting in respiratory compromise, cardiovascular collapse, and emergency gastrostomy have been reported. Therefore maintenance of spontaneous ventilation has been recommended until the fistula has been surgically ligated. In some centers, rigid bronchoscopy is performed before tracheal intubation to fully delineate the site of the fistula, and verify that only a single fistula is present. When necessary, a balloon-tipped catheter can be placed in the fistula to limit gastric insufflation and facilitate positive-pressure ventilation. Placement and dosing of a caudal catheter advanced to a thoracic location (tip at T6) allows a lower concentration of the inhaled anesthetic agent and avoidance of opioids to better maintain spontaneous ventilation. A combination of IV or inhaled anesthetic agents can be administered and titrated to a

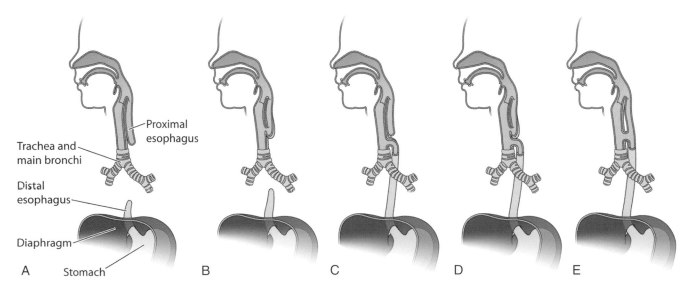

• Fig 24.2. Tracheoesophageal Fistulas (Gross Classification). Panels A through E depict the five different types of tracheoesophageal fistulas. Illustration by Rob Fedirko. (*Illustration by Rob Fedirko.*).

sufficient depth of anesthesia to allow endotracheal intubation while maintaining spontaneous ventilation. However, because of loss of functional residual capacity and high oxygen consumption in newborn infants, it is unusual to be able to preserve spontaneous ventilation while avoiding hypoxemia. Therefore many pediatric anesthesiologists[7] will gently provide assisted or controlled positive-pressure ventilation before endotracheal intubation, and may even administer a neuromuscular blocker if required. Others recommend a rapid sequence induction of general anesthesia as a first-line approach to minimize possible pulmonary aspiration of secretions retained within the proximal esophageal pouch while avoiding positive-pressure ventilation until the endotracheal tube is advanced distal to the fistula. Awake endotracheal intubation in these infants (and other newborns) is no longer considered to be the standard of care, unless the infant is critically ill.

To minimize gastric inflation after tracheal intubation, the tip of the endotracheal tube should be placed between the fistula and the carina. This may be accomplished by advancing the endotracheal tube into the right main bronchus and then gradually pulling it back while auscultating over the left thorax. The endotracheal tube is then positioned at the point where breath sounds are first heard on the left side, indicating that the tip of the tube is above the carina and probably below the position of the fistula. To further minimize the possibility of gastric inflation through the fistula, the bevel of the endotracheal tube is turned anteriorly because the fistula exits on the posterior surface of the trachea toward the esophagus. Use of a Magill or Microcuff (non-Murphy eye) endotracheal tube avoids inadvertent ventilation of the fistula through the Murphy eye. If the fistula exits the trachea close to the carina, it may be necessary to position the endotracheal tube above the fistula to avoid main bronchial intubation. As long as pulmonary inflation pressures are kept low, ventilation will generally not go into the fistula. However, if the infant has lung disease that necessitates relatively high inflating pressures, then the endotracheal tube may need to be positioned in the bronchus of the nonoperative lung until the fistula is ligated.

In the case of high inflating pressures, other methods[8] have been described to accomplish blockage of the fistula, including insertion of an embolectomy catheter[9] balloon from a cephalad approach or from a caudad gastric approach[10] if a gastrostomy has been performed. Both approaches require bronchoscopic guidance and substantial expertise and training.

Intraoperatively, if neuromuscular blockers have not been administered, spontaneous ventilation can be continued until surgical ligation of the fistula, at which time the infant may be safely paralyzed and positive-pressure ventilation initiated. There are many instances during spontaneous ventilation when hypoxemia intervenes because of surgical lung compression on the operative side. It then becomes necessary to begin controlled ventilation to improve ventilatory function and alleviate hypoxemia. Before chest wall closure, the lung on the operative side should be reexpanded under direct vision to minimize the risk for postoperative atelectasis.

After TEF repair most infants are awakened and extubated in the operating room upon completion of the procedure. Because manipulation and suture ligation of the fistula may result in the presence of blood in the tracheobronchial tree, the endotracheal tube should be gently suctioned before tracheal extubation. On occasion, a small volume of saline irrigation is required to clear the blood and secretions. A theoretical risk in extubated infants is disruption of the esophageal repair from bag-mask ventilation and head extension or laryngoscopy in the event that tracheal reintubation is necessary postoperatively. Additional complications of early extubation include hypoxemia and hypoventilation because of airway plugging from secretions, blood, and atelectasis, or inability of smaller infants to maintain increased work of breathing because of decreased compliance related to parenchymal disease.

Infants with evidence of pulmonary aspiration before surgery, or those with parenchymal lung disease because of prematurity, may require postoperative mechanical ventilation. In these cases, the endotracheal tube should be positioned in the upper trachea, 1 cm or more away from the fistula site to allow healing of the fistula repair. In addition, the length between the patient's lips and the site of the esophageal repair should be determined for use as a guide for determining the uppermost limit to which a suction catheter can be advanced postoperatively without risking disruption of the esophageal anastomosis, although some surgeons forbid suctioning beyond the oropharynx.

Some surgeons are now using thoracoscopic[11] techniques for ligation of TEF and esophageal repair in which case lung isolation is required, totally avoiding ventilation of the fistula and stomach. Some surgeons prefer prone or semiprone positioning for these procedures. Epidural analgesia is not necessary for this approach, but a catheter may be inserted via the caudal approach at the end of surgery if conversion to open thoracotomy has occurred.

References

1. Cohen DE, McCloskey JJ, Motas D, Archer J, Flake AW. Fluoroscopic-assisted endobronchial intubation for single-lung ventilation in infants. *Paediatr Anaesth*. 2011;21(6):681–684. https://doi.org/10.1111/j.1460-9592.2011.03585.x.

2. Wald SH, Mahajan A, Kaplan MB, Atkinson JB. Experience with the Arndt paediatric bronchial blocker. *Br J Anaesth*. 2005;94(1):92–94. https://doi.org/10.1093/bja/aeh292.

3. Biswas A, Luginbuehl I, Szabo E, Caldeira-Kulbakas M, Crawford MW, Everett T. Use of Serratus Plane Block for Repair of Coarctation of Aorta: A Report of 3 Cases. *Reg Anesth Pain Med*. 2018;43(6):641–643. https://doi.org/10.1097/AAP.0000000000000801.

4. Holland EL, Bosenberg AT. Early experience with erector spinae plane blocks in children. *Paediatr Anaesth*. 2020;30(2):96–107. https://doi.org/10.1111/pan.13804.

5. Guruswamy V, Roberts S, Arnold P, Potter F. Anaesthetic management of a neonate with congenital cyst adenoid malformation.

Br J Anaesth. 2005;95(2):240–242. https://doi.org/10.1093/bja/aei171.

6. Mochizuki K, Obatake M, Taura Y, et al. A modified Foker's technique for long gap esophageal atresia. *Pediatr Surg Int.* 2012;28(8):851–854. https://doi.org/10.1007/s00383-012-3151-1.

7. Broemling N, Campbell F. Anesthetic management of congenital tracheoesophageal fistula. *Paediatr Anaesth.* 2011;21(11):1092–1099. https://doi.org/10.1111/j.1460-9592.2010.03377.x.

8. Hammer GB. Pediatric Thoracic Anesthesia. *Anesth Analg.* 2001;92(6):1449–1464. https://doi.org/10.1097/00000539-200106000-00021.

9. Filston H, Chitwood Jr WR, Schkolne B, Blackmon LR. The Fogarty balloon catheter as an aid to management of the infant with esophageal atresia and tracheoesophageal fistula complicated by severe RDS or pneumonia. *J Pediatr Surg.* 1982;17(2):149–151. https://doi.org/10.1016/s0022-3468(82)80199-1.

10. Templeton Jr JM, Templeton JJ, Schnaufer L, Bishop HC, Ziegler MM, O'Neill Jr. JA. Management of esophageal atresia and tracheoesophageal fistula in the neonate with severe respiratory distress syndrome. *J Pediatr Surg.* 1985;20(4):394–397. https://doi.org/10.1016/s0022-3468(85)80226-8.

11. Krosnar S, Baxter A. Thoracoscopic repair of esophageal atresia with tracheoesophageal fistula: anesthetic and intensive care management of a series of eight neonates. *Paediatr Anaesth.* 2005;15(7):541–546. https://doi.org/10.1111/j.1460-9592.2005.01594.x.

Suggested Reading

van Hoorn CE, Costerus SA, Lau J, et al. Perioperative management of esophageal atresia/tracheo-esophageal fistula: An analysis of data of 101 consecutive patients. *Paediatr Anaesth.* 2019;29(10):1024–1032. https://doi.org/10.1111/pan.13711.

25

Orthopedic Surgery

WALLIS T. MUHLY*

Musculoskeletal Trauma

General Considerations

Whether via monkey bar falls or trampoline accidents, children often find a way into the operating room for the treatment of musculoskeletal injuries. Approximately 40% of boys and 25% of girls[1] will have at least one fracture before the age of 16. Upper extremity fractures account for two-thirds of fractures in children with the radius being the most commonly involved[2]. Surgical repair or reduction under general anesthesia is indicated in approximately 20% patients; the indications for emergent operative repair include neurovascular compromise and open fractures. Non-emergent operative repair is often required for fractures that include the growth plate, fractures that cannot be effectively reduced noninvasively, or complex fractures of the leg and ankle. Surgical repair ranges in complexity from closed percutaneous pinning (e.g. for supracondylar fractures) to open pelvic or femoral fracture repairs with the potential for significant blood loss.

Children who require emergent surgical reduction for acute fractures are considered to have "full stomach" status and should be managed with a rapid sequence technique (or modified rapid sequence depending on the clinical situation) and tracheal intubation. Children who present for elective repair and have adhered to standard fasting guidelines are at low risk for pulmonary aspiration of gastric contents, unless there are other reasons for delayed gastric emptying such as recent opioid administration. Therefore, any anesthetic or airway management technique is feasible. Pelvic and lower extremity fractures may be associated with a significant amount of blood loss. Obtaining a baseline hemoglobin level may be prudent depending on the magnitude of the injury or the risk for intraoperative bleeding. Postoperative pain management for surgical repair of acute fractures can be facilitated through a variety of approaches including nonsteroidal antiinflammatory medications (e.g., ibuprofen, ketorolac, etc.), acetaminophen, muscle

relaxants (e.g., diazepam, tizanidine, baclofen, etc.), or opioids for a limited period of time. Peripheral nerve blockade with or without a continuous catheter technique may also be advantageous. If a regional anesthetic is used, appropriate monitoring is vital to ensure early detection of compartment syndrome.

Supracondylar Fractures

The most common elbow injury in children requiring surgical repair is the supracondylar humeral fracture. It is associated with neurologic injury (10%–15%) and vascular injury (20%). Neurologic injury is typically traction neuropraxia and resolves over time. Vascular compromise of the brachial artery[3] can result in diminished or absent distal pulses which must be treated emergently if blood flow fails to improve with closed reduction. Closed reduction and pinning is the preferred mode of treatment for displaced elbow fractures. However, open reduction with vascular exploration may be required when the fracture is associated with diminished or absent pulses. The anesthetic management is dictated by the acuity of the injury and the presence of neurovascular compromise. Patients brought to the operation room (OR) emergently for operative reduction should be treated as a full stomach and intubated with a rapid sequence technique. Conversely, an appropriately fasted child, with a stable fracture, can be managed with a supraglottic airway device.

Spica Cast Placement

One strategy for management of acute lower extremity fractures in children is the spica cast, which extends from above the hip bones down to variable locations of the lower extremities. A spica cast can be used to immobilize fractures or deformities involving one or both lower extremities or stabilize fractures of the pelvis. Because it is typically used for preschool-aged children, general anesthesia is required to optimize proper fitting. The child is placed upon an elevated "spica box" during the procedure; therefore airway management usually consists of tracheal intubation or placement of a securely fitting supraglottic airway. The surgeon may request muscle relaxation to assist with skeletal reduction. As the surgeon begins to apply the spica cast, a folded towel

*Many thanks to Dr. Mary Theroux, who wrote the original orthopedic chapter and whose original thoughts form the basis of all subsequent revisions.

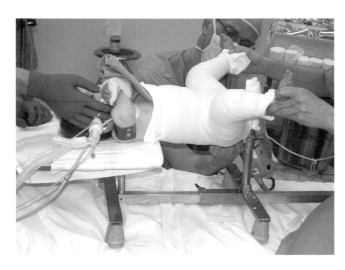

• **Fig 25.1.** Bilateral spica cast placement. For spica cast placement, we prefer tracheal intubation or supraglottic airway placement because the child will be situated upon a platform and moved several times during the procedure.

is placed under the upper portion of the cast to ensure sufficient space between the child's anterior abdominal wall and the cast (Fig. 25.1). Severe postoperative pain or discomfort should prompt examination for a tight or poorly fitted cast.

Slipped Capital Femoral Epiphysis

A unique pediatric musculoskeletal disorder that can present acutely is slipped capital femoral epiphysis (SCFE). Although not specifically a traumatic injury, this hip disorder involves displacement of the femoral head relative to the femoral neck and shaft and most commonly affects obese prepubertal children. It is likely that the combination of physical weakness and/or abnormally large physiologic loads (e.g., obesity) across the physis contribute to the development of this condition. SCFE is associated with pain and the potential for osteonecrosis of the femoral head as the blood supply to the femoral head can be compromised by the displacement of the femoral head. Surgical intervention is typically performed soon after diagnosis. The most common approach involves percutaneous fixation of the femoral head and neck with a cannulated screw to prevent further displacement.

Developmental Dysplasia or Dislocation of the Hip

Developmental dysplasia or dislocation of the hip (DDH) includes all cases of dysplasia, subluxation, or dislocation of the hip joint. The term *DDH* has gradually replaced the term *congenital dysplasia* or *dislocation of the hip* because it is more representative of the range of hip abnormalities that can present in infancy or childhood. DDH has both genetic and environmental factors and it is more common among females (80%) and infants born in the breech presentation.

DDH should be treated early in infancy with bracing techniques that immobilize the affected hip and stabilize the relationship between the femoral head and the acetabulum to facilitate normal development. If the hip remains unstable or if the pelvic anatomy is not amenable to closed reduction, surgical correction consisting of an open reduction with a femoral or pelvic osteotomy may be indicated. Adductor muscle release may also be performed.

Correction of DDH in infants is not associated with significant blood loss. Placement of an endotracheal tube should be considered as patients are typically placed in a spica cast or brace at the conclusion of the procedure, which may necessitate patient movement. Regional anesthesia for postoperative pain control is not necessary if reduction of the hip has been accomplished without invasive surgery. Depending on the extent of the surgery, postoperative analgesia can be accomplished by intraoperative infiltration of a local anesthetic or administration of peripheral or neuraxial block with or without a catheter in addition to systemic analgesic medications.

Spinal Deformity

Spinal disorders can range from the otherwise healthy adolescent presenting for correction of slowly progressing scoliosis to the critically ill infant presenting with restrictive lung disease and pulmonary hypertension secondary to thoracic insufficiency syndrome.[4] Careful surgical and anesthetic planning tailored to patient-specific anatomy and physiology is critical to ensuring positive patient outcomes.

Scoliosis is characterized by a curve of the spine in the frontal plan, which can include the thoracic vertebra, lumbar vertebra, or both. This leads to rotation of the spine and corresponding ribs which produces the characteristic chest wall asymmetry. In mild forms, scoliosis can produce a marked deformity of the trunk which, if allowed to progress, can lead to significant cardiopulmonary impairment. Scoliosis can be congenital, early onset, or idiopathic (typically presenting in adolescence), secondary to neuromuscular disease (cerebral palsy, Duchenne muscular dystrophy, and others) or secondary to systemic disease or syndromes (Marfan syndrome, neurofibromatosis, and others). The etiology of the scoliosis, rate of progression, and age at onset will influence the surgical management.

Early onset scoliosis and adolescent idiopathic scoliosis (AIS) are initially managed with bracing to prevent progression of the deformity. When this is unsuccessful, surgical interventions may be indicated. For scoliosis in younger children who have not yet achieved skeletal maturity, the spine can be stabilized with growing rods that allow for future sequential expansions to ensure adequate thoracic development. Once these patients have achieved skeletal maturity, they typically require posterior spinal fusion. Conversely, adolescents, who have reached skeletal maturity and failed bracing, will be managed with spine fusion primarily. A common measurement of spinal deformity is the Cobb angle, which represents the greatest angulation in a region of the spine. It is measured by drawing intersecting lines from the superior endplate of vertebrae at the top of the curve and the inferior endplate of the vertebrae at the bottom of the curve. A Cobb angle of 10 degrees is required for a diagnosis of scoliosis and when a curve progresses to 45 to 50 degrees or higher, surgical intervention is typically indicated.

Children with neuromuscular diseases such as cerebral palsy or various muscular dystrophies will commonly present for spinal fusion. The combination of diffuse muscle weakness and static or progressive limitations in the ability to ambulate leads to a high rate of scoliosis, with up to 95% patients with Duchenne muscular dystrophy developing progressive scoliosis during their lifetime. The primary reason for repairing the spines of these debilitated children is to allow them to sit upright without assistance, thus decreasing the incidence of chronic pulmonary aspiration, increasing their quality of life, and possibly extending their life expectancy. The most extensive surgical procedure performed in these children is when the spine is instrumented from T1 to the sacrum. These procedures typically involve greater blood loss than for idiopathic repair with the potential for patients to lose 1 to 3 blood volumes. The reason for this increased blood loss in patients with cerebral palsy is not fully understood but it may be related to abnormalities in factor levels and abnormalities in platelet function. Real-time coagulation with assessment of coagulation function with thromboelastography can help guide replacement therapy, and these patients may benefit from the early use of blood and fresh frozen plasma.

Preoperative Considerations

For otherwise healthy patients presenting with early onset scoliosis or AIS, routine pulmonary function testing or cardiac evaluation are likely not necessary as long as there are no concerning functional limitations and the spinal curve is less than 80 degrees. Conversely, patients with severe cerebral palsy or muscular dystrophy may suffer from preoperative respiratory insufficiency and require supplemental respiratory support preoperatively (bilevel positive airway pressure [BiPAP], continuous positive airway pressure [CPAP], etc.). In those patients, pulmonary function testing can help identify patients at risk for postoperative respiratory complications. Coordination with the patient's pulmonologist can help guide postoperative respiratory care and minimize acute respiratory complications (failed extubation, atelectasis, and others). Similarly, providers should have a low threshold for assessing cardiac function in the patient populations at high risk for cardiomyopathy, including Duchenne muscular dystrophy and Friedreich ataxia. Routine echocardiography in all patients with cerebral palsy presenting for spine fusion is unlikely to reveal clinically relevant cardiac abnormalities.[5]

Preoperative laboratory evaluation can include a complete blood count, blood chemistry, coagulation studies, and a type-and-cross though there is little consensus on the relative value of perioperative laboratory assessments such as blood chemistry and coagulation studies in AIS patients. Historically, autologous or directed-donor blood donation[6] was used to reduce the risk for allogenic blood transfusion in this population and, in recent years, the use of intraoperative cell salvage[7] and antifibrinolytic therapy[8] have been shown to reduce the need for allogenic transfusion.

A thorough discussion should take place with the family and patient about the nature and risks of the anesthetic, the surgical procedure, and any neurophysiologic monitoring. If an intraoperative "wake-up" test is planned, the procedure is discussed in detail with the patient to facilitate intraoperative success. The patient and family should also be told that it is common for their face to be swollen postoperatively, and that it will subside over the first two postoperative days.

Intraoperative Considerations

Patients can undergo either an inhalation or IV induction depending on patient and provider preference. Patients are usually induced on the transport bed to simplify turning the patient to a prone position on the OR table (Fig. 25.2). Tracheal intubation can be facilitated with a bolus of propofol and an opioid so as to avoid neuromuscular blockade in anticipation of neuromonitoring. After tracheal intubation,

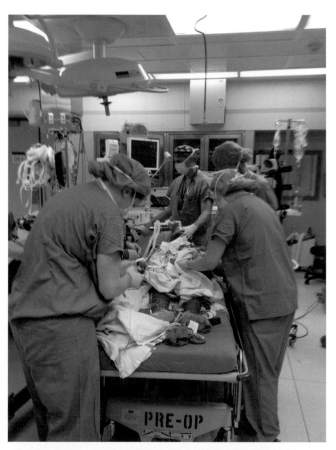

• **Fig 25.2.** Preparing for the spine fusion patient. After induction of general anesthesia, while one member of the anesthesia team manages the airway, the lines are placed, a urinary catheter is inserted, and the neurophysiologist attaches monitoring electrodes.

and before turning the patient prone, all the necessary monitors and lines are inserted. This includes a urinary catheter, orogastric tube, esophageal temperature probe, two peripheral IV lines, arterial line, and neuromonitoring leads. An arterial line is used for close hemodynamic monitoring and laboratory assessments. The ulnar artery should not be cannulated if the radial artery on the same side was punctured or if a hematoma of the radial arterial site develops. Early decision to abandon a failed site because of arterial spasm or hematoma and move to the contralateral side can help save time and avoid injury. A central line is not usually required for AIS patients but may be necessary for children with neuromuscular disease because of underlying medical conditions or challenges with securing adequate peripheral access. Finally, careful attention should be paid to securing the endotracheal tube and protecting the eyes. A soft bite block should be placed between the teeth to prevent trauma to the tongue.

Once all the team members are satisfied that the patient has been optimized for surgery, a soft-foam prone pillow is placed over the patient's face, and the patient is carefully turned prone onto the OR table (different varieties of tables are used depending on the preference of the surgeon) by all members of the team, including the orthopedic surgeons. The responsibility to ensure adequate positioning with proper padding of all vulnerable points (with special attention to the face and around the eyes) is shared between the anesthesiology and surgical teams (Fig. 25.3). The abdomen should remain free to ensure adequate ventilation. An increase in intraabdominal pressure may increase bleeding in the epidural venous plexus. For males, the genitalia should be inspected to be sure there are no points of compression, and for females, the chest roll should be placed at the top portion of the breasts to ensure lack of compression. Use of a forced-air warming device can be used to maintain normothermia and reduce hypothermia-induced coagulopathy and/or delayed awakening.

The choice of anesthetic agents used for maintenance of anesthesia is determined by the use of evoked potentials to monitor spinal cord integrity intraoperatively. A variety of neurophysiologic techniques will be used during

spinal fusion procedures, depending on the preference of the surgeon and the neurophysiologist. Most commonly, somatosensory evoked potentials (SSEPs) and motor evoked potentials (MEPs) are used. The use of low concentrations of volatile agents is variable and will depend on the preference of the neurophysiologist. At this author's institution, a total IV anesthetic without volatile agents is used when SSEP and MEP monitoring is used and the infusion is started as soon as IV access is obtained. General anesthesia is typically maintained with propofol and an opioid (remifentanil or fentanyl) infusion. A variety of other maintenance techniques have been used including long-acting opioids (methadone), neuraxial opioids (intrathecal morphine), and infusions including ketamine, magnesium, and lidocaine to optimize patient post-operative comfort.

Attention to hemostasis is critical to reduce the need for intraoperative or postoperative transfusion. As discussed previously, use of an intraoperative antifibrinolytic (tranexamic acid), cell salvage, and preoperative autologous blood donation have all been used to reduce the need for allogenic blood transfusion. Normotension (mean arterial pressure 60–65) is maintained during the dissection phase to limit blood loss. This can be achieved by deepening the anesthetic or infusing a vasodilator (e.g., nicardipine).

The surgical procedure involves a midline posterior incision and dissection that exposes the spinous processes at the apex of the curve and clears the subperiosteal tissue posteriorly. Intraoperative imaging is used to verify the correct surgical levels. Depending on the type of curve and the preference of the surgeon, pedicle screws, laminar hooks, and/or sublaminar wires are placed on both sides of the spine. An O-arm (360-degree CT scan) may be used to verify the trajectory and length of the screws. Bone graft is placed along the spine to promote fusion between the affected vertebrae. The rods are placed while performing a manual translation followed by derotation maneuvers to complete the straightening of the spine (Fig. 25.4).

The time of correction is critical as this is the point in the procedure where the spinal cord is most vulnerable to ischemia by compression of the local arterial supply and by direct damage from insertion of wires or screws. Mean arterial pressures should be maintained above 70 mm Hg with or without vasoconstrictors (e.g., phenylephrine, dopamine, etc.) and the hemoglobin level should be near 9 g/dL. During and after the distraction, the neurophysiologist continually monitors the patient's evoked potential signals to detect any abnormalities that indicate spinal cord compression. A sudden loss of evoked potentials (loss of MEP, or 50% decrease in SSEP) is a critical event. All surgical manipulation is stopped and, if necessary, the last instrumentation is reversed (e.g., loosening of a pedicle screw or sublaminar wire). The anesthesiologist should increase the mean arterial pressure to at least 90 mm Hg. If improvement in the evoked potentials is not observed, the patient can be treated with steroids (30 mg/kg bolus of methylprednisolone followed by an infusion at 5.4 mg/kg/h for 23 hours[9]), though evidence for the efficacy of this intervention is unclear.[10] If

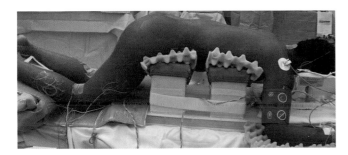

• **Fig 25.3.** Prone positioning for scoliosis repair. Once all lines and monitoring sensors are placed, the child is turned prone into position for optimal surgical access. All pressure points are well padded, especially around the head and neck. Careful attention is paid to the area around the eyes to prevent pressure-induced ischemic injury.

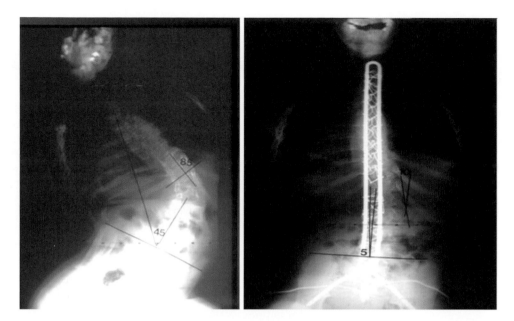

• **Fig 25.4.** Extensive surgical repair from T1 to sacrum. Before and after radiographs.

signals continue to be diminished, the instrumentation may be removed and the patient awakened.

Some surgeons still prefer using a Stagnara wake-up test, in which the patient is transiently awakened immediately after spinal cord distraction and asked to wiggle their toes to demonstrate spinal cord integrity. Preparation of the patient is the key to its success. A useful approach is to practice with the child as he or she is being anesthetized by simply asking the child to wiggle their toes several times just before losing consciousness. Even if the wake-up test is not performed, a child who was properly prepared will emerge from anesthesia and wiggle their toes on command, thus expediting tracheal extubation.

Anterior Spinal Fusion

Both idiopathic and neuromuscular scoliosis patients may require a combined anterior and posterior spinal fusion. The indications for combined fusion include: (1) a curve >75 degrees, (2) a rigid curve, (3) and patients at risk for crankshaft deformity. A crankshaft deformity is a condition where anterior spinal growth continues despite successful posterior spinal fusion, causing a rotational deformity. This occurs in skeletally immature patients who have potential for further spinal bone growth. Anterior spinal fusion consists of anterior disk excision, release of the anterior longitudinal ligament, removal of the annulus fibrosis and nucleus pulposus, and excision of the vertebral endplate cartilage through a thoracic approach with the patient positioned laterally. Some surgeons prefer a thoracoscopic approach, particularly when the number of disks to be released is minimal. This approach may require placement of an endotracheal tube that allows single-lung ventilation. Most surgeons, however, will employ an open approach that may not involve opening the thoracic cavity. Although the procedure is often done in combination with a posterior fusion on the same day, some

surgeons may schedule them as separate procedures with several days in between.

Postoperative Considerations

The postoperative care of patients undergoing posterior spine fusion has changed dramatically over the last decade especially for the AIS population. Historically, patients stayed in the hospital for 5 to 7 days after surgery. In recent years, surgical teams have allowed for early mobilization and dietary advancement which, in addition to the incorporation of broad multimodal analgesic approach, has led to a consistent reduction in length of stay that approaches 3 days at many institutions. Many spine recovery protocols now include the routine administration of gabapentin, nonsteroidal antiinflammatories, and muscle relaxants, in addition to traditional management with IV patient-controlled anesthesia. Reframing expectations and preparing the child to expect a level of discomfort postoperatively can help decrease the anxiety and fear that can accompany this procedure in children. Patients are told that they will be expected to move and participate in physical therapy early in the postoperative period; this likely has a role in improving the patient's functional status in the early and late recovery period.

A comprehensive review article on anesthetic management of pediatric spine surgery can be found here.[11]

References

1. Landin LA. Epidemiology of children's fractures. *J Pediatr Orthop B.* 1997;6(2):79–83. https://doi.org/10.1097/01202412-199704000-00002.

2. Cooper C, Dennison EM, Leufkens HG, Bishop N, van Staa TP. Epidemiology of childhood fractures in Britain: a study using the general practice research database. *J Bone Miner Res.* 2004;19(12):1976–1981. https://doi.org/10.1359/JBMR.040902.

3. Badkoobehi H, Choi PD, Bae DS, Skaggs DL. Management of the pulseless pediatric supracondylar humeral fracture. *J Bone Joint Surg Am*. 2015;97(11):937–943. https://doi.org/10.2106/JBJS.N.00983.

4. Campbell Jr RM, Smith MD. Thoracic insufficiency syndrome and exotic scoliosis. *J Bone Joint Surg Am*. 2007;89(Suppl 1):108–122. https://doi.org/10.2106/JBJS.F.00270.

5. DiCindio S, Arai L, McCulloch M, et al. Clinical relevance of echocardiogram in patients with cerebral palsy undergoing posterior spinal fusion. *Paediatr Anaesth*. 2015;25(8):840–845. https://doi.org/10.1111/pan.12676.

6. Murray DJ, Forbes RB, Titone MB, Weinstein SL. Transfusion management in pediatric and adolescent scoliosis surgery. Efficacy of autologous blood. *Spine (Phila Pa 1976)*. 1997;22(23):2735–2740. https://doi.org/10.1097/00007632-199712010-00007.

7. Bowen RE, Gardner S, Scaduto AA, Eagan M, Beckstead J. Efficacy of intraoperative cell salvage systems in pediatric idiopathic scoliosis patients undergoing posterior spinal fusion with segmental spinal instrumentation. *Spine (Phila Pa 1976)*. 2010;35(2):246–251. https://doi.org/10.1097/BRS.0b013e3181bdf22a.

8. Goobie SM, Zurakowski D, Glotzbecker MP, et al. Tranexamic Acid Is Efficacious at Decreasing the Rate of Blood Loss in Adolescent Scoliosis Surgery: A Randomized Placebo-Controlled Trial. *J Bone Joint Surg Am*. 2018;100(23):2024–2032. https://doi.org/10.2106/JBJS.18.00314.

9. Bracken MB, Shepard MJ, Collins WF, et al. A randomized, controlled trial of methylprednisolone or naloxone in the treatment of acute-spinal cord injury. Results of the Second National Acute Spinal Cord Injury Study. *N Engl J Med*. 1990;322(20):1405–1411. https://doi.org/10.1056/NEJM199005173222001.

10. Liu Z, Yang Y, He L, et al. High-dose methylprednisolone for acute traumatic spinal cord injury: A meta-analysis. *Neurology*. 2019;93(9):e841–e850. https://doi.org/10.1212/WNL.0000000000007998.

11. Soundararajan N, Cunliffe M. Anaesthesia for spinal surgery in children. *Br J Anaesth*. 2007;99(1):86–94. https://doi.org/10.1093/bja/aem120.

26

Neurosurgery

CHRISTOPHER SETIAWAN AND RONALD S. LITMAN

Pediatric neurosurgical patients present a unique set of anesthetic challenges that include treatment of increased intracranial pressure (ICP), the frequent use of lateral and prone positions, and the anesthetic implications of neurophysiologic monitoring. These and other considerations for the neurosurgical patient are addressed in the first part of this chapter, followed by a discussion of anesthetic techniques for common pediatric neurosurgical procedures.

Pathophysiology and Treatment of Increased ICP

It is important to understand the pathophysiology of increased ICP in the child. The rigid cranial vault contains 80% brain tissue, 10% cerebrospinal fluid (CSF), and 10% blood. The Monro–Kellie doctrine states that, for the ICP to remain normal, alterations in the volume of one compartment must be compensated for by opposite changes in another compartment. Once these compensatory measures have been maximized, the ICP will rise dramatically[1] with only a small increase in blood volume (Fig. 26.1). Clinical manifestations include hypertension, bradycardia, and irregular respirations with alterations in mental status.

Autoregulation is the brain's ability to maintain cerebral blood flow (CBF) despite changes in blood pressure (Fig. 26.2).

In the adult uninjured brain, CBF remains relatively constant when arterial pressures are between 50 and 150 mm Hg. In the traumatized brain, this regulatory ability may be lost, and CBF may increase or decrease as the blood pressure increases or decreases, respectively. CBF remains constant when the Pao_2 is above 60 mm Hg but increases dramatically with hypoxemia. A linear relationship exists between CBF and $PaCO_2$ in that blood flow increases as carbon dioxide increases. Furthermore, CBF is closely linked to the cerebral metabolic rate of oxygen ($CMRO_2$) consumption; it will increase if $CMRO_2$ increases, as may occur with seizures, pain, fever, or agitation.

Intracranial hypertension is usually defined as an ICP above 20 mm Hg for more than 5 minutes, and in children is most commonly caused by traumatic brain injury. Neuroresuscitative goals are the prevention of secondary brain injury and limitation of further damage to surrounding neurons.

Structural and functional differences in cranial anatomy between children and adults influence cerebral physiology and management of increased ICP. Normal ICP in small children ranges from 2 to 4 mm Hg compared with the normal adult ICP between 8 and 18 mm Hg. The newborn skull does not completely fuse until the latter part of the first year of life. The intracranial space is relatively compliant and the dura is able to expand when the brain becomes edematous as a result of trauma, hemorrhage, or space-occupying lesions. Thus neonates and small infants may not develop signs and symptoms of the early stages of pathologic processes that increase brain mass. An important clinical correlate is that signs and symptoms of increased ICP in a small infant or neonate may be evidence of already advanced disease. When increased ICP is suspected in these patients, clinical findings of irritability, tense fontanels, psychomotor delay, papilledema, seizures, or characteristic thumb-printing on a plain skull film may aid in the diagnosis. Later in childhood, after fusion of the cranial sutures, children may exhibit less intracranial compliance than adults. This may be caused by a relatively higher percentage of brain tissue to CSF and blood vessels in children. Thus children may be at higher risk for dangerous increases in ICP with relatively less edema, hemorrhage, CSF accumulation, or tumor mass.

The major goal in the management of intracranial hypertension is to ensure adequate oxygen and substrate delivery to the brain to prevent tissue metabolic crisis and neuronal injury. This is achieved at the macrocellular level by ensuring adequate oxygenation and ventilation, lowering the intracranial pressure, and maintaining an adequate cerebral perfusion pressure by optimizing systemic blood pressure.

In cases of increased ICP, the general management goal is to achieve an ICP <20 mm Hg in all ages. The cerebral perfusion pressure (CPP) is the difference between mean arterial pressure (MAP) and the ICP (or central venous pressure [CVP], whichever is greater). Numerous studies have verified that CPP varies directly with age. In children less than 8 years old, a CPP >40 mm Hg is recommended, whereas in older children the CPP should be >60 mm Hg. There is insufficient evidence as to whether it is more important to decrease ICP or optimize CPP during conditions of acutely

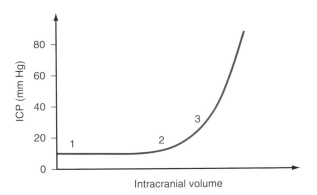

• **Fig 26.1.** Idealized intracranial compliance curve for intracranial pressure (ICP) plotted against intracranial volume. The shape of the curve depends on the time over which the volume increases and the relative size of the compartments. At normal intracranial volumes (point 1), ICP is low but compliance is high and remains so despite small increases in volume. If volume increases rapidly, compensatory abilities are surpassed, and further increases in volume are reflected as increases in pressure. This can occur when the ICP is still within normal limits but the compliance is low (point 2). If the ICP is already increased, further volume expansion causes a rapid increase in ICP (point 3). (From McClain CD, Soriano SG. Pediatric neurosurgical anesthesia. In: Coté CJ, Lerman J, Anderson BJ, eds. *A Practice of Anesthesia for Infants and Children*. 6th ed. Elsevier; 2019:604-628.e5.)

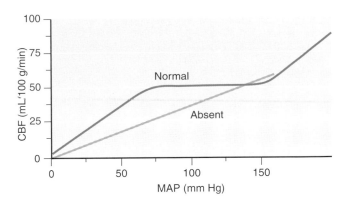

• **Fig 26.2.** Normal and absent autoregulation curves. The "absent" curve indicates a pressure-passive condition in which CBF varies in proportion to cerebral perfusion pressure (CPP). This curve is drawn to indicate subnormal CBF values during normotension, as have been shown to occur immediately after head injury and subarachnoid hemorrhage. The potential for modest hypotension to cause ischemia is apparent. *CBF*, Cerebral blood flow; *MAP*, mean arterial pressure. (From Lemkuil BP, Drummond JC, Patel PM, Lam A. Anesthesia for neurologic surgery and neurointerventions. In: Gropper M, Eriksson L, Fleisher L, et al, eds. *Miller's Anesthesia*, 9th ed. Elsevier; 2020:1868-1910.e9.)

increased ICP, and whether such manipulation affects neurologic outcome. Nevertheless, in pediatric patients, CPP values <40 mm Hg are strongly correlated with worse outcomes[2] at any ICP.

Intracranial pressure can be monitored using extradural, intraparenchymal, or intraventricular catheters. Intraventricular catheters have the additional therapeutic benefit of CSF drainage for ICP elevation management. The main indication for placement of an ICP monitor is a depressed Glasgow Coma Scale in the setting of acute brain injury.

Recently, brain tissue oxygen tension monitors have been used more frequently to guide neuroresuscitative strategies. These probes are placed in the white matter of the brain parenchyma, often in vulnerable brain tissue at risk for tissue hypoxia, cellular injury, and neuronal death. Brain tissue oxygen tension ($PbtO_2$) levels of 10 to 15 mm Hg correlate with poor outcome, while values of 25 to 26 mm Hg are observed in an uninjured brain. Augmenting CBF to target the $PbtO_2$ allows for additional goal-directed targets for cerebral resuscitation.

Fundamental methods to lower ICP are the same in children as in adults. These include elevating the head >30 degrees, avoiding jugular kinking by keeping the head positioned in the midline, ensuring adequate analgesia and sedation (caution in spontaneously ventilating patients with a natural airway), controlling ventilation with avoidance of excessive hyper or hypocapnea (i.e., which may result in unintended cerebral vasodilation or vasoconstriction and thus unintended effects on CBF), avoiding excessive ventilating pressures if positive-pressure ventilation and positive end-expiratory pressure (PEEP) are used, and optimizing arterial oxygenation.

Tracheal intubation is indicated if airway protective reflexes are absent or if there is a depressed level of consciousness Glasgow Coma Scale (GCS ≤8). Aside from risks of aspiration and worsening hypoxemia, acute hypoventilation can result in cerebral vasodilation, which can increase ICP and decrease CPP. Short-term hyperventilation is one of the most potent therapies to lower elevated ICP. However, prolonged hyperventilation or excessive hypocapnea is associated with worsening cerebral ischemia and is not recommended.

Recent studies indicate that application of PEEP does not increase intracranial pressure. Therefore, PEEP should be used to minimize alveolar collapse and optimize adequate oxygenation if clinically indicated. The current cardiovascular management strategy consists of volume resuscitation and vasopressor support as needed to maintain CPP. Administration of inhaled anesthetics will cause generalized cerebral vasodilation. In adults, an acute increase in ICP will render the patient more susceptible to the deleterious effects of volatile anesthetics. This is probably true in the pediatric population as well. Furthermore, neonates and infants appear to maintain the same degree of cerebral vasoconstriction in response to decreased Pco_2, as seen in adults. However, there is evidence that in anesthetized infants and children, cerebral vasodilation may occur at lower levels of Pco_2 than observed in adults.

Additional principles of ICP management include avoidance of hyperthermia, maintenance of normoglycemia, and seizure prophylaxis if indicated. Hyperthermia increases $CMRO_2$ and may cause a mismatch between metabolic demand and supply. Hyperglycemia will exacerbate neuronal injury and therefore should be aggressively treated with insulin. Additionally, seizure activity (especially if uncontrolled) can greatly increase $CMRO_2$ and cerebral metabolic demand, potentially worsening neuronal injury.

Hyperosmolar therapy continues to be an important component of ICP management. Mannitol (0.25–1 g/kg infused intravenously over 10–30 minutes) creates an osmotic gradient that draws extracellular brain water across the blood–brain barrier into the intravascular space. It is also thought to decrease blood viscosity, thereby enhancing oxygen delivery. The prophylactic use of mannitol is not recommended because of its volume-depleting diuretic effect, which can increase risk for systemic hypotension as well as acute kidney injury in susceptible patients. Mannitol should be reserved for critical patients with increased ICP and signs of transtentorial herniation, or intraoperatively, to assist the neurosurgeon with brain relaxation. Hypertonic saline is being used more frequently to control ICP. It reduces cerebral swelling by producing an osmolar gradient to decrease cerebral water content. Continuous infusion of 3% NaCl through a central line will prevent swings in osmolality and maintain intravascular volume. It is not unusual to have serum sodium concentrations between 150 and 160 mEq/L. Side effects of hyperosmolar therapy include renal failure (especially if the serum osmolality is >320 mEq/L), hemolysis, and subarachnoid hemorrhage related to tearing of bridging vessels caused by rapid brain shrinkage. Rapid increases in serum sodium are also associated with development of central pontine myelinolysis, so 3% saline boluses should be carefully administered.

Barbiturate coma (burst suppression on EEG) is indicated when intracranial hypertension is not controlled with conventional therapies. Barbiturates lower ICP by reducing $CMRO_2$, which then results in cerebral vasoconstriction and a reduction in CBF and volume. Barbiturates produce respiratory depression and a dose-dependent decrease in arterial blood pressure and cardiac output that often requires significant volume resuscitation and inotropic therapy. When the above measures fail, decompressive craniectomy can be considered in patients with reversible injury. The long-term neurologic benefit in patients with severe traumatic brain injury managed with decompressive craniectomy in pediatrics is unclear.

There has been a major shift in the way Pco_2 is managed during adult neurosurgery, and this has extended into pediatric practice. Adult guidelines conclude that prophylactic hyperventilation ($Paco_2$ <35 mm Hg) can theoretically compromise cerebral perfusion during a time when CBF is already reduced and may thus promote cerebral ischemia. Moreover, studies have shown that hyperventilation does not consistently lower CBF and may cause loss of autoregulation. Studies on hyperventilation in the pediatric population have yielded similar findings. Thus in pediatric patients, prophylactic hyperventilation is not recommended for fear of vasoconstriction-induced aggravation of cerebral ischemia, especially in situations of compromised regional CBF. Rather, mild hyperventilation to the lower end of eucapnia (Pco_2 in mid 30s) is most often used, the major reason being to offset the possible vasodilatory effects of general anesthetics. In the face of acute, dangerously increased ICP (i.e., sudden decline in mental status in patient with suspected increased ICP), lowering the Pco_2 below the previous level will usually result in cerebral vasoconstriction and, at least temporarily, decrease ICP. This principle may extend to Pco_2 levels below 30 mm Hg. When managing increased ICP, the fractional inspired oxygen concentration should always be set to 1.0 to maximize oxygen delivery to the brain cells.

Preoperative Assessment

The preoperative evaluation of the neurosurgical patient is critical because it can directly impact intraoperative planning, choice of anesthetic technique, physiologic goals, and ultimately disposition. Many children presenting for neurosurgery may have been hospitalized for evaluation of a recently diagnosed brain mass, vascular malformation, intracranial bleed, or malfunctioning shunt. During the course of this hospitalization, baseline laboratory values and trends, abnormal physical exam findings, and intracranial imaging should be available and evaluated. Other children with known brain pathology may have had their evaluation and imaging as an outpatient and may be admitted to the hospital on the day of the surgery. Required blood tests include a hemoglobin, and in most tumor or neurovascular cases, a type-and-screen or crossmatch if significant blood loss is anticipated. Electrolytes should be obtained if there is a possibility of hormonal alterations of sodium homeostasis, such as cerebral salt wasting, diabetes insipidus, acid–base disturbances, or syndrome of inappropriate antidiuretic hormone secretion (SIADH). These lab values may require intervention in critical patients, whether encountered preoperatively or during the course of the anesthetic. Many neurosurgical patients are often on an antiepileptic drug regimen, whether prophylactically (i.e., brain mass) or therapeutically. Unless the drug regimen is changing, or the child's seizures are uncontrolled, preoperative anticonvulsant levels are typically not indicated. In addition to consultation with the neurosurgical team, prior computed tomography (CT), magnetic resonance imaging (MRI), or angiography imaging should also be evaluated preoperatively, as these can aid in determining the surgical approach, patient positioning, and preoperative planning.

Documentation of a neurologic examination that focuses on function of the cranial nerves, brachial plexus and lumbar/sciatic plexus (especially in patients with focal neurologic deficits) is essential in the preoperative period, as these values can be compared with postoperative exams, if there is concern for an intraoperative complication. In patients with concern for severe ICP and risk for impending herniation, a focused cranial nerve evaluation with emphasis on the pupillary light reflex should be considered and routinely assessed.

The majority of children presenting for neurosurgery will benefit from preoperative anxiolysis. Because most of these children already have indwelling intravenous (IV) catheters, midazolam can be titrated to effect in the preoperative holding area. Oral or intranasal midazolam may also be administered in children without IV access. In patients presenting with ongoing pain, opioids such as fentanyl can be administered, but should be done cautiously as excessive sedation will result in hypoventilation and hypercarbia, which contribute to potential worsening of increased ICP; this situation, however, is unusual in children. Those children with acutely increased ICP will present emergently and are often obtunded or too ill to benefit from preoperative anxiolysis. In patients with acute presentation of neurosurgical pathology (acute subdural hematoma, sudden change in mental status or neurologic examination), airway protection and ventilation must be frequently assessed, and if necessary, secured before arrival in the operating room (OR) to optimize cerebral perfusion and minimize secondary insult.

It is commonly thought that increased ICP slows gastric emptying and renders the patient at risk for aspiration of gastric contents. Yet very few data exist, especially in children, to substantiate this belief. In addition, clinical experience has shown that aspiration is rare in this population. Therefore, premedication with H_2-antagonists and metoclopramide is not indicated unless the procedure is emergent and the child had a recent meal, or if there are other reasons to suspect that the child has abnormally increased gastric contents.

Anesthetic Techniques

A modified rapid sequence induction of general anesthesia is the preferred technique because of the small possibility of increased gastric contents in patients with increased ICP. Any IV induction agent can be used, along with a nondepolarizing neuromuscular blocker, while an assistant provides cricoid pressure during gentle bag-mask ventilation to minimize excessive hypercarbia. Succinylcholine is usually avoided because of its propensity to increase ICP, yet, if a reasonable risk for pulmonary aspiration of gastric contents exists, a full rapid sequence induction using succinylcholine or high-dose rocuronium is indicated. In the subset of patients with prior history of upper or lower motor neuron deficits (i.e., stroke, paraplegia, etc.), succinylcholine is contraindicated out of concern for uncontrolled hyperkalemic response because of potential upregulation of acetylcholine receptors throughout the muscle membrane. With the recent introduction of sugammadex, which has been shown to have a good safety profile in the pediatric population, rapid sequence induction with rocuronium is a good alternative. If the child does not have an indwelling IV catheter, and there is no reasonable risk for pulmonary aspiration of gastric contents, then an inhaled induction can be performed. Cricoid pressure is applied as soon as the child loses consciousness, and IV access is rapidly attained to permit continuation of a modified rapid sequence technique. The benefit of cricoid pressure here is questionable, and some practitioners may choose to omit it.

The mechanism by which succinylcholine causes transient increases in ICP is unknown. Some evidence suggests

that it is caused by afferent neuronal muscle spindle activity that results from muscle fasciculations. In adults, pretreatment with a small dose of a nondepolarizing muscle relaxant may prevent this increase in ICP from succinylcholine. Because small children tend not to exhibit muscle fasciculations, this effect of succinylcholine may not be observed. Nevertheless, unless succinylcholine is indicated based on the child's risk for aspiration or airway status, it is best avoided during induction of general anesthesia.

When avoidance of potential acute increases in ICP is of concern during induction of anesthesia, additional therapies are indicated. These include IV opioids, lidocaine, and even dexmedetomidine, which will help blunt the hemodynamic response to laryngoscopy and tracheal intubation, and thus help minimize dangerous increases in ICP. In addition, scalp infiltration with a local anesthetic[1] will limit the hemodynamic response to the surgical incision. Traditionally, the bulk of the opioid dose is given toward the beginning of the neurosurgical case, because tracheal intubation, cranial pin application for head immobilization, positioning, scalp incision, and craniotomy are the most painful and stimulating events. Furthermore, residual opioid effect is undesirable at the end of the procedure when the goals are the rapid attainment of consciousness and tracheal extubation to facilitate an immediate neurologic exam. Fentanyl, 2 to 6 µg/kg, is commonly used during induction and can be used intraoperatively as an infusion with careful consideration for context-sensitive half-time. Remifentanil is a reasonable alternative and can be used as a continuous infusion throughout the procedure. Some adult studies have suggested that alfentanil and sufentanil may increase ICP by either increasing CSF volume or increasing CBF. A study[1] in children examined the effect of alfentanil (10–40 µg/kg) on ICP in children with moderately elevated ICP presenting for revision of VP shunts. Alfentanil consistently produced a decrease in CPP that was largely accounted for by decreases in blood pressure. Increases in ICP were not observed. Ketamine is usually avoided in high-risk situations because of its propensity to increase ICP.

Any inhaled volatile agent can be used for maintenance of general anesthesia; in adults, this choice does not affect the outcome of neurosurgical procedures. All volatile general anesthetic agents can cause cerebral vasodilation and increase ICP by increasing CBF and volume, yet there is some reduction in $CMRO_2$ that may offset this augmentation. Studies in children have used the transcranial Doppler technique to measure the blood flow velocity of the middle cerebral artery, which in turn may represent overall CBF and volume. In children, isoflurane appears to have minimal effects on CBF and cerebrovascular reactivity to CO_2 between 0.5 and 1.5 minimum alveolar concentration (MAC). Furthermore, administration of a constant concentration of isoflurane over time does not affect cerebral hemodynamic variables. Sevoflurane appears to have similar effects as isoflurane, although it has not been well studied in children. Desflurane has been shown to increase ICP in adults despite application of hypocarbia but has not been directly studied in children.

Nitrous oxide (N_2O) increases CBF when used alone and in combination with propofol or sevoflurane.[5] However, it does not appear to increase CBF when combined with desflurane. This lack of effect may be explained by the potent baseline cerebrovascular dilation effect of desflurane. Overall, the vasodilatory cerebrovascular effects of all inhaled anesthetics in children are similar to that of adults. With normal levels of ICP, there is probably no clinical difference between agents. In conditions of increased ICP, although effects on CBF are mitigated by moderate hyperventilation for all volatile anesthetic agents, a balanced anesthetic technique should be employed with minimal concentrations of inhaled agents combined with an opioid-based technique.

Normally, fentanyl 1 to 5 µg/kg/h or remifentanil 0.1 to 0.3 µg/kg/min is continued throughout the procedure and targeted to desired hemodynamic parameters. As part of the preanesthetic planning, one should consider the gradual increase in the context sensitive half-time of fentanyl if used as an infusion during a prolonged procedure, especially when extubation and prompt neurologic evaluation is planned at the end of the case. In adults, studies that have examined the role of remifentanil as the primary anesthetic agent to facilitate early extubation have not demonstrated any differences in short- or long-term outcome. Similar studies have not been performed in children. Neuromuscular blockade throughout the procedure is encouraged to facilitate positioning, especially if Mayfield pins secured to the cranium are used, and to assure lack of patient movement during brain dissection. Children on chronic anticonvulsant therapy will require more frequent dosing of aminosteroidal muscle relaxants. If the child has a preexisting hemiparesis, the twitch monitor should be placed on the nonhemiparetic side.

Use of N_2O is controversial in neurosurgery because there is evidence that it raises $CMRO_2$ and may increase CBF and ICP. No outcome studies exist that influence the decision whether to include it in the anesthetic management of children. However, because N_2O is not essential for any reason in neuroanesthesia, it should not be used when increased ICP is a possibility. In addition, N_2O is contraindicated in any child who returns for a repeat craniotomy within 1 month because of the possible development of pneumocephalus[6] secondary to air remaining within the ventricles or cisternal system.

A general rule in pediatric neuroanesthesia is that if a child's trachea was not intubated on arrival to the OR, then he or she should be awakened at the completion of the procedure with the intent of tracheal extubation and immediate neurologic evaluation. Exceptions include cases where adverse intraoperative events occurred that would likely cause postoperative cardiorespiratory depression, need for immediate postoperative imaging, or if there is concern with the ability of the child to protect their airway from obstruction or aspiration. Children with acute head trauma who underwent tracheal intubation in the field or the emergency department are also potential candidates for tracheal extubation after a successful evacuation of a blood clot or hemorrhage,

assuming all cardiorespiratory parameters have normalized. Children in whom life-threatening increased ICP is expected to persist into the postoperative period should receive continuous sedation and neuromuscular blockade, and should be managed postoperatively in the intensive care unit (ICU) with controlled mechanical ventilation.

Positioning Children for Neurosurgery

Positioning pediatric patients for neurosurgery entails proactive attention to detail that will prevent complications or problems during the procedure. This includes careful fixation of the endotracheal tube and securing of circuit, atraumatic placement of an orogastric tube and esophageal temperature probe, administration of petroleum-based eye lubrication, careful securing of arterial and IV catheters/lines, and careful positioning of an indwelling urinary catheter. Most often the patient will be positioned supine with the head turned to the side, but many procedures require prone, lateral, head-up (i.e., semi-sitting, reverse trendelenburg) or even sitting (rarely) positioning. All anesthetic monitors and access lines should be placed and their adequacy confirmed before draping. In addition, the anesthesiologist must plan the workspace so as to include adequate access to the patient during the surgery. Padding pressure points will help prevent compression injuries. If the patient is prone, free and easy abdominal movement with ventilatory movements should be confirmed by inspection of the abdomen and confirmation that ventilatory compliance is unchanged from baseline.

Though declining in frequency, the sitting position may occasionally be used in pediatric patients for surgical access to the posterior fossa; it entails the same monitoring and safety considerations as for adults in the sitting position. Similarly, in children there is also the risk for venous air embolism from entrainment of air into open vessels. A retrospective audit[7] of complications associated with the sitting position in children reported the incidence of venous air embolism to be about 9%. All were detected and treated appropriately, and none directly caused morbidity or mortality. Other pediatric studies have reported an incidence of venous air embolism in the sitting position as high as 37%. Some evidence exists that children have higher dural sinus pressures than adults, and may account for the generally lower incidence of venous air embolism in children compared with adults. However, some studies suggest that venous air embolism is more likely to result in hypotension in pediatric patients because, in theory, the same-sized air bubble would be larger relative to the smaller blood volume of children and, therefore, cause greater hemodynamic instability. Overall, outcome studies in children in the sitting position do not show greater risk than in adults. If one is planning to use the sitting position in a child, it is strongly recommended to obtain a preoperative echocardiograph to rule out any interatrial or interventricular communications. Even when the standard sitting position is not used, the risk of venous air embolism[8] via open venous channels in the bone and dural sinuses still exists, especially when the head of the table is elevated to improve surgical access and cerebral venous drainage. In addition to invasive blood pressure monitoring transduced at the level of the brain and vigilant hemodynamic monitoring, the standard use of a well-positioned and tested precordial Doppler for these situations is recommended to rapidly detect the presence of a venous air embolism. Although some institutions may place central venous catheters for the purpose of theoretical management of a venous air embolism, there is little data in children to suggest that the benefits of this indication outweigh the potential risks of its placement and use.

Manipulation of the head and cervical spine is frequent during neurosurgical positioning and complications of such positioning (i.e., brain ischemia, paraplegia) can be disastrous. Rotation of the cervical spine can result in some decrease in ipsilateral carotid blood flow. Extreme flexion of the neck can compromise vertebral and carotid arterial blood flow as well venous drainage, and positioning should be checked to ensure that there is sufficient thyromental distance (2–3 fingerbreadth). Given the inherent risks, patient positioning should be a joint effort between surgical and anesthesia teams, and the final position should be agreed upon before incision.

When a child is positioned for neurosurgery in a head frame fixation device (e.g., Mayfield or Sugita) there is often flexion of the neck. This maneuver may result in downward displacement of the endotracheal tube within the trachea and cause the endotracheal tube to enter the right main bronchus. Therefore in anticipation of neck flexion, the endotracheal tube should be positioned on the higher side within the trachea, to compensate for its descent. Once positioning is finalized, bilateral breath sounds should be confirmed; in children with healthy lungs, any unexplained oxygen saturation below 96% (especially if accompanied with increased inspiratory pressures and decreased breath sounds to left lung fields) should prompt an exploration for a right main bronchial intubation.

When an invasive head fixation device is used to secure the patient's head, one must take into consideration the stimulation from placement of the device throughout the anesthetic. Pin placement may serve as a highly stimulating part of the anesthetic, especially if lower levels of maintenance are used during line placement and initial positioning at the start of the case. At the end of the case, the anesthetic should be planned to maintain adequate depth until the pins are removed, while planning for a rapid emergence thereafter for extubation and neurologic evaluation.

Neurophysiologic Monitoring

Many neurosurgeons employ the use of intraoperative neurophysiologic monitoring to evaluate the function of neurologic pathways and to prevent potential cerebral or spinal cord ischemia. This may include electrocorticography (ECoG), electroencephalography (EEG), somatosensory evoked potentials (SSEP), motor evoked potentials (MEP), and brainstem auditory evoked potentials (BAEP). When these modalities are used, the anesthesiologist should proactively discuss with the neurophysiologist the implications of anesthetic management on the accuracy of the monitoring. Because many anesthetic agents (i.e., clinically required concentrations of volatile agents) have impact on the sensitivity and quality of neurophysiologic signals, the anesthetic goal in these situations is to maintain steady-state levels of anesthetic agents. The technique most frequently employed is total intravenous anesthesia without neuromuscular blockade, often with a titratable analgesic (i.e., remifentanil, fentanyl, sufentanil) and use of a propofol infusion or low-dose volatile agent for hypnosis. Use of remifentanil is advantageous in these situations, as it will be rapidly eliminated at the end of the procedure to allow prompt return of spontaneous ventilation and emergence. Additionally, significant changes in physiologic variables (temperature, hemodynamics, ventilation, electrolytes, glucose levels) have been associated with changes in evoked potentials.

Sevoflurane, isoflurane, and desflurane can increase signal latency and decrease amplitude in a dose-dependent manner and can abolish MEPs to a greater degree than SSEPs. As a sole agent, N_2O reduces amplitude and increases latency without changing wave morphology but does so to a greater effect when combined with halogenated agents. Conversely, ketamine can increase SSEPs and MEPs and can be used as a bolus or infusion, especially for surgeries at risk for significant postoperative pain (i.e., multilevel spinal fusion, scoliosis surgery); in patients with increased ICP, however, this medication should be used with caution. Similarly, etomidate has been shown to increase cortical SSEPs and a negligible MEP depression. Dexmedetomidine, an alpha-2 agonist, can be safely used as it has been shown to have clinically nonsignificant impact on neurophysiologic signals.

Fluid Management

Except for neonates or other children who may be at risk for development of hypoglycemia, glucose-containing solutions are generally avoided during neurosurgical procedures. Though definitive outcome studies are lacking, hyperglycemia has been associated with worse neurologic outcomes during episodes of brain ischemia. Isotonic solutions such as normal saline or Plasma-Lyte are typically advocated during neurosurgery to lessen the risk for excess brain water, but Lactated Ringer's solution can also be used if ICP is not increased.

Common Pediatric Neurosurgical Procedures

Ventriculoperitoneal Shunt Insertion or Revision

Ventriculoperitoneal (VP) shunt insertion or revision is probably the most commonly performed pediatric neurosurgical procedure. A shunt is initially placed to palliate disorders that cause hydrocephalus. The proximal end of the shunt is placed within the lateral ventricle of the brain, and the shunt is tunneled underneath the scalp and skin of the neck, chest, and abdomen, where it inserts into the peritoneal cavity to drain CSF. Some children may have their shunt terminate into the atrium via one of the large veins of the neck or chest. Children with existing shunts will periodically require revisions because of a variety of reasons that include growth, obstruction, and infection. Occasionally, these revisions will be performed on an emergent basis if the child exhibits signs or symptoms of acutely increased ICP.

There are a variety of causes of hydrocephalus. The most common cause of congenital hydrocephalus is narrowing of the aqueduct of Sylvius. Acquired hydrocephalus is most commonly a result of intracranial hemorrhage in prematurely born infants. Other causes of hydrocephalus that require shunting include Arnold-Chiari compression associated with myelomeningocele, infections, tumors, and head injury.

Preoperative assessment consists of evaluation of comorbidities and the severity of increased ICP. Premedication with an anxiolytic such as midazolam is usually indicated, but when a child is deemed to have clinically important increased ICP, an IV catheter should be placed before surgery, and premedication is then carefully titrated under direct supervision. There is no routine preoperative blood work except evaluation of electrolytes if protracted vomiting is present preoperatively.

Perioperative fluids should consist of normal saline solution or Lactated Ringer's solution. Insensible losses usually range from 2 to 4 mL/kg/h. Standard monitors are appropriate, and one IV access line is usually sufficient.

In children with preoperative signs and symptoms of increased ICP, a modified rapid sequence IV induction is indicated. A moderate amount of opioid is used to facilitate induction and tracheal intubation but should be tailored toward tracheal extubation at the completion of the procedure. Any volatile or IV anesthetic agent is appropriate for maintenance of general anesthesia. N_2O should be avoided if the child has had a craniotomy within the past month, because of the possibility of expanding an existing pneumocephalus. After tracheal intubation, the stomach should be suctioned with an appropriate large-diameter (i.e., 14-16 French) orogastric tube, and an esophageal temperature probe is recommended.

The surgical procedure for initial insertion consists of two small incisions: one on the lateral side of the head, and the other on the skin of the abdomen, with which to retrieve the tunneled shunt and insert it into the peritoneum. Ordinarily the entire unilateral area from the head to the abdomen is prepared and draped. The child lies supine with the head turned away from the operative side. The OR table is turned 90 degrees away from the anesthesiologist (Fig. 26.3A and B).

The most commonly used VP shunt is made of Silastic and contains a bubble reservoir with a one-way valve that

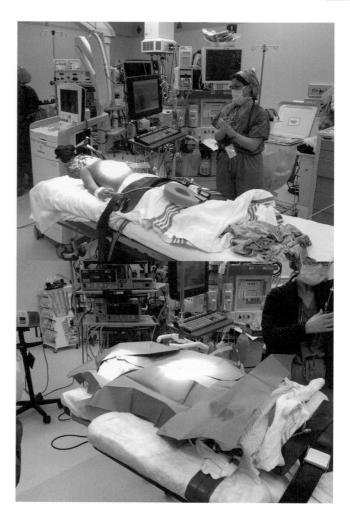

• **Fig 26.3.** (A) Ventriculoperitoneal (VP) shunt. Positioning 90° from anesthesia machine. (B) Ventriculoperitoneal (VP) shunt. Prepped, draped, and ready for incision. Photo credit to Ronald S. Litman.

allows passive flow of CSF out of the brain. With existing shunts that require revision because of malfunction and increasing hydrocephalus, the obstruction can be located either proximally between the lateral ventricle and the valve, or distally between the valve and the tip of the shunt in the peritoneal cavity.

Postoperative concerns include observation for neurologic changes that may be a signal of impending shunt malfunction or intracranial bleeding. Opioids are occasionally required for moderate pain; significant postoperative headache should initiate an investigation of an additional cause.

Anesthesia for Central Nervous System Tumor Resection

Most intracranial tumors in children (more than 60%) are cerebellar and brainstem malignancies of the posterior fossa. Preoperative presentation can include vomiting, headache, and gait and balance abnormalities. Laboratory evaluation consists of hemoglobin, type-and-screen, and electrolytes, which may be altered by chronic vomiting or hormonal effects of tumors. Preoperative anxiolytic medications are tailored to the condition of the child.

There is insufficient data to suggest that patients with brain tumors are at an increased risk for pulmonary aspiration during induction of general anesthesia. Therefore any method of induction and tracheal intubation is acceptable, without the need for modified or strict rapid sequence induction. After tracheal intubation, the stomach should be suctioned with an orogastric tube, and an esophageal stethoscope and temperature probe are recommended. An additional large-bore IV cannula is placed, and an arterial line (depending on the length and invasiveness of the procedure, see below) is inserted to monitor blood pressure changes closely and facilitate access to blood for periodic measurement of hemoglobin, electrolytes, and acid–base status. Isotonic IV fluids (e.g., normal saline, Plasma-Lyte) are recommended, and should be compatible with concomitant blood administration. Ventilation is adjusted to maintain the P_{CO_2} in the normocapnic (35 ± 5 mm Hg) range.

Major craniotomies will require direct blood pressure measurement by arterial cannulation. Beat-to-beat arterial pressure is required when there is the possibility of rapid hemodynamic changes that may result from blood loss, venous air embolism, or unexpected effects from manipulation of the cranial nerves or the brainstem. An arterial catheter will also provide a method to easily obtain blood gas samples when using mild hyperventilation, or when the anesthesiologist needs rapid determination of hemoglobin.

Intraoperative risks include the possibility of unpredictable and sudden blood loss (from the area surrounding the tumor, or from a venous sinus tear), brain herniation, venous air embolism, positioning-related complications, and airway edema. Stimulation of brainstem structures in the posterior fossa can cause sudden hypertension, hypotension, and/or bradycardia. Adjuvant therapies include antibiotics, mannitol, hypertonic saline, prophylactic anticonvulsants, and glucocorticoids (i.e., dexamethasone), depending on the preferences of the surgeon. If the patient was administered acetazolamide preoperatively, expect a baseline metabolic acidosis (and unusually low $P_{ET}CO_2$). Blood loss during tumor removal in small children and infants can be unexpected, rapid, and life-threatening. Before beginning a major craniotomy, two intravenous lines should be established in the extremities. Central access is unnecessary, unless dictated by the child's underlying medical condition or when massive blood loss is expected, as is usually the case of a neonatal brain tumor that occupies much of the brain. If adequate peripheral access is difficult, the femoral approach to venous cannulation is a feasible alternative because it avoids the risk for pneumothorax associated with subclavian or internal jugular vein puncture and will not interfere with cerebral venous return.

Mannitol is often administered during craniotomies at doses that range from 0.25 to 1.0 g/kg, and is almost always used in the setting of increased ICP; many neurosurgeons, however, will ask that it be administered during routine cases. By transiently raising serum osmolality, mannitol will draw free water out of the brain and into the circulation. Because of its diuretic effect, urine output will increase for approximately 1 hour after its administration. It should be given no faster than 0.5 g/kg over 20 to 30 minutes because of the possibility of hypotension and decreased CPP if given at a faster rate. Furosemide (0.25–1 mg/kg) is also useful for decreasing cerebral edema and has been shown *in vitro* to prevent rebound swelling because of mannitol. When diuretics are administered, urine output and electrolytes are rendered unreliable for diagnosing hypovolemia, and hormonal imbalances of sodium, such as diabetes insipidus, or SIADH. Dexamethasone is commonly administered to children to decrease brain swelling associated with intracranial masses but does not possess acute effects. Although hypertonic saline is finding increasing popularity in the pediatric population as an adjuvant treatment for increased ICP, it is less commonly utilized in the OR for elective cases.

Assuming there are no intraoperative events that would warrant postoperative ventilation, tracheal extubation at the completion of the procedure should be planned. The neurosurgeons will want to evaluate the child's neurologic status as soon as possible after regaining consciousness. In fact, the child is often kept in the OR until a superficial neurologic exam is completed. Unexpected deficits or delayed awakening will warrant an immediate head CT scan to detect unanticipated brain herniation or bleeding.

Postoperative considerations include frequent neurologic assessments to detect intracranial events and careful monitoring of cardiorespiratory parameters. Analgesic requirements are variable and some children require opioids. Significant head pain should warrant an investigation for intracranial complications.

Myelomeningocele Repair

Myelomeningocele (also known as spina bifida) is the most common congenital defect of the central nervous system, with a prevalence rate of approximately 4 per 10,000 live births. A myelomeningocele is a fetal malformation involving a posterior protrusion of the spinal cord and meninges through a defect in the spinal column and back, usually at the lumbar level (Fig. 26.4A). Because of the risk for meningitis, it is considered a surgical urgency and infants are almost always operated on within 24 hours of birth. Most infants born with myelomeningocele have an accompanying Arnold-Chiari malformation, resulting from downward displacement of the hindbrain into the foramen magnum, and thus receive a VP shunt before discharge home in the newborn period.

Preoperative assessment includes careful documentation of all neurologic deficits and a review of other organ systems to rule out additional congenital malformations (i.e., congenital heart defects). Blood work should include a hemoglobin and type-and-screen. Premedication is not indicated for this age group.

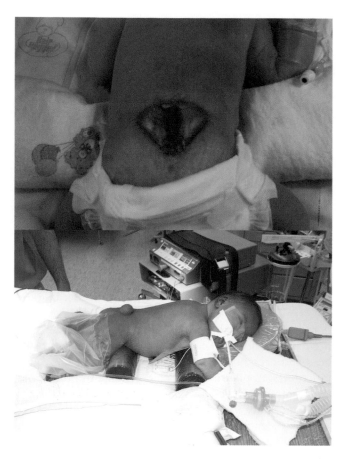

• **Fig 26.4.** (A) Open myelomeningocele. (B) Closed myelomeningocele covered by intact skin.

Positioning during induction of general anesthesia and tracheal intubation is challenging. A cushion is formed and placed under the back to prevent contact injury to the dural sac. The surgical repair is performed in the prone position, with appropriate cushioning that provides ample room for abdominal excursion during ventilation (see Fig. 26.4B). Avoidance of latex-containing products is begun at birth to prevent eventual development of sensitization.

Two IV catheters are inserted for glucose maintenance solution and volume replacement with warmed normal saline or Lactated Ringer's solution, up to 25 mL/kg in the first hour and 6 to 8 mL/kg/h thereafter. Blood loss is usually minimal, unless the skin is undermined and rotation of a myocutaneous flap is required. Therefore packed red blood cells should be immediately available for the procedure.

Standard monitors are indicated before turning the infant prone. The risk for intraoperative hypothermia is significant. A forced-air warming blanket should be placed underneath and around the infant, and all infused fluids should be warmed.

All standard IV and inhaled anesthetic agents are acceptable for use during induction and maintenance of general anesthesia, while planning for tracheal extubation at the completion of the procedure if clinically indicated (i.e., consider potential risks of postopertive apnea in premature infants). Infants born with myelomeningocele have an increased incidence of an abnormally short trachea. Therefore, the endotracheal tube position and its relation to the carina should be precisely measured to determine the appropriate length of insertion. Regional anesthesia is usually not possible, although reports exist[1] of the sole use of spinal anesthesia administered by the surgeon throughout the procedure.

Latex Allergy

Latex allergy is one of the most frequent causes of intraoperative anaphylaxis in children. It occurs in children who have become sensitized to latex by virtue of their frequent exposure to latex-containing medical products, such as rubber gloves and urinary drainage equipment. The most common type of patient with latex allergy is the child with a history of myelomeningocele and neurogenic bladder requiring daily frequent bladder catheterizations. Up to 70% of children with myelomeningocele are reportedly allergic to latex, in contrast to approximately 1% to 5% in the general population of healthy children. Chronic exposure to latex early in life appears to be an important predecessor to the development of latex allergy.

An intraoperative reaction to latex usually occurs 30 to 60 minutes after the start of the surgical procedure. It may manifest as a spectrum of clinical findings that range from mild anaphylactoid reactions (e.g., rash) to severe anaphylaxis consisting of bronchospasm and hypotension. It is indistinguishable from other sources of anaphylaxis and may be difficult to diagnose during a complicated surgical procedure, where these types of clinical findings may be because of any number of causes. Other common offenders, such as recently administered muscle relaxants, antibiotics, or blood products, should also be considered in the differential. Allergic reactions to latex are thus often a diagnosis of exclusion.

Immediate treatment of anaphylaxis consists of epinephrine and volume replacement while removing the suspected latex-containing products. Histamine-1 and histamine-2 antagonists and steroids are administered as well. Bronchodilators may be included in the treatment regimen if bronchospasm persists. Once treatment is established, a workup to identify the exact allergen is recommended, as these patients may ultimately require future anesthetic encounters.

Prevention of intraoperative latex reactions is accomplished by identifying susceptible patients and maintaining a completely latex-free OR environment. Children with myelomeningocele are automatically considered latex-sensitive from birth; thus latex-containing products are not used in their care. Prophylactic medications before surgery are no longer used because their use does not necessarily protect against development of a reaction upon exposure. Furthermore, large case series have shown that children with latex allergy will not develop reactions when cared for in a latex-free environment.

Central Nervous System Trauma

Surgery for pediatric head trauma most often involves evacuation of a subdural or epidural hematoma, or evacuation of an intracerebral hemorrhage that is causing an increased mass effect and increased ICP. Other injuries of the head and neck should be strongly suspected, as emergent cases may still have an ongoing trauma survey. Until cervical spine injuries are completely ruled out, appropriate precautions should be observed during induction of anesthesia and tracheal intubation. Clinically important head trauma is usually associated with systemic hypertension and either obtundation or combativeness. When significant hypotension is present, other injuries causing major blood loss should be sought to fit the clinical scenario. The most common sites of significant blood loss in pediatric trauma are the intraabdominal organs, the pelvic bones, and the femur. Other etiologies of profound hypotension, including cardiogenic, neurogenic, or spinal shock should be considered.

In 2019[10] the Brain Trauma Foundation updated their most recent Guidelines for the Management of Pediatric Severe Traumatic Brain Injury. Anesthesia providers in a trauma center should be familiar with these most up-to-date recommendations regarding neuroimaging, ventilation therapies, hyperosmolar therapy with hypertonic saline, temperature control/hypothermia, use of analgesics and sedatives, seizure prophylaxis, and nutrition. These interventions will be critical in the perioperative period. The most recent update[1] provides quick access to current evidence and links to a comprehensive set of guidelines/algorithms to aid providers.

The preoperative assessment should include review of the child's medical history, physical exam with emphasis on airway anatomy and cardiorespiratory status and review of laboratory tests. Review of primary and secondary trauma surveys and any imaging studies should be carefully reviewed to evaluate extent of other associated injuries. If time is available, blood tests should include hemoglobin, platelets, clotting factors, and a type-and-crossmatch. In the event of a severe acute event causing life-threatening increased ICP, these lab specimens can be sent from the OR and O-negative blood can be administered emergently if necessary.

At least two large-bore IV cannulas should be placed, preferably in the upper extremities. Lower extremity and femoral access is acceptable in the absence of intraabdominal trauma, which may include disruption of the inferior vena cava. An arterial line is preferable before induction of general anesthesia in cases where there is a reasonable threat of hemodynamic compromise or brain herniation. Otherwise, in most cases, it is inserted after induction of general anesthesia.

Intraoperative fluids should consist of isotonic crystalloid solutions such as normal saline or Plasma-Lyte, and blood products when indicated. An indwelling urinary catheter is almost always required and can be removed at the end of the procedure if no longer necessary. Pediatric patients should be maintained within normothermic range. There is currently no indication for hypothermia during surgery for pediatric head trauma.

A modified rapid sequence induction is most often performed, using propofol (2–4 mg/kg), rocuronium (1.2–1.6 mg/kg) or vecuronium (0.2–0.4 mg/kg), lidocaine (1 mg/kg), and fentanyl (3–5 μg/kg) or remifentanil (bolus 1 μg/kg over 2 minutes, and followed by a continuous infusion at 0.1–0.3 μg/kg/min titrated to hemodynamic values). In obtunded patients with signs of significant midline shift and at risk for herniation, the induction technique should be controlled to minimize exaggerated increases in ICP or significant drops cerebral perfusion with systemic hypotension. Gentle hyperventilation with cricoid pressure will minimize the deleterious effects of hypercarbia during this period. If the child has a known full stomach and thus has a reasonable risk for pulmonary aspiration of gastric contents during induction, then a rapid sequence technique is indicated. Cervical spine precautions should be observed during tracheal intubation. This consists of manual in-line neck stabilization by an assistant, and maintenance of the head and neck in a neutral position during all subsequent procedures. Application of cricoid pressure to prevent passive regurgitation is controversial and may not be indicated.

Maintenance agents can include any volatile anesthetic agent, avoidance of N_2O if pneumothorax or pneumocephalus is considered, and titration of opioids with the intent of tracheal extubation at the completion of the procedure. In some cases, the neurosurgeon will request an immediate postoperative CT scan; the child should then remain anesthetized until the CT has been completed and the surgeon confirms that it is safe to awaken the patient.

Children with head trauma will almost always be transferred to an ICU postoperatively. Since postoperative bleeding and intracerebral swelling are possible, children who manifest acute neurologic changes should receive an immediate head CT, neurosurgical consultation, and possible reexploration.

References

1. Intracranial pressure. *Anaesthesia UK*. Updated 6/8/2021. Accessed 28/06/2021. https://www.frca.co.uk/article.aspx?articleid=100755.
2. Downard C, Hulka F, Mullins RJ, Piatt, Joseph MD, et al. Relationship of cerebral perfusion pressure and survival in pediatric brain-injured patients. *J Trauma*. 2000;49(4):654–659. https://doi.org/10.1097/00005373-200010000-00012.
3. Hartley EJ, Bissonnette B, St-Louis P, Rybczynski J, et al. Scalp infiltration with bupivacaine in pediatric brain surgery. *Anesth Analg*. 1991;73(1):29–32. https://doi.org/10.1213/00000539-199107000-00006.
4. Markovitz BP, Duhaime AC, Sutton L, Schreiner MS, et al. Effects of alfentanil on intracranial pressure in children undergoing ventriculoperitoneal shunt revision. *Anesthesiology*. 1992;76(1):71–76. https://doi.org/10.1097/00000542-199201000-00011.
5. Wilson-Smith E, Karsli C, Luginbuehl I, Bissonnette B. Effect of nitrous oxide on cerebrovascular reactivity to carbon

dioxide in children during sevoflurane anaesthesia. *Br J Anaesth.* 2003;91(2):190–195. https://doi.org/10.1093/bja/aeg171.

6. Reasoner DK, Todd MM, Scamman FL, Warner DS. The incidence of pneumocephalus after supratentorial craniotomy. Observations on the disappearance of intracranial air. *Anesthesiology.* 1994;80(5):1008–1012. https://doi.org/10.1097/00000542-199405000-00009.

7. Harrison EA, Mackersie A, McEwan A, Facer E. The sitting position for neurosurgery in children: a review of 16 years' experience. *Br J Anaesth.* 2002;88(1):12–17. https://doi.org/10.1093/bja/88.1.12.

8. Harris MM, Yemen TA, Davidson A, Maureen A. Strafford, et al. Venous embolism during craniectomy in supine infants. *Anesthesiology.* 1987;67(5):816–819. https://doi.org/10.1097/00000542-198711000-00036.

9. Viscomi CM, Abajian JC, Wald SL, Rathmell JP, et al. Spinal anesthesia for repair of meningomyelocele in neonates. *Anesth Analg.* 1995;81(3):492–495. https://doi.org/10.1097/00000539-199509000-00011.

10. Kochanek PM, Tasker RC, Bell MJ, Adelson, P. David, et al. Management of Pediatric Severe Traumatic Brain Injury: 2019 Consensus and Guidelines-Based Algorithm for First and Second Tier Therapies. *Pediatr Crit Care Med.* 2019;20(3):269–279. https://doi.org/10.1097/PCC.0000000000001737.

11. Reuter-Rice K, Christoferson E. Critical Update on the Third Edition of the Guidelines for Managing Severe Traumatic Brain Injury in Children. *Am J Crit Care.* 2020;29(1):13–18. https://doi.org/10.4037/ajcc2020228.

Suggested Reading

Bhalla T, Dewhirst E, Sawardekar A, Dairo O, Tobias JD. Perioperative management of the pediatric patient with traumatic brain injury. *Paediatr Anaesth.* 2012;22(7):627–640. https://doi.org/10.1111/j.1460-9592.2012.03842.x.

27

Ophthalmologic Surgery

RONALD S. LITMAN

This chapter covers general considerations for ophthalmologic procedures in children, specific anesthetic considerations for the more commonly performed pediatric ophthalmologic procedures, and several unique anesthetic complications that occur in pediatric ophthalmologic procedures.

Although the vast majority of children presenting for surgery on the eye are healthy, some ophthalmologic conditions are accompanied by coexisting morbidities. The majority of infants presenting for cataract surgery in the newborn period do not have coexisting diseases, but a variety of pediatric syndromes include cataracts in the constellation of anomalies. Some examples include intrauterine viral infection (e.g., rubella or toxoplasmosis) and metabolic disorders such as Lowe syndrome (developmental delay, hypotonia, and renal dysfunction). Infants with congenital glaucoma are less likely than those with cataracts to have coexisting abnormalities. Infants with retinopathy of prematurity (RoP) who present for laser photocoagulation will often have multisystem abnormalities associated with extreme prematurity, and they should be thoroughly evaluated preoperatively. Some children with strabismus may have a myopathic disease.

Preoperative Considerations

For children without traumatic disorders of the eye, age-appropriate anxiolytic premedication is indicated. If the child has an intravenous catheter, midazolam should be titrated to the child's comfort. In the absence of intravenous access, oral midazolam 0.5 mg/kg (max 10 mg) can be administered.

Procedural Considerations

The major anesthetic implication for ophthalmologic procedures is the avoidance of factors that acutely increase intraocular pressure (IOP), especially in cases of ocular trauma where the integrity of the eye contents is at risk.

Normal IOP in children ranges from 10 to 21 mm Hg. Acute increases of IOP during intraocular surgery can cause extrusion of the vitreous humor, lens prolapse, and/or hemorrhage into the eye (Table 27.1).

Anesthesia providers should be familiar with the types of topical ophthalmic medications used in the perioperative period and the possible related systemic effects (Table 27.2).

Anesthetic Plan

Unless the child has significant comorbidities, standard monitors are sufficient for virtually all eye surgeries. Fluid and blood losses are minimal. Hypothermia does not usually occur, except in the smallest infants. In fact, in most cases, because most of the child's body is covered, their temperature tends to rise by the end of the procedure. Most intravenous and inhaled agents will tend to lower IOP (in a dose-dependent manner), so they can safely be used for induction and maintenance of general anesthesia (see Table 27.1). There are, however, some notable exceptions. Ketamine has been shown to acutely increase IOP in children. Administration of intramuscular ketamine is associated with both increased and decreased IOP, depending on the study one reads. Nevertheless, other associated effects of ketamine such as blepharospasm and nystagmus render it undesirable during eye procedures. If intramuscular ketamine is required for an older uncooperative child who requires emergency eye surgery, then its advantages probably outweigh the risks; this decision should be made on a case-by-case basis. Administration of etomidate has been shown to reduce IOP, but in one case it was associated with loss of eye contents from a ruptured globe as a result of myoclonic movements that occurred after its administration. Nitrous oxide (N_2O) should be avoided if the ophthalmologist plans to inject sulfur hexafluoride gas, because N_2O can then diffuse into the eye and increase IOP. This also applies if sulfur hexafluoride gas was injected into the eye in the previous 2 weeks.

Succinylcholine causes a 7 to 12 mm Hg increase in IOP that lasts 5 to 6 minutes. The mechanism of this phenomenon is controversial: originally, it was thought that succinylcholine uniquely caused contraction of the extraocular muscles, but one study[1] demonstrated an increase in IOP in an in vitro isolated eye model without extraocular muscles attached. Different induction regimens have been reported to attenuate the effects of succinylcholine before tracheal intubation, but none consistently decreases IOP. Therefore, most pediatric anesthesiologists prefer to avoid succinylcholine in open globe procedures, unless its benefit (i.e., rapid paralysis) clearly outweighs its risks. In other words, one would have to believe that the risk for pulmonary aspiration is sufficiently high so as to risk the loss of sight that would occur if succinylcholine caused extrusion of eye contents. On the other hand, proponents of succinylcholine cite the fact that there are no reported cases of succinylcholine-induced loss of sight, and an often-cited article[2] described the use of succinylcholine in 71 patients with an open globe without a single instance of eye content extrusion. Fortunately, reasonable alternatives to succinylcholine exist, such as rocuronium or high-dose vecuronium. If a situation arises whereby the anesthesiologist believes that succinylcholine is required to relieve acute life-threatening airway obstruction, then it should be used immediately.

Lidocaine, in doses of 1 to 2 mg/kg, has been evaluated for attenuating the increase in IOP seen after laryngoscopy and intubation during halothane/N$_2$O anesthesia, or after administration of succinylcholine. All doses of lidocaine were effective in decreasing, but not abolishing, the increase in IOP. Although there are no data evaluating the optimal timing of lidocaine administration, it is logical to administer it 1 to 3 minutes before intubation.

Unless specifically contraindicated, nondepolarizing neuromuscular blockers should be used during the maintenance phase of the anesthetic to ensure lack of movement that could endanger the contents of the eye. In an American Society of Anesthesiologists (ASA) closed claims analysis,[3] lack of neuromuscular blockade and subsequent patient movement was commonly cited as the primary reason for vision loss. An additional safety procedure is the use of a skin-tight barrier across the bridge of the nose to prevent nasal secretions from entering the eye during an open procedure and introducing potential infectious organisms.

In many cases, a deep extubation may be warranted to avoid acute increases in IOP during emergence, assuming there are no contraindications (e.g., full stomach, difficult airway). Lidocaine may attenuate the acute increase in IOP that may occur during emergence when the child reacts to the endotracheal tube, but no studies have specifically examined this issue.

Postoperative Considerations

Except for lacrimal duct probing, most children who undergo eye surgery either have their operative eye patched or have some impairment of vision in the immediate postoperative period. This can cause a great deal of confusion and annoyance for the child. Parents should be allowed to comfort their children as soon as possible in the postanesthesia care unit (PACU). For hospitalized patients, mild sedatives and anxiolytics can be titrated to effect. Postoperative pain can be disabling. Eye surgery patients describe this feeling as having a foreign object stuck in their eye. Therefore, the child should be comforted and ongoing pain or agitation treated with oral or parenteral opioids, nonsteroidal antiinflammatory drugs (NSAIDs) such as ketorolac, or dexmedetomidine to induce sleep.

Anesthetic Management of Common Pediatric Ophthalmologic Procedures

Lacrimal Duct Probing and Irrigation

Many infants are born with a blocked nasolacrimal (tear) duct, but more than 90% of cases resolve with conservative management (external massaging of the duct) by 1 year of

TABLE 27.1	Perioperative Factors That Potentially Affect IOP

FACTORS INCREASING IOP

- Coughing, straining, bucking, crying, vomiting, head flexion, Valsalva maneuver
- Succinylcholine administration
- Ketamine (possibly)
- Laryngoscopy and endotracheal intubation
- Hypoxia, hypercarbia
- External pressure on the eye
- Acute hypertension
- Contraction of the extraocular muscles or orbicularis oculi
- Eyelid closure

FACTORS DECREASING IOP

- Intravenous lidocaine
- Most sedative or general anesthetic agents
- Hypothermia
- Retrobulbar block
- Head-up position
- Diuretics
- Systolic blood pressure <85 mm Hg
- Hypocarbia
- Deep inspiration

TABLE 27.2	Commonly Used Topical Ophthalmologic Medications		
Medication	Concentration and Dose	Ocular Effects	Possible Systemic Effects
Phenylephrine HCl	2.5%; 1–2 drops in each eye	Preoperative mydriatic: dilates the pupil and constricts the blood vessels of the eye	Hypertension and reflex bradycardia
Cyclopentolate HCl	0.5%–1%; 1 drop in each eye every 5 minutes (2 doses)	Preoperative cycloplegic: dilates the pupil and prevents lens accommodation	Usually none

age. Some families may choose to undergo this procedure earlier than 1 year of age because of constant eye irritation or recurrent infections. The procedure, which usually takes less than ten minutes to complete, involves the placement of a fine metal probe from the opening of the duct through to its exit in the nasal cavity, followed by irrigation to confirm that it is patent (Fig. 27.1). Occasionally, the probing includes moving a portion of the inferior turbinate, which can result in minor bleeding. In refractory cases, a silicone stent is placed into the duct, or balloon dilatation is performed.

The only anesthetic consideration for this procedure is the choice of airway management. The oculocardiac reflex is possible but unlikely (see below). Many anesthesiologists will be comfortable using a mask anesthetic throughout the procedure, with intermittent removal during the probing. However, it is possible that irrigation fluid or blood may enter the back of the pharynx and precipitate laryngospasm. A small suction probe is placed into the nasal canal to evacuate fluid and blood during the irrigation. It seems that a laryngeal mask would be ideal for this procedure, but some providers may choose endotracheal tube placement instead. Postoperative pain from this procedure is usually not severe, and is treated with acetaminophen or ibuprofen.

Open Globe Injuries

A ruptured globe occurs from a blunt or penetrating injury into the eye and includes the potential loss of vitreous humor, which entails permanent blindness, if severe. Therefore, it is usually a surgical emergency. Increases in IOP will potentially cause or exacerbate loss of the vitreous. The anesthesiologist should do everything possible to avoid acute increases in IOP (see Table 27.1). Preoperatively, the child should be sedated to prevent excessive crying and protect the eye from further injury. A full stomach should be assumed if the injury occurred within 8 hours after food ingestion. Preoperative sedation should not be so heavy as to

compromise the child's airway reflexes that protect against pulmonary aspiration.

Anesthetic induction is accomplished using a rapid sequence technique that is modified by avoiding succinylcholine and using a nondepolarizing muscle relaxant. An acceptable recipe is propofol 3 to 5 mg/kg and rocuronium 1.2 to 1.6 mg/kg. Intravenous fentanyl 1 to 3 µg/kg (or other opioid of choice) and intravenous lidocaine 1.5 mg/kg will help prevent acute increases in IOP from propofol-associated pain and during laryngoscopy and tracheal intubation. Once the endotracheal tube is inserted, an orogastric tube should evacuate remaining gastric contents. Anesthetic maintenance can be accomplished with any technique that sufficiently controls hemodynamic responses to surgical stimulation. Mild hypocarbia may help keep IOP low. At the completion of the surgical procedure, arm restraints will prevent the child from reaching up and disrupting the surgical repair.

During emergence, it will be important to avoid increases in IOP that may be caused by acute hypertension or coughing on the endotracheal tube. Strategies to avoid this include administration of intravenous lidocaine 1.5 mg/kg, or deep extubation. In addition, antiemetic prophylaxis is indicated (ondansetron 0.05 to 0.1 mg/kg plus dexamethasone 0.1 to 0.5 mg/kg) to avoid emesis-induced increases in IOP postoperatively.

Strabismus Repair

The indications for strabismus repair include congenital esotropia or intermittent exotropia. The surgery, which is primarily performed for cosmetic reasons, consists of measuring and shortening the affected extraocular muscles (Fig. 27.2). There are various anesthetic considerations for strabismus repair. Its occurrence is associated with different pediatric medical disorders, the most important of which are myopathies. Other common coexisting disorders include cerebral palsy, hydrocephalus, meningomyelocele, and many other different types of congenital syndromes and chromosomal aberrations. In

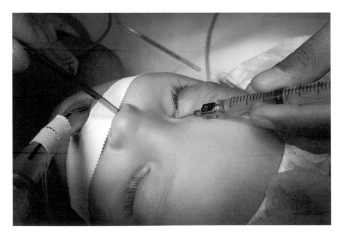

• **Fig 27.1.** Probing and irrigation. Using laryngeal mask anesthesia, the surgeon injects fluorescein dye to assess patency of the nasolacrimal duct. Photo credit to Ronald S. Litman.

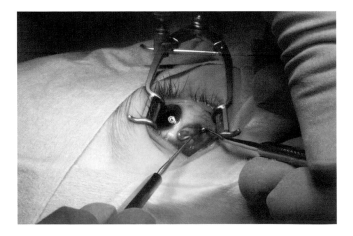

• **Fig 27.2.** Strabismus repair. Although the eyelids are retracted, the extraocular muscles are measured and shortened during strabismus repair. Photo credit to Ronald S. Litman.

previous years it was thought that children with strabismus may be at a higher risk than average for development of masseter muscle rigidity and malignant hyperthermia, but this has not been substantiated. This is probably an aberration because strabismus is often associated with myopathies.

Aside from investigation of comorbidities, children presenting for strabismus repair require routine preoperative assessment. Oral midazolam is the most common anxiolytic premedication used. Acetaminophen or ibuprofen syrup can be added to the premedication for their contribution to postoperative analgesia. Intraoperatively, fluid and blood losses are minimal, and active warming measures are unnecessary, as children tend to get warm beneath the covers. The unique aspects of the intraoperative anesthetic management for strabismus repair include occurrence of the oculocardiac

reflex and postoperative nausea and vomiting (PONV). The oculocardiac reflex usually occurs during the initial stages of the repair (during pressure on the globe or traction on the extraocular muscles), and is easily treated with administration of intravenous glycopyrrolate or atropine. Induction and maintenance of general anesthesia with propofol may result in less PONV than if an inhaled agent is used. Children undergoing strabismus repair should receive combination antiemetic therapy with a serotonin antagonist such as ondansetron (0.05 to 0.1 mg/kg, maximum 4 mg), plus dexamethasone (0.1 to 0.5 mg/kg, maximum 10 mg).

Airway management for strabismus repair consists of either a flexible laryngeal mask airway (LMA) or oral RAE endotracheal tube, depending on the preference of the anesthesia provider.

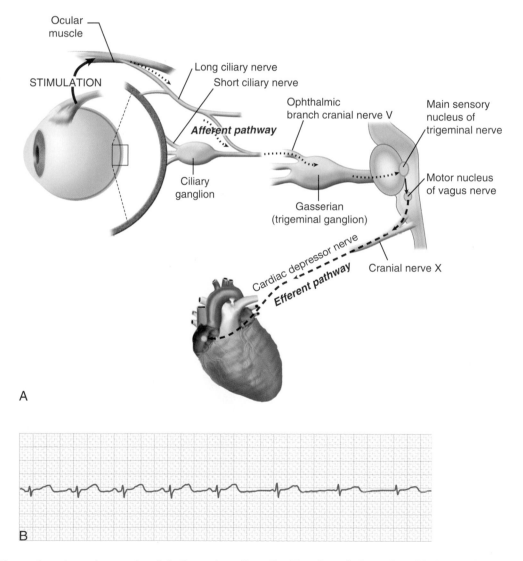

• **Fig 27.3.** Traction on the extraocular muscles elicits the oculocardiac reflex. The afferent limb consists of the long and short ciliary nerves, which synapse in the ciliary ganglion *(dotted arrows)*. The ophthalmic division of the trigeminal nerve (cranial nerve V) carries the impulse to the gasserian ganglion, and the arc continues to the sensory nucleus of cranial nerve V in the brainstem. Fibers in the reticular formation synapse with the nucleus of the vagus nerve (cranial nerve X). Efferent fibers from the vagus nerve terminate in the heart *(dashed arrow)*. The neurotransmitter from the vagus nerve to the sinoatrial node is acetylcholine, and the reflex is blocked by antimuscarinic pharmacologic agents (i.e., atropine and glycopyrrolate). (From: Tobin JR, Weaver RG. Ophthalmology. In: Coté CJ, Lerman J, Anderson BJ, eds. *A Practice of Anesthesia for Infants and Children. 6th ed.* Elsevier;2019:790–803.e4.)

Postoperative pain can be significant. Administration of intravenous ketorolac has been associated with postoperative pain relief for up to 5 hours after strabismus surgery. Intense pain that is unresponsive to opioids should prompt a reexamination by the ophthalmologist.

Exam Under Anesthesia

Children with glaucoma routinely require careful IOP measurements that cannot be accurately measured in the ophthalmologist's office. These children are often scheduled for IOP measurement under general anesthesia (Fig. 27.3), with the intention of going forward with the glaucoma surgery at the same time if the IOP is found to be too high. Knowing that anesthetic agents lower IOP, the goal is to do the measurement as quickly as possible after loss of consciousness to keep the effects of the anesthetic agent on IOP to a minimum. Shortly after the infant loses consciousness, we allow the ophthalmologist to obtain their measurements, which only takes a few moments. If the pressures are within normal limits, the infant is then allowed to awaken. If the pressures are high, and glaucoma surgery will proceed, we then place an intravenous catheter and conduct a routine general anesthetic with an oral RAE endotracheal tube.

Retinopathy of Prematurity

Retinopathy of prematurity (RoP) is a vasoproliferative disorder of the retina that occurs in premature infants and is one of the leading causes of blindness in children. The disorder is primarily related to the immaturity of the retina and is exacerbated by high oxygen concentrations or fluctuations in oxygen concentration.[4] Laser photocoagulation has replaced cryotherapy as the surgical treatment of choice for this disorder. The procedure is commonly performed in the first few months of life to the avascular part of the retina, and usually takes 30 to 60 minutes to perform. These infants should be thoroughly screened for comorbidities associated with prematurity. There are no other unique aspects to the anesthetic management. As with strabismus, an LMA is an acceptable alternative to an endotracheal tube. Anesthesiologists should never withhold oxygen for fear of causing or exacerbating RoP. On the other hand, in an otherwise healthy infant, there is no reason to maintain the oxyhemoglobin saturation greater than 97%. Postoperatively, residual pain is often not significant, but prematurely born infants are at risk for developing central apnea and should be monitored for at least 12 hours before discharge home according to institutional guidelines.

Unique Complications During Pediatric Ophthalmologic Procedures

Oculocardiac Reflex

The oculocardiac reflex (OCR) is defined as a decrease in pulse rate associated with traction on the extraocular muscles or compression of the eyeball. The bradycardia that ensues may be severe; asystole and ventricular dysrhythmias have been reported. The afferent arc of the reflex consists of the ophthalmic division of the trigeminal (V_1) nerve, whose constituents include the short and long ciliary nerves from the eye. The efferent arc consists of the vagus (X) nerve, which originates in the brainstem and terminates in the sinus node of the heart (Fig. 27.4).

The OCR can be prevented by prophylactic administration of intravenous atropine 0.02 mg/kg, or glycopyrrolate 0.01 mg/kg shortly before eye manipulation. If prophylaxis has not been administered, OCR-induced bradycardia can be treated with the same dose of intravenous atropine. Alternative treatments include cessation of the offending stimulus and instillation of local anesthetic into the eye muscles.

Postoperative Nausea and Vomiting

PONV is a common complication after ophthalmic procedures, especially strabismus, with an incidence as high as 75% in some reported studies. A variety of regimens have been studied in an attempt to decrease its occurrence. The incidence of PONV is decreased by using propofol[5] instead of inhaled anesthetics for maintenance of general anesthesia, and decreasing the amount of opioids used intraoperatively.

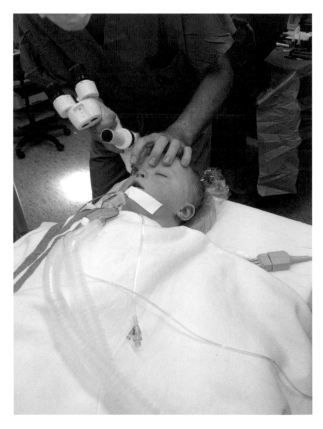

• **Fig 27.4.** Congenital glaucoma. Children with congenital glaucoma often require exams under anesthesia for accurate measurements of intraocular pressure and a more detailed look at the structures of the eye. Photo credit to Ronald S. Litman.

Prophylactic antiemetics are routinely administered. This includes a combination[6] of a serotonin antagonist and dexamethasone. Optimal doses and the time to administer the antiemetics have not been precisely determined, but differences in these factors probably do not alter the incidence significantly. The level of inspired oxygen during the procedures does not influence the incidence of PONV after strabismus repair.[7] For most eye procedures, the opioid dose can be minimized by using topical tetracaine 1%[8] drops at the completion of the surgery.

References

1. Kelly RE, Dinner M, Turner LS, Haik B, Abramson DH, Daines P. Succinylcholine increases intraocular pressure in the human eye with the extraocular muscles detached. *Anesthesiology*. 1993;79(5):948–952. https://doi.org/10.1097/00000542-199311000-00012.
2. Libonati MM, Leahy JJ, Ellison N. The use of succinylcholine in open eye surgery. *Anesthesiology*. 1985;62(5):637–640. https://doi.org/10.1097/00000542-198505000-00017.
3. Gild WM, Posner KL, Caplan RA, Cheney FW. Eye injuries associated with anesthesia. A closed claims analysis. *Anesthesiology*. 1992;76(2):204–208. https://doi.org/10.1097/00000542-199202000-00008.
4. Hartnett ME, Penn JS. Mechanisms and management of retinopathy of prematurity. *N Engl J Med*. 2013;368(12):1162–1163. https://doi.org/10.1056/NEJMc1301021.
5. Watcha MF, Simeon RM, White PF, Stevens JL. Effect of propofol on the incidence of postoperative vomiting after strabismus surgery in pediatric outpatients. *Anesthesiology*. 1991;75(2):204–209. https://doi.org/10.1097/00000542-199108000-00006.
6. Tramèr M, Moore A, McQuay H. Prevention of vomiting after paediatric strabismus surgery: a systematic review using the numbers-needed-to-treat method. *Br J Anaesth*. 1995;75(5):556–561. https://doi.org/10.1093/bja/75.5.556.
7. Treschan TA, Zimmer C, Nass C, Stegen B, Esser J, Peters J. Inspired oxygen fraction of 0.8 does not attenuate postoperative nausea and vomiting after strabismus surgery. *Anesthesiology*. 2005;103(1):6–10. https://doi.org/10.1097/00000542-200507000-00005.
8. Anninger W, Forbes B, Quinn G, Schreiner MS. The effect of topical tetracaine eye drops on emergence behavior and pain relief after strabismus surgery. *J AAPOS*. 2007;11(3):273–276. https://doi.org/10.1016/j.jaapos.2007.01.124.

28

Plastic Surgery

GRACE HSU, PAUL STRICKER, AND RONALD S. LITMAN

In this chapter we review plastic surgery procedures that pose a wide range of perioperative challenges for the anesthesiologist, including difficult airway management, significant intraoperative blood loss, and comorbidities secondary to an underlying genetic syndrome. We also review considerations for subcutaneous administration of epinephrine.

Craniofacial Anomalies

The Committee on Nomenclature and Classification of Craniofacial Anomalies of the American Cleft Palate Association has organized facial anomalies into five categories: cleft, synostosis, hypoplasia, hyperplasia, and unclassified. Each of these categories of craniofacial anomalies are potentially associated with difficult airway management.

Clefts can involve the lip, palate, or both. Craniosynostosis occurs when there is premature closure of one or more cranial sutures. Some of the most common craniosynostosis syndromes include Apert, Pfeiffer, Crouzon, Saethre-Chotzen, Carpenter, and Muenke syndromes, and all are associated with difficult intubation. Examples of syndromes associated with craniofacial hypoplasia include Pierre Robin sequence and Goldenhar syndrome. Ease of intubation tends to improve with age in children with hypoplastic craniofacial dysmorphisms. Mucopolysaccharidoses, including Hunter and Hurler syndromes and vascular malformations, are examples of hyperplastic anomalies.

Cleft Lip Repair

A cleft lip is a unilateral or bilateral split of the upper lip between the mouth and nose. It can range from a slight notch to a complete separation of one or both sides of the lip extending up and into the nose and is often accompanied by a cleft palate (Fig. 28.1). The overall incidence of cleft lip is approximately 1 in 800 live births. Although the majority of cleft lips are not associated with any predisposing factors, a history of maternal smoking or phenytoin use increases the risk. Associated defects such as congenital heart disease occur in approximately 10% of affected children. Feeding difficulties in the newborn period may lead to poor growth and anemia. Surgical repair is usually performed at 3 to 6 months; some centers are correcting these lesions in the first 30 days of life with findings that high levels of estrogen found in neonates aid in the surgical repair and recovery. Older children may return for subsequent cosmetic repairs of the lip or nasal tip.

In infants with cleft lip/palate as an isolated defect, preoperative evaluation and intraoperative management is no different from that for other healthy infants undergoing elective procedures. Because cleft lip repair is often performed around 3 months of age, a preoperative hemoglobin level may be checked as this coincides with the physiologic nadir of infancy.

A mask induction of general anesthesia is most often performed, followed by endotracheal intubation with an oral Ring, Adair, and Elwyn (RAE) endotracheal tube. Special care must be taken in selecting the proper size oral RAE tube, as the location of the preformed bend on these tubes varies according to the tube size. The patient's eyes may be protected with ophthalmic ointment and covered by a transparent adhesive covering to preserve visible surgical landmarks. The operating room (OR) table is turned 90 degrees away from the anesthesia provider to facilitate surgical repair from the head or side of the table. A small amount (usually <1 mL) of local anesthetic with epinephrine is injected into the surgical field to facilitate hemostasis at the incision site. Blood and fluid losses are minimal. Therefore, maintenance and preoperative deficit fluid replacement is sufficient. A small amount of opioid may be administered intraoperatively. The intravenous (IV) administration of acetaminophen may also be helpful to decrease opioid requirements. Bilateral soft arm restraints are used to keep the infant from handling the repair postoperatively.

Some pediatric anesthesiologists advocate regional anesthesia for cleft lip repair. An infraorbital nerve block[1] with a long-acting local anesthetic can provide up to 18 hours of pain relief and decrease postoperative administration of opioids.

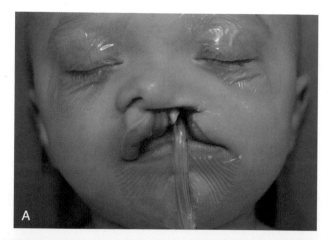

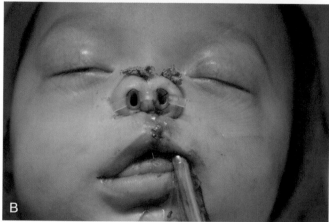

• **Fig 28.1.** Cleft lip and palate repair. (A) Unilateral cleft lip and palate repair. The surgeon is situated behind the child when performing a cleft lip or palate repair. An oral Ring, Adair, and Elwyn (RAE) tube is used for ventilation. (B) Completion of the cleft lip and palate repair. Nasal conformers and tip bolsters are notable in this picture and are used during a concomitant nasal tip rhinoplasty, a procedure that may but not always accompany a cleft lip and palate repair. (From: Jonathan M Sykes. Cleft Lip Rhinoplasty. In: Azizzadeh B, Murphy MR, Johnson CM Jr, Numa W, eds. *Master Techniques in Rhinoplasty*. Saunders Elsevier; 2011:431–445.)

Cleft Palate Repair

A cleft palate occurs when the roof of the mouth (i.e., hard and/or soft palate) has not unified completely during fetal development. A cleft palate can range from a small bifid uvula to a complete separation of both the soft and hard palate. Associated congenital defects occur in up to 50% of infants born with a cleft palate. The velocardiofacial syndrome, also known as *DiGeorge syndrome*, is the most common syndrome associated with a cleft palate. About 1 in 3000 children per year are born with it. Cleft palate can also exist as a component of the Pierre Robin sequence (triad of cleft palate, glossoptosis, and micrognathia). Early concerns in the newborn period relate to feeding difficulties and airway compromise.

In children with cleft palate and upper airway obstruction caused by micrognathia and glossoptosis, mild cases of obstruction can often be managed by prone positioning. In more severe cases, life-threatening upper airway obstruction may result, mandating surgical intervention. Surgical options in these cases include glossopexy (tongue-lip adhesion, to prevent glossoptosis), mandibular osteotomies and placement of distractor hardware (to elongate the mandible via distraction osteogenesis), and tracheostomy. These procedures are typically done early in infancy, months before the palatoplasty is performed.

Surgical correction of cleft palate is usually performed at 9 to 12 months of age. Older children may present for subsequent procedures such as correction of velopharyngeal incompetence, or repair of residual palatal defects with a bone graft. If a child is born with both cleft lip and cleft palate, the lip repair is performed first because the repaired lip helps decrease the expanding width of the palatal defect as the infant grows. Repairing the lip defect also facilitates bottle feeding using a specially molded nipple.

Preoperative considerations for children presenting for cleft palate repair are focused on delineation of coexisting medical problems and assessment of airway patency. Infants older than about 9 months of age and without airway compromise are candidates for anxiolytic premedication. Unless intravenous access is previously established, inhaled induction of general anesthesia is performed. Upper airway obstruction during this phase is common and is often relieved by placement of an oral airway to prevent the tongue from becoming lodged in the cleft. Endotracheal intubation by direct laryngoscopy may be complicated by the presence of micrognathia or unintentional placement of the laryngoscope blade into the cleft during laryngoscopy. Some pediatric anesthesiologists prefer to place gauze material into the cleft before laryngoscopy attempts. If this is done, caution must be taken to ensure that the gauze does not become dislodged and cause airway obstruction. An oral RAE tube is inserted and the OR table turned 90 degrees to facilitate surgical repair from behind the head of the infant.

Surgical exposure is achieved by placing the supine infant on a small shoulder roll, extending the neck, and inserting a Dingman retractor into the mouth. Neck extension is associated with cephalad movement of the tracheal tube tip, so proper positioning of the tube should be confirmed after final patient positioning. Care must be taken to avoid pinching the tracheal tube (usually presenting as a sudden increase in airway resistance) during placement of the Dingman retractor. Neck extension may need to be avoided in children with abnormalities of the cervical spine. Local anesthetic containing epinephrine is then infiltrated into the surgical field to facilitate intraoperative hemostasis; typically, the amount injected is well within the calculated toxicity dose limit for these children (discussed at the end of the chapter). Blood and fluid losses are minimal but somewhat greater than for cleft lip repair, and may not always be readily apparent. A throat pack may be placed by the surgeon to absorb blood and prevent it from passing into the esophagus and stomach.

A balanced anesthetic of inhaled and intravenous agents is chosen for maintenance of general anesthesia. The primary concern after emergence from anesthesia and tracheal extubation is the potential for upper airway obstruction caused by surgical closure of the palatal defect combined with soft tissue swelling. A conservative dose of opioids before emergence is prudent, and perioperative dexamethasone is administered to decrease soft tissue edema. Intravenous acetaminophen may be administered to reduce opioid requirements. Before tracheal extubation, the oropharynx should be gently suctioned to remove retained blood and secretions while taking care not to disrupt the delicate suture lines. In some cases, the surgeons will place a loop suture through the anterior portion of the tongue, which can then be pulled anteriorly if the tongue is causing postoperative upper airway obstruction. This suture is then usually removed within several hours after the procedure when the child has demonstrated the ability to maintain airway patency without assistance.

The primary postoperative concerns after cleft palate repair are airway patency and pain control. Prone or lateral positioning is often helpful to alleviate obstruction by the tongue. If indicated, small doses of morphine or hydromorphone are administered while monitoring upper airway patency. Children with the combination of cleft palate and micrognathia (e.g., Pierre Robin sequence) are at increased risk for postoperative airway obstruction after palatoplasty procedures. In these cases, the surgeon may insert a soft nasopharyngeal airway and secure it with a suture during the operation. Placement of an oral airway postoperatively is relatively contraindicated because it may disrupt the surgical repair. A nasal airway or nasotracheal tube is also relatively contraindicated in future anesthetics if a posterior pharyngeal flap was used to repair the cleft. If nasotracheal intubation is needed for a future anesthetic, flexible bronchoscopic guided intubation is necessary for careful guidance of the tracheal tube around the pharyngeal flap because flap damage and subsequent hemorrhage can occur.

Significant postoperative hemorrhage is infrequent but does occur and may initially be unrecognized as the blood may be swallowed. Postoperative hemorrhage requires immediate surgical exploration, and airway management can be challenging because of blood in the airway. Transfusion may be necessary, and restoration of an adequate circulating volume should occur before induction of anesthesia.

Bilateral suprazygomatic maxillary nerve blocks[2] have been shown to decrease postoperative opioid requirements in infants undergoing cleft palate repair and can be performed with the classical landmark technique or with ultrasound guidance.

Craniosynostosis Repair

Types of Craniosynostosis

At birth, the skull consists of distinct cranial bones separated by malleable strips of connective tissue that are known as cranial sutures. During the first 2 years of life, the sutures serve as growth sites for the deposition of additional cranial

bone with eventual formation of the adult skull. Primary craniosynostosis, which occurs in approximately 1 in 2000 live births, results when one of these sutures closes prematurely, thus restricting growth of the adjacent cranial bones in a perpendicular direction (Fig. 28.2A–G). The remaining cranial bones that are adjacent to normal sutures continue to grow unchecked, producing a misshapen head that may affect facial anatomy, brain structure, and brain function. Elevated intracranial pressure may also occur. Secondary craniosynostosis results from an abnormal progression of brain growth and expansion. Most forms of craniosynostosis are diagnosed in the first several months of life, after the completion of normal cranial molding that is attributed to the birth process.

In most infants with craniosynostosis that involves only a single suture, the primary concern is cosmetic: surgery will prevent a permanent craniofacial deformity. However, increased intracranial pressure has been reported to occur in as many as 14% of children with single-suture craniosynostosis. Although primarily "cosmetic," normalization of skull morphology and appearance has a significant psychosocial impact that is lifelong. More severe forms of craniosynostosis (which involve multiple cranial sutures) may occur as part of a genetic syndrome and are more likely to be associated with increased intracranial pressure, neurologic deficits, and ophthalmologic problems, including vision-threatening

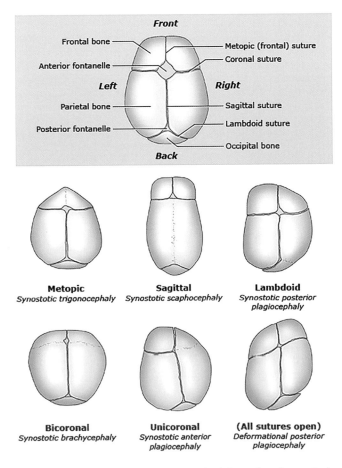

• **Fig 28.2.** Newborn skull and sutures, and variations of craniosynostosis.

sequelae of amblyopia, strabismus, and exposure keratopathy. Malar hypoplasia and midface retrusion are common features of these craniosynostosis syndromes, which manifest as upper airway obstruction. Surgical correction of craniosynostosis is usually performed as early as 3 to 6 months of age to prevent permanent craniofacial deformities and secondary brain abnormalities. Optimal results are achieved when these procedures are performed in infancy because incomplete ossification of cranial vault defects after surgery is more likely in older children, leaving bony gaps in the skull after correction. These procedures are extensive, typically requiring wide scalp dissections and multiple cranial osteotomies, and have been associated with significant morbidity. Reported complications include massive blood loss, intraoperative cardiac arrest, transfusion reactions, venous air embolism, hypotension, coagulopathy, bradycardia, postoperative seizures, surgical site infections, facial swelling, and unplanned postoperative mechanical ventilation. Many of the most severe and commonly seen problems are associated with the rate and extent of blood loss.

Scaphocephaly (dolichocephaly) is the most common type of craniosynostosis (50%) and results from premature closure of the sagittal suture. The cranial bones continue to grow in an anteroposterior direction and produce an elongated skull with frontal bossing and occipital protrusion. Although the transverse dimension of the head is narrow, head volume is normal; therefore, increased intracranial pressure and neurologic deficits are not usually observed.

A number of surgical procedures have been developed to correct scaphocephaly. Open surgical procedures involving complete reconstruction of the infant skull are often performed to achieve satisfactory cosmetic results. The frontal, parietal, and occipital bones are excised and then trimmed, reshaped, and relocated with the objective of restoring a normal biparietal diameter and reducing the severity of frontal bossing and occipital protrusion. These procedures are typically done between three and 6 months of age. Because of the large scalp dissection to achieve adequate exposure and the extensive craniotomies that are performed, these procedures are associated with significant hemorrhage, making transfusion nearly universal.

In an effort to minimize blood loss, transfusion, and length of hospital stay, surgeons are increasingly employing less invasive approaches in the treatment of craniosynostosis. The most common of these techniques in the United States is endoscopic strip craniectomy. Endoscopic strip craniectomies are most commonly performed for the surgical repair of sagittal craniosynostosis, though they can be done for other types of craniosynostosis as well. In these procedures, two small incisions are made in the scalp perpendicular to the fused suture (the anterior and posterior fontanelles, in sagittal craniosynostosis). Using endoscopic guidance, the scalp is dissected from the skull, osteotomies are performed to remove the strip of cranial bone containing the fused suture, which is then separated from the dura and removed. Significant blood loss can occur if the sagittal sinus is inadvertently entered. Additional osteotomies

(barrel staves) in the surrounding bones may also be performed neuroendoscopically. Rather than the immediate correction that occurs with a complex intraoperative reconstruction, normalization of skull shape is achieved through postoperative cranial helmet molding. Customized helmets (cranial molding orthotics) are worn by these infants for at least 6 months with regular follow-up visits to monitor response and make adjustments.

A major disadvantage of endoscopic correction of craniosynostosis is the need for prolonged helmeting to achieve and maintain correction. Another minimally invasive technique that is used in the treatment of sagittal synostosis is spring-mediated cranioplasty. In this procedure, a small scalp incision exposing the synostotic sagittal suture is made, and a small strip of bone containing the fused suture is excised. Two to three springs are then placed along the edges of the strip craniectomy site, which apply approximately five to seven N of force in a direction perpendicular to the natural axis of the sagittal suture. The incisions are then closed, and over the following months the forces applied by the springs allow for normalization of skull shape during growth. After 3 to 4 months, the infant returns to the operating room for removal of these springs. Like endoscopic strip craniectomy, these procedures have the advantage that they can be performed with minimal blood loss. The principal disadvantage is the need for a second operation to remove the springs.

Plagiocephaly (18%) results from a unilateral synostosis of a coronal suture, producing a unilateral "tilting" forehead and orbital anomalies. Brachycephaly (9%) results from a bilateral coronal synostosis and causes a broadened skull and midface hypoplasia. Brachycephaly occurs in Apert and Crouzon[3] syndromes. Brachycephaly is associated with a higher incidence of neurologic complications, including increased intracranial pressure, optic atrophy, and cognitive impairment. These deformities are corrected surgically by advancement of the frontal bone and orbital segments of the skull.

Trigonocephaly (9%) is the result of premature closure of the metopic suture, resulting in a triangular-shaped head and hypotelorism, with an increased risk for associated anomalies of the forebrain. It is often accompanied by additional congenital deformities including cleft palate and urinary tract anomalies. Trigonocephaly is surgically corrected by incision, reconstruction, and replacement of the frontal bone.

Anesthetic Management for Craniosynostosis Repair

Preoperative assessment of the infant presenting for craniosynostosis repair should include a thorough investigation of all comorbidities, congenital anomalies, and the possibility of increased intracranial pressure. In particular, examination of the facial structure and upper airway may reveal the possibility of a difficult airway, including difficult mask ventilation and/or intubation. In children with syndromic forms of craniosynostosis, a history of obstructive sleep apnea should be sought, and plans for postoperative airway management should be adjusted accordingly. A complete blood count, coagulation studies, and a type-and-crossmatch should be obtained. A preoperative anxiolytic may be indicated in some infants older than about 9 months. Infants presenting for craniofacial surgery are usually admitted from home on the day of surgery.

Most infants with craniosynostosis receive an inhaled induction of general anesthesia. A muscle relaxant is administered in the absence of suspicion of a difficult airway. Direct visualization of the larynx may not be possible in infants with syndromic midface hypoplasia. In these cases, fiberoptic bronchoscopy or video laryngoscopy is required to achieve endotracheal intubation via the nasal or oral route, depending on the site of the surgery and the preferences of the anesthesiologist and surgeon. The endotracheal tube should be carefully taped (or even sutured) in place so as not to become dislodged during critical portions of the surgical procedure.

Maintenance of general anesthesia can be accomplished with an inhaled agent supplemented with opioids and a neuromuscular blocker. Administration of opioids by continuous infusion is useful to maintain effective plasma concentrations during longer procedures and those with extensive blood loss. Intraoperative N_2O is avoided because of the risk for venous air embolism (see below). Dexmedetomidine is a useful anesthetic adjunct, as it decreases intraoperative anesthetic requirements and facilitates a smooth emergence from anesthesia by providing both sedation and analgesic properties without depressing respiratory drive.

Two large-bore (at least 22-gauge) intravenous catheters are inserted after anesthetic induction, followed by insertion of an arterial catheter. The arterial catheter provides continuous assessment of blood pressure and facilitates frequent sampling of blood for hemoglobin and blood gas determinations. Intravascular volume status is monitored using invasive systemic blood pressure measurement, together with continuous vigilant assessment of the surgical field and responses to fluid challenges. Central venous pressure monitoring is used routinely at some centers, while others reserve central venous catheter insertion for children with inadequate peripheral venous access. We demonstrated[4] that in young children undergoing craniofacial reconstruction, tachycardia does not occur in these infants during periods of blood loss and hypotension.

Anesthetic management for endoscopic synostosis repair and for spring-mediated cranioplasty is similar to that for other cranial vault reconstruction procedures except that an arterial catheter is usually omitted. Although significant hemorrhage and transfusion are uncommon, packed red blood cells should be immediately available and anesthesiologists should be prepared to replace large volume blood loss as accidental dural venous sinus tears are possible during these procedures.

A rectal temperature probe is inserted because exposure of the infant and a large amount of administered crystalloid and blood can result in hypothermia. Normothermia is maintained by using fluid- and blood-warming devices, a forced warm-air blanket over the unexposed portions of the infant, a heating mattress between the infant and the OR table, a heated and humidified breathing circuit, and, when necessary, heating the OR environment. Even mild hypothermia can increase blood loss and need for transfusion; with meticulous attention, this complication is avoidable in these children. An indwelling urinary catheter is inserted and maintained postoperatively.

During the craniotomy portions of the surgical procedure, rapid and significant blood loss is expected as a result of bleeding from the scalp incisions, osteotomy sites, and the dural venous sinuses. Accurate estimation of blood loss during these procedures is difficult and results in imprecise replacement, which may result in hypovolemia, hypotension, and metabolic acidosis. Life-threatening hypovolemia may occur because of the small total blood volume of these infants. All attempts should be made to prepare for this eventuality by keeping pace with blood loss, maintaining a hemoglobin level >7.5 g/dL, though preferably at least 10 g/dL. During a large craniofacial reconstruction over several hours, blood product transfusion of large amounts (50–100 mL/kg) are common. Fresh frozen plasma administration is often necessary after one blood volume has been lost and replaced, and platelet transfusion may be needed with losses exceeding $1\frac{1}{2}$ to 2 blood volumes. Supplemental calcium administration is also indicated with red cell transfusions.

At our institution, blood lost during complex cranial vault reconstruction is replaced with either whole blood or reconstituted[5] blood, which is made by combining a unit of packed red blood cells and a unit of fresh frozen plasma derived from the same blood donor. With this approach, coagulopathy from dilution of soluble clotting factors is avoided, while also limiting blood donor exposures.

Blood Conservation Strategies

Various strategies have been employed in this population to limit blood loss and transfusion requirements. These strategies broadly fall into two categories: those that decrease bleeding, and those that increase the volume of blood loss that can be safely tolerated. Variations in surgical technique, deliberate hypotension, and the administration of antifibrinolytics are among those strategies that aim to decrease actual bleeding. Current evidence supports both the efficacy and safety of antifibrinolytics in this population and they should be administered in the absence of any specific contraindication. The greatest reductions in blood loss have been achieved through the development of new surgical techniques, such as endoscopic strip craniectomy[6] and spring-mediated cranioplasty.[7] Strategies that have been used to increase the amount of tolerable blood loss in these children include the use of cell saver technology, acute preoperative normovolemic hemodilution, and preoperative erythropoietin therapy.

Venous Air Embolism

Venous air embolism (VAE) has been reported to occur in up to 83% of infants undergoing craniosynostosis repair because the noncollapsible veins of the skull at the operative site are often above the level of the heart and are exposed to air. It can also occur during endoscopic strip craniectomy.[8] VAE is reported to be responsible for life-threatening hemodynamic instability and death intraoperatively. Some centers routinely use a precordial Doppler ultrasonic probe to detect the occurrence of a VAE and will attempt to aspirate air using an inserted central venous catheter. However, the majority of detected VAEs do not cause clinical consequences and attempted aspiration though a central venous catheter has not been shown to influence outcome during this complication. We believe that continuous and vigilant expansion of the intravascular space leads to a low incidence of clinically apparent VAE.

Postoperative Course

After craniosynostosis repair, most children are awakened and their tracheas extubated in the OR. All children are routinely admitted to the intensive care unit because of concerns for ongoing blood loss and hemodynamic instability, and for monitoring for upper airway obstruction, which may occur from the large amount of swelling that occurs in the facial region. Postoperative mechanical ventilation is not often required, except in those children with syndromic craniosynostosis associated with preexisting obstructive sleep apnea.

Subcutaneous Epinephrine Use in Children

Subcutaneous administration of a local anesthetic containing epinephrine is common in plastic surgical procedures with the goal of attaining epinephrine-mediated vasoconstriction and minimization of blood loss. In anesthetized patients, the epinephrine may induce ventricular dysrhythmias, and is exacerbated in the presence of an inhaled anesthetic agent. The alkane anesthetic agents (i.e., halothane) are characterized by their propensity to "sensitize" the myocardium to endogenous or exogenously administered catecholamines. The ethers (i.e., isoflurane, sevoflurane, desflurane) do not sensitize the myocardium to the same extent as that for the alkane anesthetics.

The maximum amount of epinephrine that may be safely administered is unknown. A retrospective study[9] in children undergoing cleft palate repair reported the safe use of subcutaneous administration of epinephrine in doses reaching a maximum of 10 mcg/kg, administered as needed at 30-minute intervals.

References

1. Bösenberg AT, Kimble FW. Infraorbital nerve block in neonates for cleft lip repair: anatomical study and clinical application. *Br J Anaesth*. 1995;74(5):506–508. https://doi.org/10.1093/bja/74.5.506.
2. Chiono J, Raux O, Bringuier S, et al. Bilateral Suprazygomatic Maxillary Nerve Block for Cleft Palate Repair in Children: A Prospective, Randomized, Double-blind Study versus Placebo. *Anesthesiology*. 2014;120:1362–1369. https://doi.org/10.1097/ALN.0000000000000171.
3. Br0therM0nkey. "It's Frankensteen": Dr. Frederick Frankenstein meets Igor for the first time. Accessed 28/06/2021. https://youtu.be/nxxSIX3fmmo.
4. Stricker PA, Lin EE, Fiadjoe JE, Sussman EM, Jobes DR. Absence of tachycardia during hypotension in children undergoing craniofacial reconstruction surgery. *Anesth Analg*. 2012;115(1):139–146. https://doi.org/10.1213/ANE.0b013e318253708c.
5. Stricker PA, Fiadjoe JE, Davis AR, et al. Reconstituted blood reduces blood donor exposures in children undergoing craniofacial reconstruction surgery. *Paediatr Anaesth*. 2011;21(1):54–61. https://doi.org/10.1111/j.1460-9592.2010.03476.x.
6. Meier PM, Goobie SM, DiNardo JA, Proctor MR, Zurakowski D, Soriano SG. Endoscopic strip craniectomy in early infancy: the initial five years of anesthesia experience. *Anesth Analg*. 2011;112(2):407–414. https://doi.org/10.1213/ANE.0b013e31820471e4.
7. Ririe DG, Smith TE, Wood BC, et al. Time-dependent perioperative anesthetic management and outcomes of the first 100 consecutive cases of spring-assisted surgery for sagittal craniosynostosis. *Paediatr Anaesth*. 2011;21(10):1015–1019. https://doi.org/10.1111/j.1460-9592.2011.03608.x.
8. Tobias JD, Johnson JO, Jimenez DF, Barone CM, McBride Jr. DS. Venous air embolism during endoscopic strip craniectomy for repair of craniosynostosis in infants. *Anesthesiology*. 2001;95(2):340–342. https://doi.org/10.1097/00000542-200108000-00013.
9. Kinsella Jr CR, Castillo N, Naran S, et al. Intraoperative High-Dose Epinephrine Infiltration in Cleft Palate Repair. *J Craniofac Surg*. 2014;25(1):140–142. https://doi.org/10.1097/SCS.0000000000000376.

Suggested Reading

Morris LM. Nonsyndromic Craniosynostosis and Deformational Head Shape Disorders. *Facial Plast Surg Clin North Am*. 2016;24(4):517–530. https://doi.org/10.1016/j.fsc.2016.06.007.

29

Urologic Surgery

KATHERINE H. LOH AND RONALD S. LITMAN

Most urologic procedures are simple surgical repairs in healthy children and are performed on an outpatient basis. Some children require complex repairs, and it helps to understand the repair to tailor the anesthetic technique.

Circumcision

Children beyond the newborn period may present for circumcision under general anesthesia as an elective procedure for cosmetic reasons, or as a treatment for recurrent phimosis.

Preoperative assessment should include assessment for sedative premedication. An oral analgesic agent such as acetaminophen 15 mg/kg or ibuprofen 10 mg/kg may also be included. Most children undergo inhalational induction and maintenance with sevoflurane. Airway management is provided by face mask or supraglottic airway. Tracheal intubation is usually reserved for small children in whom a supraglottic airway may not be suitable because of the imperfect fit, and because the child may be situated further down the operating room (OR) table where the airway is not readily accessible. Regional analgesia should be provided by a penile block, caudal epidural block (see Chapter 20), or pudendal block. Postoperative fever is very common after circumcision, especially in children with preexisting phimosis.

Hypospadias Repair

Hypospadias is a congenital defect that consists of an abnormal positioning of the penile meatus. It occurs in approximately 1 out of every 350 male births. It ranges from a very mild defect, in which the urethral opening is located along the underside (ventral aspect) of the penis, to a severe defect where the opening is located on the underside of the scrotum. The severity of the lesion will determine the type of surgical procedure. Surgery is necessary to allow normal urination, to correct the deformation for cosmetic reasons, and to ensure normal sexual functioning in the case of a severe chordee. Repair is often performed during the first year of life.

There are several types of surgical procedures, depending on the severity of the lesion. In general, the more severe the lesion, the longer and more extensive the surgery. Preoperative

assessment is routine and includes screening for other congenital anomalies, and optimizing coexisting medical conditions. Laboratory studies are not indicated. Anxiolytic premedication should be ordered if the child is older than 10 or 11 months, and an oral analgesic may be included. Induction and maintenance of general anesthesia are provided by inhalational agents. Airway management consists of a supraglottic airway or tracheal intubation, depending on the age of the child and the length of the procedure. Regional anesthesia with a caudal epidural block or pudendal block is standard pain management, especially because the more involved repair is expected to cause prolonged pain and analgesic needs. Systemic analgesics may also be necessary.

Over the past several years there has been a controversy brewing[1] about whether the inclusion of caudal anesthesia increases the chances that the child will develop a postoperative urethral fistula. There is no plausible mechanism, and at this point, no convincing evidence[2] that there is an association.

Testicular Torsion Repair

Testicular torsion manifests as acute scrotal pain and results from a twisting of the spermatic cord with vascular compromise of the testicle. If the problem is not surgically corrected within about 6 to 8 hours, testicular ischemia can result. This is generally considered a surgical emergency. Temporizing treatment involves manual detorsion; this may alleviate ischemia but orchidopexy is still required.

Preoperatively, the patient should be prepared for emergency surgery. An intravenous (IV) catheter should be inserted to provide hydration and to prepare for a rapid sequence induction of general anesthesia. Adolescents may be offered spinal anesthesia with sedation. Intraoperative analgesia is provided by local infiltration at the surgical site and small doses of opioids. Postoperative concerns include pain and nausea/vomiting, which are treated by standard therapies.

Orchidopexy

Orchidopexy (also known as orchiopexy) is performed to repair cryptorchidism (also known as *undescended testicle*). During fetal development, the testicles develop in the abdomen and descend into the scrotum during the last trimester. In a small percentage of newborns (3%), one or both testicles fail to descend. Approximately half then descend within the first year of life. The remaining must undergo surgical intervention because of the increased risk for infertility and malignancy in testicles that remain undescended within the abdominal cavity during childhood.

Children with undescended testicles are usually healthy, although there is a higher incidence of prematurity. A number of congenital syndromes are assoicated with undescended testicles and include Noonan's and Prader-Willi syndromes, among many others. Prune-belly syndrome consists of undescended testicles, absent anterior abdominal musculature, and dilatation of parts of the urinary tract.

This rare syndrome may be accompanied by impaired renal function.

Preoperative assessment is routine and will depend on any coexisting medical conditions. Induction and maintenance of general anesthesia are routine. Airway management consists of a supraglottic airway or tracheal intubation. The procedure consists of two incisions: one in the lower groin to retrieve the testicle, and the other at the bottom of the scrotum to anchor the testicle. Blood and insensible fluid losses are minimal. Regional analgesia is provided by an ilioinguinal block (with surgical local infiltration of the scrotal incision) or caudal epidural block (see Chapter 20). Postoperative concerns include pain and nausea/vomiting.

A DEEPER DIVE: THE PUDENDAL NERVE BLOCK

The pudendal nerve block has been used for many applications in adults, and more recently has emerged as a regional technique for analgesia in pediatric urologic surgery. Pudendal blocks can offer notable advantages over traditional caudal blocks. Adverse effects associated with caudal blocks such as lower extremity motor blockade, are avoided by specifically targeting the innervation of the perineal space. Contraindications to neuraxial techniques may be circumvented. In terms of pain control, pudendal blocks have been shown to confer analgesia of better quality and longer duration compared with caudal block, when used for hypospadias repairr.[3]

The pudendal nerve provides sensory innervation to the external genitalia and perineal space, and motor innervation to the transverse perineal muscles and rectal and urethral sphincters. After originating from the anterior rami of S2 through S4, the pudendal nerve courses through the pudendal canal alongside the internal pudendal artery and vein. Its distal branches land within the ischioanal fossa, a fat-filled space between the rectum and ischium (Fig. 29.1). The transperineal approach is a field block that relies on the spread of local

anesthetic within the ischioanal fossa to reach to branches of the pudendal nerve.

The child is placed in lithotomy or frog leg position, and the needle is inserted between the rectum and ischial tuberosity, palpated laterally. Ultrasound is useful for visualizing local anesthetic spread within the ischioanal fossa, between the hypoechoic rectum and hyperechoic ischial tuberosity, and for avoiding rectal or vascular puncture (Fig. 29.2). If neurostimulation is used, conventional responses include (1) anal sphincter contraction from stimulation of the inferior rectal nerve, followed by (2) penile up-and-down movement from stimulation of the perineal nerve. A dose of 0.3 to 0.5 mL/kg of 0.2% ropivacaine or 0.25% bupivacaine with a maximum of 10 mL is injected on each side. Local anesthetic containing epinephrine is avoided to prevent terminal arterial ischemia.

As the pudendal nerve block is a relatively new technique to pediatric anesthesia, complication rates remain to be determined. Inherent to the block, there is a risk for injury to the rectum, vasculature, somatic and autonomic nerves, and a risk for infection. However, the block is generally superficial and relatively safe with the use of ultrasound.

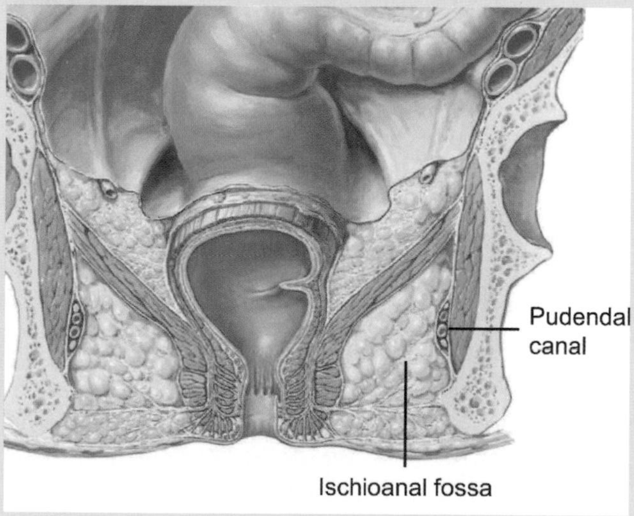

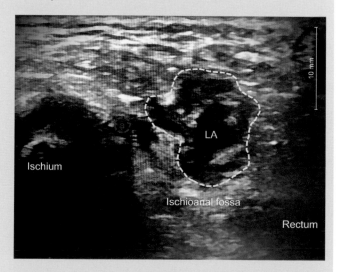

• **Fig 29.1.** Anatomy of the pudendal nerve within the pudendal canal. (From Hansen JT. Pelvis and perineum. In: *Netter's Clinical Anatomy*, 4th ed. Elsevier; 2019:233–289.)

• **Fig 29.2.** Ultrasound-guided pudendal nerve block. Local anesthetic (LA) is deposited within the ischioanal fossa, avoiding the pudendal artery (a).

Ureteral Reimplantation

Ureteral reimplantation is the surgical correction of vesico-ureteral reflux (VUR), which is a congenital incompetence at the site where the distal ureter implants into the bladder. This results in the retrograde flow of urine from the bladder up into the ureter and kidneys during micturition. If undiagnosed or untreated, VUR may cause dilatation of the ureter and hydronephrosis. Long-term effects include pyelonephritis, hypertension, and progressive renal failure. Many children with severe VUR are diagnosed in utero by a fetal ultrasound that demonstrates hydronephrosis. Milder forms may manifest during childhood as recurrent urinary tract infections.

Preoperative assessment includes evaluation of renal function. Premedication and fasting guidelines are age-appropriate.

Traditionally the procedure is performed in the supine position, with a low transverse incision, but advances in robotic surgical techniques have resulted in nearly all our repairs now done robotically with the patient in the lateral position. The procedure involves reimplantation of the distal ureter into the bladder wall. Several surgical methods have been described to prevent VUR and are beyond the scope of this discussion. Cystoscopic injection of an anti-reflux material (Deflux) into the bladder wall is employed in selected cases. Intraoperative anesthetic considerations include maintenance of normothermia and administration of sufficient fluid to avoid stasis of blood within the bladder that can obstruct bladder outflow.

Induction and maintenance of general anesthesia are routine. Intraoperative and postoperative pain control can be accomplished using opioids and ketorolac, especially if the robotic technique is used, in which there are only several small incisions to accommodate the telescopic arms of the robot. Regional anesthesia is preferred in some centers. In recent years, we have found[4] that intrathecal morphine 5 µg/kg instead of epidural local anesthesia provides excellent postoperative analgesia. Postoperative pain from bladder spasms can be troublesome. Treatment includes ketorolac[5] and bethanechol.

Pyeloplasty

A pyeloplasty is a procedure to repair ureteropelvic junction (UPJ) obstruction, the most common cause of congenital hydronephrosis. In most cases it is diagnosed by fetal ultra-sonography. Older children may present with urosepsis, nausea/vomiting, failure to thrive, flank pain, abdominal mass, or hematuria. The most common surgical therapy is a robotic pyeloplasty, which involves excision of the narrowed segment of the UPJ and a reanastomosis of the ureter to the renal pelvis.

Preoperative assessment includes confirmation of normal renal function. Induction and maintenance of general anesthesia are standard with endotracheal intubation performed for the procedure. The infant will be placed in the semilateral position with flexion of the OR table. Blood loss should be minimal. Routine monitors will suffice.

Intraoperative and postoperative analgesia can be accomplished with epidural analgesia, intrathecal morphine, or neither because of the minimally invasive robotic technique. Systemic analgesia can include opioids and ketorolac. There are no unique postoperative anesthetic issues for these children.

Wilms Tumor

Wilms tumor is the most common renal tumor in children. Most cases are sporadic, but some are inherited. It is most commonly diagnosed in preschool children. Presenting signs and symptoms may include an abdominal mass, abdominal pain, hypertension, fever, hematuria, and anemia. An associated, acquired von Willebrand disease has been reported in some of these children. In advanced disease, the tumor most commonly spreads to the liver and lungs, and may spread contiguously to the inferior vena cava and aorta. Treatment consists of a radical nephrectomy of the involved kidney, chemotherapy, and possibly radiation (also see Chapter 8). The prognosis depends on the extent of spread and histology of the tumor.

Preoperative assessment should include a complete blood count, electrolytes, liver and renal function studies, coagulation studies, and a type-and-crossmatch. Radiologic studies should assess the extent of spread of the tumor and presence of metastases. Cardiac function should be assessed in children who have received chemotherapy with anthracyclines (e.g., doxorubicin). Children with a large intraabdominal mass that impedes gastric emptying should have preoperative placement of an IV catheter for rehydration and to prepare for a rapid sequence induction of general anesthesia. Anxiolytics should be administered as appropriate.

The procedure is performed with the child supine. Standard monitors are sufficient unless there is significant tumor involvement of the aorta or inferior vena cava IVC. If this is the case, a central venous catheter may be inserted for monitoring central venous pressure and ease of large volume infusions. In addition, an arterial catheter may be indicated for direct blood pressure measurement and facilitation of intraoperative blood tests. Two large-bore IV catheters should be placed in the upper extremities and red blood cells should be immediately available for transfusion if necessary. Intraoperative risks include sudden or massive blood loss, tumor embolism, or hypotension from IVC compression and loss of preload. Insensible fluid losses may exceed 10 mL/kg/h, depending on the extent of the surgical procedure. Hypothermia is common and should be prevented by warming the OR, use of a forced-air warming blanket, and warming of IV fluids and blood products.

Unless the tumor is very large (indicating the need for rapid sequence intubation RSI), induction of general anesthesia is routine. Maintenance of general anesthesia should consist of a balanced technique using neuromuscular blockade to enhance surgical exposure. If coagulation studies are normal, an epidural catheter may be placed after induction to provide intraoperative and postoperative analgesia. Unless the surgical procedure involved large blood losses or clinically significant hemodynamic changes, these children are awakened and extubated in the OR. Postoperative admission to the intensive care unit is dependent on the medical condition of the patient and the extent of the surgery. Postoperative concerns include oliguria that may be caused by impaired renal function or hypovolemia if bleeding is continuing. Poor pain control may result in splinting, and cause atelectasis and hypoxemia.

References

1. Braga LH, McGrath M, Farrokhyar F. Dorsal penile block versus caudal epidural anesthesia effect on complications post-hypospadias repair: Dilemmas, damned dilemmas and statistics. *J Pediatr Urol*. 2020;16(5):708–711. https://doi.org/10.1016/j.jpurol.2020.08.009.

2. Splinter WM, Kim J, Kim AM, Harrison MA. Effect of anesthesia for hypospadias repair on perioperative complications. *Paediatr Anaesth*. 2019;29(7):760–767. https://doi.org/10.1111/pan.13657.

3. Kendigelen P, Tutuncu AC, Emre S, Altindas F, Kaya G. Pudendal Versus Caudal Block in Children Undergoing Hypospadias Surgery: A Randomized Controlled Trial. *Reg Anesth Pain Med*. 2016;41(5):610–615. https://doi.org/10.1097/AAP.0000000000000447.

4. Ganesh A, Kim A, Casale P, Cucchiaro G. Low-dose intrathecal morphine for postoperative analgesia in children. *Anesth Analg*. 2007;104(2):271–276. https://doi.org/10.1213/01.ane.0000252418.05394.28.

5. Park JM, Houck CS, Sethna NF, et al. Ketorolac suppresses postoperative bladder spasms after pediatric ureteral reimplantation. *Anesth Analg*. 2000;91(1):11–15. https://doi.org/10.1097/00000539-200007000-00003.

30

Remote Anesthetizing Locations

RONALD S. LITMAN

More and more pediatric anesthesia cases are scheduled in non operating room (OR) locations. These locations are often far from the main surgical area, and some anesthesiologists feel out of place in these environments because they may not have easy access to anesthesia equipment and helpful personnel. This chapter will review the implications for anesthetizing children in the most common non-OR areas so that you will now feel "in place" when you are assigned there.

The location of the anesthetic does not alter the standard of care with regard to safety standards of monitoring and personnel. At all times, the American Society of Anesthesiologists Guidelines for Nonoperating Room Anesthetizing Locations applies. When total intravenous (IV) anesthesia is administered, it is not necessary to also have a full anesthesia machine with inhaled anesthetics. Children with anticipated difficult airways (ventilation or intubation) should first have their airway safely secured in the main operating room area where there is a full complement of equipment and personnel, and then be transported to the location of the procedure with an endotracheal tube and continuous capnography.

The cost efficiency of anesthetizing children in remote areas may also present an additional challenge. The daily schedule should take into account the time it takes to transport patients between anesthetizing locations and the postanesthesia care unit (PACU). Unexpected delays are common and should be incorporated into the normal scheduling times (so they become expected delays). Ideally, in any given institution, a subset of anesthesiologists will make up the "off-site team" so that differences in preferences and techniques will be minimized and a trusting relationship can develop between members of the team and staff in these areas.

Magnetic Resonance Imaging

General anesthesia for magnetic resonance imaging (MRI) has become easier to accomplish with the advent of MRI-compatible anesthesia machines, monitoring stations, and electronic infusion pumps, which are nonferromagnetic. MRI-compatible temperature monitors are especially indicated for neonates and small infants because the relatively cold environment in the scanner room predisposes this population to hypothermia. These patients should be covered with several layers of blankets and the MRI fan should be turned off. Limiting the volume of IV fluids administered will also minimize hypothermia. There are many possible anesthetic techniques for pediatric MRI. If the child is an outpatient and does not have preexisting IV access, general anesthesia is induced by inhaled sevoflurane. This may occur within the MRI scanner room or at a nearby separate anesthetizing location, depending on the location of the anesthesia machine and supplies.

At our institution, children for MRI undergo induction of general anesthesia by sevoflurane inhalation in an area separate from the scanner, to optimize the use of ferromagnetic equipment that cannot be used in the immediate scanner vicinity. We maintain two induction rooms and two anesthesia machines in a central location between MRI magnets. Maintenance of general anesthesia is most often accomplished using a laryngeal mask airway and sevoflurane in oxygen. This technique reliably eliminates upper airway obstruction that may occur with a propofol infusion and natural airway technique, and administration of ondansetron eliminates nearly all post-operative nausea and vomiting (PONV). Endotracheal intubation is preferred for small infants and neonates. Intubated children who require scans of the head or neck will benefit from the use of an oral RAE tube, because of its lower profile when using a head coil.

The most important anesthetic consideration in MRI is to ensure that no ferromagnetic objects are accidentally brought into the MRI scanner room. In the presence of a strong magnetic field, these objects become dangerous projectile missiles that can maim or fatally injure[1] the patient or personnel (Fig. 30.1). This includes all types of anesthesia equipment, oxygen tanks, IV poles, gurneys, etc. All oxygen tanks in the MRI facility should be made of aluminum. Each MRI facility must have strict safety precautions that limit the number and types of personnel allowed into the scanner area, and protocols should be established to detect metallic objects transported into the facility. We typically monitor the child using a remote access monitor in an adjacent room (Fig. 30.2).

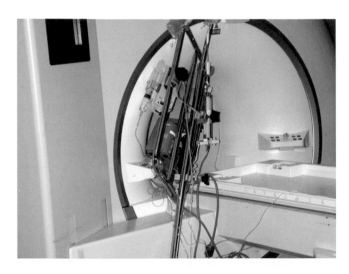

• **Fig 30.1.** Ferromagnetic IV pole with infusion pumps drawn into magnet (Courtesy of Ronald S. Litman).

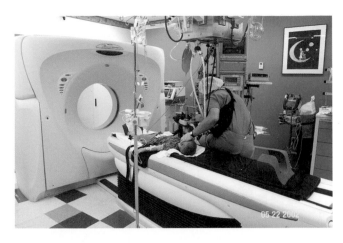

• **Fig 30.3.** Anesthesia for CT scan. The anesthesia provider applies mask ventilation with sevoflurane and leaves the room during the scan if the airway is patent (Courtesy of Ronald S. Litman).

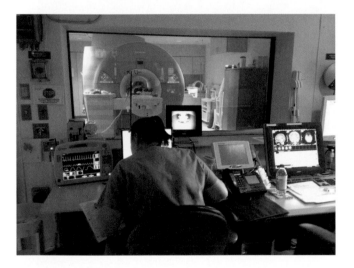

• **Fig 30.2.** During MRI the anesthesia provider monitors the patient from an adjacent room (Courtesy of Ronald S. Litman).

Computerized Tomography

Computerized tomography (CT) scan technology has improved to the point where most scans are so brief that the need for sedation or anesthesia in children has decreased considerably. However, children with severe anxiety or significant medical disease will still require our services. There are few anesthetic implications for the child who requires general anesthesia for a CT scan. Standard anesthesia machines and monitoring devices can be used in close proximity to the child. The anesthesia provider may remain near the child during the scan (with lead protection) (Fig. 30.3) or may leave the room during the brief scan as long as the child's airway is patent.

There are two important anesthetic-related issues in children presenting for CT. The first is the timing of the administration of oral contrast before abdominal CT. Although decreasing in frequency, some centers use Diatrizoate Meglumine (Gastrografin, Gastroview, Hypaque, etc.), a water-soluble iodinated substance with an osmolality of 1900 mmol/L. Radiologists prefer that contrast be administered within an hour of the time of the scan to enhance visualization of the upper gastrointestinal tract. However, this violates generally accepted fasting guidelines, and may predispose the child to aspiration of the contrast after onset of general anesthesia (or sedation) with an unprotected airway. The gastric emptying time of diatrizoate is not known, but it can be assumed to empty with the same speed as a clear liquid because there is no ingredient (fat or protein) that delays gastric emptying. Nevertheless, pulmonary aspiration of this agent is dangerous because its high osmolality renders it toxic to the lung. Therefore many pediatric anesthesiologists choose to perform rapid sequence induction of general anesthesia with tracheal intubation after contrast administration, instead of "deep sedation" without airway protection. Alternatively, the contrast material can be administered via an orogastric tube after routine administration of general anesthesia and endotracheal intubation. This latter method then requires a waiting period for the contrast to pass into the intestinal tract while the patient is anesthetized in a separate area from the CT scanner (so as not to interfere with patient throughput). In each institution, anesthesiologists and radiologists should agree on a standard protocol that best meets their patients' needs.

The second issue concerns children with cancer undergoing chest CT for detection of (usually metastatic) lung tumors. The onset of general anesthesia and immediate loss of functional residual capacity, and development of atelectasis may often mask small lung nodules (Fig. 30.4). Therefore, it may be necessary for the anesthesiologist to provide positive pressure, either by endotracheal tube or laryngeal mask, to expand and reveal all possible lung fields. Usually, the addition of 5 cmH$_2$O of positive end expiratory pressure (PEEP) will attenuate atelectasis. One may also provide transient PEEP and positive pressure ventilation using a bag-mask technique in unintubated children under deep sedation.

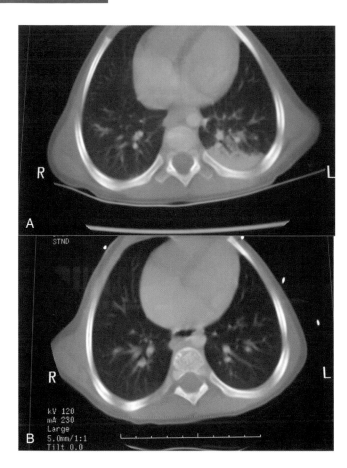

• **Fig 30.4.** Diagnostic chest CT for metastases in child with Wilms tumor. (A) Spontaneous ventilation without positive pressure during general anesthesia often results in atelectasis (posterior left lung). (B) Positive pressure expands lungs and removes atelectasis to reveal all lung fields (Courtesy of Ronald S. Litman).

TABLE 30.1	Unique Anesthetic Considerations of Radiation/Proton Treatment

The child must remain absolutely motionless.

Children undergoing treatment to the brain must wear a constrictive hard plastic mask that adheres tight to their face.

For treatment of posteriorly located brain tumors, the child is turned prone, with their chin resting on a platform that pushes the mandible posteriorly, sometimes causing obstruction of the breathing passage behind it (Fig. 30.5).

For brain tumors, the child undergoes this treatment every weekday for a period of up to 6 weeks; abdominal radiation usually lasts 1–2 weeks.

In some centers, total body irradiation (TBI) necessitates that the child lies prone, and sometimes, on the floor.

With the burden of having a child with cancer, and the necessity of traveling far from home, parents have no tolerance for minor day-to-day inconsistencies.

The anesthesia provider must monitor the child from another room.

Radiation Oncology

The radiation treatment suite is a unique environment for anesthetizing children. It is usually located far from the main OR suite, sometimes in a remote building. There are a number of important considerations that differ from any other anesthetic (Table 30.1).

Most radiation treatments last approximately 20 to 30 minutes, depending on the nature of the tumor and the specific radiation protocol. Radiographs are also obtained weekly. The anesthesia provider monitors the patient's vital signs, oxyhemoglobin saturation and capnograph by observing a monitor outside the treatment room, or by watching a

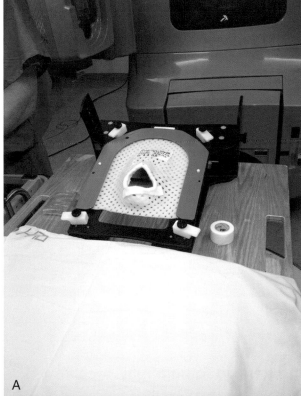

A

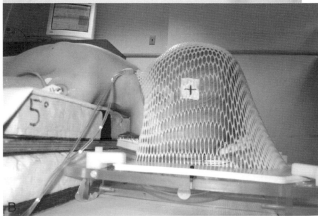

B

• **Fig 30.5.** (A) Hard plastic facemask to accommodate the patient's face during prone radiation treatment. (B) Patient is positioned prone for radiation treatment (Courtesy of Ronald S. Litman).

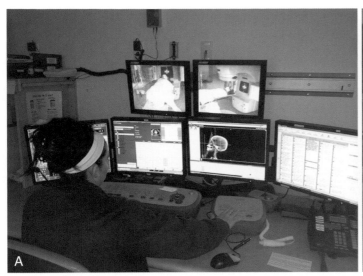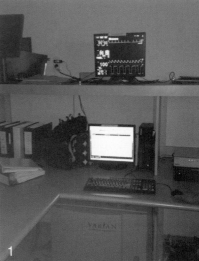

• **Fig 30.6.** (A) The radiation technologist programs the treatment and directly observes the patient in an adjacent room. (B) Remote monitoring of the radiation treatment patient outside the treatment room (Courtesy of Ronald S. Litman).

video screen connected to a camera focused on the monitor inside the room (Fig. 30.6). Additional video cameras are used to observe the patient, to detect patient movement.

We have found that the most practical method for rapid induction and recovery of general anesthesia after radiation treatment is a propofol-based technique, with a supraglottic airway. The tones of the pulse oximeter should be heard via a microphone inside the treatment room that is transmitted to speakers located in the observation area.

Most children have tunneled central venous catheters or implanted venous access ports. If not, every attempt is made at the first visit to place a long intravenous catheter that can remain for the duration of the treatment (i.e., PIC line). This enables the child to become anesthetized each day without the emotional trauma of a mask inhaled induction or the need for midazolam premedication. Parents should be counseled about proper fasting guidelines and encouraged to offer their child clear liquids 1 hour before each daily treatment. To minimize fasting, these treatments should be scheduled as early in the day as possible.

The Oncology Clinic

General anesthesia is often provided in the oncology clinic, where children require painful procedures such as bone marrow biopsy, and lumbar puncture for administration of intrathecal chemotherapy. These procedures are performed with the child lying prone or in the lateral position (Fig. 30.7), depending on the preference of the practitioner performing the procedure. Oral premedication may not be necessary because most children who are currently receiving chemotherapy will have some type of existing IV catheter.

The anesthetic should be tailored for a severe but brief painful stimulus. Some anesthesiologists prefer a sedative technique using a combination of a benzodiazepine (e.g.,

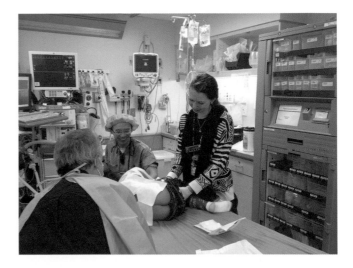

• **Fig 30.7.** Anesthesia in the oncology clinic (Courtesy of Ronald S. Litman).

midazolam) and an opioid (e.g., fentanyl or remifentanil). However, this technique will rarely ensure complete loss of consciousness and immobility and may prolong time to discharge and worsen nausea and vomiting. If this technique is used, antiemetic prophylaxis is indicated.

Some anesthesiologists prefer a propofol-based technique, which renders the patient unconscious and is not associated with prolonged recovery or emesis. However, the depth of propofol anesthesia that is required to induce immobility in the face of a severely painful stimulus, almost always causes apnea, thus necessitating assisted ventilation.

In our oncology clinic, we prefer an inhaled agent-based technique. We maintain an anesthesia machine in the procedure room, with a fully stocked anesthesia equipment cart and an experienced anesthesia technician on site at all times (Fig. 30.7). We use propofol for induction of general anesthesia (or sevoflurane if the child does not have existing IV access), and then maintain general anesthesia with sevoflurane by mask or supraglottic airway. This technique provides immobility, analgesia, and maintenance of spontaneous ventilation with relatively short emergence and discharge times.

References

1. ABC News. (2006). *Boy, 6, killed in freak MRI accident.* https://abcnews.go.com/US/story? id=92745&page=1. Accessed 21.06.28.

Suggested Reading

Committee on Standards and Practice Parameters (CSPP). (2018). Statement on nonoperating room anesthetizing locations. *American Society of Anesthesiologists* [Last update 2018]. https://www.asahq.org/standards-and-guidelines/statement-on-nonoperating-room-anesthetizing-locations; Accessed 21.10.5.

31

Postoperative Considerations

RONALD S. LITMAN

The pediatric postanesthesia care unit (PACU) is a noisy and chaotic environment. Nurses are attempting to calm crying toddlers, parents are being educated, physicians are being summoned for discharge orders, and the phones ring continuously with reports of available inpatient beds. Monitor alarms are artifactually ringing, and entire families gather in their child's room to watch the latest reality television show. But lying beneath the din, some children are in pain, or nauseated, or unconsciously screaming for no reason whatsoever. Some children may even become deeply hypoxic. Such is the daily routine in a busy children's hospital PACU.

Routine Postoperative Care

Each child's vital signs shall be fully monitored until they have regained their baseline neurologic and cardiorespiratory status. Continuous pulse oximetry is vital because the most important postoperative complication is upper airway obstruction, which rapidly leads to hypoxemia. Upper airway obstruction can be detected even faster using continuous capnography, but most PACUs do not yet use the technology to monitor end-tidal carbon dioxide in an awake and spontaneously breathing child. Continuous electrocardiogram (ECG) monitoring is only necessary in select cases, depending on the patient's clinical status. The child's temperature should be obtained on arrival in the PACU and monitored at regular intervals until discharge. Hypothermia is common in small children who may require a warming blanket postoperatively. Hyperthermia is occasionally seen in some children as a result of iatrogenic overheating in the operating room (OR), or other unknown factors related to the surgical procedure. It is never an initial presenting feature of malignant hyperthermia, unless accompanied by other signs and symptoms of hypermetabolism. Supplemental oxygen administration should be guided by pulse oximetry. In some centers, children are discharged from the phase 1 acute PACU to the phase 2 recovery area (day surgery unit) after regaining consciousness and maintaining stability of vital signs without oxygen supplementation. In other centers, these two phases are combined into one area where the patient stays until discharge home or to an inpatient care area.

Discharge Criteria

Many pediatric centers have established specific physiologic parameters that classify the stages of emergence after general anesthesia. These criteria are used to determine readiness for discharge to the hospital ward or to home. Most pediatric centers use discharge criteria first described[1] in 1975 by David Steward, who modified the standard Aldrete recovery score[2] for use in children (Table 31.1).

The Steward score uses levels of consciousness and airway patency, to a total score of six used to establish appropriate readiness for discharge. However, the relationship of this score to other outcome variables, such as oxyhemoglobin value, has not been established. In most pediatric centers, there are additional discharge requirements that include adequate hydration, pain control, and control of nausea and vomiting. Gradual oral intake of fluids is allowed but not encouraged or required for discharge home. Urinary voiding is also not required for discharge home unless specified by the surgeon based on the procedure.

Postoperative Complications

Nausea and Vomiting

Postoperative nausea and vomiting (PONV) are probably the most common complications after general anesthesia in children. Although PONV is not life-threatening, it causes profound discomfort to the child and their family and has been demonstrated to be a primary factor in patient dissatisfaction. Certain types of procedures, such as ENT, ophthalmologic, and orthopedic, increase the risk for PONV. Anesthetic risk factors include use of inhaled anesthetics and opioids. Patient-related factors include previous PONV, history of motion sickness, and age greater than about 3 years. The incidence of PONV can be decreased by use of propofol instead of inhaled agents, avoidance of opioids, use of regional anesthesia, limiting postoperative oral intake, increasing intravenous hydration, and prophylactic administration of antiemetic medications. Combination (multimodal) therapy with different classes of antiemetics more successfully prevents PONV than one type of antiemetic alone. Intraoperative evacuation of gastric contents does not

TABLE 31.1	Steward Postanesthetic Recovery Score	
Patient Sign	**Ocular Effects**	**Score**
Consciousness	• Awake	2
	• Responds to stimuli	1
	• Does not respond to stimuli	0
Airway	• Actively crying or coughs on command	2
	• Maintains airway patency	1
	• Requires assistance to maintain airway patency	0
Movement	• Moves limbs purposefully	2
	• Moves limbs randomly	1
	• Not moving	0

reduce PONV in adults but has not been studied in pediatric patients. Children with protracted PONV are admitted to continue IV access to provide fluids and analgesics.

Serotonin Antagonists

Serotonin (5-HT$_3$) antagonists significantly reduce the incidence and severity of vomiting in the first 24 hours after surgery and are the first-line medications because of their favorable benefit-to-risk ratio. Although there are several different varieties of serotonin antagonists, ondansetron is the oldest and most widely studied in children and is available as a generic preparation. Newer variants may have a longer duration of action than ondansetron. Doses of ondansetron probably do not need to exceed 0.05 mg/kg.[3] Children that develop PONV despite receiving ondansetron prophylaxis usually do not respond to additional doses but may respond to another type of serotonin antagonist.

Dexamethasone

Dexamethasone is a glucocorticoid steroid that effectively prevents and treats PONV. Combination therapy along with a serotonin antagonist is more effective than when either is administered alone, and is indicated in children at high risk for PONV. Dose ranging studies demonstrate inconsistent results. Most pediatric anesthesiologists use a dose of 0.1 to 0.5 mg/kg. Side effects of dexamethasone include hyperactivity, insomnia, and increased appetite. Dexamethasone may cause tumor lysis syndrome[4] in patients with leukemia, and thus, should be avoided in these patients.

Nonpharmacologic Treatment of PONV

Acupuncture, acupressure, and electrical stimulation at the Nei-Guan (P6) point on the wrist (slightly proximal to the distal skin crease of the wrist on the ulnar side) have been shown to decrease the incidence of PONV in children but these methods have not been adopted in most centers.

Stridor

Inspiratory stridor in the postoperative period (also called postintubation or postextubation croup) is an indication of upper airway swelling, usually below the glottis. It is presumed to be caused by tracheal mucosal edema related to pressure from a cuffed or uncuffed endotracheal tube. The exact location of the swelling is unknown but presumed to be located at the level of the rigid cricoid ring. In a past era (before the 1990s), the incidence of postintubation croup was about 1%, but in the present era, it is much less than that. This decrease is largely because of the use of nonreactive endotracheal tubes, recognition of keeping the endotracheal tube cuff pressure low, and increased use of the laryngeal mask instead of an endotracheal tube. When it occurs, it rarely causes oxyhemoglobin desaturation. If the child with stridor underwent surgery of the upper airway or neck, immediate surgical consultation is warranted. Initial management strategies include administration of supplemental oxygen, repositioning the head or neck, administration of dexamethasone (if not already given for PONV prophylaxis), and, if severe, or if oxygen saturations are declining, nebulized racemic epinephrine. If stridor is progressive and associated with a worsening SpO$_2$ despite the aforementioned therapies, tracheal intubation is indicated, and ENT consultation is required to help with diagnosis and further management. In mild cases that require minimal intervention, the child can be discharged home when the stridor has abated, as long as there is no evidence of oxyhemoglobin desaturation (e.g., below 96%) without oxygen supplementation.

Inhaled racemic epinephrine (supplied as a 2.25% solution) provides topical vasoconstriction and shrinks edematous tracheal tissue. The dose is 0.05 mL/kg (maximum dose 0.5 mL) diluted in 3 mL of normal saline. It is administered as a nebulized solution every hour if needed, based on clinical symptoms and sympathomimetic side effects. Administration of racemic epinephrine usually constitutes mandatory overnight or prolonged hospital observation because of its limited duration of effects and possible recurrence of airway obstruction.

Emergence Delirium

Emergence delirium (ED) is a state of inconsolable agitation shortly after waking up from general anesthesia. It is characterized by unremitting crying, tachycardia, pupillary dilatation, disinterest in drinking, and the inability to be consoled by the presence of parents. Although essentially a benign condition, it is extremely disconcerting to parents and even PACU staff. The Pediatric Anesthesia Emergence Delirium (PAED) scale[5] was created and validated to measure ED in children, and has mainly been used as a research tool. It consists of five reliable indicators of ED: (1) lack of eye contact with the caregiver; (2) nonpurposeful actions; (3) lack of awareness of surroundings; (4) restlessness; and (5) inconsolability.

The precise cause is unknown but is thought to represent a state of residual anesthetic agent in the brain that causes disinhibition. "Stormy inductions" and maintenance of general anesthesia with sevoflurane or desflurane increase the incidence of emergence delirium. Administration of intraoperative propofol,[6] fentanyl,[7] morphine, and α_2-adrenergic agonists (e.g., clonidine[8] and dexmedetomidine[9]) have been shown to decrease the incidence of ED. Once ED occurs, it is treated by having the child fall asleep by reducing external stimuli (e.g., lights out) and swaddling the child in a warm blanket. This may be facilitated by administration of small amounts of morphine, propofol, or dexmedetomidine. Once asleep, these children will typically awaken in about an hour in a more normal state of grogginess.

The most important aspect of emergence delirium is to differentiate it from serious events, such as hypoxemia and pain that need prompt treatment.

Hyponatremia

In some children, postoperative dilutional hyponatremia (<125 mEq/L) results from hypotonic fluid administration combined with high antidiuretic hormone (ADH) levels. Acute hyponatremia can lead to the development of cerebral edema. Symptoms include confusion and lethargy but can be as severe as seizures, coma, or death if sodium levels drop below 115 mEq/L. Because postoperative hyponatremia is associated with the use of hypotonic intravenous maintenance fluid, only isotonic fluids[10] are recommended in children in the immediate postoperative period, unless otherwise indicated by the clinical situation.

References

1. Steward DJ. A simplified scoring system for the post-operative recovery room. *Can Anaesth Soc J.* 1975;22(1):111–113. https://doi.org/10.1007/BF03004827.
2. Antonio AJ, Kroulik D. A Postanesthetic Recovery Score. *Anesth Analg.* 1970;49(6):924–934.
3. Watcha MF, Bras PJ, Cieslak GD, Pennant JH. The dose-response relationship of ondansetron in preventing postoperative emesis in pediatric patients undergoing ambulatory surgery. *Anesthesiology.* 1995;82(1):47–52. https://doi.org/10.1097/00000542-199501000-00007.
4. Chanimov M, Koren-Michowitz M, Cohen ML, Pilipodi S, Bahar M. Tumor lysis syndrome induced by dexamethasone. *Anesthesiology.* 2006;105(3):633–634. https://doi.org/10.1097/00000542-200609000-00042.
5. Sikich N, Lerman J. Development and psychometric evaluation of the pediatric anesthesia emergence delirium scale. *Anesthesiology.* 2004;100(5):1138–1145. https://doi.org/10.1097/00000542-200405000-00015.
6. Aouad MT, Yazbeck-Karam VG, Nasr VG, El-Khatib MF, Kanazi GE, Bleik JH. A single dose of propofol at the end of surgery for the prevention of emergence agitation in children undergoing strabismus surgery during sevoflurane anesthesia. *Anesthesiology.* 2007;107(5):733–738. https://doi.org/10.1097/01.anes.0000287009.46896.a7.
7. Cravero JP, Beach M, Thyr B, Whalen K. The effect of small dose fentanyl on the emergence characteristics of pediatric patients after sevoflurane anesthesia without surgery. *Anesth Analg.* 2003;97(2):364–367. https://doi.org/10.1213/01.ane.0000070227.78670.43.
8. Pickard A, Davies P, Birnie K, Beringer R. Systematic review and meta-analysis of the effect of intraoperative α_2-adrenergic agonists on postoperative behaviour in children. *Br J Anaesth.* 2014;112(6):982–990. https://doi.org/10.1093/bja/aeu093.
9. Guler G, Akin A, Tosun Z, Ors S, Esmaoglu A, Boyaci A. Single-dose dexmedetomidine reduces agitation and provides smooth extubation after pediatric adenotonsillectomy. *Paediatr Anaesth.* 2005;15(9):762–766. https://doi.org/10.1111/j.1460-9592.2004.01541.x.
10. Moritz ML, Ayus JC. Hyponatraemia: Isotonic fluids prevent hospital-acquired hyponatraemia. *Nat Rev Nephrol.* 2015;11(4):202–203. https://doi.org/10.1038/nrneph.2014.253.

Suggested Reading

Vlajkovic GP, Sindjelic RP. Emergence delirium in children: many questions, few answers. *Anesth Analg.* 2007;104(1):84–91. https://doi.org/10.1213/01.ane.0000250914.91881.a8.

32

Pediatric Pain Assessment

F. WICKHAM KRAEMER III*

The next several chapters are dedicated to teaching trainees about pediatric pain and the various options for pain management in children. In this first of five chapters, we introduce the topic of pediatric pain assessment. Because expression of pain is related to age and development, practitioners must use specially developed and validated tools for assessing and measuring pain in different age groups. You cannot manage what you cannot measure.

Pediatric pain is often not recognized and not effectively managed. Perhaps this is caused by the inability of children to effectively describe the location and severity of their pain, especially those with cognitive impairment. But health care workers may also unknowingly contribute to the inadequate treatment of pain in children. The basis for this is speculative and may include a lack of knowledge about pathophysiology of pediatric pain or pharmacology of analgesics in pediatric patients. Other possible explanations include ignorance of appropriate pediatric pain assessment tools and available treatment options and an inability to recognize the large variability in pain experienced by different patients with similar types of pain.

Many health care professionals still believe that pain is an inevitable, expected consequence of illness and injury, and that pain is less harmful than the risks associated with the analgesic interventions. Many parents believe that their child's pain is unavoidable or they fear side effects of analgesics. Inflexible prescribing practices that use PRN regimens with inappropriately low or infrequent analgesic doses still occur. Fear of side effects such as nausea, vomiting, respiratory depression, and fear of long-term sequelae (e.g., drug dependence and addiction) also cause inadequate treatment of pain in children. The fact is, however, that a variety of analgesic therapies can be provided safely to children, even prematurely born neonates.

Lack of adequate pain treatment in children is partially caused by the lack of approved labeling of potent analgesics. Pharmaceutical companies have been unwilling to fund necessary studies to obtain pediatric labeling because the market size is limited. This has resulted in a paucity of pharmacokinetic and pharmacodynamic data and a lack of information about adverse effects.

At What Age Are Children Capable of Experiencing Pain?

To experience pain, one must possess the ability to perceive a peripheral noxious stimulus via a functioning nociceptive system and to develop a motor, autonomic, metabolic, psychological, behavioral, or emotional response. Neonates sense noxious stimuli and routinely demonstrate all these responses. In the developing fetus, cutaneous sensation begins in the 7th week of gestation in the perioral region and soon spreads to the face, hands, feet, and trunk. By the 15th week of gestation, cutaneous sensation has spread to the extremities, and by the 20th week of gestation, sensory perception is present in all cutaneous and mucosal regions. Substance P appears in fetal nerve tissue by the 10th week and endogenous opioids are detected at the 22nd week of gestation. Synapses begin to form between peripheral sensory neurons and dorsal horn neurons by this time. Myelination of nerve tracts in the spinal cord and brainstem begins during the 22nd week of gestation and is complete by the third trimester. Peripheral nerve myelination is not fully completed until after birth. However, one of the major nociceptive neurons is unmyelinated (C-fibers) and the other is thinly myelinated (A-δ fibers). This does not mean that noxious signals are not transmitted, but that they are transmitted more slowly.

Centrally, the cerebral cortex begins to develop at 8 weeks and will contain 10 billion neurons by the 20th week of gestation. Fetal electroencephalographic patterns, though intermittent and unsynchronized, appear by the 22nd week; by the 27th week, signals are synchronized in both hemispheres. By the 30th gestational week, cortical evoked potentials can be detected. At the beginning of the third trimester, all elements of the nociceptive system required to process noxious stimulation are present. The only component of the nociceptive system that is not present at birth is the descending inhibitory pathway, which develops during the first 6 months of antenatal life. Thus the neonate is not capable of attenuating nociceptive signals. The dorsal horn cells of the neonate that are responsible for transmitting nociceptive signals centrally have wider receptive fields and lower excitatory thresholds than in older subjects. These properties mature quickly in the postnatal period. Excitatory thresholds of dorsal horn neurons are further lowered by repetitive minor injuries such as daily heel lancing. Neonates may experience more pain in response to a given noxious stimulus than older children or adults.

Some practitioners erroneously assume that, because neonates cannot remember a painful event, it is of no consequence. But the metabolic and behavioral stress response that accompanies neonatal pain is associated with increased morbidity and mortality. This response can be reduced by using regional anesthesia, opioids, or general anesthesia before painful procedures.

Though little is known about neonatal consciousness and the perception of pain, there is evidence of complex, integrated cortical responses to nociceptive stimulation. Neonates that are subjected to noxious events (circumcision, repeated heel lancing, phlebotomy, etc.) demonstrate abnormalities in short-term behavior such as periods of increased crying, and feeding and sleeping abnormalities. Furthermore, painful experiences during early infancy affect future responses to painful events. In some instances, physiologic responses are enhanced, while behavioral responses are blunted. Opposite changes may occur under different circumstances. For example, infants who were circumcised at birth without anesthesia will demonstrate an exaggerated pain response to immunizations[1] in the first year of life compared with infants who received some form of pain control during newborn circumcision.

To summarize, neonates may not be able to interpret or remember painful events but even premature newborns are capable of perceiving noxious events and mounting a variety of physiologic and behavioral responses. These responses may translate into short- and long-term behavioral changes during subsequent painful stimuli. Because these stress responses and adverse outcomes can be reduced by the judicious use of analgesics, pain should be anticipated whenever possible, recognized when present, and treated appropriately.

Assessing Pain in Children

One of the challenges of pediatric pain management is the assessment and treatment of pain in preverbal children and patients with neurologic or cognitive impairment who cannot communicate their experience of pain.

Pain assessment is most accurate when the child can describe its location, nature, and severity. With appropriate words and tools, children over 3 years of age can reliably communicate their pain and may be able to relate their pain to a number or face on a scale (see below). In children under 3 years, one must rely on a combination of behavioral clues and physiologic signs. Many of these signs are also seen in conditions other than pain, such as parental separation, hunger, fear, and anxiety. Thus misinterpretation is common. Parents can often determine whether their child is in pain by learning specific behaviors in their child that distinguish pain from distress or anxiety.

Piaget described four developmental stages of childhood. During the initial *sensorimotor stage* (up to approximately 2 years of age), children have little or no understanding of pain and no language ability. During this stage, we rely on behaviors (posture, activity, crying, feeding, sleeping, etc.) and physiologic signs (e.g., tachycardia, hypertension, diaphoresis, and oxyhemoglobin saturation) to determine the severity of an infant's pain. We primarily rely on five different types of pain scales that are used in different age groups. For the neonatal population[2] (up to approximately 3 months of age), we use the Neonatal Infant Pain Scale (Table 32.1). It is primarily used to assess pain associated with medical procedures and includes assessment of facial expression, severity of crying, breathing patterns, movement of arms and legs, and state of arousal.

The CRIES score is also used in infants and uses five parameters: severity of crying, oxygen requirement, increased heart rate and blood pressure, facial expression, and degree of sleeplessness, each of which are graded from zero to two; this gives a total between zero and 10 (Table 32.2). A score over four indicates that additional analgesics are required.

The second Piaget developmental stage is the *preoperational stage* (approximately 2 to 7 years), in which children acquire some language ability and can localize pain, differentiate "a little" and "a lot," and can use simple terms to describe their pain such as "boo-boo," "ouch," "hurt," and "ow-ee." For this age group, we commonly use the Wong-Baker FACES (Fig. 32.1) scale or the FLACC scale (Table 32.3). This FACES scale has recently been updated to include more realistic facial expressions. Mature children in this stage may be able to use patient-controlled analgesia.

The FLACC (Face, Legs, Activity, Cry, Consolability) scale was initially designed for younger patients who are

TABLE 32.1	Neonatal Infant Pain Scale	
Parameter	Finding	Points
Facial Expression	Relaxed	0
	Grimace	1
Cry	No cry	0
	Whimper	1
	Vigorous crying	2
Breathing Patterns	Relaxed	0
	Change in breathing	1
Arms	Restrained	0
	Relaxed	0
	Flexed	1
	Extended	1
Legs	Retrained	0
	Relaxed	0
	Flexed	1
	Extended	1
State of Arousal	Sleeping	0
	Awake	0
	Fussy	1

TABLE 32.2 CRIES Scale for Postoperative Pain

	0	1	2
Crying	No	High-pitched	Inconsolable
Requires $SpO_2 > 95\%$	No	$F_1O_2 < 30\%$	$F_1O_2 < 30\%$
Increased vital signs	Heart rate and blood pressure equal to or less than preoperative values	Less than 20% of preoperative values	Greater than 20% of preoperative values
Expression	None	Grimace	Grimace/grunt
Sleeplessness	No	Awakens Frequently	Awake

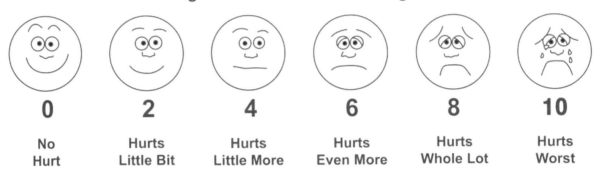

Wong-Baker FACES® Pain Rating Scale

0	2	4	6	8	10
No Hurt	Hurts Little Bit	Hurts Little More	Hurts Even More	Hurts Whole Lot	Hurts Worst

• **Fig 32.1.** Wong-Baker FACES scale. Source: Originally published in Whaley & Wong's Nursing Care of Infants and Children. © Elsevier Inc.

TABLE 32.3 FLACC Scale

Criteria	0	1	2
Face	No particular expression or smile	Occasional grimace or frown, withdrawn, disinterested	Frequent to constant quivering chin, clenched jaw
Legs	Normal position or relaxed	Uneasy, restless, tense	Kicking, or legs drawn up
Activity	Lying quietly, normal position, moves easily	Squirming, Shifting back and forth, tense	Arched, rigid, or jerking
Cry	No cry (awake or asleep)	Moans or whimpers; occasional complaint	Crying steadily, screams or sobs, frequent complaints
Consolability	Content, relaxed	Reassured by occasional touching, hugging, or being talked to, distractible	Difficult to console or comfort

nonverbal, preverbal or unable to self-report their own pain. The scale is structured into 5 categories and a care provider scores the patient 0 to 2 in each category, to achieve a cumulative score of 0 to 10. Also commonly used is the Revised-FLACC (rFLACC) scale, which is a modification of the FLACC scale aimed to better evaluate pain in pediatric patients with cognitive impairments, in addition to those who are unable to report their pain score because of age or have difficulty with oratory or motor skills. As such, rFLACC was modified to include several additional behavioral descriptors, including: verbal outbursts, tremors, increased spasticity, jerking movements, and respiratory pattern changes, such as breath holding or grunting.

During Piaget's *concrete operations stage* (approximately 8 to 12 years), children think logically and can be taught methods of cognitive and behavioral pain control such as distraction, relaxation, guided imagery, and hypnosis. They can relate details about their pain such as how the pain varies with activity or time of day. For children in this age range, we use FACES, or a simple verbal numeric 11-point scale

(0–10) on which 0 represents no pain and 10 represents the worst pain imaginable. Patient-controlled analgesia is often used during this developmental stage.

Licensing opportunities for the Wong-Baker FACES® Pain Rating Scale can be found at wongbakerfaces.org.

In the final stage of child development, Piaget's *formal operations stage*, abstract thought is possible. Adolescents can more precisely characterize their pain with adjectives like burning, stinging, throbbing, or stabbing. They can articulate subtle changes in severity of pain with different treatments. For this age group, we can use numeric pain scores and patient-controlled analgesia. A variety of nonpharmacologic techniques can be used as adjuncts to control pain, including imagery, hypnosis, distraction, relaxation, and biofeedback.

There are children with intellectual disability who do not go through the four developmental stages of childhood. For example, they might remain in the first stage with no understanding of pain and very limited ability to communicate the pain in terms of location, severity, and character. Multidimensional measurement approaches that include physiologic factors and pain behaviors are useful in recognizing pain in this vulnerable population. Family members often have knowledge about unique pain indicators for an individual. One commonly used scale is the rFLACC discussed earlier. Another scale, the Individualized Numeric Rating Scale (INRS)[3] uses the patient's specific pain indicators and behaviors to create a unique pain scale for a nonverbal child with severe intellectual disability, which can be used by hospital caregivers to guide pain management therapy.

References

1. Taddio A, Katz J, Ilersich AL, Koren G. Effect of neonatal circumcision on pain response during subsequent routine vaccination. *Lancet*. 1997;349(9052):599–603. https://doi.org/10.1016/S0140-6736(96)10316-0.
2. Suraseranivongse S, Kaosaard R, Intakong P, et al. A comparison of postoperative pain scales in neonates. *Br J Anaesth*. 2006;97(4):540–544. https://doi.org/10.1093/bja/ael184.
3. Solodiuk JC, Scott-Sutherland J, Meyers M, et al. Validation of the Individualized Numeric Rating Scale (INRS): a pain assessment tool for nonverbal children with intellectual disability. *Pain*. 2010;150(2):231–236. https://doi.org/10.1016/j.pain.2010.03.016.

Suggested Readings

Anand KJ, Hickey PR. Pain and its effects in the human neonate and fetus. *N Engl J Med*. 1987;19(21):1321–1329. https://doi.org/10.1056/NEJM198711193172105. 317.
Maxwell LG, Fraga MV, Malavolta CP. Assessment of Pain in the Newborn: An Update. *Clin Perinatol*. 2019;46(4):693–707. https://doi.org/10.1016/j.clp.2019.08.005.

33

Analgesic Medications

F. WICKHAM KRAEMER III

Insufficient knowledge about the pharmacology of analgesic medications in the pediatric age group has led to inadequate treatment of pediatric pain partly related to the fluctuating pharmacokinetic and pharmacodynamics properties of analgesics during development.

Although all analgesic medications have undergone thorough pharmacologic investigation in adults, similar studies have not always been performed in children. Only since 2001 has the Food and Drug Administration (FDA) required studies of all new pharmaceuticals in the pediatric population. All of the medications discussed in this chapter gained FDA approval before this time.

Pharmacokinetic Considerations

Because of the physiologic changes that occur between infancy and adulthood, the pharmacokinetics of many medications administered to pediatric patients differ from those of adults. Differences in body compartment composition, plasma protein binding capacity, enzyme and renal function, metabolism, and respiratory function result in varied medication absorption, distribution, metabolism, clearance, and response.

Drug absorption in the pediatric patient differs from adults in many ways. The gastric pH of an infant is relatively less acidic leading to a potential for decreased bioavailability of orally administered medications that are weakly acidic. On the other hand, there is a similar potential for an increase in the bioavailability of weakly alkaline oral medications. Infants also demonstrate prolonged gastric emptying and abbreviated intestinal transit time, which can delay the absorption of medications. Biliary and pancreatic enzymatic function are not fully developed initially, and resultantly neither is the pediatric patient's ability to solubilize and absorb drugs, which are lipophilic and rely on these functions. Because of the increased hydration of the epidermis, greater perfusion to subcutaneous regions, and greater body surface area to body mass ratio, transdermal applications may be absorbed more rapidly in the pediatric patient. Furthermore, a reduction in blood flow to skeletal muscle provides for a theoretical risk in delayed absorption of intramuscular medications.

The percentage of free drug available for action in the serum relies on the extent to which it is bound to plasma proteins. In neonates, there is a reduction in protein binding compared with older children and adults. This is because of several factors. First, there is a decreased amount of albumin produced in the neonatal period. This factor, in combination with a qualitative difference in the albumin itself, leads to a decrease in both the effectiveness and occurrence of protein binding. Second, the level of alpha-1-acid glycoprotein is markedly decreased in infancy. Opioids and local anesthetics are heavily bound to these proteins, and deficiency leads to increased plasma levels of unbound drug. This causes a potential increase in not only analgesic effect, but also potential for increased respiratory and neurologic depression, and cardiotoxicity. Conversely, there are various disease states that are associated with increased levels of alpha-1-acid glycoprotein, including burns, malignancy, infection, and trauma. This leads to increased drug binding and subtherapeutic effects at normal medication dosages.

Body composition also changes the way in which the pediatric patient responds to medications. The total body water percentage of an infant is 85% which decreases to 60% total body composition by adulthood. In the pediatric patient, this equates to an increased volume of distribution, an increased duration of action, and an increased dosing interval required for many water-soluble drugs. Muscle and fat proportions in the neonate are significantly decreased compared with the older patient, which results in decreased amount of drug uptake into these pharmacodynamically inactive sites. This results in higher drug concentrations at active sites, and a potential for supratherapeutic drug levels. Finally, the relative increase in blood flow to the neonatal brain and immature blood-brain barrier can lead to increased drug concentrations in the brain.

Metabolism plays a critical role in the termination of action of medications into hydrophilic, metabolically inactive compounds, which can then be excreted primarily by the kidneys and—to a lesser degree—by the biliary system. There are two stages of metabolism that occur primarily at the liver. Phase I metabolism includes oxidation, reduction, hydrolysis, and hydroxylation reactions. The most important enzyme family in this stage is the cytochrome P450 system, which is a mixed oxidase system that uses nicotinamide adenine dinucleotide phosphate (NADPH) and oxygen. This system is responsible for the reduction and oxidation of many medications including acetaminophen, nonsteroidal antiinflammatory diseases (NSAIDs), and opioids. Phase II metabolism uses glucuronidation, sulfation, and acetylation reactions to increase the water solubility of a drug, thus converting parent molecules into more polar, water-soluble, inactive metabolites. These drugs may then undergo renal excretion.

Hepatic enzymes are severely deficient at birth but rapidly develop and approach adult levels by a few months of age. This development continues, and between approximately 2 and 6 years of age, hepatic function actually exceeds that of an adult. It then declines to again reach levels similar to those of adulthood by puberty. However, during this period of increased function, the patient may require increased dosing, shorter interval dosing, and higher infusion rates to accomplish equianalgesic effects. Metabolism can also be influenced by pressure gradients within the body compartments themselves. For instance, hypotension or increase in intraabdominal pressure—as can be seen in an infant in the immediate postoperative period status postclosure of an omphalocele—may result in a decrease in renal and hepatic blood flow and, therefore, a decrease in the function of the kidneys and liver, respectively.

Excretion of water-soluble metabolites and, to a lesser extent, parent compounds is primarily completed by the renal system. In neonates, the glomerular filtration rate is decreased, which can lead to an accumulation of these products. This can result in metabolite-associated toxicity with many drugs. An example is the highly potent metabolite of normeperidine, which can lead to seizure activity in the patient with renal impairment.

When administering opioids to pediatric patients, respiratory function must be considered to avoid potential issues with atelectasis, airway obstruction, and respiratory failure.

Pediatric patients have an increased work of breathing secondary to compliant chest walls, poor respiratory muscle tone, smaller caliber airways, compliant laryngeal and tracheal cartilage, and decreased presence of fatigue-resistant, type 1 muscle fibers. Furthermore, their respiratory drive is diminished, especially in the neonatal period, as the ventilatory response to carbon dioxide and oxygen is decreased. When combined with their significantly increased relative oxygen consumption, typically negligible doses of opioids can result in a decrease in respiratory drive that can result in hypoventilation, hypercarbia, acidosis, respiratory arrest, and cardiac arrest.

Antipyretic, Analgesic, and Nonsteroidal Antiinflammatory Drugs

Cyclooxygenase (COX) inhibitors used for pain in pediatric patients include acetaminophen and NSAIDs. They are used to treat mild to moderate pain and can be used concomitantly with opioids in treatment of severe pain. Unlike opioid analgesics, these medications do not have the unwanted side effects of respiratory depression and sedation. They also have little to no dependence and abuse potential.

COX is an enzyme that is responsible for the metabolism of arachidonic acid into prostanoids, including prostaglandins and thromboxanes (Fig. 33.1). These substances contribute to pain via sensitization of peripheral nerve endings. They also act as vasodilators, contributing to erythema and swelling associated with the inflammatory response.

There are two isozymes of cyclooxygenase. COX-1 is found in tissues throughout the body, in the presence or absence of disease. It plays an integral role in the mediation of physiologic functions such as gastric mucosa protection, renal blood flow regulation, and platelet aggregation. It is inhibition of this isozyme that is associated with the negative effects attributed to COX inhibitors (including gastric ulceration, coagulation disturbance, renal blood flow compromise, and bronchoconstriction). COX-2 is the inducible isozyme,

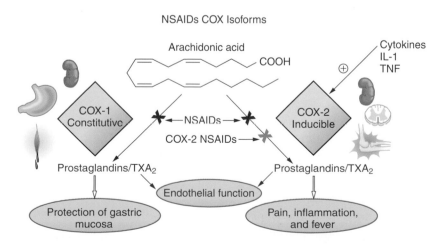

NSAIDs COX Isoforms

• **Fig. 33.1** Mechanism of action of nonsteroidal antiinflammatory drugs (NSAIDs), with comparison of cyclooxygenase (COX)-1 and COX-2 inhibition effects. *IL-1*, Interleukin-1; *TXA$_2$*, thromboxane A$_2$; *TNF*, tumor necrosis factor. (From Brogan SE, Mandyam S, Odell DW. Nonopioid analgesics. In: Hemmings HC Jr, Egan TD, eds. *Pharmacology and Physiology for Anesthesia*. 2nd ed. Elsevier; 2019:369–389.)

which is produced by the cell in response to trauma or inflammation. It is inhibition of this enzyme that is responsible for the therapeutic effects of COX inhibitors.

The majority of COX inhibitors are nonselective, preventing the action of both COX-1 and COX-2, thus interfering with desirable physiologic effects in addition to those that are associated with inflammation. The development of COX-2 inhibitors, such as celecoxib and rofecoxib, has provided the antiinflammatory and analgesic benefits of nonselective COX inhibitors without contributing to gastric ulceration and other undesired associated effects. These medications are not yet well studied in pediatric patients.

Acetaminophen is the most common antipyretic and analgesic medication currently used in pediatrics. This drug came to the forefront in pediatric pain management in the 1980s, when aspirin was determined to be a contributing factor to Reye syndrome. Acetaminophen quickly gained traction as one of the primary analgesic medications because of its relatively low side-effect profile and its analgesic and antipyretic efficacy. The effects of acetaminophen are thought to be exclusively mediated by central COX inhibition, and thereby the negative effects of peripheral COX inhibition commonly associated with NSAIDs are avoided. However, acetaminophen offers no peripheral antiinflammatory action.

Though optimal analgesic plasma concentrations are variable and not well-defined, antipyretic effects of acetaminophen are seen at 10 to 20 µg/mL. This therapeutic range is accomplished at oral doses of 10 to 15 mg/kg at 4-hour dosing intervals. With oral dosing, peak effects are noted at 30 minutes after administration. Rectal bioavailability is much lower and more variable and for these reasons it is used less at the author's institution. However, initial rectal dosing of 35 to 45 mg/kg will achieve therapeutic range with peak effect at 2 to 3 hours. Because of the delayed effect of rectal acetaminophen, the dosing interval is increased to every 6 to 8 hours. After initial administration, subsequent rectal dosages of 10 mg/kg are sufficient. The maximum daily dose relies on the patient's age, ranging from 40 mg/kg in premature neonates of 28 to 32 weeks of age to 75 mg/kg in children and adults.

Acetaminophen is also available in IV form, which is dosed similar to the oral form. Although IV administration results in more predictable pharmacodynamics and pharmacokinetics with 50% higher cerebrospinal fluid (CSF) peak concentration compared to oral or rectal administration, evidence of significant benefit of IV over oral acetaminophen dosing is lacking except in specific circumstances, such as during gastrointestinal compromise where absorption via oral dosing may not be possible.

At therapeutic doses, the metabolism of acetaminophen is primarily hepatic, yielding primarily nontoxic, inactive metabolites that can be excreted by the kidneys. This is accomplished via three pathways: glucuronidation (45%–55%), sulfate conjugation (20%–30%), and N-hydroxylation and dehydration, typically followed by glutathione conjugation. The last pathway results in an intermediate metabolite, N-acetyl-p-benzoquinone imine (NAPQI), which is potentially toxic and the primary culprit for the destructive effects seen in acetaminophen overdose. At usual doses, NAPQI is detoxified by glutathione conjugation and minimal amounts are oxidized by the cytochrome P450 pathway. In the setting of overdose, the glutathione pathway is overwhelmed and oxidation is enhanced. This leads to high levels of oxidation byproducts, which are associated with fulminant hepatic failure and necrosis. The treatment for acetaminophen overdose is N-acetylcysteine (NAC), which serves to replenish glutathione reserves and thereby enhance nontoxic metabolism.

Aspirin (acetylsalicylic acid) is the oldest NSAID. It is an irreversible inhibitor of COX-1 and is a modifier of COX-2 activity. Because of its association with Reye syndrome—a rare disorder characterized by brain and liver damage—it is not often used in pediatrics except in certain populations, such as those with juvenile rheumatoid arthritis and various other rheumatic diseases. Oral dosing of aspirin is 10 to 15 mg/kg every 4 hours with a maximal daily dose of 90 mg/kg.

There are many other NSAIDs with little variability among their benefit and side-effect profiles (Fig. 33.2). These are selected based on desired dosing interval and the patient's fasting status. Ibuprofen is the most widely used NSAID in pediatric patients. It is available in multiple pediatric formulations and has few adverse effects. Oral dosing is 15 mg/kg for a single dose, with decreased repeated doses of 10 mg/kg. For a maximum of 40 mg/kg per day.

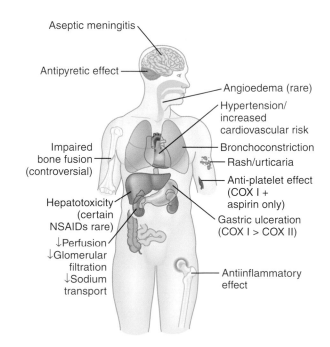

• **Fig. 33.2** Overview of the common pharmacokinetic and pharmacodynamic effects of nonsteroidal antiinflammatory agents. *COX*, Cyclooxygenase; *NSAID*, nonsteroidal antiinflammatory drug. (From Brogan SE, Mandyam S, Odell DW. Nonopioid analgesics. In: Hemmings HC Jr, Egan TD, eds. *Pharmacology and Physiology for Anesthesia*. 2nd ed. Elsevier; 2019:369–389.)

The dosing interval for repeated doses is every 6 hours. Naproxen has a longer half-life than ibuprofen and is dosed at 5 to 10 mg/kg PO every 8 to 12 hours up to a maximum daily dose of 20 mg/kg. The safety of naproxen in neonates is not well established.

Ketorolac is unique in that it is currently the only non-steroidal antiinflammatory drug in the United States that is available for oral, intramuscular, and intravenous dosing. This medication should be used for no longer than 5 days because of risk for gastric ulceration and hemorrhage and renal dysfunction. Because of its effect on platelet function, it should be avoided in patients at high risk for issues with bleeding. Ketorolac is dosed at 0.5 mg/kg every 6 hours with a maximum of 30 mg per dose, and the maximum daily dose is the lesser of 120 mg or 2 mg/kg.

Ketamine

Ketamine is a phencyclidine derivative that is used most commonly as a dissociative anesthetic at doses of 1 to 5 mg/kg IV (see also Chapter 19). Potent analgesia is demonstrated at subanesthetic doses (0.25–0.5 mg/kg IV), and it can be administered in oral, IV, intramuscular, or rectal form. It is useful in pain settings in which there is a large neuropathic component. In high doses, ketamine can be given orally or intramuscularly to induce general anesthesia when IV access is not an option, such as in pediatric patients who are severely behaviorally challenged. In addition to providing anesthesia and analgesia during short, stimulating procedures, ketamine can be administered as a prolonged infusion that can result in analgesic effects for up to 3 months after discontinuation.

Ketamine provides its analgesic effects primarily by antagonism of the N-methyl-D-aspartate (NMDA) receptor (Fig. 33.3).

It is also thought to enhance descending neurologic inhibition and cause antiinflammatory effects at central sites. This compound possesses a high affinity for central muscarinic receptors and exerts significant cholinergic effects.

Opioids

Opioids are the primary treatment for moderate to severe nociceptive pain. Although they are still used for neuropathic pain, they are not as effective. Opioids exert their effect by binding centrally to both pre- and postsynaptic cell membranes. Upon agonistic binding to an opioid receptor, G-protein coupled calcium channels are deactivated. This deactivation results in a decrease in intracellular calcium (Fig. 33.4).

At the same time, G-protein coupled potassium channels are activated, which leads to hyperpolarization of the neuron's cell membrane. Combined, there is a decrease in calcium-related activity. Presynaptically, this results in a decrease of excitatory neurotransmitter release (substance P and glutamate). Postsynaptically, there is an associated increase in induction of spinal adenosine release. These neurotransmitters are paramount to pain signal transmission, and a strong analgesic effect is the result.

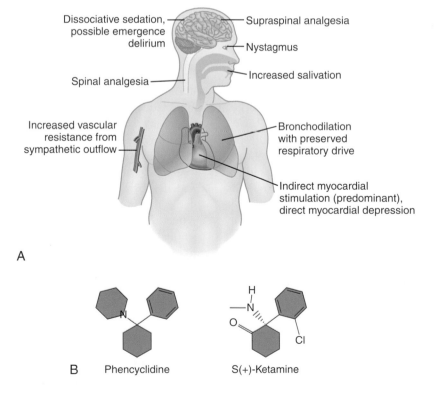

• **Fig. 33.3** (A) Selected effects of ketamine. (B) Structures of S(+) ketamine and its parent drug phencyclidine. Ketamine is usually supplied as a racemic mixture but the more active S(+) isomer is available in some countries. (From Garcia PS, Whalin MK, Sebel PS. Pharmacology of intravenous anesthetics. In: Hemmings HC Jr, Egan TD, eds. *Pharmacology and Physiology for Anesthesia*. 2nd ed. Elsevier; 2019:193–216.)

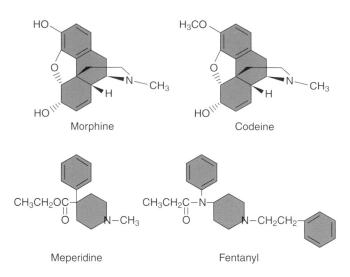

• **Fig. 33.4** The molecular structures of morphine, codeine, meperidine, and fentanyl. Note that codeine is a simple modification of morphine; fentanyl and its congeners are more complex modifications of meperidine, a phenylpiperidine derivative. (From Ogura T, Egan TD. Intravenous opioid agonists and antagonists. In: Hemmings HC Jr, Egan TD, eds. *Pharmacology and Physiology for Anesthesia.* 2nd ed. Elsevier; 2019:332–353.)

Opioids act on a variety of specific receptors. The μ receptor—named because of its affinity for morphine—is located predominantly in the cerebral cortex, thalamus, periaqueductal gray matter, and substantia gelatinosa of the spinal cord. This receptor is responsible for supraspinal analgesia, dysmotility, bradycardia, dependence, respiratory depression, and sedation. Systemic action is primarily caused by supraspinal μ receptors while neuraxial opioids work additionally on μ and κ receptors, which are located in the substantia gelatinosa of the spinal cord.

There are various other opioid receptors, including the κ receptor, which is associated with analgesia and sedation, respiratory depression, hallucinations, miosis, dysphoria, and, by inhibition of antidiuretic hormone, diuresis. The δ receptor contributes to analgesic and antidepressant effects, convulsions, and physical dependence. It is also thought to be associated with modulation of μ-mediated respiratory depression. Other receptor subtypes contribute to opioid effects to a lesser extent.

Most opioids undergo extensive first-pass hepatic metabolism before reaching systemic circulation, resulting in reduced bioavailability. Opioids are generally lipophilic, which allows crossing of cell membranes to the desired site of action. However, this decreases the ability of the compound to be renally excreted. For this reason, metabolism is necessary, rendering the molecule more hydrophilic and amenable to excretion by the kidneys. This is accomplished by phase I and II metabolism, as mentioned above (see also Chapter 2). In the case of opioids, phase II is primarily accomplished by the process of glucuronidation, catalyzed by uridine diphosphate glucuronosyltransferase (UGT), which results in the highly hydrophilic opioid metabolite. This by-product is then easily excreted by the kidneys.

Opioids can be classified by their potency, means of derivation (naturally occurring, semisynthetic, or synthetic), or by their mechanism of action. The latter is perhaps the most useful, and includes the following classifications: agonists, partial agonists, mixed agonist-antagonists, or pure antagonists. Agonists bind to the receptor of interest and result in a change of cellular function, resulting in the characteristic pharmacologic effect. Agonists include drugs such as morphine, meperidine, hydromorphone, methadone, oxycodone, codeine, fentanyl, and remifentanil. Partial agonists, such as buprenorphine, bind to the receptor and cause a less-than-maximal response than full agonism.

Conversely, antagonists bind to the receptor, prevent binding of the agonist, and result in the antagonism of the pharmacologic effects of the agonist. Opioid antagonists include naloxone, naltrexone, and nalmefene. Mixed agonist-antagonists demonstrate agonistic and antagonistic effects when they bind to multiple receptor subtypes, and include nalbuphine and pentazocine.

There are many side effects associated with opioid medications. Nausea and vomiting are common and associated with the rostral spread of the opioid to the medullary vomiting center. It is important to consider the clinical context and rule out potentially dangerous causes of these signs and symptoms, such as hypotension secondary to sympathectomy associated with neuraxial techniques. When appropriate, multiple therapies can be effective, such as opioid rotation, phenothiazines, 5-HT3 antagonists (such as ondansetron), antihistamines, various antipsychotics at low doses, and anticholinergic medications.

Urinary retention is another unwanted, dose-independent side effect of opioids. It is more commonly associated with neuraxial than systemic opioid administration but frequently occurs in either setting. The mechanism for urinary retention involves parasympathetic outflow inhibition at the sacral spinal cord resulting in increased urinary bladder capacitance and decreased tone of the detrusor muscle involved in bladder emptying. This is addressed with continuous or intermittent catheterization, or with low-dose naloxone administration.

Opioid-associated pruritus is histamine independent and mediated by opioid receptors in the brainstem at the level of the trigeminal nucleus. For this reason, the pruritus is frequently most concentrated in the distribution of the trigeminal nerve. Treatment can include naltrexone, naloxone, mixed agonist-antagonist opioids, or serotonin antagonists. Though frequently used, antihistamines offer relief only to the extent of providing sedation.

Constipation and miosis are the two opioid-related side effects most resistant to tolerance. Opioid therapy requires bowel prophylaxis in both the acute and chronic setting. If constipation is left untreated, ileus may result.

The most dangerous side effect of opioids is respiratory depression. Concomitant administration of medications with the side effect of sedation can lead to an increased risk for severe respiratory depression. At the population-based level, benzodiazepines are highly correlated with opioid-associated overdose mortality. Even medications such as gabapentin which are not known respiratory depressants by themselves but rather are described as sedating, have been shown to increase respiratory depression when given with opioids. Opioid analgesic response and level of side effects are highly variable by individual, and careful monitoring and appropriate titration on a patient-to-patient basis is paramount to avoiding these unwanted, potentially lethal effects.

Morphine

Morphine is a naturally occurring opioid derived from the poppy straw of the opioid poppy. It is the prototypical opioid, against which the potency of all other opioids is measured.

A multitude of formulations exist, including IV, oral, buccal, sublingual, intranasal, subcutaneous, intramuscular, and neuraxial. When administered IV, peak effect is seen at 20 minutes, while oral dosages peak around 30 to 60 minutes. When taken orally, morphine undergoes an extensive first-pass metabolism and only about 50% reaches the site of action.

Morphine is primarily metabolized in the liver, and to a far lesser extent in the kidneys and in the brain, by glucuronidation. The result of the second phase of this metabolism results in an active metabolite (morphine-6-glucuronide) and an inactive compound (morphine-3-glucuronide), which both undergo renal excretion. Morphine-6-glucuronide has a potency 100 times greater than that of its parent compound; however, because of its decreased lipophilicity, it is minimally capable of traversing the blood-brain barrier in patients with normal renal function. In neonates and those with reduced glomerular filtration rate, this metabolite may accumulate and result in respiratory depression.

Though the above pathway of metabolism is present in the neonatal period to some extent, it develops to a much greater capacity over the course of the first few weeks of life. Morphine's volume of distribution and clearance increase rapidly with age during this initial period of life. Levels have reached those of an adult by the age of 2 weeks to 2 months of age, and vary from individual to individual.

Fentanyl

With a potency 100 times that of morphine and a strong affinity for μ-opioid receptor agonism, fentanyl is the most widely used synthetic opioid in medicine. Fentanyl demonstrates a wide therapeutic index and can be safely used in many medical settings in which strong analgesia is indicated.

The highly lipophilic compound rapidly crosses cell membranes and has been successfully used in IV, epidural, intrathecal, transdermal, intranasal, and other transmucosal applications. Because of its lipophilicity and membrane permeability, neuraxial fentanyl acts more locally at the spinal level at which it is administered, though it is largely absorbed to the systemic compartment and exerts significant systemic effects. It can be used intranasally in short, ambulatory procedures in which IV access is not necessary, such as myringotomy and tube insertion. The bioavailability

of intranasal delivery is 70% to 90%. Transmucosal modes of delivery include fentanyl lollipops, oral disintegrating tablets, and sublingual sprays.

Fentanyl patches are made from a semipermeable membrane with a drug reservoir. These come in dosages of 25 to 100 mcg/h released, and reach peak affect 12 to 24 hours after application. Offset is prolonged because of drug deposition into the skin and subcutaneous tissue. Uptake of the drug from the reservoir is dependent on the patient's temperature, body fat composition, and the patch placement location. Alterations in any of these factors, such as an increase in body temperature, can result in unpredictable drug levels and the potential for increased risk for adverse and potentially dangerous side effects. For this reason, and because of the delayed analgesic effects with the inability to rapidly and carefully titrate drug levels, this delivery system is not indicated for the opioid naïve patient. Fentanyl patches are reserved for cancer pain or palliative patients who have been treated with opioids in the past, and are especially useful in the setting of renal failure, swallowing hindrances, or intolerable side effects from other oral opioids.

Fentanyl has a rapid onset and short duration of action, making it ideal for clinical situations in which a high level of analgesia is required for a short duration of time. With single bolus dosing, action is generally terminated secondary to redistribution from active sites, rather than metabolism. Fentanyl demonstrates a variable, prolonged context sensitive half-time: when high, repeated, or continuous doses are administered and compartments are saturated, termination of action will rely on metabolism and elimination. This leads to a less predictable time until offset.

While in the serum, fentanyl is highly bound to alpha-1-glycoproteins. In newborns, less of these glycoproteins are formed and therefore a higher percentage of the drug is unbound. Fentanyl undergoes hepatic metabolism by glucuronidation and is excreted by the kidneys.

Though relatively safe in the clinical setting by a well-trained practitioner, there are occasional deaths related to medical use of fentanyl. More commonly, however, overdose is related to recreational use. This is a particular problem in the setting of the recent opioid epidemic. A Schedule II drug in the United States, fentanyl demonstrates a high dependence potential, and is an increasingly common substance of abuse. Fentanyl analogs with up to 10,000 times the potency of morphine are synthesized for recreational sale. These formulations are frequently combined with heroin or other illicit drugs and are ingested, smoked, or taken intranasally or IV. In 2016 alone, there have been over 20,000 deaths from fentanyl-related overdose, which is over 5 times those which occurred in 2013. Of these, 82% involved illegally manufactured fentanyl, while only 4% are thought to arise from prescribed medication.

Hydromorphone (Dilaudid)

Hydromorphone is a hydrophilic hydrogenated ketone which is synthesized from morphine. Its potency is approximately

5 times greater than that of morphine. When administered IV, peak analgesia is seen at 15 to 30 minutes and analgesic effect remains for 2 to 3 hours. Hydromorphone has a low oral bioavailability. When administered in oral form, dosage is increased by a factor of approximately four. It is a dehydroxylated phenanthrene opioid; one which lacks a hydroxyl group at position 6. This structural difference is thought to be associated with the decreased incidence of nausea and vomiting associated with hydromorphone compared with hydroxylated opioids, such as morphine.

Methadone

Methadone is a synthetic opioid with a potency roughly equivalent to morphine and the unique added characteristic of NMDA antagonism. This latter feature makes it useful in the setting of pain with a neuropathic component. It is used for analgesia in both the acute and chronic settings, and for opioid weaning in the setting of dependence. In the acute setting, methadone can be used for moderate to severe pain, with analgesic properties, respiratory depression, and sedation persisting for 12 to 36 hours after a single dose. With IV dosing, peak analgesia is seen as soon as 10 to 15 minutes. Methadone has one of the most variable half-lives among the opioids, ranging between 12 and 100 hours. The maximal analgesic benefit from methadone is seen when steady state is reached, which occurs around 5 days after initiation of treatment.

Dosing for methadone should be initiated at 0.05 to 0.1 mg/kg, given every 30 minutes, and titrated to effect. Once desired analgesia is obtained, maintenance dosage is 0.05 to 0.1 mg/kg every 12 hours. The bioavailability of methadone when dosed orally ranges from 65% to 95%. Conversion of morphine to methadone varies with daily morphine dose, with a conversion of 2:1, respectively, at dosages less than 30 mg a day. This conversion increases up to 20:1 with daily morphine equivalent doses over 1000 mg. When initially titrating, the practitioner should avoid methadone dosages higher than 30 mg/day.

Methadone has been associated with QT interval prolongation in some patients, predisposing such individuals to arrhythmias such as torsades de pointes. Pre- and intratherapeutic electrocardiographic monitoring of QT is recommended in the setting of rapid titration, large dosages, potential decrease in clearance, coadministration of QT-prolonging medications, and premorbid conditions which all independently increase risk for cardiac arrhythmia in the setting of methadone administration.

Oxycodone

Oxycodone is a semisynthetic opioid derived from the alkaloid compound thebaine, which is found in the opium poppy. This medication expresses full agonism at the μ receptor, and partial κ and δ activity. Its potency is approximately 1.5 times that of morphine.

Oxycodone is available as an oral solution and tablet form in immediate release, extended release, and tamper-resistant formulations. It is also combined with acetaminophen with the combined intention of both improved analgesia and decreased abuse potential. As one of the most commonly abused oral opioid medications, combinations with naloxone have also been created in attempts to deter abuse, though effectiveness has yet to be proven.

The onset of action of the immediate release formulation is 10 to 30 minutes, with peak plasma levels occurring at 30 to 60 minutes. It is metabolized via the CYP3A4 and CYP2D6 pathways in the liver, and undergoes renal clearance. Although the active metabolite, oxymorphone, is only responsible for 10% to 15% of the drug's action, it can accumulate and cause a pronounced level of respiratory depression and sedation. In the setting of decreased renal and hepatic function, dosages must be adjusted.

Nalbuphine

Nalbuphine is a unique complete κ receptor agonist and μ receptor antagonist. Because of the associated μ antagonism, it is often used to counteract the μ-mediated side effects of opioids which include nausea, vomiting, pruritus, and urinary retention. In opioid-tolerant individuals, nalbuphine is capable of producing withdrawal symptoms if a patient is transitioned abruptly from μ agonistic opioid therapy. Though the contribution of nalbuphine to respiratory depression is minimal, the sedating effect of this medication is well-described and, when used in conjunction with other sedatives, decreasing dosage is recommended.

Nalbuphine exhibits analgesic properties with a potency roughly equivalent to that of morphine. A ceiling effect is seen at approximately 200 mcg/kg, over which dose minimal additional analgesic benefit is seen. Compared with strict μ antagonists, nalbuphine causes less significant elevation in biliary tract pressure and is useful in the treatment of pain associated with biliary tract pathology. The plasma half-life of nalbuphine is 3 to 6 hours, and it is metabolized primarily by the liver. As the oral bioavailability of nalbuphine is only around 20%, it is typically administered IV.

Naloxone

Naloxone is a potent antagonist at the μ receptor but also has moderate antagonistic properties at the δ and κ receptors. At doses up to 10 mcg/kg IV, it reverses respiratory depression and oversedation in the setting of opioid overdose. All μ effects are coincidentally reversed with naloxone administration, such as analgesia, urinary retention, nausea and vomiting. Assuming adequate ventilatory support, careful titration in incremental doses of 0.5 to 1 mcg/kg is paramount to avoiding opioid withdrawal symptoms in chronic opioid users or opioid-dependent patients. Such potential effects include restlessness, agitation, tachycardia, hypertension, ventricular fibrillation, dyspnea, pulmonary edema, diaphoresis, nausea, and vomiting. In low doses of 0.25 to 2 mcg/kg/h, naloxone is also useful in the reversal of opioid-induced pruritus.

Naloxone undergoes rapid hepatic metabolism to naloxone-3-glucuronide, which then undergoes renal excretion. With a half-life of 60 to 90 minutes, the effects of naloxone commonly wear off well before the causative μ agonist has been eliminated. For this reason, continual monitoring of patients and redosing as necessary are recommended to prevent recurrence of sedation and respiratory depression.

In the setting of the current opioid overdose epidemic, naloxone has recently become a topic of political debate. Though still considered a prescription medication, it is becoming increasingly available from pharmacies in the majority of states without prescription. This medication is available in multiple forms for administration, including nasal spray. Single-use filled syringe kits are also being made increasingly available to law enforcement and first responders, with the hopes that increased availability will decrease the number of deaths from opioid overdose.

Codeine

Codeine is a pain medication which deserves a brief description and significant warning about its use in the practice of pediatric pain medicine. There are many safer and more effective medications and modalities in the treatment of pain. The passé/outdated idea that one opioid medication is less dangerous or addictive than any other has unfortunately been proven wrong over the past two decades of the opioid epidemic. All opioids which interact with opioid receptors have the potential to cause dependence, leading to addiction and possibly overdose death.

Codeine is a pro drug which is metabolized by CYP2D6 into morphine. Codeine itself is a very weak agonist of opioid receptors. Therefore, almost all the pain relief activity of codeine is based on its conversion to morphine. It is often noted that codeine is a weak pain reliever and this is attributed to the fact that only 10% of codeine is metabolized into morphine for most people. However, there are patients with increased CYP2D6 activity (ultrarapid metabolizers) who can convert 90% of codeine into morphine. The ultrarapid metabolizers are estimated at 1–2% of the population. Conversely, approximately 7–10% of the US population do not have the ability to metabolize codeine into an active form, providing no pain relief. This wide variability in efficacy should worry prescribers as the side effects, namely respiratory depression, of the opioid agonism will correspondingly vary as well. In addition, in 2013 the Food and Drug Administration (FDA) issued a boxed warning for codeine against its use in postop pain management in children after tonsillectomy/adenoidectomy. This warning was updated to a *contraindication* in 2017 to state that codeine should not be used in children under 12 years old to treat pain or cough. Due to the FDA contraindication, demonstrated variability of metabolism and efficacy and the availability of other pain-relieving modalities, the author does not recommend using codeine in pediatric pain management.

Suggested Readings

King MR, Wu RL, De Souza E, Newton MA, Anderson TA. Nonopioid analgesic usage among pediatric anesthesiologists: a survey of Society for Pediatric Anesthesia Members. *Paediatr Anaesth.* 2020;30(6):713–715. https://doi.org/10.1111/pan.13891.

Papacci P, De Francisci G, Iacobucci T, et al. Use of intravenous ketorolac in the neonate and premature babies. *Paediatr Anaesth.* 2004;14(6):487–492. https://doi.org/10.1111/j.1460-9592.2004.01250.x.

Rauch DA. Use of ketamine in a pain management protocol for repetitive procedures. *Pediatrics.* 1998;102(2 Pt 1):404–405. https://doi.org/10.1542/peds.102.2.404.

Wong I, St John-Green C, Walker SM. Opioid-sparing effects of perioperative paracetamol and nonsteroidal anti-inflammatory drugs (NSAIDs) in children. *Paediatr Anaesth.* 2013;23(6):475–495. https://doi.org/10.1111/pan.12163.

34

Local Anesthetics and Adjuvant Analgesics

F. WICKHAM KRAEMER III

Local anesthetics are synthetic derivatives of cocaine, a plant alkaloid obtained from the leaves of the South American coca plant, and the first local anesthetic to be discovered. Cocaine is a benzoic acid derivative coupled to a tertiary amine compound by an ester linkage. It is a weak base that is poorly soluble in water. Similarly, all local anesthetics contain a lipophilic benzoic acid derivative linked to a hydrophilic tertiary amine by an ester or amide chain and exist in ionized (cationic) and unionized forms (weak base). The lipophilic and hydrophilic components of local anesthetics enable their penetration into both lipid and aqueous membranes. It is this property that permits local anesthetics to traverse perineurium and axonal walls and block neural transmission without affecting cellular function or metabolism. Sodium conductance (i.e., depolarization) is prevented when an adequate concentration and volume of local anesthetic surround the nerve. The external opening of the Na+ channel is not the site of action of local anesthetics. Rather, the lipophilic, uncharged base form of the local anesthetic penetrates the neuronal cell wall and reaches the axoplasm where it exists in equilibrium as both a charged ionized salt and an uncharged base. The relative concentration of these forms depends on the tissue pH and the pKa of the compound. Once in the axoplasm, the charged base or cationic form enters the internal opening of the sodium channel and blocks Na+ conductance.

Local anesthetic metabolism is determined by the chemical linkage (Fig. 34.1). Those with an ester linkage are metabolized by plasma esterases and those with an amide linkage are metabolized in the liver. Compounds with ester linkages are more likely to cause allergic reactions. The degree of lipid solubility of a local anesthetic determines its potency because the neuronal cell wall is a lipid structure. However, the relationship between lipid solubility and potency is not linear. The onset of action of a local anesthetic is correlated with its specific dissociation constant, or pKa, the pH at which 50% of the drug is present as the uncharged base and 50% as the cationic form. Only the unionized base can penetrate the cell wall. All local anesthetics have a pKa greater than 7.4. The lower the pKa of a local anesthetic, the greater the number of uncharged molecules available to traverse the lipid cell membrane, and the more rapid its onset of action.

The duration of action of a local anesthetic is determined by its protein binding capacity. After traversing lipid membranes, the local anesthetic enters the Na+ channel, a protein structure, to exert its pharmacologic effect. Therefore duration of action is directly correlated with degree of protein binding.

Frequency-dependent blockade is another important characteristic of local anesthetics. Most local anesthetics enter the Na+ channel only when it is open during depolarization. Thus neurons with high-frequency depolarization (i.e., sensory and pain fibers) are more readily blocked than fibers that have low-frequency depolarization (i.e., motor nerves).

Local anesthetic systemic toxicity (LAST) is the most feared complication of using regional anesthesia as it may result in side effects ranging from mild, transient symptoms to permanent disability or even death. Other reactions to local anesthetics include allergies and neurotoxicity. The best treatment of these problems is through prevention. However, this might not always be possible, so it is important to know the consensus statements[1] published by the American Society of Regional Anesthesia and Pain Medicine.

Rare allergic reactions are mainly associated with ester local anesthetics, which are metabolized by plasma esterases to form para-aminobenzoic acid (PABA), the probable allergenic component. PABA is present in sunscreens and it is recommended that ester local anesthetics not be administered to patients with a history of sunscreen allergy. Skin testing is available to diagnose true local anesthetic allergy. The amide local anesthetics are safe in

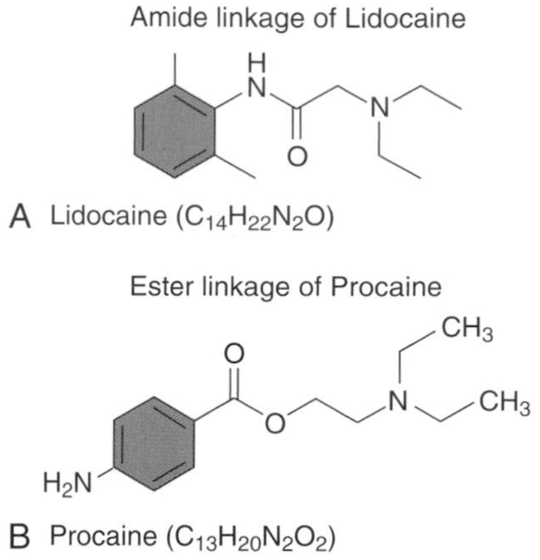

Fig. 34.1 Local anesthetic structural classification. (A) Amide linkage of lidocaine (B) and ester linkage of procaine. (From Suzuki S, Gerner P, Lirk P. Local anesthetics. In: Hemmings HC Jr, Egan TD, eds. *Pharmacology and Physiology for Anesthesia*. 2nd ed. Elsevier: 2019:390–411.)

patients with a true allergy to ester anesthetics as cross-reactivity between ester and amide local anesthetics has not been demonstrated.

Every local anesthetic is capable of producing neurotoxicity. However, this complication is rare. True local anesthetic neurotoxicity is usually mild and resolves completely over time. More common is a neuropathy that follows a nerve injury because of needle trauma or a direct intraneural injection of epinephrine-containing local anesthetics in high concentrations. Lidocaine 5% for spinal anesthesia has been a particular concern because of its association with transient neurologic symptoms (TNS). This syndrome is characterized by the appearance of back pain that radiates to the buttocks within 24 hours of the block, the absence of motor and sensory deficits, and resolution within 3 to 10 days. The lowest effective concentration of local anesthetic should be used when performing any regional block.

Pharmacology of Local Anesthetics

Tetracaine

Tetracaine is an ester local anesthetic with a high pKa of 8.5, slow onset, and long duration of action (60–360 minutes). It is among the most potent local anesthetics in clinical use today. It is also among the most toxic. The maximum dose is 1 mg/kg. Tetracaine is most commonly used for spinal anesthesia (usual dose 0.2–0.6 mg/kg) and topical anesthesia of the eye. For spinal anesthesia in children, it comes in two forms: a lyophilized crystal that is reconstituted or a 1% solution that is diluted with distilled water, cerebrospinal fluid, or dextrose to produce hypobaric, isobaric, or a hyperbaric solution, respectively. The duration of action of tetracaine is prolonged by addition of epinephrine. It is also available as an ophthalmic solution as tetracaine hydrochloride 0.5%. The usual dose is 1 to 2 drops per eye. Long-term

use of the drops is not recommended as damage to the surface of the eye may occur.

2-Chloroprocaine

2-Chloroprocaine is gaining popularity for pediatric epidural analgesia because it is rapidly metabolized by plasma esterases, its accumulation in the plasma is unlikely, and systemic toxicity is rare.[2] Although neonates and infants have half the plasma esterase level of adults, there is no clinical difference in metabolism of 2-chloroprocaine. Chloroprocaine has a relatively high pKa of 9 and only about 5% of the drug is present in the unionized form at physiologic pH. Chloroprocaine has a rapid onset of action (5 to 10 minutes) because of its high tissue penetration. It has a short duration of action (45 minutes) that can be prolonged (to 70–90 minutes) with addition of epinephrine. It has roughly a quarter of the potency of tetracaine or bupivacaine.

Use of epidural chloroprocaine decreased in the 1980s because of neurotoxicity associated with its 0.2% bisulfite preservative. Currently, chloroprocaine is available without preservatives for epidural use. Even with preservative-free chloroprocaine, a syndrome of back pain after large epidural doses has been described in adults. Epidural anesthesia[3] is achieved by administering up to 1 mL/kg of 2-chloroprocaine (2% or 3%) with epinephrine 1:200,000 (maximal dose of chloroprocaine, 20–30 mg/kg). Continuous epidural analgesia has been used in infants aged less than 6 months using 1.5% chloroprocaine at 0.4 to 0.8 mL/kg/h.

Lidocaine

Lidocaine was the first amide local anesthetic introduced and remains a popular local anesthetic still in use today. Lidocaine has a relatively low pKa of 7.9 and 25% of the drug is nonionized at physiologic pH. It has a rapid onset and an intermediate duration of action (60–90 minutes) that is prolonged by adding epinephrine. It has one-eighth the potency of bupivacaine or tetracaine. The maximum dose of 5 mg/kg can be increased to 7 mg/kg by adding epinephrine. In addition to epidural and peripheral nerve blockade, lidocaine can be administered transcutaneously in the form of a skin patch (Lidoderm). It is also available as an oral formulation (mexiletine) for the treatment of neuropathic pain, and it is the only anesthetic recommended for IV regional blockade.

Bupivacaine

Bupivacaine has a relatively high pKa of 8.1 and is only 15% nonionized. Therefore the time to onset is relatively slow. Bupivacaine is highly protein bound and thus has a long duration of action, which is not prolonged by adding epinephrine. However, addition of epinephrine will reduce the rate of systemic absorption, and thus lower the peak plasma concentration, which is an important consideration given the potential toxicity of bupivacaine. Bupivacaine is one of the most potent local anesthetics in use today. Its l-enantiomer, levobupivacaine, may have less cardiac toxicity but it has equal anesthetic potency. The maximum dose of both bupivacaine and levobupivacaine is 3 mg/kg. Severe cardiovascular depression at plasma levels slightly above those considered necessary to produce signs and symptoms of neurotoxicity has been observed with bupivacaine. Bupivacaine has more depressant effects on the cardiac conduction system than lidocaine, but is no more toxic than lidocaine with regard to its effects on blood pressure and cardiac output. Bupivacaine can reduce conduction time and increase the potential for reentrant rhythms. Its duration is long because it is highly protein-bound and thus takes a long time to "wash out" from the sodium channel. Thus resuscitation can be prolonged but is not impossible.

Ropivacaine

Ropivacaine is the newest of the amide local anesthetics and was developed because of the cardiotoxicity associated with bupivacaine. It is chemically similar to bupivacaine, having a propyl side-chain whereas bupivacaine has a butyl side-chain. Its pKa is 8.0 and a slightly greater percentage of the drug is present in the nonionized form at physiologic pH. Ropivacaine is slightly less protein-bound than bupivacaine, so it is not surprising that it has a faster onset but slightly shorter duration of action (150–300 minutes). Like bupivacaine, the duration of blockade is not prolonged by adding epinephrine.

Ropivacaine is produced only as the l-enantiomer. One feature common to all the amide anesthetics is that their l-form possesses less cardiotoxicity. Ropivacaine appears to possess more sensorimotor discrimination than bupivacaine when administered to produce equivalent analgesia. It is estimated that ropivacaine is about three-quarters as potent as bupivacaine. It is available as 0.2% and 0.5% solutions and is dosed for epidural and peripheral nerve block with a maximum dose of 4 mg/kg for single injections and 0.4 mg/kg/h for continuous infusions.

Pharmacology of Adjuvant Analgesics

Clonidine

Clonidine is an α-2-adrenergic agonist that was developed primarily as a nasal decongestant because of its peripheral vasoconstrictor properties. It was soon recognized to have hypotensive effects and was primarily then used as an antihypertensive agent in adults. More recently, its anxiolytic and antinociceptive effects have been useful in the perioperative setting. For sedation and anxiolysis, clonidine, 2 to 4 µg/kg, can be administered orally. It possesses the ability to reduce intraoperative anesthetic requirements, reduce postoperative opioid consumption, and stabilize hemodynamic responses to laryngoscopy and surgery.

Clonidine is used as an analgesic adjuvant in the management of acute and chronic pain in children. In peripheral and epidural[4] nerve blocks, clonidine prolongs both sensory and motor blockade of the local anesthetic. Clonidine alone can produce analgesia when injected in the epidural or intrathecal space, or in the proximity of peripheral nerves. However, because of the large doses required, side effects of hypotension, bradycardia, and sedation limit its utility as a sole analgesic agent. Clonidine has proven useful to control withdrawal symptoms in children with opioid or benzodiazepine dependence.

The mechanism by which clonidine exerts its analgesic effects are uncertain. In the superficial laminae of the dorsal horn of the spinal cord and in certain brain stem nuclei, α-2-receptors are abundant. Central sympatholysis is believed to be responsible for its antihypertensive effect. The prevention of norepinephrine release from presynaptic nerve terminals by clonidine is believed to be partially responsible for producing analgesia. However, there is evidence that clonidine increases acetylcholine release from neurons in the dorsal horn of the spinal cord, thus activating spinal acetylcholine receptors. This may enhance local anesthetic blockade of C and Aδ fibers by augmenting potassium conductance.

Clonidine can be administered by a variety of routes. As an epidural additive, the bolus dose is 1 µg/kg, which may be followed by an infusion of 0.05 to 0.2 µg/kg/h. When given orally, it is almost totally absorbed from the GI tract. Once in the systemic circulation, its high lipid solubility allows it to penetrate the spinal cord and brain. Clonidine comes in an injectable form and in a tablet (0.1, 0.2, and 0.3 mg) and transdermal patch (0.1, 0.2, and 0.3 mg). The patches need to be changed every 7 days. The patches should not be cut, and an alternative delivery method should be employed. The oral starting dose is 2 to 4 µg/kg/day and transdermal dose of clonidine is 4 to 8 µg/kg/day, both with a maximum of 0.3 mg/day. The oral dose is usually administered in two divided doses. Clonidine cannot be abruptly discontinued after prolonged administration, because severe hypertension and other symptoms similar to an abstinence syndrome may occur.

Anticonvulsants

Anticonvulsants are useful for managing a variety of neuropathic pain conditions including complex regional pain syndrome, phantom limb pain, and postherpetic neuralgia. However, few studies in children exist and the use of this class of drugs in children is based on extrapolation from adult literature and from growing anecdotal pediatric experience. Although early adult experience established the efficacy of phenytoin, carbamazepine, and valproic acid as analgesic adjuvants, gabapentin is now the first-line anticonvulsant used for this purpose.

Gabapentin

Gabapentin was developed as a gamma aminobutyric acid (GABA) analog for relief of muscle spasticity but was later recognized to be more effective as an anticonvulsant. The mechanism of action of gabapentin has not been clearly delineated. It does not appear to interact with receptors or sodium channels, and may enhance extracellular GABA concentrations by altering GABA transport. Gabapentin is not metabolized and is entirely dependent on renal excretion for elimination. It is not protein-bound and has a half-life of 5 to 9 hours. The most common adverse effects include abdominal pain, dizziness and ataxia, tremor, nystagmus, somnolence, and mood and behavior disturbances. However, gabapentin is generally well tolerated and the side effects can be largely avoided by slowly increasing the dose of gabapentin on a daily basis until analgesia results or intolerable side effects disappear. In the author's institution we start with 5 mg/kg (maximum dose 300 mg) at bedtime on the first day, 5 mg/kg twice-daily on the second day, and then 5 mg/kg thrice-daily. We continue to increase the daily dose in this fashion by 5 mg/kg/day. If somnolence is bothersome, we administer half the daily dose at bedtime. The maximum daily dose is 80 mg/kg/day, or the adult dose of 3600 mg.

Carbamazepine

Carbamazepine is an anticonvulsant that is believed to produce analgesia by sodium-channel blockade. Carbamazepine is metabolized by the liver. Therapy is initiated in children aged over 6 years with an oral dose of 10 mg/kg/day divided in two to four doses and increased to the usual maintenance dose of 15 to 30 mg/kg/day. Severe adverse effects including aplastic anemia, agranulocytosis, congestive heart failure, sedation, fatigue, ataxia, slurred speech, and hepatitis have been reported. A complete blood count and liver function studies should be obtained before and during therapy.

Valproic Acid

Valproic acid is an adjuvant treatment for neuropathic pain accompanied by a mood disturbance, and prophylactic therapy for migraine headaches. At least three mechanisms of action have been proposed for valproic acid: (1) increased production and release of GABA in central neurons; (2) reduced neuronal excitation initiated by N-methyl-D-aspartate (NMDA)-type glutamate receptors; and (3) direct membrane stabilizing effects. The usual oral starting dose of 10 to 15 mg/kg/day may be increased to 60 mg/kg/day in two to three divided doses. Anorexia, nausea and vomiting, weight gain or loss, and sedation are common side effects. The most serious side effects include hepatotoxicity, hyperammonemia, platelet dysfunction, and pancreatitis.

Tricyclic Antidepressants

When added to an analgesic regimen, tricyclic antidepressants (TCAs) improve sleep, mood, and daily functioning. Studies of its use for chronic pain in children have not been performed. These drugs are believed to produce analgesia by central serotonin and norepinephrine reuptake inhibition, thus augmenting descending inhibitory pathways. This class of drugs causes anticholinergic side effects: dry mouth, sedation, orthostatic hypotension, constipation, urinary retention, and tachycardia. Sudden death from arrhythmias has been reported in children on tricyclic antidepressants for treatment of depression. Before initiating TCA therapy, we obtain a history for palpitations, syncope, and cardiac conduction disturbances. An electrocardiogram should be obtained to rule out prolonged QT interval. Nortriptyline may produce less daytime somnolence and fewer anticholinergic effects than amitriptyline. However, when insomnia accompanies chronic neuropathic pain, we prefer to use amitriptyline. Therapy with amitriptyline or nortriptyline is initiated at 0.1 to 0.2 mg/kg at bedtime and increased by 0.1 to 0.2 mg/kg every 3 to 4 days to a maximum of 1 mg/kg/day or 50 mg.

Local Anesthetics

Lidocaine and its oral formulation (mexiletine) are referred to as membrane stabilizers because they block sodium channels, prevent membrane depolarization, and block excitatory impulses along neural pathways. They are used to treat neuropathic pain in adults and have been used in children with mixed results. To determine its usefulness, we administer an IV bolus of 1 mg/kg followed by an infusion at 1 mg/kg/h, with gradual increases to achieve a plasma lidocaine concentration of 2 to 5 μg/mL. If this test regimen produces adequate analgesia, oral therapy with mexiletine is begun. Adverse side effects of mexiletine include nausea and vomiting, ataxia, diplopia, and sedation; these frequently limit its use.

References

1. American Society of Regional Anesthesia and Pain Medicine. Checklist for treatment of local anesthetic systemic toxicity. Updated November 1, 2020. https://www.asra.com/guidelines-articles/guidelines/guideline-item/guidelines/2020/11/01/checklist-for-treatment-of-local-anesthetic- systemic-toxicity. Accessed 03.08.21.
2. Cladis FP, Litman RS. Transient cardiovascular toxicity with unintentional intravascular injection of 3% 2-chloroprocaine in a 2-month-old infant. *Anesthesiology*. 2004;100(1):181–183. https://doi.org/10.1097/00000542-200401000-00030.
3. Tobias JD, Rasmussen GE, Holcomb GW III, et al. Continuous caudal anaesthesia with chloroprocaine as an adjunct to general anaesthesia in neonates. *Can J Anaesth*. 1996;43(1):69–72. https://doi.org/10.1007/BF03015961.
4. Singh R, Kumar N, Singh P. Randomized controlled trial comparing morphine or clonidine with bupivacaine for caudal analgesia in children undergoing upper abdominal surgery. *Br J Anaesth*. 2011;106(1):96–100. https://doi.org/10.1093/bja/aeq274.

35
Acute Pain Management

F. WICKHAM KRAEMER III

"Acute pain" in the pediatric setting is generally nociceptive pain arising from tissue injury, inflammation, or infection. It is typically most pronounced immediately after the insult and gradually improves as the tissues repair. This type of pain usually responds to regional techniques, opioid medications, nonsteroidal antiinflammatory drugs (NSAIDs) and nonpharmacologic interventions, such as cognitive behavioral therapy and acupuncture; it rarely progresses to chronic pain.

Nociception involves the transduction of an inflammatory, mechanical, or thermal stimulus into a neural impulse, the transmission of the neural impulse from the periphery to the central nervous system (CNS), the modulation of that impulse, and the perception of the stimulus. The patient's perception of pain is the most variable of the above components and relies heavily on a combination of psychological, behavioral, and environmental factors.

Pathophysiology of Acute Pain

Trauma to tissue results in the release of arachidonic acid from cellular membranes and its conversion by cyclooxygenase and lipoxygenase into multiple inflammatory substances. These pain-inducing substances include: substance P, histamine, bradykinin, serotonin, leukotrienes, potassium, and hydrogen ions. Substance P is a neurotransmitter and neuromodulator of key importance in the pain response. It is a peptide compound produced in the spinal and Gasserian ganglia which is stored in somatic and visceral neurons. Its release results in nitric oxide dependent vasodilation, bronchoconstriction, further cytokine release, resultant inflammation, and an increase in vascular permeability, which leads to increased edema and erythema at the site of injury. Substance P is associated with the development of denervation hypersensitivity, which is a state of postsynaptic overactivity caused by the increased formation of postsynaptic receptors in response to decreased neurotransmitter release after trauma-associated denervation of substance P nerve terminals. This cascade results in an increased response to any release of substance P into the synaptic cleft.

Nociceptors are sensors located at the sensory neurons axonal terminus, which responds to a variety of noxious mechanical and thermal stimuli. These noxious impulses are carried by A-δ (thinly myelinated) and C (unmyelinated) afferent nerve fibers to the CNS for processing. These are different from other sensory nerves in that periods of prolonged nociceptor stimulation result in a reduction of the excitatory threshold and, consequentially, peripheral sensitization.

A-α and A-β fibers transmit nonnoxious afferent signals, which then have the potential to be transformed in the CNS into pain signals through various mechanisms. This can result in peripheral or central sensitization. Peripheral sensitization includes the phenomena of hyperalgesia (an increased response to normally noxious stimuli) and allodynia (a painful response to a typically nonnoxious stimulus).

Central sensitization, or "wind-up," is the result of repeated stimulation of C fibers in the peripheral nervous system that results in increased electrical activity. There is also an associated dysfunctional remodeling that occurs at the convergence of peripheral afferent nerve fibers where signals are typically processed and modified. This activity is most concentrated at the dorsal horn of the spinal cord and involves NMDA receptor response priming. This priming results in an amplification of pain intensity and duration. For this reason, patients who undergo repeated, painful procedures may experience an increased perception of pain in the absence of increased stimulation.

The spinal cord is separated into multiple layers, referred to as the Rexed laminae. Most pain signal transmission—via A-δ and C fibers—involves laminae I and V, with a lesser degree of involvement from laminae III, IIo, and II (substantia gelatinosa). Lamina I is the most dorsal aspect of the dorsal horn of the spinal cord. It receives pain and temperature signals primarily from the dorsolateral tract. The sensation relayed at this level is not modulated.

Lamina V is located at the neck of the dorsal horn and receives signals from cutaneous, muscular, and joint mechanoreceptors, and from visceral afferents. This layer contains a large number of wide dynamic range neurons which are involved in sensory discrimination and associated with the wind-up phenomenon, viscerosomatic pain referral, and chronic neuropathic pain.

After signals are processed and modified in the dorsal horn, second-order neurons transmit to the CNS after traveling via tracts in the anterior and anterolateral aspects of the spinal cord. With regard to pain signal transmission, the spinothalamic tract is the most important of these tracts. The spinothalamic tract consists of two pathways: the anterior spinothalamic tract (transmitting signals pertaining to crude touch) and the lateral spinothalamic tract (involved in pain and temperature signals). The spinoreticular tract and spinomesencephalic tracts also play a role in pain transmission, presumably to a lesser extent.

Peripheral nociceptive signal transmission is regulated centrally to some degree by the inhibitory descending pathway. This pathway arises in the cerebral cortex and involves motor neurons which are located in the Rexed laminae I, IIo, and V. Serotonin and norepinephrine are the primary neurotransmitters involved in this pathway and the action of medications like tricyclic antidepressants, tramadol, and clonidine are thought to exert their effects, to some degree, by their modification of the activity at the inhibitory descending pathway.

The transduction, transmission, modulation, and perception of pain involves a complex network of nociceptive pathways involving the limbic system, frontal cortex, and medial thalamus. The patient's pain experience is further influenced by their emotional state, behavior, past experience, and other cultural and societal factors. The successful management of the acute pain patient requires careful consideration of many different variables and a resultantly balanced and appropriately tailored treatment plan.

Setting Pain Expectations

The many modalities of pain management employed in the acute pain setting are enhanced by discussions of expected procedural pain and management strategies before the patient even arrives at the hospital. The surgical visit is the first step in setting a patient's and family's expectations for the hospital experience and management of pain. At the author's institution, a collaboration between the pain team, surgeons, nurses, and staff has resulted in pathways and order sets which reduce a patient's length of stay while maintaining or decreasing pain scores. These pathways have focused mainly on orthopedic procedures such a posterior spinal fusion, hip procedures, and sports medicine surgeries that use regional anesthesia and opioids through multimodal analgesia and continued home management with a reduced number of prescriptions. Although it is difficult to tease out which particular aspect or medication in the pathway is responsible for the reductions in length of stay, the establishment of the pain expectation for the patient has been translated into other procedures, including the Nuss procedure for pectus excavatum repair. Consistent use of order sets on the pathway reduce practice variation and maintain a uniform pain management

plan to the patient and family. This compliance improves the quality of care delivered and can increase patient and family satisfaction.

Patient-Controlled Analgesia

Patient-controlled analgesia (PCA) has been used for the management of pediatric pain since the 1980s and has become the most common mode of analgesia for the treatment of acute, moderate-to-severe pain in children over the age of about 6 years. PCA is most commonly used in the postoperative period when the patient is still NPO and in patients who have experienced trauma or burns. PCAs, in general, are considered to be safe, effective, and highly satisfactory for patients and their families.

The use of a PCA allows for self-titration of IV opioids, which allows for patient-driven tailoring of medication administration based on the individual patient's pain experience. Because of more frequent, smaller dosing of opioids, this method of administration leads to a narrower range of opioid levels in the blood compared with IV nurse-administered bolus dosing. Patients avoid pronounced peak drug levels that are associated with side effects such as oversedation and respiratory depression and relatively low trough levels, which result in an increase in pain levels.

PCA can also be used for epidural, peripheral nerve catheter, and transdermal medication administration. Compared with IV routes, epidural administration of PCA-delivered opioids has consistently shown to provide more effective analgesia, particularly in situations of severe pain. IV PCA consists of a pump that is attached to a reservoir of medication and controlled by a hand held remote button, by which demand doses are requested. This reservoir is connected to the patient through IV tubing allowing for delivery of medication straight into the patient's circulation. The pump itself is programmed to record utilization, allowing for monitoring and trending of overall drug usage.

Though the name implies control by the patient, PCA can also be controlled by the parent, nurse, or a combination thereof. Selection relies on a variety of factors which include the patient's age (school-age is generally the age at which the patient is developmentally appropriate and self-aware enough to begin assisting with their pain control), cognitive ability, physical ability (the patient must be physically able to press the PCA button), and parental involvement in patient care. The immediate analgesic effect offered by PCA provides the administrator some degree of control over the pain experience, which is particularly useful for parents or patients with a high level of pain-associated anxiety.

When the infusion pump is controlled by the patient alone, there is minimal risk for overdose resulting in CNS and respiratory depression. However, with parental or nurse control, this is a potential risk if demands are requested when the patient is already sedated. Though seemingly intuitive, it is important to educate parents and nursing staff on the importance of ensuring that the patient is awake before demands are requested and that the PCA not be used to treat natural sleep-associated movements or vocalizations. With overly concerned parents, it is helpful to affirm that if the patient is asleep, an adequate level of analgesia has been achieved. At the author's institution, all patients receiving PCA are monitored by heart rate, respiratory rate, and pulse oximetry for at least the first 24 hours and after any increases to the PCA for 24 hours more to ensure continued safety.

The infusion pump used for PCA employs a few basic settings. These include the demand dose, lockout interval, continuous infusion rate, and 1- or 4-hour total medication limits. Additionally, one should administer an initial loading dose of the medication to obtain adequate levels of analgesia before relying solely on the PCA as it can take significant periods of time to obtain these levels when using the low, demand dose from the PCA. This initial bolus should be given in a highly monitored environment in which respiratory resuscitation equipment is immediately available, (e.g., PACU = post-anesthesia care unit). In this way, the physician can ensure proper dosing and absence of medication allergy or intolerance.

The demand dose is the amount of medication delivered via the pump with each push of the PCA button. This is given at a frequency determined by the dosing interval which is a predetermined lockout that typically ranges from 6 to 12 minutes depending on the medication and clinical setting. Because of this safety feature, regardless of how many times the button is pushed, there will only be one demand dose delivered per lockout interval. One can also set a 1-hour or 4-hour limit to predetermine the maximum amount of medication that can be given over that respective time period.

In some situations, such as in the postoperative period after a procedure with anticipated severe levels of pain, a continuous basal infusion can be added to the PCA program. This continuous infusion is administered to the patient independent of demand usage and can be continuous throughout the entire day or adjusted to be given over a specific time period. For instance, a night time infusion can be started to help prevent the troughs associated with decreased button use during sleep. Basal rates are associated with increased side effects and minimal associated improvement in analgesia. Furthermore, there is an association between continuous infusions and sleep disturbances.

A rescue dose should also be assigned—usually a larger dose of the same medication in the PCA—to be administered on an as-needed basis in cases of severe pain for which the demand dose is not sufficient. These are particularly useful in situations where blood drug levels have decreased significantly, such as upon awakening with minimal overnight demand use with no background continuous infusion. Rescue doses are also important for incident pain: periods of time with higher levels of stimulation, such as dressing changes or bodily rotation.

Naloxone, 10 μg/kg, should be immediately available to treat respiratory depression. Because of the high incidence of nausea and vomiting with opioid administration, ondansetron 0.1 mg/kg every 8 hours as needed is also frequently used. Nalbuphine 50 μg/kg can be given every 4 hours for pruritus. Nalbuphine is also effective in the treatment of mild to moderate pain and can be scheduled or used on an as-needed basis. Of note, this and similar mixed agonist-antagonists can precipitate withdrawal symptoms in patients who are on preexisting μ-agonistic opioid therapy.

Selection of the medication for use in patient-controlled analgesia relies on preexisting disease, clinical setting, and patient response (Table 35.1). One must consider the metabolites and routes of elimination of each option. Though morphine is the most well-studied and most commonly used opioid in PCA, hydromorphone is associated with less nausea and vomiting. Furthermore, morphine's active metabolite, morphine-6-glucuronide, makes it a poor choice in the setting of renal insufficiency. Morphine is also avoided in patients whose neurologic status must be frequently assessed because of its long duration of action. Nalbuphine can be useful in patients with primary GI illness where the maintenance of gut motility is important such as with patients who have Crohn disease.

The side effects of patient-controlled analgesia with opioid medications include those typically associated with opioids. In addition to those mentioned above, these include urinary retention, confusion, and myoclonus. Opioids also interfere with intestinal coordination and activity, and therefore can contribute to postoperative ileus.

TABLE 35.1	**PCA Dosing Guidelines**				
Drug	Demand Dose (μg/kg)	Lockout Interval (min)	Basal Infusion (μg/kg)	1-Hour Limit (μg/kg)	IV Rescue Dose (μg/kg)
Morphine	20	8–10	0–20	100	50
Hydromorphone	4	8–10	0–4	20	10
Fentanyl	0.5	6–8	0–0.5	2.5	0.5–1.0
Nalbuphine	20	8–10	0–20	100	50

Continuous Intravenous Opioid Infusion

Continuous intravenous opioid infusions (CIVs) can be used in situations in which patient-controlled analgesia is not appropriate, such as young age, cognitive impairment, and physical incapacity to operate the demand button. This method is ideal in situations which involve minimal fluctuation in level of stimulation, such as an intubated and sedated postoperative patient in the ICU. By adding a bolus PRN dose, it can also be used in many settings in which a PCA is not indicated and when it is important to avoid fluctuations in plasma drug concentrations.

Compared with a PCA, continuous intravenous opioid infusions require minimal maintenance by nursing staff and minimal involvement by family. However, they do not adjust in response to an increase or decrease in analgesic needs and intermittent bolus dosing is commonly required. CIVs should not be dosed to eliminate all of the patient's pain, for at such a dose of opioid the patient will likely experience significant side effects including respiratory and CNS depression.

The strategy for opioid selection in a continuous infusion is similar to the selection criteria for patient-controlled analgesia. The dosing rates assigned should take into consideration a patient's comorbidities, history of opioid exposure, age, and weight. If the patient is at a high risk for depression of the respiratory or CNS, the dosage should be significantly decreased (by 25%–50%). Morphine is the most common opioid chosen for continuous opioid infusions, though when given in the neonatal period, it comes with an increase in risk for respiratory depression; the infusion rate must therefore be adjusted accordingly (Table 35.2).

When used alone, continuous IV opioid infusion will result in steady state levels of opioid within 4 to 5 half-lives of the medication administered. A bolus dose can be used up front to shorten the amount of time until steady state is achieved. At high infusion dosages, opioids, most notably fentanyl, may eventually rely on metabolism and excretion for termination of action, rather than redistribution. This is known as context sensitive half-life, which can result in a much longer than typical drug duration of action. This feature must be considered in various clinical situations such as planning for extubation.

Continuous Epidural Analgesia

Continuous epidural analgesia is an effective means of pain control for nociceptive pain experienced below the level of the fourth thoracic dermatome (Table 35.3). It can be achieved using a single local anesthetic agent and in combination with a variety of adjunctive medications, which include opioids (agonists or agonist-antagonists), clonidine, ketamine, and other medications. The use of adjuncts offers the advantage of enhanced or prolonged local anesthetic effects and a resultant decrease in risk for toxicity associated with higher doses of a single agent.

An epidural catheter is often placed preoperatively so the anesthesia provider has the option to dose the epidural throughout the procedure, resulting in the treatment of pain, blunting the stress response, and reducing general anesthetic load. The catheter should be placed at approximately the level of the middle of the surgical area. Postoperatively, maintenance of epidural analgesia has been shown to result in decreased thromboembolic complications and improved

TABLE 35.2 Continuous Morphine Infusion Dosing

Age Range	Dose (µg/kg/h)
Newborns (0–2 months)	5–10
Infants (3–6 months)	10–15
Infants >6 months	15–20
Children >1 year	20–30

TABLE 35.3 Epidural Infusions in Different Age Groups

	Bupivacaine		Ropivacaine				
	Concentration (mg/ml)	Max. Rate (mg/kg/h)	Concentration (mg/ml)	Max. Rate (mg/kg/h)	Morphine (mg/ml)	Fentanyl (µg/ml)	Clonidine (µg/ml)
Newborns	0.5–1	0.2, limit 48 hours	1–1.5, limit 72 hours	0.2	Not recommended	2	Not recommended
Infants 30–90 days	0.5–1	0.25, time limit to 48 hours	1–1.5, limit 72 hours	0.25	Not recommended	2	Not recommended
Infants >90 days	0.5–1.25	0.3, limit 48 hours	1–2	0.3	25	2	0.6 (use >6 months)
Children >1 year	0.5–1.25	0.3	1–2	0.4	25–50	2–5	0.6

immune function (in part because of a decrease in dosage of IV opioid medication) and respiratory function in certain populations.

When continuous epidural analgesia is in use, a pain management service should be immediately available to address dose adjustments and other problems. Hypotension is a common side effect of epidural analgesia, in part because of the sympathectomy that results in peripheral vasodilation and reduced capability for venous return. Other complications include nausea and vomiting (secondary to hypotension or epidural opioids), motor blockade, urinary retention, epidural site infection, or, with high blockade, respiratory or CNS depression.

In the patient receiving epidural opioids, there should be a standing order restricting IV opioids except when directly ordered by the acute pain service managing the epidural. The patient should receive continuous hourly respiratory rate monitoring for the first 24 hours after placement and every 4 hours subsequently. Pain scores, blood pressure, heart rate, and mental status should be measured every 4 hours while the epidural is in place. Continuous IV access should also be maintained in case of urgent need for rescue medication. Respiratory equipment, oxygen supplementation, and naloxone 0.01 mg/kg should be immediately available to treat oversedation or severe respiratory depression associated with high blockade or opioid overdose.

Ineffective blockade is a common concern with epidural analgesia. If associated with unilateral blockade (because of migration of the catheter down one side and too far from the midline within the epidural space) it can sometimes be corrected by withdrawal of the catheter of a few mm, which may result in a more midline placement of the catheter tip. If the patient requires frequent epidural boluses to maintain adequate blockade, the infusion can be increased. Dense motor blockade can be improved with a decrease in medication concentration. If there is no block regardless of adequate dosing, replacement of the epidural catheter may be required. Other potential issues with continuous epidural analgesia include kinked, obstructed, leaking, or broken catheters, and failure of the pump itself. There is also a risk for local anesthetic toxicity through systemic absorption, though this risk is low when dosed according to guidelines.

Patient-Controlled Epidural Analgesia

Patient-controlled epidural analgesia (PCEA) is useful in patients who are about 7 years of age and above who have an epidural in place and who are capable of using a PCA demand button appropriately. The precautions for PCEA are similar to those for continuous epidural analgesia and similar rules apply. The patient alone should press the demand button to avoid potentially serious side effects. PCEA has been compared with continuous epidural infusions, demonstrating a decrease in overall local anesthetic dosage and a decrease in motor blockade without an associated decrease in analgesic effect. There is also an associated increase in patient satisfaction, and patients with PCEA are less likely than those using CEI = continuous epidural infusion to require further anesthetic interventions. Initial PCEA pump parameters include a demand dose of 0.05 to 0.1 mL/kg, a lockout interval of 20 to 30 minutes, a basal infusion of 0.1 to 0.2 mL/kg, and a 1-hour limit of 0.2 to 0.4 mL/kg up to a maximum hourly dose of 19.9 mL/hr.

Drug Transition

Transition from the above specialized techniques to an oral analgesic regimen more appropriate for outpatient maintenance requires close patient monitoring and careful titration. Oral opioids can be initiated in the acute pain pediatric patient once they are tolerating other oral medications and, preferably, oral feeds without significant nausea or vomiting. When starting oral opioids, it is preferable to administer with food to try to decrease the associated potential for abdominal discomfort and increase in nausea. Typical oral regimens include oxycodone 0.1 mg/kg every 4 hours, hydromorphone 0.03 to 0.08 mg/kg every 4 hours, or morphine 0.3 to 0.5 mg/kg every 6 hours.

When weaning patients from epidural analgesia, it is useful to bridge analgesia with oral opioids, administering the initial doses before discontinuation of the epidural infusion and thereby avoiding significant increases in pain. Once oral analgesics are started and a baseline level of analgesia is obtained, the PCA continuous dose is discontinued and the demand dosage progressively decreased. During this weaning process an IV opioid rescue medication should be immediately available to treat moderate to severe pain. Common rescue dosages include morphine 0.05 mg/kg IV every 4 hours, hydromorphone 0.01 mg/kg IV every 4 hours, or nalbuphine 0.05 mg/kg IV every 3 hours. Adjunctive oral medications are also frequently useful during this period and include acetaminophen 10 to 15 mg/kg every 6 hours (maximum dose of 3000 mg daily), ibuprofen 10 mg/kg every 4 hours, or ketorolac 0.5 mg/kg every 6 hours for a maximum daily dose of 60 mg and for a maximal duration of 5 days (Table 35.4).

TABLE 35.4	Adjuvant Medications for Patients Receiving Epidural Analgesia
Symptom	**Medication**
Nausea or vomiting	Ondansetron 0.1 mg/kg IV every 8 hours
Breakthrough pain, pruritus, nausea, or vomiting	Nalbuphine 50 µg/kg IV every 4 hours
Breakthrough pain	Ketorolac 0.5 mg/kg IV every 6 hours (maximum 20 doses)
Muscle spasm	Diazepam 0.1 mg/kg PO/PR every 6 hours

PO = per os; PR = per rectum.

Additional Therapies

Adjunct therapies, such as anxiolytics, antispasmodics, anticonvulsants, and nonpharmacologic interventions, are of key importance in the acute setting. Procedure-associated anxiety, musculoskeletal dysfunction, and neuropathic pain components can play a large role in the acute pain experience and failure to address one or all of the above can represent the difference between effective and unsatisfactory pain management.

Muscle spasms contribute significantly to the acute pain experience. Surgical manipulation of musculoskeletal structures oftentimes results in a response of muscular tightening. The resultant pain is oftentimes described as a "cramping," "dull," or "throbbing" type of discomfort. Analgesics, such as opioids, may be ineffective at alleviating this type of pain. Diazepam, a member of the benzodiazepine class, can be used on an as-needed or scheduled basis in conjunction with other antispasmodics to address this muscular component. Methocarbamol, a central muscle relaxant, is generally scheduled 3 to 4 times daily. It is generally considered to be less sedating than other muscle relaxants, which include tizanidine and baclofen.

In patients with a psychological propensity for highly anxious states, the perioperative period can represent a time of heightened anxiety levels and decreased ability to cope with the associated emotional distress. If unaddressed, this can lead to an altered response to nociceptive stimulation and an intensification of the patient's pain experience. Benzodiazepines with greater psychotropic action, lorazepam, for example, are frequently used in low doses to successfully de-escalate such responses in patients who are unsuccessful with nonpharmacological interventions, such as cognitive behavioral therapy. It is important to titrate dosages and avoid concurrent administration of benzodiazepines with other sedating medications.

Neuropathic pain can play a significant role in both chronic and acute pain experiences. Gabapentin and pregabalin are two anticonvulsants that are commonly used to address neuropathic pain in the acute setting. This can provide better analgesia with decreased opioid consumption and improved gut motility.

Nonpharmacologic modalities can also play a significant role in the acute setting. Studies of electroacupuncture suggest that the intervention is associated with an increase of β-endorphin, encephalin, and endomorphin release, which then affects μ- and δ-opioid receptor agonism. Though the mechanism is otherwise largely unknown, acupuncture has been successfully used in treatment of acute, chronic, and neuropathic pain. Acupuncture can be performed pre- or postoperatively and is associated with a decreased incidence of nausea and vomiting, decreased incisional and visceral pain, reduced analgesic requirements, reduced sympathetic system activation with surgical stimulus, and a more rapid recovery to baseline musculoskeletal function after surgery.

Suggested Readings

Gibbs A, Kim SS, Heydinger G, et al. Postoperative analgesia in neonates and infants using epidural chloroprocaine and clonidine. *J Pain Res.* 2020;13:2749–2755. https://doi.org/10.2147/JPR.S281484.

Martin LD, Adams TL, Duling LC, et al. Comparison between epidural and opioid analgesia for infants undergoing major abdominal surgery. *Paediatr Anaesth.* 2019;29(8):835–842. https://doi.org/10.1111/pan.13672.

McNicol ED, Rowe E, Cooper TE. Ketorolac for postoperative pain in children. *Cochrane Database Syst Rev.* 2018;7(7). https://doi.org/10.1002/14651858. CD012294. Published 2018 Jul 7. CD012294.pub2.

Sun Y, Gan TJ, Dubose JW, et al. Acupuncture and related techniques for postoperative pain: a systematic review of randomized controlled trials. *Br J Anaesth.* 2008;101(2):151–160. https://doi.org/10.1093/bja/aen146.

Veneziano G, Tobias JD. Chloroprocaine for epidural anesthesia in infants and children. *Paediatr Anaesth.* 2017;27(6):581–590. https://doi.org/10.1111/pan.13134.

Walker SM. Pain in children:recent advances and ongoing challenges. *Br J Anaesth.* 2008;101(1):101–110. https://doi.org/10.1093/bja/aen097.

36

Chronic Pain

F. WICKHAM KRAEMER III

Pain is considered chronic when it is constant or recurrent and lasts for more than 3 months. It may persist because of ongoing tissue inflammation, as seen in children with inflammatory bowel disease or juvenile rheumatoid arthritis.

It may also occur without tissue inflammation when peripheral or central nervous system neurons become abnormally modified by disease or lesion, or neuropathic pain. Neuropathic pain syndromes are an enigmatic and heterogeneous group of disorders that have been recognized by a variety of names for over 100 years and continue to baffle physicians, patients, and their families. This perplexity stems from the lack of known precise pathophysiologic mechanisms responsible for the debilitating symptoms. Neuropathic pain syndromes are likely caused in part by abnormalities of the peripheral, central, and autonomic nervous system. Other contributory factors include myofascial dysfunction and/or psychological distress. Neuropathic pain conditions are best understood through a biopsychosocial framework wherein multiple factors contribute to the manifestation of this complex pain presentation.

Neuropathic pain is not as uncommon during childhood as once thought. The most common type of neuropathic pain in children is complex regional pain syndrome type 1 (CRPS-1), which is the focus of this chapter.

Complex Regional Pain Syndrome

In 1993, the International Association for the Study of Pain (IASP) recommended that neuropathic pain syndromes should be grouped together and called complex regional pain syndrome (CRPS). CRPS is divided into two different types depending on the initiating injury: CRPS type 1 (formerly called reflex sympathetic dystrophy) follows a soft tissue injury, and CRPS type 2 (formerly called causalgia) follows a peripheral nerve injury. CRPS-2 is rare in children and will not be discussed further in this chapter.

The differential diagnosis of a painful condition involving the distal extremity is long (see Table 36.1).

It is usually possible to eliminate most conditions based on the results of prior diagnostic evaluations, history, and physical examination. Furthermore, the diagnosis of CRPS-1 is excluded by the existence of conditions that would otherwise account for the degree of pain and

dysfunction. Unfortunately, there are no tests that can confirm the diagnosis of CRPS-1. The IASP has established and validated diagnostic criteria for CRPS-1 called the "Budapest Criteria[1]" after an international consensus meeting was held there in 2003. However, it still remains a diagnosis of exclusion.

Delayed diagnosis of CRPS-1 is common and may exceed a year from the time symptoms begin. Diagnostic delays lead to prolonged pain, suffering, and disability, and may result in harmful therapies such as splinting or casting. Immobilization of the effected extremity may exacerbate the condition.

There are several aspects of CRPS-1 in children that may provide clues to the proper diagnosis. As with adults, females are affected more than males by a ratio of 4:1, but unlike adults, the lower extremities are most often affected. A history of trauma, albeit trivial, can be elicited in many children. Frequently the trauma occurs during an organized sporting event. At the time of diagnosis, many of these children are disabled and unable to attend school or participate in normal activities. Some children with lower-extremity CRPS-1 are able to ambulate with crutches, but in more extreme cases children are bedridden or wheelchair bound.

Children diagnosed with CRPS-1 will often manifest psychological symptoms that contribute to their pain and disability. These include fear, anxiety, anger, depression, maladaptive coping skills and behaviors, and sleep disturbances. In three large pediatric reports, psychological disorders were identified in 25% to 77% of patients.

Clinical Signs and Diagnosis

The clinical presentation of children with CRPS is heterogeneous and starts with pain that can be out of proportion to any inciting event, which in many instances is minor or even absent. The individual should report change in the following four categories: sensory, vasomotor, sudomotor, and motor changes. They should also report these changes during examination. Per the Budapest Criteria, the individual should report a constellation of at least one symptom from three of the four categories and the physician should document at least one sign in two or more categories during the physical exam. Lastly, as CRPS remains a diagnosis of

TABLE 36.1	Differential Diagnosis of Distal Limb Pain in a Child

- Osteomyelitis
- Septic arthritis
- Cellulitis
- Lyme disease and other rheumatologic conditions
- Bone fracture or sprain
- Neoplasm
- Osteoid osteoma
- Entrapment neuropathy
- Small fiber neuropathy (i.e., diabetic neuropathy)
- Deep venous thrombosis
- Vascular insufficiency
- Lymphedema
- Erythromelalgia
- Psychiatric etiologies (e.g., somatization or conversion disorders)

exclusion, no other disease process should better explain all the signs and symptoms of the child.

The sensory symptoms of allodynia (defined as pain caused by a stimulus that does not normally provoke pain) or hyperesthesia (defined as increased sensitivity to stimulation) are usually the most obvious cues to the child that something is amiss. A wool sock might be so scratchy that the child must remove it immediately, or the pressure of a bed sheet on the affected extremity causes extreme pain. Often, these unusual sensations cause the child to sleep with an extremity propped in the air so that nothing touches or stimulates the affected extremity. Hygiene can become difficult if the temperature of warm water used in bathing is felt as scalding water on the child's affected body part. These sensory changes are not often in a dermatomal distribution and can be described as "burning, sharp, or achy." On examination, pinprick may provoke hyperalgesia while vibration or light touch or joint movement may provoke allodynia.

The vasomotor changes relate to color or temperature changes in the skin. This can be asymmetric color or temperature changes between the affected and unaffected extremity or skin color changes over the affected body part. An adolescent may mention or display periods of redness and warmth followed by other periods of mottled or pale skin. Infrared thermometry can confirm temperature differences which in some studies vary by 0.6°C between the colder affected limb and the unaffected limb.

The sudomotor changes described by the child may consist of edema or sweating. Often these reports will consist of asymmetric changes that have no apparent provocation. The affected limb will have edema or unusual sweating. A swollen, discolored extremity has been the classic presentation of CRPS. Direct examination and comparison with the unaffected limb can yield signs of sudomotor changes.

Finally, motor and trophic changes can have the most significant effect on the functional ability of the adolescent. There could be complaints of hair loss over a distal extremity or brittle nails. Other trophic changes can involve the bones losing density and wasting of the skin, tissue, and muscle. The adolescent may complain that she is unable to complete simple tasks because of weakness or that tremors affect her handwriting. Problems using the affected area often limit participation in activities such as sports, dance, music playing, and social events. Often, routine activity such as school attendance is abandoned because of the functional disability associated with CRPS.

Therapies

Reported therapies include nonsteroidal antiinflammatory drugs (NSAIDs), tricyclic antidepressants, opioids, anticonvulsants, corticosteroids, sympathetic blocks, physiotherapy, transcutaneous electrical nerve stimulation (TENS), and psychological therapies, particularly cognitive-behavioral therapies. Although most of these achieve modest success, none has proven effective in prospective, controlled, clinical trials. Yet children with CRPS-1 appear to be more responsive to therapy than adults. Combinations of the above therapies result in resolution of symptoms in 46% to 69% of children, the average recovery time being 7 weeks (range 1 to 140 weeks). In recent years, several intensive interdisciplinary pain rehabilitation programs using inpatient and day-hospital models[2] have demonstrated large improvements in functioning and reductions of pain in children treated with a combination of intensive physical therapy, occupational therapy, and cognitive-behavioral therapies, with or without medications or sympathetic blocks.

Children with CRPS are best cared for by an experienced multidisciplinary team of individuals that includes a physician, a psychologist, and a physical therapist. The physician confirms the diagnosis, coordinates physical and psychological therapies, and when appropriate starts medications or performs sympathetic blocks to facilitate participation in physical therapy.

Daily physical therapy is the cornerstone of treatment for children with CRPS-1. It should focus on desensitization, full weight-bearing, and functional usage of the extremity. The goal is to return the affected extremity to normal functioning, rather than only pain relief. The therapist should acknowledge the presence of pain during initial treatments but continue nonetheless. It is thought that the pain of CRPS-1 results when the body misinterprets sensory information and responds as though an acute injury is in progress. Physical therapy halts this inappropriate response and reestablishes normal neuronal responses. The central nervous system is bombarded with "normal" sensory information such as the perception of touching or weight-bearing by using the affected body part in functional activities.

Additional therapies such as hot and cold packs, TENS, and ultrasound are not usually effective. Immobilization of the affected limb is contraindicated because it may enhance progression of the disease.

Psychological Assessment

The purpose of psychological assessment is to estimate the severity of the child's and the family's pain-related distress and dysfunction and to assist in treatment planning. The psychologist will attempt to gain an understanding of their expectations for treatment, their coping styles and skills, recent stressful events and other life changes, and developmental and social histories. The psychologist will help the child and family understand the mechanism of the pain in general terms and will teach coping strategies, relaxation techniques, techniques that maximize function, and cognitive restructuring techniques to address negative thinking. The psychologist will evaluate symptoms of depression and anxiety and will teach the child and family how to increase their sense of self-control over the pain and disability.

Some families may resist psychological involvement because they view it as an indication that the pain is psychosomatic. Therefore the medical team should present psychological therapy as an integral component of the global pain management program and inform families of the ways in which psychological techniques are useful in pain management. The treatment team should emphasize the mind-body connection so that patients understand that pain is not necessarily a medical or psychological entity, but rather that pain treatment requires a combination of medical and psychological approaches.

There is a growing consensus in chronic pain research that the immune system is clinically involved in the mechanistic changes that occur between acute and chronic pain. Through the communication between neurons and immune cells, the immune system has the ability to propagate and maintain a chronic pain state including neuropathic pain such as CRPS. The immune system can work both peripherally and centrally to release mediators that sensitize neurons which provide a positive feedback loop which can perpetuate chronic pain. This might in part explain why many current medications are poor at treating chronic pain as almost none slow this immune-mediated-positive feedback loop while multidisciplinary programs have some success by focusing on improved function and exercise, regulated sleep, improved diet, and psychological stress reduction, which are all demonstrated to improve immune system function.

Clinical Course and Progression

The clinical course and progression of CRPS-1 is highly variable and difficult to predict with reasonable accuracy. Most children will experience a remission of symptoms but about 30% will relapse at the original site or at a new location. Outcomes are variable, with some children returning to their premorbid activities and others having a chronic, progressive course with severe pain and disability.

In summary, CRPS-1 is a chronic pain disorder associated with significant morbidity. Its inciting factors and pathophysiology are not fully known. Prompt intervention by an experienced multidisciplinary team can lead to resolution of severe symptoms in most children. However, remissions marked by persistent pain and disabilities are common.

References

1. Harden RN, Bruehl S, Perez RSGM, et al. Validation of proposed diagnostic criteria (the "Budapest Criteria") for Complex Regional *Pain Syndrome. Pain.* 2010;150(2):268–274. https://doi.org/10.1016/j.pain.2010.04.030.
2. Logan DE, Carpino EA, Chiang G, et al. A day-hospital approach to treatment of pediatric complex regional pain syndrome: initial functional outcomes. *Clin J Pain.* 2012;28(9):766–774. https://doi.org/10.1097/AJP.0b013e3182457619.

37

Trauma and Burn Management

ALISON PERATE AND ADITEE AMBARDEKAR

With approximately 15,000 deaths per year, trauma is the leading cause of death in children over 1 year of age in the United States. Anesthesiologists and anesthetists in nearly every type of hospital setting will eventually be exposed to the multiply injured child. In this chapter, we review in detail the anesthetic considerations for trauma and burn management in the pediatric population.

The most common causes of traumatic injury in children are based on age. In infants, the most common cause is child abuse. In toddlers, it is falls from heights, and in school-aged children motor vehicle and bicycle accidents.

Pediatric Trauma

Traumatic Brain Injury

Severe traumatic brain injury (TBI) is the most common cause of death in injured children. An acceleration or deceleration injury can result in a cerebral contusion, which may be located on the same side as the impact, on the opposite side of the impact (contra-coup injury), or both. Blunt or penetrating trauma may cause an intracranial hemorrhage. A tear of the middle meningeal artery produces an epidural hematoma, and trauma that causes rupture of bridging veins results in a subdural hematoma. Any of these aforementioned injuries may produce a condition known as diffuse axonal injury (DAI), which is associated with permanent disability. Children are more susceptible to TBI because of less central nervous system (CNS) myelination, thinner and more compliant cranial bones, and a larger head-to-body ratio than adults.

Contusions and intracranial bleeds are diagnosed by computed tomography (CT). Patients with DAI and abnormal neurologic exams may initially have a normal CT scan. Cerebral edema may be evident on a subsequent scan.

TBI should be suspected in children with head trauma despite an absence of neurologic abnormalities. Indicators of occult TBI include loss of consciousness any time after the event, and multiple episodes of emesis. Sedated children with multiple injuries should be considered to have TBI because of their inability to perform a reliable neurologic exam.

Child Abuse

TBI resulting from child abuse is the leading cause of death in children under 1 year of age. This diagnosis should be considered when the child's injuries are out of proportion to the history or the child's developmental level. Common presenting signs include irritability, emesis, decreased level of consciousness, seizures, and coma. There may be multiple injuries at different stages of healing. Injuries may be severe and include subdural hematoma, subarachnoid hemorrhage, skull fracture or DAI with or without cerebral edema. Although state law varies, all physicians must report suspected child abuse to the proper authorities (i.e., social services, child protective services, police, etc.). Careful documentation of the history, physical examination and intraoperative findings is helpful if legal testimony is required at a later date.

Suffocation

While this category includes chocking, Sudden Infant Death Syndrome (SIDS) is the leading cause of death in children from 1 month to 1 year of age. According to the Centers for Disease Control and Prevention (CDC), 26% of SIDS deaths are caused by accidental suffocation or strangulation in bed (ASSB). In 1994 a national "Safe to Sleep Campaign" was launched to combat this epidemic. Since the initiation of "Safe to Sleep," SIDS deaths have decreased by 50% in the United States. Over half of all infants that present with SIDS will require escalation of care and most will proceed to have significant neurologic injury from hypoxia.

Cervical Spine Injury

The incidence of spinal cord injury (SCI) in pediatric trauma is estimated to be 1%, which is lower than the adult population because of greater flexibility of the pediatric cervical spine. Any child with an unknown mechanism of injury, multisystem trauma, brain injury, or a known injury above the clavicle should be suspected to also have SCI. Approximately 50% of children with SCI have concomitant TBI. Conversely, the presence of TBI substantially increases the risk for SCI.

SCI in children is diagnosed and managed in a similar manner to adults. Radiographs of the cervical spine should include anteroposterior and lateral views that include the cervicothoracic junction ("swimmer's view"), and views of the odontoid process of C2. However, the cervical spine cannot be "cleared" by radiographic examination without a normal neurologic exam. Therefore children with normal cervical spine radiographs should be kept immobilized until thoroughly examined because spinal cord instability and neurologic deficits may occur without a fracture. A neurologic deficit without a fracture is called *SCIWORA* (spinal cord injury without radiologic abnormalities). The term was coined in the pre-MRI era. We now know that most of these children will have demonstrable abnormalities on magnetic resonance imaging (MRI). SCIWORA can occur in the cervical or thoracic spinal cord, mainly in children less than 8 years of age. In about one-quarter of children with SCIWORA, the onset of the neurologic deficit is delayed. These children will initially have minor sensory or motor deficits that progress over time. The majority of SCIWORA injuries are caused by severe flexion or extension injuries of the neck that cause ligamentous stretching or disruption without bony injury. Continued immobilization and cervical spine precautions are necessary because of the possibility of evolving injury.

Other Common Injuries

The majority of thoracic trauma in children consists of blunt injuries caused by motor vehicle accidents. Adults struck by cars typically experience pelvic or lower extremity fractures because of the level of the bumper of a car. For most school age and younger children, the level of the bumper corresponds to the thorax or head. Therefore children are more likely to suffer thoracic injuries and TBI when struck by a car. Thoracic injuries are the second leading cause of death despite accounting for less than 5% of pediatric trauma. Pulmonary contusion is the most common type of thoracic injury; rib fractures are less common than in adults. Because of the relatively high compliance of the chest wall of young children (noncalcified rib cage) severe intrathoracic injuries can occur without obvious external injuries or rib fractures. As in adults, pneumothorax, hemothorax, and lung laceration are important sequelae of penetrating thoracic trauma.

Blunt abdominal trauma is primarily associated with injuries to the spleen and liver, but renal, pancreatic, and hollow viscous injuries can also occur. When a child restrained by a lap belt presents with abdominal or flank ecchymosis (lap belt sign), there is likely an abdominal injury or a horizontal fracture of a lumbar vertebral body (Chance fracture). Management of solid organ injury is largely expectant unless the child demonstrates hypotension unresponsive to resuscitative measures. Penetrating abdominal injuries usually result in intestinal injury and require surgical intervention. Extremity injuries with or without underlying vascular tears are common in children, as are complex lacerations and growth plate injuries. Simple scalp lacerations may be the cause of a significant amount of blood loss.

Attention to the quantity and quality of the urine output is important. Head trauma is associated with development of diabetes insipidus or SIADH. Direct muscle injury may result in rhabdomyolysis, which may cause myoglobinuria and lead to renal damage.

Assessment and Resuscitation

Primary Survey

The initial management period (the "golden hour") after an injury is focused on cardiorespiratory resuscitation and transport to an appropriate facility. As with adult trauma, there is controversy concerning the most appropriate care facility for pediatric trauma victims; outcome studies that provide a definitive answer are lacking. Pediatric trauma patients treated in adult hospitals had higher in-hospital mortality[1], and longer lengths of stay.

Management during this period is guided by the principles of advanced trauma life support (ATLS). The initial approach involves primary and secondary surveys, followed by definitive care of all injuries. The primary survey consists of optimizing oxygenation and ventilation, recognizing potentially life-threatening injuries and stabilizing the cervical spine. All life-threatening conditions are identified and managed simultaneously. Once the primary survey is completed, a thorough head-to-toe examination (secondary survey) is performed to identify all injuries.

Ventilatory Management

The most critical aspect of successful management of pediatric trauma is adequate oxygenation and ventilation. The lucid and hemodynamically stable child can be managed conservatively; oxygen can be delivered by facemask as required. In the child with depressed consciousness, chin-lift and jaw-thrust maneuvers may be required to maintain upper airway patency while simultaneously stabilizing the child's neck in the neutral position. Additional interventions may include oropharyngeal suctioning, insertion of an oral airway, and if the child is unstable, positive pressure ventilation using bag-mask ventilation or insertion of a laryngeal mask. Bag-mask ventilation can be effective and, in some children, may be an alternative to endotracheal intubation in the prehospital setting (depending on the training and experience of the prehospital provider). Indications for tracheal intubation in injured children include the following:

- Decreasing level of consciousness (Glasgow Coma Scale <8; Table 37.1)
- Marked respiratory failure secondary to chest trauma or other causes
- Hemodynamic instability despite initial fluid resuscitation

TABLE 37.1 Glasgow Coma Scale Modified for Infants

GLASGOW COMA SCALE		INFANT COMA SCALE	
RESPONSE	SCORE	RESPONSE	SCORE
Eye Opening		**Eye Opening**	
Spontaneous	4	Spontaneous	4
To Speech	3	To Speech	3
To pain	2	To pain	2
None	1	None	1
Best motor response		**Best motor response**	
Obeys verbalcommand	6	Normal spontaneousmovements	6
Localizes pain	5	Withdraws to touch	5
Withdraws in response to pain	4	Withdraws to pain	4
Abnormal flexion	3	Abnormal flexion	3
Extension posturing	2	Extension posturing	2
None	1	None	1
Best verbal response		**Best verbal response**	
Oriented and converses	5	Coos, babbles, interacts	5
Confused	4	Irritable	4
Inappropriate words	4	Cries to pain	4
Incomprehensible Sounds	3	Moans to pain	3
None	1	None	1

- Difficult bag-mask ventilation or the anticipated need for prolonged assisted ventilation, and to facilitate hyperventilation during management of increased intracranial pressure
- Loss of protective airway reflexes

Endotracheal intubation may be difficult or in some cases impossible in conscious or semiconscious children. Unless consciousness is severely depressed, endotracheal intubation is accomplished by induction of general anesthesia using a modified rapid sequence technique with application of cricoid pressure and hyperventilation with 100% oxygen.

There are no universal recommendations regarding the most appropriate approach to maintain cervical spine stabilization during tracheal intubation. As in adults, manual in-line stabilization by a trained assistant is used most often, with care taken to keep the cervical spine in the neutral position during direct laryngoscopy, or fiberoptic-guided tracheal intubation. Flexible fiberoptic bronchoscopy is an option in pediatric trauma patients but pediatric-sized bronchoscopes are not available in all facilities and often have poor optical resolution and limited suctioning capabilities. Tracheal intubation with video-laryngoscopy can be used to minimize cervical spine movement. Nasotracheal intubation may be easier using fiberoptic bronchoscopy but is contraindicated in patients with basilar skull fractures. Characteristics of a basilar skull fracture include periorbital (raccoon's eyes) and mastoid (Battle's sign) ecchymosis, and cerebrospinal spinal (CSF) drainage from the nose or ear canals.

Additional precautions during airway manipulation are warranted for the pediatric trauma patient with possible head or neck injury. These include avoidance of the Trendelenburg position, and keeping the neck in the neutral position at all times to avoid jugular kinking. In infants less than 6 months of age, the head and cervical spine should be immobilized using a spine board with tape across the infant's forehead, and blankets or towels around the neck. In older infants and children, the head should be immobilized in the manner described above or by using a small rigid cervical collar. Children older than about 8 years of age require a medium-sized cervical collar. In infants with a prominent occiput, a roll placed under the shoulders provides neutral alignment of the spine and avoids excessive flexion that often occurs in the supine position. These maneuvers will help prevent further cervical spine injury. A rigid collar will effectively prevent cervical spine distraction. A soft collar will permit a five to seven mm distraction of the cervical spine during laryngoscopy; hence it is not routinely recommended.

Cardiovascular Management

Primary cardiac arrest is unusual in pediatric trauma unless the child has suffered direct cardiothoracic trauma.

Commotio cordis is the term given to the development of ventricular fibrillation after a sudden, intense, nonpenetrating impact on the chest wall over the anatomic location of the left ventricle. Animal studies demonstrate that the timing of this impact in relation to the cardiac cycle (between the QRS complex and the T wave) is crucial for development of this fatal complication.[2]

Pediatric trauma commonly causes shock, which is usually classified as hypovolemic, cardiogenic, neurogenic, or septic. The traumatized, hypovolemic child presents unique physiologic patterns, in that children tend to compensate for blood loss and may retain normal vital signs until 30% to 40% of their blood volume has been lost. In other words, blood pressure may remain normal during clinically significant anemia and hypovolemia. The systolic and diastolic blood pressures may be maintained by vasoconstriction and the pulse pressure may be narrow, rather than wide, as observed during general anesthesia and neurogenic shock (owing to loss of arterial and venous peripheral tone). Hypotension and decreased urine output are more ominous signs of hypovolemic shock; however, they may not occur in children until more than 30% blood volume has been lost. Bradycardia in this setting is life-threatening, as heart rate is a major component of cardiac output in small children.

TBI can be associated with hypotension. The hypertensive component of Cushing's triad may not be present and cerebral perfusion pressure (CPP; mean arterial pressure minus ICP or CVP, whichever is higher) may not be maintained. The minimum CPP necessary to meet metabolic demands in infants and children has not been established and is largely extrapolated from adults. In children under 6 years of age, cerebral blood flow averages 106 mL per 100 g of brain tissue, and cerebral metabolic rate averages 5.2 mL/min per 100 g of brain tissue. This is in contrast to 58 mL and 3.3 mL per 100 g of brain, respectively, in the adult, and indicates greater cerebral blood flow and metabolic requirements in children. As cerebral autoregulation can also be impaired in children with TBI, systemic blood pressure should be maintained above normal in the absence of ICP monitoring. In injured children, an increased ICP (>20 mm Hg) and decreased CPP (<50 mm Hg) are associated with a poor outcome. Additional risk factors in brain-injured children include Pao_2 <60 mm Hg, $Paco_2$ <25 mmHg or >45 mm Hg, and a systolic blood pressure <90 mm Hg.

Vascular access is an important and often challenging component of pediatric trauma management. A 22-gauge or larger peripheral IV catheter will suffice for induction of general anesthesia but may not be adequate for resuscitation of the child with major trauma. In the latter scenario, at least two large-bore IV catheters are recommended. Saphenous veins are larger than the peripheral veins of distal extremities and thus are commonly used to secure vascular access, either percutaneously or by surgical exposure. In an emergent situation, if peripheral access is unobtainable after three rapid attempts or duration greater than 90 seconds in young children, intraosseous (IO) access[3] should be inserted using any large-bore needle, EZ IO or bone marrow needle.

Any nontraumatized long bone may be used. The preferred site is the anteromedial surface of the proximal tibia, 2 cm below and 1 to 2 cm medial to the tibial tuberosity on the flat part of the bone. Other possible sites of insertion include the distal femur 3 cm above the lateral condyle in the midline, and the medial surface of the distal tibia 1 to 2 cm above the medial malleolus. The insertion technique entails the advancement of a large-bore needle until the periosteum of the bone is contacted. With a twisting, boring motion the needle is advanced until it is felt to penetrate into the marrow cavity by a loss of resistance. Negative aspiration of marrow does not preclude use of the intraosseous line provided that infused fluids do not extravasate into the subcutaneous tissues. If marrow is obtained, it may be sent for routine lab investigation and type-and-crossmatch. Any type of crystalloid or colloid solution may be infused into the marrow, and higher than normal infusion pressures may be required. This route of access is temporary until more definitive access can be secured.

It is important to recognize the risk for hyperkalemia in significant blood transfusion in pediatric trauma patients. Because of smaller caliber intravenous catheters, the risk for hemolysis from shearing forces is greater. This can lead to increase in the release of intracellular potassium as the cell membrane is compromised. The age of the O negative blood used must also be considered as both length of storage and irradiation can cause leaking of the intracellular potassium in to the supernatant. In infants and toddlers this potassium load from rapid infusion can quickly cause cardiac compromise and even asystole.

Central venous catheters are acceptable routes of venous access in children. The femoral vein is preferred in children with head or neck injuries; however, it is contraindicated in abdominal trauma with suspected inferior vena cava injury.

In the immediate post injury phase, aggressive fluid resuscitation is critical, as hypoperfusion and hypoxia can induce anaerobic cellular metabolism resulting in the formation of inflammatory mediators that can have significant systemic effects. There are no evidence-based data to unequivocally support either crystalloid or colloid as preferred resuscitative fluid in pediatric trauma. Initial fluid resuscitation in children consists of warmed isotonic crystalloids solution (e.g., Lactated Ringer's) as a bolus of 20 mL/kg. If there is no physiologic response or there is evidence of persistent volume loss, a second bolus should be administered. The goal of initial crystalloid resuscitation is to rapidly achieve normal age-appropriate hemodynamic values and to restore adequate tissue perfusion. Children with evidence of hemorrhagic shock who fail to respond to initial crystalloid resuscitation efforts should receive a red blood cell transfusion (at least 10 mL/kg) and undergo immediate surgical evaluation for possible operative interventions. Hypotonic dextrose-containing crystalloid solutions should be avoided and hydroxyethyl starch administration is discouraged because it may exacerbate a coexisting coagulopathy when administered in amounts greater than 20 mL/kg. Hypertonic saline lowers intracranial pressure and improves cerebral blood flow in patients with TBI, but further study is ongoing to determine its role in pediatric trauma resuscitation.

Neurologic Assessment

In infants, the Glasgow Coma Scale (GCS) has a modified verbal component to allow a developmentally appropriate evaluation. The trend in GCS is more important than the absolute number. Pupillary examination is also an important component of the neurologic assessment. For example, pinpoint pupils indicate pontine herniation and dilated pupils suggest uncal herniation.

In the final phase of the primary survey, the entire body must be examined while avoiding hypothermia. Normothermia is maintained by increasing the room temperature, and using overhead warming lights and forced warm-air blankets.

Secondary Survey

Once the child is in stable condition, a secondary survey should be considered. The secondary survey includes a complete history and detailed full body examination to rapidly identify and begin to treat all nonlife-threatening injuries. The mnemonic AMPLE can be helpful in quickly obtaining a relatively comprehensive history of the injury mechanism, as well as preexisting medical conditions:

- **A**llergies (medications, including anesthetics)
- **M**edications currently used (including steroid use)
- **P**ast illnesses and medical history (including recent viral illnesses)
- **L**ast meal or oral intake (assume full stomach unless otherwise confirmed)
- **E**vents/Environment related to the injury scene

Because of age-related communication limitations with children, such history must often be obtained from family members, others present at the injury scene, or prehospital personnel with knowledge of the injury scene and medical care provided during transport. Priorities for treatment and further diagnostic investigations (e.g., imaging and laboratory studies) can then be determined, including appropriate subspecialist consultation and decisions for operating room intervention. If the child becomes unstable at any point during the secondary survey, return to the primary survey and resuscitation.

Patient examination during the secondary survey involves exposing the child by fully undressing to assess for any hidden injuries, but with special care to avoid hypothermia. Key portions of the physical examination in injured children include the following:

- Palpation of the skull and face for pain or deformities.
- Careful assessment of the cervical spine for tenderness while maintaining cervical immobilization until the spine is "cleared" by a combination of physical exam and radiographic assessment; because of their more cartilaginous spine structure, young children have a higher incidence than adults of SCIWORA, and may require CT or MRI imaging rather than plain film imaging, in cases of high concern.

- Assessment for flail chest segments, chest wall tenderness, and crepitance, as well as auscultation for poorly transmitted or asymmetric breath sounds, and for heart murmurs.
- Abdominal examination for external signs of internal injury (e.g., "seatbelt sign"), distention, tenderness, open wounds, and presence of bowel sounds; crying children often "swallow" significant amounts of air that can lead to abdominal distention that can limit the utility of the abdominal palpation exam, and increases the risk for vomiting and aspiration.
- Rectal examination for anal sphincter tone (e.g., absence of tone in complete spinal cord injury), prostate position, and presence of blood in the stool.
- Perineal examination for hematoma or blood in the urethral meatus (e.g., urethral injury).
- Careful examination of all extremities for deformity, open wounds, distal pulses, and motor/sensory function.

After the history and physical examination, blood samples are collected for hemoglobin and electrolyte assessments, and should also include coagulation studies, type and cross-match, and an arterial blood gas in the case of more severe injuries or intubated children. In older children, possible use of drugs or alcohol should be assessed by blood or urine toxicology, particularly if urgent surgical intervention and general anesthesia are planned. Hemoglobin levels sampled early in hypovolemic shock patients are not always a sensitive indicator of blood loss because hemodilution from crystalloid resuscitation may not yet have occurred.

As in adult trauma management, the recommended radiologic examination during initial assessment and stabilization of major blunt trauma include plain films of the chest, pelvis and cervical spine. In stable patients with intraabdominal injuries, the diagnostic test of choice is a rapid abdominal CT scan. Diagnostic peritoneal lavage (DPL) and "focused abdominal sonography for trauma" (FAST) can also be used to assess intraabdominal injuries, but requires operators with special expertise and training to perform and interpret these exams properly in children. Other radiologic examinations (e.g., extremity plain films) are performed based on the physical examination findings. Children with suspected child abuse injuries less than 2 years of age generally require a more complete skeletal survey including radiographs of the skull, chest, abdomen and long bones.

Preoperative Considerations

After initial resuscitation in the emergency room, children may require emergent surgical interventions to control ongoing bleeding or craniotomy for TBI. In addition, some children with acute injuries who are otherwise stable may require procedural sedation in the emergency room for diagnostic or therapeutic procedures, or for radiologic examination. Still other children may require more elective (nonemergent) surgical interventions for management of their traumatic injuries.

Because of the critical nature of certain injuries, a focused preanesthetic evaluation with a brief history should elicit information regarding allergies, medications, time of the last meal, and events (AMPLE mnemonic, see above) surrounding the injury. Except in emergent surgical cases, a thorough anesthesia-oriented physical examination should be performed with the main focus on airway, breathing, and circulation, and the extent of associated injuries and their possible impact on the conduct of the anesthetic. A general principle is that the true fasting interval is the time between the most recent meal and the traumatic event. Patients who have fasted for at least 8 hours from the time of the injury are still considered to be at risk for pulmonary aspiration of gastric contents during induction of general anesthesia because gastric emptying may be delayed by a variety of factors that include catecholamine release, opioid administration, and abdominal trauma.

Hemodynamically stable children should receive sedation and analgesia in the emergency department. Unstable children who receive only muscle relaxants to facilitate tracheal intubation may have recall of the event and should receive amnestic agents as tolerated.

Anesthetic Techniques

Before transport, the operating room should be adequately staffed and contain all age-appropriate equipment and medications, including those to facilitate the adequate management of hypovolemic shock, such as IV and intraosseous access supplies, fluid and blood warmers, a rapid transfusion system, and an age-appropriate infusion pump. The operating room should also be equipped with a defibrillator with appropriately sized paddles for both internal and external defibrillation. The ambient operating room temperature should be warmed, preferably to 26°C for infants and young children.

Premedication is avoided in children who are hemodynamically unstable or if increased ICP is suspected. However, in stable children, a small dose of IV midazolam can be given to facilitate separation from parents and placement of monitors before induction.

In pediatric trauma, general principles of airway management are followed, with the focus on the possibility of a difficult ventilation or intubation. Preoxygenation may be difficult to achieve in the frightened or agitated child. One has to weigh the risks and benefits of forcing preoxygenation in this setting. As in adult trauma, an IV induction technique is preferred. The choice of induction agent will depend on the child's clinical condition and provider familiarity. Etomidate 0.2 to 0.3 mg/kg will provide a rapid onset, hemodynamic stability, and decrease the cerebral metabolic rate of oxygen consumption, which ultimately decreases cerebral blood flow and ICP. Etomidate is known to cause transient suppression of adrenocortical function; however, many providers believe its short-term benefits outweigh its potential long-term risks. Ketamine 1 to 2 mg/kg is an alternative induction agent that does not usually cause hemodynamic depression; however, it is avoided in children with possibly increased ICP. Succinylcholine should be used to rapidly obtain endotracheal intubation. Although succinylcholine has been shown to transiently increase ICP, this effect has not been shown to adversely affect the outcome in children with associated TBI. Alternatively, rocuronium 1.2 to 1.6 mg/kg may be used but will entail a greater duration of action.

A balanced anesthetic technique is most often selected for maintenance. Nitrous oxide is avoided because of its diffusion into closed spaces and exacerbation of pneumocephalus, pneumothorax, and bowel distention, and the possibility that it may increase intracranial pressure. Isoflurane and sevoflurane have similar effects on cerebral autoregulatory capacity. IV fentanyl 2 to 20 µg/kg, or morphine 0.1 to 0.2 mg/kg, may be administered as a bolus during induction of general anesthesia, or in divided doses or continuous infusion (fentanyl 1–4 µg/kg/h; morphine 10–40 µg/kg/h) during maintenance. Remifentanil is more easily titratable during periods of hemodynamic instability. Neuromuscular blockade can be achieved with any nondepolarizing neuromuscular blocker. It is important to consider possible awareness as the child's depth of anesthesia is balanced with his or her hemodynamic status.

Monitoring

In the severely traumatized child, direct arterial access is recommended for continuous monitoring of blood pressure and facilitation of blood sampling. Central venous pressure monitoring can be used to follow trends in intravascular volume status. Urine volume and content should be continuously monitored. Intracranial pressure monitoring can be useful for detecting and monitoring increased ICP, but outcome studies of its use in children have not been performed. A study[4] in adults did not demonstrate a benefit in overall survival. Continuous temperature monitoring is essential because of the high likelihood of hypothermia in trauma patients. Intentional hypothermia as a brain protection strategy is not currently advocated in children. Coagulopathy occurs early in severe trauma and should be treated expectantly.[5]

Glucose

When cerebral ischemia occurs in the presence of hyperglycemia, anaerobic metabolism produces accumulation of excess lactic acid, which can worsen neurologic injury. In a retrospective study[6] of the relationship between serum glucose on admission and outcome after TBI in children, hyperglycemia (glucose >250 mg/100 mL) was associated with worse outcomes. There are no prospective controlled trials that have determined the relationship between serum glucose and outcome in pediatric trauma patients. However, sustained hyperglycemia should be treated aggressively.

Because of the increased metabolic demand of the pediatric patient, nutrition should be started as soon as possible in the postoperative period. Enteral feeding has demonstrated superior metabolic matching compared with parenteral feeding, but is not always feasible with bowel or thoracic injuries.

If possible, placement of feeding tubes (nasogastric) as soon as safely possible to minimize lean muscle mass loss is critical.

Pediatric Burn Management

Burns are a leading cause of morbidity and mortality in children. Scald injuries tend to be the most common type of burn in children, followed by flame and then contact burns. Infants who are not yet walking are often burned when placed in contact with hot surfaces or as a result of a hot liquid spill. Mobile toddlers are able to pull a cup containing hot liquid off a table, chew on an electrical cord, or accidentally step on a hot surface. Adolescent burns usually involve gasoline and fire. Overall, 70% of pediatric burns are associated with hot liquids.

Classification

Burns are classified according to percentage body surface area (BSA) involved and depth (Fig. 37.1). The total percentage BSA derives from the "Rule of Nines," which is different in children than in adults because the pediatric head accounts for a larger percentage of BSA. The depth of the burn is classified as first-, second-, or third-degree (Table 37.2).

Morbidity and mortality increase with increasing size and depth of the burn but inhalational injury, nonaccidental trauma, and early shock are associated with greater risk for short-term mortality. The risk for mortality increases when the burn extends to greater than 60%; yet patients who have survived with a 90% burn have been reported. Severely burned patients may survive the initial insult, only to succumb to a secondary complication (e.g. infection).

TABLE 37.2	Classification of Burns by Depth
Classification	**Depth and Description**
First degree	• Only epidermis involved; painful and Erythematous
Second-degree	• Epidermis and dermis involved, but dermal appendages spared • Superficial 2nd-degree burn is blistered and painful • Any blistering qualifies • Deep 2nd-degree burn may be white and painless, require grafting, and progress to full-thickness burn with wound infection
Third-degree	• Full-thickness burn involving epidermis and all of the dermis, including dermal appendages • Leathery and painless • Requires grafting

The age of the burned child is important for their survival because of better prognosis with increasing age.

A *major burn* is defined as (1) a second-degree burn >10% BSA (20% for children over 10 years); (2) a third-degree burn >5% BSA; or (3) a second- or third-degree burn of the face, hands, feet, perineum, or major joints, electrical or chemical burns, inhalational injury, or burns in patients with preexisting medical conditions. After initial resuscitation, children with major burns should be transferred to a regional burn center for further management. The American Burn Association has published guidelines and criteria[7] for burn center referrals.

Electrical Burns

Electrical injury occurs in a bimodal distribution with highest incidence in children under 6 years and in young adulthood. Patients with electrical burns may sustain deep tissue injuries despite a superficial point of current entry on the skin. Seemingly superficial and small injuries may overlie devitalized muscle. Electrical burns can also cause dysrhythmias and brain or spinal cord injury.

Initial Management of the Burned Child

The anesthetic management of the pediatric burn patient involves paying attention to all organ systems that are directly or indirectly affected by the burn injury. Burns have serious implications for anesthesiologists and involve airway and respiratory management, circulatory concerns and pain management.

Airway Management, Oxygenation, and Ventilation

The initial management of the burned child should focus on airway evaluation and management for the provision of

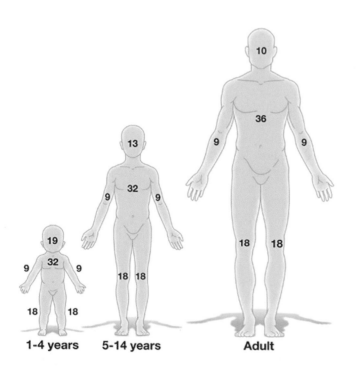

• **Fig. 37.1** Body surface areas by age. Illustration by Rob Fedirko.

adequate oxygenation and ventilation and stabilization of circulatory volume. Wound care is deferred until after the acute resuscitation phase. Tracheal intubation is indicated if there is evidence of inadequate ventilation, singed nasal hair, facial or upper airway edema, hoarseness, or stridor. Patients with stridor or other signs of upper airway obstruction should have tracheal intubation performed before the development of facial and upper airway edema, which can complicate airway management. Total body edema can occur in the setting of large volume resuscitation without airway burns or smoke inhalation and should prompt early intubation. In adults and older children, awake fiberoptic intubation is preferred if upper airway edema or injury is suspected; the extent of airway injury can be examined at the same time. Uncooperative young children, who will not tolerate an awake fiberoptic intubation, will require tracheal intubation after induction of general anesthesia.

Respiratory failure and asphyxia may result from inhalation of toxic fumes, chemical injury from smoke, upper airway edema and, in the later stages, eschar formation on the chest wall. Inhalation of toxic chemicals can cause increased airway secretions, irritability, capillary leaking, and pulmonary edema. Clinical manifestations include hypoxia, hypercapnia, dyspnea, bronchospasm, cough, and stridor. Circumferential burns of the chest wall can cause restrictive respiratory failure for which an escharotomy may be required.

Carbon monoxide (CO), which is a prominent byproduct of combustion, and present in smoke, is responsible for the majority of deaths from smoke inhalation (Table 37.3). Carbon monoxide poisoning should be suspected in patients with inhalation injury or with burns from fires in an enclosed space. Carbon monoxide has a 250 times greater affinity for hemoglobin than oxygen, displaces oxygen from hemoglobin binding sites, and shifts the oxygen dissociation curve to the left. Although the arterial partial pressure and saturation of oxygen is read as normal, the oxygen content of the blood is decreased. Thus carboxyhemoglobin must be specifically measured as a component of blood gas analysis. Clinical symptoms are directly proportional to CO levels.

Low CO levels cause mild CNS symptoms; high CO levels cause coma. The 4-hour half-life of CO can be decreased to 40 minutes with 100% oxygen therapy. Severe CO intoxication can be treated with hyperbaric oxygen therapy; however, there is little evidence that it prevents permanent neurologic deficits.

Smoke from the burning of plastic materials with elevated nitrogen content may contain large amounts of hydrogen cyanide. Cyanide toxicity should be suspected in patients exposed to open fires involving nitrogen-containing plastics. Cyanide binds to cytochrome oxidase and impairs tissue oxygenation by converting intracellular aerobic metabolism to anaerobic metabolism. An elevated venous oxygen level and a lactic acidosis that does not improve with oxygen administration are suggestive of cyanide toxicity. Children who sustain cyanide poisoning as a result of inhalational injury may succumb from asphyxiation and should be treated with sodium thiosulfate or sodium nitrite if seizures, cardiopulmonary failure, or persistent lactic acidosis occurs.

Circulation and Intravascular Volume Resuscitation

During the acute phase of a burn, patients have a transiently decreased cardiac output because of depressed myocardial function, increased blood viscosity, and increased systemic vascular resistance from the release of vasoactive substances. Burn shock can occur because of hypovolemia from the loss of intravascular volume to extravascular space. During the hypermetabolic phase, tissues and organ blood flow is increased because of increased cardiac output and decreased systemic vascular resistance.

Administration of IV fluids is indicated when the burn is >10% BSA. Several formulas have been proposed to estimate fluid requirements in children. The Parkland formula describes use of Lactated Ringer's solution, which is administered at the child's maintenance rate plus 4 mL/kg per 1% total BSA burn for the initial 24 hours. At some institutions, half the total fluid is given over the first 8 hours with the other half given over the next 16 hours. The Cincinnati and Galveston formulae were designed later to be more specific to the fluid needs of children, especially those less than 30 kg. These "two-figure" formulae consider the insensible loss and the hourly, maintenance requirements of children. Dextrose-containing maintenance fluids may be required in the very young or in those children unable to maintain normal blood glucose levels. Fluid requirements are greatest during the first 24 hours after injury.

Established formulae should be used as guides only; fluid administration should be based on parameters of adequate tissue perfusion. Urine output should be maintained at a minimum of 0.5 to 1.0 mL/kg/h. Oliguria in burned patients is usually the result of inadequate fluid resuscitation and not renal insufficiency. Other commonly followed parameters include lactate and base excess, heart rate and systolic blood pressure, and sensorium although these can be challenging to assess during the hypermetabolic state.

After the first day, fluid losses occur by evaporation through denuded skin and as a component of the burn exudate. Maximum weight gain caused by edema occurs on the second or third day and is followed by a diuresis and return to normal weight by day 14. Protein loss through the burn exudate occurs until all wounds are grafted and healed.

TABLE 37.3	Carbon Monoxide Levels and Clinical Symptoms
CO Level	**Symptoms**
<20%	Headache
30%–50%	Irritability, confusion, visual disturbances, emesis, fainting
50%–80%	Convulsions, respiratory failure, coma, death

During graft harvesting, the surgeon may infuse crystalloid solution under the donor skin to facilitate harvesting and decrease blood loss. The amount infused can sometimes be large and should be accounted for in the total volume of fluids given. The use of colloids as a component of fluid resuscitation in children remains controversial; small studies have emerged to show that colloid administration within 8 hours of burn injury decreased overall volume delivered, reduced volume overload, and decreased length of stay.

Other Organ Systems

During the acute phase of injury, the glomerular filtration rate is decreased because of decreased cardiac output and increased vascular tone from circulating catecholamines, vasopressin, and activation of the renin-angiotensin-aldosterone system. The child with a major burn is at higher risk for renal failure secondary to rhabdomyolysis, myoglobinuria, and hypotension. Neurologic dysfunction can result from hypoxia, hyperthermia, electrolyte imbalance, and hypertension. Hematologic abnormalities may include anemia from red cell hemolysis and decreased red cell survival, and thrombocytopenia caused by platelet aggregation at wound sites and at damaged microvasculature. A hypercoagulable state, with possible disseminated intravascular coagulation (DIC) can develop from increasing clotting factor production. The burned child is susceptible to development of sepsis secondary to the loss of skin and intestinal mucosal barriers, and an impaired immune response. Early enteral nutrition minimizes the intestinal mucosal barrier damage and decreases endotoxemia. Liberal application of topical antibiotic ointment has decreased the mortality from infection. Children with major burns are at risk for hypothermia from evaporative losses through large areas of exposed skin. Duodenal and gastric stress ulcers may cause chronic occult bleeding; therefore H_2-antagonists are routinely administered. Nearly all patients will develop an ileus and will require gastric decompression with a nasogastric tube.

Hypermetabolism: Stress Response and Major Organ Effects

Children with approximately 30% BSA burn or more will demonstrate a hypermetabolic response that consists of release of stress hormones, including catecholamines, antidiuretic hormone, renin, angiotensin, aldosterone, glucagon, and cortisol. This hypermetabolic state lasts until all wounds are healed (possibly many months), and generally declines during the first 9 to 12 months postinjury. The degree of hypermetabolism depends on the severity of the burn. The mechanisms involved in this response are complex and may include increased adrenergic output, gut-induced endotoxemia, and endogenous resetting of energy production. The hypermetabolic state manifests as increased catabolism, nitrogen wasting, hyperthermia, hyperglycemia, increased CO_2 production, and increased oxygen utilization. Approximately 8 hours after the burn, the hypothalamic-pituitary thermoregulatory set point resets to a higher than normal body temperature. During the hypermetabolic phase, high caloric nutritional support will help prevent protein breakdown and promote wound healing. Because hypermetabolism increases oxygen consumption and CO_2 production, minute ventilation should be increased, and a warm ambient temperature ($\geq 30°C$) should be maintained to help prevent catabolism caused by hypothermia.

Anesthetic Management of the Burned Child

Burns >30% BSA should be excised and grafted early after injury. After acute resuscitation and stabilization, studies suggest that initial grafting and excision should occur within 48 hours to improve morbidity and mortality. After initial grafting, extremely painful dressing changes are usually required regularly. Split-thickness skin grafts and scar revisions may occur weeks or months after the initial burn. The most important anesthetic and perioperative implications include airway management, vascular access, hemodynamic monitoring, blood and volume replacement, and provision of adequate analgesia.

Preoperative Evaluation

Burn injury causes physiologic changes in hemodynamics, pulmonary compliance, volume status, and metabolism. Preoperative evaluation should include an assessment of the severity and consequences of the burn such as degree and location, physiologic abnormalities, and analgesic requirements. Some patients with minor burns (BSA <10%) do not require major resuscitation but patients with major burns (BSA >30%) develop significant systemic physiologic changes that require vigorous volume resuscitation. Coexisting medical illness, such as asthma in patients with inhalational injuries may necessitate more aggressive treatment and resuscitation, even with minor burns.

A thorough examination of the face, neck, and airway must be performed to determine the likelihood of impending airway compromise as well as potential difficult airway. Burn patients may have concomitant injuries related to the initial cause, such as a motor vehicle accident. Laboratory evaluation should include hematologic, acid-base, electrolyte, coagulation, and renal function studies. A type-and-crossmatch should be obtained when blood loss is anticipated, especially early after the burn. Initial burn wound excision is associated with significant blood loss, and additional blood product availability should be ensured. Acid-base disturbances should be corrected early and continually monitored.

Adequate nutritional balance is of utmost importance in these patients. The fasting state usually required to minimize aspiration during anesthetic management should be carefully considered. Negative nitrogen and caloric balance are associated with higher mortality in burned children. Gastric feeds may be continued through the perioperative period in an already intubated child who will be in the supine position. Nasojejunal enteral feeds are an alternative to nasogastric feeds to minimize the risk for aspiration. Parenteral nutrition should be continued during the perioperative period. Because hypoglycemia is more likely during the hypermetabolic state, frequent glucose level checks should be performed during the perioperative period

Psychologically safe and developmentally appropriate interactions are imperative for these children, who often have long term psychological impairments because of the injury. Child life psychologists are important members of the burn team. In addition to premedication with intravenous anxiolytics, distraction through play and virtual reality have emerged as useful adjuncts to minimize anxiety and pain during these stressful situations. Tolerance to anxiolytics and sedatives develops soon after burn injury.

Children that require extensive excision and grafting should have early tracheal intubation (with a cuffed endotracheal tube) because of the potential for fluid shifts and blood loss, and the need for controlled ventilation because of their expected hypermetabolic state. Fiberoptic intubation may be planned for children with face and neck contractures who present weeks or months after the initial burn. If the contractures limit tracheal intubation or ventilation (chest contractures), these should be surgically released during anesthesia with mask ventilation or IV ketamine before tracheal intubation. If the patient has been previously ventilated, and has developed acute respiratory distress syndrome, the ventilator on the anesthesia machine may not be capable of delivering adequate tidal volumes, inspiratory pressures, or positive end-expiratory pressure (PEEP). Thus a more sophisticated intensive care unit (ICU) ventilator may be necessary in the operating room and anesthetic management is adjusted in favor of the use of total IV anesthesia.

Monitoring

Standard monitoring can be challenging in the burned child. Blood pressure cuffs may have to be placed over a burned area, and needle electrodes may have to be used for the electrocardiogram (ECG). Pulse oximetry readings may not be reliable with extensive burn injury, low blood pressure or hypothermia. In this case pulse oximetry probes may be placed on the ear lobe, buccal mucosa, or tongue. Children that require major burn surgery will require invasive arterial blood pressure monitoring, and possibly central venous pressure monitoring to track volume status acutely. Temperature measurement and maintenance of normothermia is essential because burned children are susceptible to hypothermia. The operating room and IV fluids should be warmed, inspired gases should be heated and humidified, and all exposed body surfaces covered.

Anesthetic Technique

The choice of anesthetic induction agent will depend on the clinical condition of the child. Propofol may be used if the child is normovolemic; ketamine or etomidate are suitable alternatives if the child is hypovolemic. Inhaled induction

is stable and effective when an endotracheal tube is already in place.

The choice of neuromuscular blocker used to intubate the trachea in burned patients depends on the time from the injury and concern for a difficult airway. After the initial 24-hour postburn period, administration of succinylcholine can cause significant hyperkalemia secondary to up-regulation of extrajunctional acetylcholine receptors on injured or burned muscle. This risk peaks between 5 days and 3 months and may persist for up to 2 years after the initial injury or until the patient has regained adequate muscle function. Burn patients may demonstrate resistance to the nondepolarizing neuromuscular blockers; thus relatively larger doses are required to achieve relaxation, especially in patients with major burns and 1 to 2 months after the initial burn. This resistance is thought to be caused by changes in postjunctional acetylcholine receptors.

Maintenance of general anesthesia can be accomplished using a balanced technique with an inhalational anesthetic agent. Titration of opioid should be based on the expectation of rapidly acquired tolerance. Burn patients have greater requirements for opioids because of both pharmacokinetic changes and development of tolerance. Because of the pharmacologic changes with burn injury, all drugs should be titrated to clinical effect and appropriate hemodynamic and oxygenation monitoring are required to detect opioid-induced respiratory depression. Large opioid needs during the intraoperative and postoperative periods are common. For example, it is not unusual for children to require IV morphine doses ≥ 0.5 mg/kg/h during the acute perioperative period. A total intravenous anesthetic should be planned if the child requires the higher support from an ICU ventilator.

Burn debridement commonly results in large blood losses because of the relatively large surface area of exposed skin from donor and graft sites. Once the burn eschar is excised and the large capillary bed is exposed, bandages soaked in epinephrine are often placed over the wound to decrease bleeding; this often manifests as tachycardia and hypertension. Consequently, because blood loss may be underestimated, early transfusion is warranted during these procedures to avoid sudden hypovolemia. It should be noted that rapid transfusion through a central line is challenging because of the length and resistance of the catheter. Large bore intravenous access, if available, allows for easier and faster large volume resuscitation.

Red blood cell transfusion is indicated when oxygen-carrying capacity is inadequate to meet cellular metabolic demands. The maximum allowable blood loss is determined using the estimated blood volume (EBV) of the child, which varies with age (see Chapter 14). There is no absolute hematocrit below which all patients require blood transfusion and most previously healthy children tolerate a hematocrit lower than 30% without adverse sequelae. In the trauma setting, the hematocrit is often unknown and estimates of EBV, blood loss, and blood needs are empiric. In life-threatening emergencies, immediate transfusion with type O blood is warranted. Some centers administer O-positive blood to boys and O-negative to girls whereas some centers administer O-negative blood to all children. Administration of large amounts of blood to small children entails risks that include hyperkalemia from lysis of stored red cells, hypocalcemia from citrate toxicity, hypothermia, and coagulopathy that results from dilution of platelets and clotting factors. Pulmonary edema and volume overload are also problematic.

Temperature Regulation

Burned children are at risk for intraoperative heat loss because of large exposed surface areas and lack of intact skin. Hypothermia can cause arrhythmias, coagulopathy, and decreased wound healing. The operating room should be warmed, overhead heating lamps should be available, and barriers should be used to decrease heat loss from radiation. Convective heat loss can be prevented by warming the operating room and by placing the patient on warming blankets. Patients can be covered with materials such as plastic sheets and forced warm air blankets, and the anesthetic gases should be humidified to decrease evaporative heat losses.

Pain Management

Pain is a major problem in burned children. In the acute period, pain can be categorized as background pain, procedural pain, and postoperative pain. Background pain is proportional to the size of the burn and is treated with oral or IV opioids. Because of rapidly developing tolerance, opioid doses need to be adjusted regularly. Adjuvant analgesics such as acetaminophen, ketamine and dexmedetomidine should also be included. Nonsteroidal antiinflammatory drugs such as ibuprofen are less often used because of concerns with bleeding or renal injury. Procedural pain is controlled with opioids, benzodiazepines (for procedure-related anxiolysis) and adjuvants such as ketamine and regional analgesia, such as central axis and peripheral nerve blocks.

Postoperative Wound Care

The adequate provision of anxiolysis and analgesia for daily wound care are challenging for providers, patients and families. Opioid-based techniques are most commonly used and the route of administration depends on the availability of IV access and the expected number of dressing changes over time, as well as the child's level of anxiety. Inhaled nitrous oxide is effective for mildly painful procedures. More painful procedures may be amenable to oral or IV ketamine, in conjunction with a benzodiazepine and a topical local anesthetic. Epidural analgesia is useful for repeated wound care of the perineum or lower extremities. In some cases, administration of general anesthesia (by facemask or supraglottic device) may be required. Nonpharmacologic techniques, such as hypnosis, distraction therapy, and virtual reality have proven very useful in some children. Child-life specialists should be intimately involved with the patient and

their family. Using the same medical and nursing personnel in a familiar environment with expectant management for repeated wound care lessens patient and family stress and improves provider conditions.

Postoperative Considerations

Most children with major trauma or burns will remain intubated while transported to an ICU. Adequate analgesia and sedation must be administered for the transport from the operating room to the ICU or other location where further diagnostic evaluation is performed. The decision to extubate the trachea will depend on clinical circumstances, including preoperative findings, intraoperative events, and the expected postoperative course. Before leaving the operating room (OR), an assessment to rule out physiologic derangements must be performed. It is important to anticipate the child's anesthetic needs for the hour after surgery since transport of the patient and handing over care to the primary medical service takes some time. On arrival at the ICU, a hematocrit, arterial blood gas, and electrolytes should be obtained as well as a chest radiograph to exclude pathophysiologic changes that might have occurred during transport.

References

1. Densmore JC, Lim HJ, Oldham KT, Guice KS. Outcomes and delivery of care in pediatric injury. *J Pediatr Surg*. 2006;41(1):92–98. https://doi.org/10.1016/j.jpedsurg.2005.10.013.
2. British Heart Foundation. Man suffers cardiac arrest and friend performs CPR to help save his life. 2019. Created on October 16, 2019. Accessed on August 25, 2021. https://youtu.be/jZusvD_9j2E.
3. Nagler J, Krauss B. Videos in clinical medicine. Intraosseous catheter placement in children. *N Engl J Med*. 2011;364(8):e14. https://doi.org/10.1056/NEJMvcm0900916.
4. Chestnut RM, Temkin N, Carney N, et al. A Trial of Intracranial-Pressure Monitoring in Traumatic Brain Injury. *N Engl J Med*. 2012;367:2471–2481. https://doi.org/10.1056/NEJMoa1207363.
5. David JS, Godier A, Dargaud Y, Inaba K. Case scenario: management of trauma-induced coagulopathy in a severe blunt trauma patient. *Anesthesiology*. 2013;119(1):191–200. https://doi.org/10.1097/ALN.0b013e31828fc627.
6. Michaud LJ, Rivara FP, Longstreth Jr WT, Grady MS. Elevated initial blood glucose levels and poor outcome following severe brain injuries in children. *J Trauma*. 1991;31(10):1356–1362. https://doi.org/10.1097/00005373-199110000-00007.
7. Burn Center Referral Criteria. American Burn Association. Accessed on August 25, 2021.http://ameriburn.org/wp-content/uploads/2017/05/burncentrcrefcrralcriteria.pdf.

Suggested Readings

Jeschke MG, Herndon DN. Burns in children: standard and new treatments. *Lancet*. 2014 29;383(9923):1168–1178. https://doi.org/10.1016/S0140-6736(13)61093-4.
Trachtenberg FL, Haas EA, Kinney HC, Stanley C, Krous HF. Risk factor changes for sudden infant death syndrome after initiation of Back-to-Sleep campaign. *Pediatrics*. 2012;129(4):630–638. https://doi.org/10.1542/peds.2011-1419.

38

The Critically Ill Child

SAMUEL ROSENBLATT, C. HUNTER DAIGLE AND DONALD BOYER

Because critically ill children may occasionally present for emergency surgery, all anesthesiologists should have a working knowledge of the most common critical illnesses and their therapies. In this chapter, we review the clinical features of these illnesses, and also describe the most current Pediatric Advanced Life Support (PALS) guidelines and the use of inotropic medications and methods of providing invasive access in children.

Pediatric Advanced Life Support

Every few years, the American Heart Association (AHA) publishes updated Pediatric Advanced Life Support (PALS) guidelines, incorporating the latest findings in pediatric resuscitation science. At the time of this writing, the most recent version was published in 2020. Since the 2010 guidelines, the focus of resuscitation is to use the "CAB" (Circulation, Airway, Breathing) approach, with an emphasis on achieving and maintaining optimum cerebral and coronary perfusion via quality cardiopulmonary resuscitation (Q-CPR). Chest compressions should begin immediately upon recognition of cardiac arrest while trying to establish airway and breathing (simultaneous but secondary actions). It is easier and faster to establish vital organ blood flow through effective chest compressions during a no-flow state of cardiac arrest before gathering equipment and securing an airway.

The PALS update in 2020 focuses on CPR quality and postresuscitation care[1]. CPR quality is assessed by the fraction, depth, and rate of chest compressions (Table 38.1). These can be measured using technologically advanced defibrillators and defibrillator pads that provide real-time feedback on CPR quality. The use of end tidal CO_2 ($EtCO_2$) and arterial blood pressure monitoring are also useful guides of CPR quality. Postresuscitation care focuses on maintaining normal core temperature, adequate blood pressure for coronary and cerebral perfusion, and normal oxygenation.

Circulation

When encountering the pulseless child, chest compressions should be initiated immediately. In infants, the best way to perform chest compressions is to encircle the chest with your hands, with the thumbs placed one finger-width below the intermammary line over the midsternum. For older children, the chest is compressed by placing the heel of your hand two-finger breadths above the lower end of the sternum and with a depth of at least 1/3 the anterior-posterior diameter of the chest (approximately 2 inches [or 5 cm]). Avoid compressions over the lower third of the sternum, which may cause trauma to internal abdominal organs. Compressions are delivered at a rate of 100 to 120 times per minute. The most important aspect of pediatric CPR is to maintain the frequency and depth of the compressions while minimizing interruptions and allowing for full chest recoil. Rotate compressors every 2 minutes to minimize fatigue and ensure effective compressions.

During CPR, peripheral venous access should be obtained, and if unsuccessful after 3 attempts or 90 seconds, whichever comes first, intraosseous (IO) vascular access[2] is indicated. Isotonic fluids, such as lactated Ringer solution

TABLE 38.1 **"Rules" of High-Quality CPR**

- *Push hard:* ≥1/3 anterior-posterior diameter of the chest
- At least 5 cm in children; at least 4 cm in infants
- *Push fast:* 100–120 compressions/min
- *Allow full chest recoil:* no residual leaning
- *Minimize interruptions:* no more than 10-second pauses for pulse checks and compressor changes
- *Optimize compression:* ventilation ratio
- Single rescuer: 30 compressions: 2 rescue breaths
- Two rescuers: 15 compressions: 2 rescue breaths
- After tracheal intubation (or supraglottic airway): 100–120 compressions/min with one breath every 2–3 seconds (20–30 breaths/min)

or normal saline, should be rapidly administered in 10 to 20 mL/kg doses, and continued until blood pressure is normalized. If unable to establish normal-for-age hemodynamics after ~60 mL/kg isotonic fluid administration, vasoactive medications should be considered with choice of agent dependent on hemodynamic profile. Children with hemorrhagic shock should receive uncrossmatched type O, Rh-negative packed red blood cells or whole blood. (Type-specific blood can be administered if the patient's blood type is already known) Medications that can be administered through the endotracheal tube and absorbed from the bronchial tree include lidocaine, atropine, naloxone, and epinephrine (mnemonic = LANE).

Pulseless electrical activity (PEA) may be seen during cardiac arrest in children and is often caused by a reversible process. Thus the differential diagnosis should be kept in mind by remembering the Hs and the Ts (Table 38.2).

Airway and Breathing

Assuming the child in cardiac arrest did not have previous airway management, it is addressed once chest compressions have begun. Proper airway positioning is important to maximize oxygenation and ventilation. Usual airway maneuvers (e.g., head tilt, chin lift, and/or jaw thrust) are performed to maintain airway patency with bag-mask ventilation; securing the airway with tracheal tube placement is preferred but a supraglottic airway may be acceptable when tracheal intubation is unobtainable or when attempts at tracheal intubation would compromise the provision of high-quality CPR. Hyperventilation is a known risk during CPR with an advanced airway and may increase intrathoracic pressure, impeding venous return and decreasing cardiac output. When an advanced airway is in place, breaths do not need to be coordinated with compressions and should be given at a rate of 20 to 30 breaths per minute (approximately one breath every 2–3 seconds). Before an advanced airway, compression and bag-mask breaths should be coordinated. In single-rescuer CPR, it should be a ratio of 30 compressions to 2 breaths; and for two-rescuer CPR in children, it should be 15 compressions to 2 breaths.

TABLE 38.2	Differential Diagnosis of PEA (H and T)	
Hypoxemia	Tamponade (pericardial)
Hypovolemia	Tension pneumothorax
Hypothermia	Thromboembolism (myocardial ischemia, pulmonary embolus)
Hyper/Hypokalemia	Toxins
Hydrogen ions (acidosis)	Trauma

Disability and Drugs

Disability

Once circulation and breathing are addressed, the child's neurologic status should be evaluated. A Glasgow Coma Scale (GCS) score is calculated while assessing for focal neurologic injury. Abnormal pupillary responses (e.g., unilateral dilated pupil) may suggest impending cerebral herniation and should be promptly evaluated and addressed. Maintaining cervical spine immobilization, especially if there is a suspected traumatic mechanism of injury, is essential until the spine can be cleared clinically or radiographically. Cervical spinal cord trauma may cause neurologic deficits and neurogenic shock, which is characterized by vasodilation and hypotension without tachycardia. Hypoglycemia should immediately be treated as it can lead to additional neurologic injury.

Drugs

Epinephrine is the most important drug in pediatric cardiac arrest. The initial resuscitation dose for pediatric cardiac arrest is 0.01 mg/kg (0.1 mL/kg of standard 1:10,000 concentration) via the IV or IO route; alternatively, 0.1 mg/kg can be administered via an endotracheal tube if vascular access is not available. This dose can be repeated every 3 to 5 minutes if there is no response to the initial dose. Amiodarone (5 mg/kg) or lidocaine (1 mg/kg) may be used for ventricular tachycardia or ventricular fibrillation that is refractory to defibrillation and consultation with a pediatric cardiologist should be considered if an arrest situation is unresponsive to epinephrine doses and alternative agents are being considered. Atropine (0.02 mg/kg) may be helpful in cases of bradycardia, but when bradycardia is caused by hypoxemia, oxygen is the most important drug to address the underlying arrest physiology.

Exposure and Environment

Once ventilation and circulation are stabilized, all the child's clothing should be removed to search for additional traumatic or toxic injuries. Hypothermia and hyperthermia should be aggressively treated to prevent clotting disorders and to prevent further focal neurologic injury. Profound hypothermia resulting in arrest may warrant extracorporeal rewarming; consultation with intensive care specialists should be pursued.

Post arrest Care

The foundation of postarrest care is focused on minimizing secondary injury and this may be required in the operative environment if the postarrest patient requires operative care or if they require anesthesia expertise to facilitate imaging or other diagnostic/therapeutic maneuvers.

After return of spontaneous circulation (ROSC) or after cannulation onto extracorporeal support during emergency CPR (E-CPR), efforts should be focused on ensuring age-appropriate physiology that minimizes metabolic demand and end organ injury. Hypertension and hypotension can both be injurious but the postarrest patient is most at risk for hypotension and blood pressure should be targeted to age-standardized norms that prevent end-organ hypoperfusion. Metabolic demand should be minimized by avoiding fevers, shivering, and seizures. This may require around-the-clock administration of antipyretic medications and temperature-regulating devices such as a thermoregulation blanket. (Pediatric studies of targeted temperature management [TTM] of the postarrest patient have not demonstrated benefit of empiric cooling)[1]. The postarrest patient may require neuromuscular blockade to limit shivering, and for arrests where neurologic status is altered from baseline after arrest, continuous electroencephalography (EEG) monitoring should be considered to monitor subclinical status epilepticus to treat quickly and minimize metabolic demand. Hypo- and hyperglycemia should be avoided and routine glucose monitoring should be instituted to minimize effects from these metabolic derangements.

Treatment Algorithms

Because it is difficult to memorize the specific treatment algorithms for the various possible dysrhythmias, anesthesiologists should have immediate access to the most current AHA guidelines. We recommend that each anesthesia practitioner have a copy (or have access to a copy in each anesthetizing location) of a PALS Pocket Reference Card[2] (AHA 20-1118) that can be easily obtained from many Internet retailers.

Common Pediatric Critical Illnesses

Status Epilepticus

Continuous seizure activity lasting for more than 5 minutes or multiple seizures without return to baseline is considered status epilepticus and should prompt immediate intervention. Common causes in children include epilepsy, head trauma, hypoxic-ischemic encephalopathy, infection (e.g., meningitis, encephalitis), medication toxicity, genetic or metabolic disease, or electrolyte disturbance (e.g., hypoglycemia, hyponatremia). The cause is unknown in approximately 50% of cases. Empiric broad-spectrum antibiotics with or without antiviral therapy should be administered if an infection is suspected. Spinal fluid should ideally be collected before antimicrobial administration, if possible. Head CT is indicated unless the diagnosis is obvious and not related to structural brain abnormalities.

If untreated, status epilepticus may result in neurologic injury or death. Common causes of injury from status epilepticus include hypoventilation and pulmonary aspiration. Immediate treatment consists of ensuring airway patency, supplemental oxygen, and administration of an anticonvulsant. Neuromuscular blockade (NMB) will facilitate endotracheal intubation but may mask recognition of continued

seizure activity; alternative approaches to assess ongoing seizure activity (e.g., EEG) should be considered if NMB has been administered. Hypotension may result from prolonged seizure activity or cardiodepressant effects of anticonvulsant drugs and should be treated with volume expansion and vasopressors. The possibility of neurologic damage is increased with persistent hypoxemia, hypotension, hypoglycemia, and metabolic acidosis. Hyperthermia should be aggressively treated to minimize cerebral metabolic oxygen consumption. Immediate EEG evaluation to evaluate for nonconvulsive status epilepticus may aid in diagnosis if a patient is not returning to baseline mental status.

Treatment guidelines[3] from the American Epilepsy Society have been published. Initial treatment should consist of an intravenous benzodiazepine such as lorazepam, midazolam, or diazepam. If vascular or intraosseous access is not rapidly obtained, midazolam can be administered via the intramuscular, buccal, intranasal, or rectal route and diazepam can be administered via the rectal route.

If an initial dose of a benzodiazepine is not effective in quieting seizure activity, most guidelines call for repeat administration with a second dose. Next-line agents may be used if patients are not responding to the initial treatment with benzodiazepines. These include levetiracetam, valproic acid, or fosphenytoin. Levetiracetam is often used as the first next-line agent because of its favorable side effect profile and minimal respiratory depression, however, a recent study[4] showed no difference between these three medications in effectiveness or adverse effects.

Phenobarbital, 15 to 20 mg/kg infused slowly, can be used as an adjunct anticonvulsant. Side effects include respiratory depression (especially when used in combination with benzodiazepines), hypotension, and prolonged sedation. In young infants, it may be more effective than other antiepileptic medications.

When status epilepticus remains unresponsive to conventional therapies, it should be aggressively managed using adjunct medication infusions in consultation with a pediatric neurologist. Common drug infusions for status epilepticus include: midazolam, pentobarbital, and ketamine; with dosing adjusted based on EEG and clinical seizure burden. Side effects of each agent can be significant and local formularies should be consulted before initiation to be vigilant about side effects such as cardiac depression (that may require inotropic therapy) and granulocytopenia. Inhalational anesthetics or propofol may also be used to suppress seizures in refractory cases, with guidance provided by pediatric neurology colleagues.

Shock

Shock describes a state of insufficient delivery of oxygen to meet the metabolic demands of the tissues. There are three progressive stages of shock: compensated, uncompensated, and irreversible.

In **compensated shock**, blood pressure and organ perfusion are maintained by activation of compensatory mechanisms, such as increasing heart rate and systemic vascular resistance (SVR). Because neonates and young infants cannot significantly increase stroke volume, cardiac output (stroke volume × heart rate) is augmented by increasing heart rate. In this initial stage, the patient may demonstrate cool, pale extremities with delayed capillary refill (>4 seconds), and decreased urine output. In **uncompensated shock**, cellular dysfunction, ischemia, and endothelial injury occur when compensatory mechanisms begin to fail. The patient will demonstrate an altered level of consciousness and decrease in urine output. The onset of tachypnea may signify the body's attempt to compensate for a new metabolic acidosis. Bradycardia is an ominous sign in an infant because it significantly decreases cardiac output and may portend impending cardiac arrest. Hypotension is a late finding of pediatric shock and places the patient at risk for multiorgan system failure. **Irreversible shock** occurs when there is unrecoverable end-organ damage.

There are four major categories of shock described by PALS:

1. **Hypovolemic shock** is the most common cause and results from decreased intravascular volume. It can be caused by water and electrolyte loss (e.g., vomiting, diarrhea, renal losses, or heat stroke), blood loss (e.g., trauma), or plasma losses (e.g., burns, nephrotic syndrome). Initial management is focused on replacing lost fluids after the initial CAB (circulation-airway-breathing) assessment of the primary survey. Fluid resuscitation is guided by normalization of heart rate, peripheral perfusion, and urine output (goal > 0.5–1 mL/kg/h). If blood loss is obvious, blood products should be the initial replacement fluid. Hypovolemic shock from blood loss is classified into four categories based on the estimated blood volume deficit. When available, fresh whole blood (<48 hours old) should be transfused because it contains red blood cells, platelets, and clotting factors. When whole blood is unavailable, a balanced resuscitation with 1:1:1 packed red blood cells (PRBCs): fresh frozen plasma (FFP): platelets should be considered in alignment with institutional massive transfusion practices, as patients transfused with large amounts of blood products will usually develop a dilutional coagulopathy if coagulation factor and platelet losses are not also corrected. If blood is needed immediately, type O, Rh-negative blood is the "universal donor" and should be used until type-matched products are available. In nonhemorrhagic, hypovolemic shock, isotonic crystalloid fluids are used as the initial resuscitation fluid, commonly normal (0.9%) saline or Lactated Ringers (LR). Patients should be given replacement of their estimated fluid losses (current weight [kg] – prior weight [kg] = estimated liters of fluid loss) with resuscitation guided by normalization of heart rate and markers of end-organ perfusion.

2. **Distributive shock** is caused by abnormalities in vasomotor tone, such as vasodilatation, and results in relative hypovolemia. Common causes include sepsis, neurogenic shock, and anaphylaxis. **Septic shock** is caused by overwhelming infection and manifests as a combination of hypovolemia, altered vascular tone, cardiac pump failure, and cellular metabolic derangements, resulting in a profound metabolic acidosis. Initially, the extremities can be warm and well-perfused or cold with high systemic vascular resistance and delayed capillary refill. In warm septic shock, patients have vasodilation which is caused by inflammatory mediators (e.g., endotoxin, tumor necrosis factor, and interleukin-1) and is manifested clinically as diastolic hypotension and a wide pulse pressure. In cold septic shock, patients present with vasoconstriction, cool extremities, normal to elevated blood pressures, and may have myocardial dysfunction. If untreated, persistent septic shock will rapidly lead to multiorgan system failure and possibly death. Septic shock requires identification and treatment of the sources of infection. These patients usually require rapid administration of isotonic fluids (>60 mL/kg) and may require vasopressors. Vasopressor selection is dictated by the clinical presentation and may require an agent that preferentially targets vascular tone (e.g., phenylephrine, norepinephrine), cardiac function (e.g., low-dose epinephrine, dobutamine), or both. For patients with vasopressor-refractory shock and those with adrenal insufficiency, consider use of hydrocortisone 2 mg/kg IV bolus (max 100 mg). Further management includes monitoring for end-organ perfusion abnormalities and supporting physiology to improve cardiac output and reverse the shock state. **Neurogenic shock** may be seen in spinal cord injury, usually at the cervicothoracic area. Loss of sympathetic vascular tone causes bradycardia, vasodilation, and hypotension. **Anaphylaxis** may manifest as an acute allergic response resulting in venodilation, arterial vasodilation, increased capillary permeability, and pulmonary vasoconstriction. Epinephrine is the firstline vasopressor in the treatment of anaphylaxis. In distributive shock, Trendelenburg positioning (head down with cervical spine immobilized if indicated) and administration of isotonic fluids may restore circulatory stability. Vasopressor drugs with direct alpha-1-adrenergic activity may be necessary to improve vascular tone and decrease risk for hypotension and myocardial ischemia.

3. **Cardiogenic shock** can be caused by congenital heart disease, prolonged arrhythmias (e.g., supraventricular tachycardia), acquired cardiomyopathies (Kawasaki disease with coronary aneurysms), infection, and drug intoxications. Central venous pressure monitoring and physical examination will guide cautious fluid administration. These patients will usually benefit from inotropic support and afterload reduction. Severe cases may require mechanical circulatory support with implanted cardiac support devices and/or extracorporeal support.

4. **Obstructive shock** is caused by extracardiac causes of circulatory failure, often caused by poor right ventricular cardiac output. Obstructive shock can occur as a result of tension pneumothorax, pulmonary embolism, pulmonary hypertension, cardiac tamponade from pericardial effusion, and restrictive pericarditis. Treatment for obstructive shock requires relief of the obstruction (e.g.,

needle decompression and chest tube placement for tension pneumothorax; anticoagulation and/or thrombectomy for pulmonary embolism, etc.). In the interim, treatment with fluid (additional preload) may help overcome the obstruction unless the right ventricle is volume overloaded and failing as seen with pulmonary hypertension. In those situations, inotropic support for the right ventricle may be useful while treating the etiology of obstructive shock.

Neonates presenting in shock in the first few days of life are unique because it may indicate undiagnosed congenital heart disease with ductal-dependent systemic circulation. These babies are asymptomatic at birth because aortic blood flow is provided by the patent ductus arteriosus (PDA). However, when the PDA closes, shock develops from inadequate systemic output. These patients usually have left-sided obstructive lesions, such as hypoplastic left heart syndrome, aortic valve stenosis, interrupted aortic arch, or coarctation of the aorta. Prostaglandin E1 (0.05–0.1 μg/kg/min) will keep the ductus open until a palliative or definitive surgical procedure is performed.

Inotropic and Vasoactive Agents in Children

Dopamine

Dopamine is mainly a central neurotransmitter but is also found peripherally in the sympathetic nervous system and in the adrenal medulla. Dopamine stimulates dopaminergic, alpha and beta receptors in the brain and peripheral vascular beds, and depending on its concentration, can produce vascular dilatation or constriction.

Dopamine is used to treat hypotension and oliguria in children with distributive, septic, or cardiogenic shock when volume resuscitation has been ineffective. Low infusion rates (1–5 μg/kg/min) stimulate dopamine receptors and increase glomerular filtration and renal blood flow. Moderate doses (5–10 μg/kg/min) increase heart rate and improve myocardial contractility via beta receptor stimulation and release of norepinephrine from nerve terminals, resulting in an increase in systolic blood pressure and minimal change in diastolic pressure. Higher doses (>10 μg/kg/min) increase SVR by alpha receptor stimulation and vasoconstriction.

Adverse effects of dopamine include tachycardia, hypertension, dysrhythmias, and increased myocardial oxygen consumption. Dopamine decreases Pao_2 by inhibiting hypoxic pulmonary vasoconstriction, and it can depress the ventilatory response to hypoxemia by as much as 60%. More recent data suggests sequelae on innate immune responses and impacts on the hypothalamic-pituitary-adrenal axis, thus it has been used sparingly at some institutions as a first-line vasoactive agent.

Dopamine clearance decreases by about 50% during the first 20 months of life, and then continues to decrease by lesser amounts throughout childhood. All studies of dopamine pharmacokinetics in seriously ill children show substantial inter individual variation in pharmacokinetic parameters. Thus there is a large variation in the dose required to achieve a desired clinical response.

Dobutamine

Dobutamine has greater selectivity for beta-1 and beta-2 receptors than dopamine. At a dose range of 5 to 20 μg/kg/min, it enhances myocardial contractility and increases stroke volume, with less increase in heart rate than dopamine. It decreases SVR and PVR, and hypotension may occur if the patient is volume depleted or has an elevated sympathetic imbalance. Dobutamine is used to treat cardiac dysfunction, as seen for example with congenital heart disease or myocarditis. Because it increases myocardial oxygen demand, it may predispose to arrhythmias.

Ephedrine

Ephedrine acts indirectly by enhancing the release of norepinephrine from sympathetic neurons. It increases heart rate and cardiac output with a variable increase in SVR. Ephedrine is used (0.2–0.3 mg/kg/dose) to treat hypotension related to administration of general or regional anesthesia.

Epinephrine

Epinephrine stimulates alpha, beta-1, and beta-2 receptors. It is useful in treating shock from all causes, and is the drug of choice to treat anaphylaxis. At low doses (0.05–0.1 μg/kg/min), epinephrine stimulates beta-1 receptors, and increases heart rate and inotropy. Beta-2 receptor stimulation causes relaxation of arterioles, which decreases SVR and diastolic blood pressure. Higher doses (0.1–0.3 μg/kg/min) cause activation of alpha receptors resulting in vasoconstriction with a resultant increase in SVR that may compromise blood flow to end organs. Epinephrine clearance rates in critically ill children are lower than clearance rates in healthy adults.

Isoproterenol

Isoproterenol is a nonselective beta-adrenergic agonist with low affinity for alpha-adrenergic receptors. It increases heart rate, enhances myocardial contractility, and decreases SVR, thus resulting in an increase in cardiac output. Isoproterenol may be used to treat hemodynamically significant bradycardia and has been used in infants after cardiac surgery to improve cardiac index.

Norepinephrine

Norepinephrine has potent alpha activity with some beta-1 activity and little beta-2 activity, thus increasing SVR. Norepinephrine improves perfusion in children with hypotension and a normal or elevated cardiac index that has not responded to volume resuscitation. Treatment with norepinephrine is beneficial in the setting of tachycardia, because it can increase SVR, arterial blood pressure, diastolic blood pressure, and urine flow without an increase in heart rate. The usual starting infusion dose is 0.05 to 0.1 μg/kg/min, which is then titrated to effect. Norepinephrine administration may improve blood pressure without improving perfusion. This is most commonly seen in children with a low cardiac index and stroke volume.

Phenylephrine

Phenylephrine is an alpha-adrenergic agonist used to treat hypotension when SVR is low. Phenylephrine increases blood pressure and causes a vagally mediated sinus bradycardia, which is less pronounced in children than adults. A typical starting dose of phenylephrine in children is 0.1 mcg/kg/min, titrated to effect.

Milrinone

Milrinone is a phosphodiesterase inhibitor that produces inotropy and vasodilatation (usually without tachycardia). It has been used in children to treat low-output states after cardiac surgery and in the management of shock when catecholamine infusions alone are unsuccessful. Children demonstrate a higher volume of distribution of milrinone and a more rapid clearance rate than adults. A loading dose of 50 to 75 µg/kg over 15 to 60 minutes is followed by a continuous infusion of 0.375–1 µg/kg/min, titrated to effect. Milrinone is associated with atrial or ventricular arrhythmias in adults but usually not in children. Children with renal dysfunction have decreased clearance and may develop hypotension due to accumulation of drug and low SVR.

Vasopressin

Vasopressin acts on vasopressin receptors to promote water reabsorption in the kidney and a direct vasoconstrictor on arterioles to increase SVR. Vasopressin can be used in settings of catecholamine-resistant hypotension (e.g., septic shock). Our usual infusion doses for catecholamine-resistant shock start at 12 milliunits/kg/h and we increase by 12 milliunits/kg/h every 10 to 15 minutes to a maximum of 240 milliunits/kg/h. Dosing of vasopressin is challenging because of the nonuniformity of units[5] used between different institutions and publications.

Vasopressor Refractory Shock

For patients that are refractory to fluid resuscitation and vasoactive medications, providers should consider giving steroids for suspected adrenal insufficiency. Hydrocortisone is the steroid of choice giving both glucocorticoid and mineralocorticoid effects. The usual initial pediatric dose is 100 mg/m² bolus dose followed by 100 mg/m²/day divided every 4 hours. The use of extracorporeal membrane oxygenation (ECMO) should be considered for refractory shock.

Hepatic Failure

Hepatic failure results from necrosis of liver cells that leads to impairment of hepatic function and possibly, hepatic encephalopathy. It can occur as a primary process in a healthy person, as an exacerbation of a chronic liver disease, or as part of multiorgan system failure. Hepatic failure can be classified into three types based on the time interval between the onset of jaundice and the development of encephalopathy: hyperacute (0–7 days), acute (1–4 weeks), and subacute (4–12 weeks). Main causes of fulminant hepatic failure in children include viral hepatitis, drug-induced liver injury, and inherited metabolic diseases.

Clinical features of hepatic failure include jaundice, enlarged liver, and encephalopathy, in conjunction with abnormal biochemical data such as hypoalbuminemia, hyperbilirubinemia, hyperammonemia, lactic acidemia, hypoglycemia, and coagulopathy with prolongation of the prothrombin time. There is no specific therapy or antidote for acute hepatic injury, with the exception of early administration of N-acetylcysteine to treat acetaminophen toxicity and as a potential antiinflammatory agent. Diagnostic tests are necessary to determine etiology and eligibility for liver transplant.

Hepatic failure can adversely affect other organ systems. Encephalopathy may result from diminished hepatic synthesis of an unknown substance(s) needed for normal brain function or diminished hepatic metabolism of an unknown substance(s) that confers neurotoxicity or promote neural inhibition. As liver function deteriorates, hepatic encephalopathy worsens. Serum ammonia levels do not correlate with the severity of encephalopathy. Advanced encephalopathy is associated with severe cerebral edema and life-threatening cerebral herniation.

Acute renal failure develops in 30% to 50% of patients with acute liver failure (hepatorenal syndrome). Contributing factors include intravascular volume depletion caused by excessive diuresis or untreated gastrointestinal hemorrhage and nephrotoxic drug administration.

Hemorrhagic complications in liver failure result from inadequate synthesis of clotting factors, thrombocytopenia from disseminated intravascular coagulation (DIC), and splenic sequestration of platelets. Blood loss may occur from stress-induced gastritis or from esophageal or gastric varices that develop secondary to portal hypertension. Vitamin K administration augments production of factors II, VII, IX, and X. Fresh frozen plasma and/or cryoprecipitate is administered when patients are bleeding or before an invasive procedure.

Hypoxemia can develop in acute liver failure for several reasons. Failure of the damaged liver to clear vasodilating humoral substances can cause intrapulmonary shunting and ventilation/perfusion mismatch. Pulmonary edema results from low oncotic pressure and fluid overload associated with antidiuretic-like activity. Atelectasis can develop from massive ascites that impedes full respiratory excursion or hypoventilation caused by encephalopathy. Ascites develops as a result of increased hepatic vascular resistance, decreased oncotic pressure, and altered aldosterone secretion creating abdominal competition.

Patients with chronic liver failure develop a high cardiac output in conjunction with a low SVR, again because of vasodilating humoral substances. Oxygen delivery is increased, but oxygen consumption is decreased because of microcirculatory disturbances that lead to tissue hypoxia.

Orthotopic liver transplantation is the most important therapy for acute liver failure. There is no clear set of indications for liver transplantation in pediatric patients, but without hepatic transplantation, acute hepatic failure carries a poor prognosis with an 80% to 85% mortality rate. Death is usually caused by cerebral herniation from intracranial hypertension or septicemia. At present, some artificial liver support systems are used in clinical practice as a bridge to liver transplantation such as molecular adsorbent recirculation system (MARS) and continuous veno-venous hemodiafiltration (CVVHDF) with or without plasmapheresis.

Renal Failure

Acute renal failure is the sudden inability of the kidney to regulate fluid, electrolyte, and solute balance, which can occur with or without a change in urine volume. Causes of acute renal failure can be categorized into three categories: prerenal disease, intrinsic renal parenchymal damage, and postrenal disease.

The prerenal type is caused by inadequate perfusion as a result of systemic hypovolemia, poor cardiac output, or vascular obstruction. Most intrinsic renal failure is caused by ischemia, nephron damage from toxins, or inflammation. Postrenal renal failure is caused by obstruction of the urinary collecting system. When the obstruction occurs at the level of the bladder or urethra, renal function is more likely to be severely affected because both kidneys will be injured. Unilateral obstruction does not result in renal failure if the other kidney is healthy.

The diagnosis of acute renal failure requires a stepwise approach that includes analysis of urinary sediment: white cell casts suggest interstitial nephritis; red cell casts are found in glomerulonephritis; and heme-positive urine without red blood cells suggest myoglobinuria. Analysis of urine osmolality, urine creatinine (Cr) and electrolytes can also aid diagnosis. Calculation of the fractional excretion of sodium (FE_{Na}) will help distinguish prerenal from renal causes:

$$FE_{Na} = 100 \times \frac{(Urine\ Na \times Plasma\ creatinine)}{(Plasma\ Na \times Urine\ creatinine)}$$

Patients with hypovolemia will usually have concentrated urine that is manifested by a urine osmolality >500 mOsm/kg, urine sodium content <20 mEq/L, and FE_{Na} <1. In patients with tubular necrosis, the urine is dilute: urine osmolality <350 mOsm/kg, urine sodium content usually >40 mEq/L, and FE_{Na} usually >1.

The primary treatment of acute renal failure is to treat the underlying cause. With prerenal causes, effective circulating volume is restored. Oliguric patients with euvolemia need replacement of fluid losses, including insensible losses calculated at 300 mL/m²/day in addition to replacing other losses such as urine output, nasogastric tube drainage, and

diarrhea. If significant volume overload exists, then fluid restriction to insensible losses or even smaller quantities is indicated.

Electrolyte and acid–base abnormalities frequently occur in renal failure. Hyponatremia is usually caused by water retention. In hospitalized patients, the administration of hypotonic fluids can contribute to or worsen hyponatremia. Restriction of free water is indicated if the patient is volume overloaded. When hyponatremia is symptomatic (e.g., seizures and obtundation), it is appropriate to administer hypertonic saline (approx. 3–5 mL/kg of 3% saline) to raise the serum sodium to 125 mEq/L. Correction of serum sodium to normal (140 mEq/L) too rapidly can lead to central pontine myelinolysis and neurologic injury. Hyperphosphatemia develops because of decreased renal phosphate clearance and is treated with dietary phosphorous restriction and agents that bind phosphate enterally (e.g., calcium carbonate). Hypocalcemia may develop because of calcium losses and calcium binding to phosphorous in the setting of hyperphosphatemia. A metabolic acidosis develops because of impaired renal excretion of acids and alterations in renal bicarbonate reabsorption and regeneration. In the case of acidosis and severe hypocalcemia, calcium must be replaced before bicarbonate replacement because alkalization will decrease the ionized calcium levels further and may exacerbate symptoms of hypocalcemia such as tetany or arrhythmias.

Hyperkalemia (potassium >6.0 mEq/L) is the major life-threatening electrolyte abnormality in acute renal failure and must be aggressively treated. ECG abnormalities include tall, peaked T-waves initially, followed by prolongation of the P-R interval and widening of the QRS complex, leading to ventricular fibrillation and cardiac arrest. Therapy involves stabilizing the myocardium with calcium administration, redistributing potassium from the extracellular to intracellular space to decrease serum potassium levels with sodium bicarbonate, insulin, and glucose, and enhancing potassium elimination from the body with medications such as diuretics (e.g., furosemide) and sodium polystyrene. Exogenously administered potassium in fluids or feeds should be stopped immediately upon recognition of hyperkalemia.

The absolute indications for dialysis in renal failure are: intractable acidosis, electrolyte abnormalities such as hyperkalemia or hyperphosphatemia, symptomatic uremia such as pericarditis, bleeding or encephalopathy, volume overload with congestive heart failure, pulmonary edema, severe hypertension, and to remove toxins that are dialyzable (e.g., ammonia, salicylates, methanol, ethylene glycol). A relative indication is to provide better nutrition or multiple blood products during periods of oliguria. Peritoneal dialysis, intermittent hemodialysis, or continuous hemofiltration are all viable options, determined in consultation with a pediatric nephrologist.

Chronic renal failure (Table 38.3) is the irreversible deterioration in the glomerular filtration rate (GFR) to a point that renal replacement therapy is necessary to sustain life. This usually occurs with a GFR below 10 to 20 mL/min/1.73 m.²

TABLE 38.3	Features of Chronic Renal Failure

Electrolyte Disorders

- Hyperkalemia
- Hyperphosphatemia
- Hypocalcemia
- Hypermagnesemia
- Hyponatremia
- Metabolic acidosis

Gastrointestinal

- Delayed gastric emptying
- Nausea and vomiting

Hematologic

- Anemia
- Platelet dysfunction secondary to uremia

Cardiovascular

- Hypertension
- Volume overload

Endocrine

- Growth failure

Respiratory Failure

Respiratory failure is the inability to maintain normal exchange of oxygen and carbon dioxide between the lungs and blood. It occurs more frequently in infants and children because of a developmentally immature respiratory system, greater oxygen consumption and carbon dioxide excretion demands, and a higher frequency of disease processes with primary or secondary respiratory complications.

Respiratory failure can be classified into two main types: hypoxemic or hypercarbic. Hypoxemic respiratory failure results from ventilation to perfusion (V/Q) mismatch leading to noncardiac mixing of venous and arterial blood. It results in hypoxemia with normal or low carbon dioxide. Hypercarbic respiratory failure results from inadequate alveolar ventilation in relation to physiologic needs and is characterized by both hypoxemia and hypercarbia. This occurs when a disease or injury leads to an imbalance between the power available to do the respiratory work and the load on the respiratory system. Diseases that affect anatomic components of the lung result in regions of low or absent V/Q ratios, leading to hypoxemic respiratory failure. Diseases of the extrathoracic airway and respiratory pump result in a respiratory power/load imbalance and hypercarbic respiratory failure.

The first-line treatment of hypoxemia is to administer supplemental oxygen. When lung disease results in significant oxygenation abnormalities (i.e., $F_iO_2 \geq 0.60$ required to maintain $PaO_2 \geq 60$ mm Hg), CPAP may be helpful. CPAP can be applied using a tight-fitting mask or nasal cannula[1]. 5 to 10 cm H_2O of CPAP increases lung volume, and enhances ventilation to areas with low V/Q ratios and

improves respiratory mechanics. An alternative to CPAP is high-flow nasal cannula (HFNC), which allows for administration of heated and humidified oxygen or blended oxygen and air at a higher flow than regular nasal cannula, while providing some degree of CPAP. If CPAP ≥ 10 cmH_2O does not relieve hypoxemia, application of bilevel positive airway pressure (BiPAP) may be useful to decrease work of breathing and hypoxemia. If hypoxemia or work of breathing persist despite noninvasive ventilation, then treatment with mechanical ventilation is indicated.

Diseases of the respiratory pump (central nervous system, respiratory muscle, or chest wall) cause hypercarbic respiratory failure. Noninvasive and invasive modes of mechanical ventilation can be instituted to decrease the work of breathing and provide adequate gas exchange. Noninvasive mechanical ventilation can be delivered via nasal prongs or face-mask. Inspiratory pressure support is a ventilator modality where the patient's effort is boosted by increased circuited pressure during inspiration. This allows the patient to initiate their own breaths and regulate inspiratory time and tidal volume. The pressure support strategy promotes patient synchrony and comfort with mechanical support, but this technique may not be suitable for children with advanced disease.

Conventional modes of mechanical ventilation are designed to assist physiologic respiratory pump function and improve lung volumes. Positive pressure is used to inflate the lungs. $PaCO_2$ levels are used to adjust minute ventilation. Minute ventilation is adjusted by modifying the respiratory rate or the tidal volume. Tidal volume can be adjusted by controlling either the delivered volume (volume-controlled ventilation) or the inspiratory pressure (pressure-controlled ventilation). The duration of inspiration is adjustable but this parameter only indirectly effects minute ventilation through its effect on expiratory time or when high airway resistance is present and some alveoli with longer time constants need longer opening times.

Principles of Pediatric Mechanical Ventilation

The goals of mechanical ventilation are to improve alveolar ventilation, reduce V/Q mismatch, re-expand collapsed lung segments, reduce work of breathing, and eliminate respiratory muscle fatigue. Indications for institution of mechanical ventilation in children include:

1. Hypoxemic respiratory failure: PaO_2 <50 mm Hg at F_iO_2 >0.5; commonly caused by alveolar diseases such as pneumonia, acute respiratory distress syndrome, or pulmonary edema[1].
2. Hypercarbic respiratory failure: $PaCO_2$ >50 mm Hg and an arterial pH <7.30, with or without hypoxemia; caused by respiratory pump failure, such as CNS abnormalities, or respiratory muscle disease. Examples include neuromuscular disease (e.g., spinal muscular atrophy) or hypoventilation (e.g., accidental narcotic overdose).
3. Circulatory failure such as shock or congestive heart failure. In this setting, mechanical ventilation can cause a reduction in metabolic expenditure, decrease respiratory

muscle dysfunction caused by hypoxia, decrease LV afterload, or decrease respiratory dysfunction associated with shock (i.e., ARDS).

4. Neurologic injury. Tracheal intubation and mechanical ventilation ensures a stable airway in patients with an acute neurologic injury who are at risk for aspiration or airway obstruction. Mechanical ventilation can control arterial $PaCO_2$, which influences cerebral blood volume and intracranial pressure.

5. Postoperative surgical conditions that require sedation and/or immobility.

6. Mechanical ventilation can be pressure or volume controlled. The main difference is the targeted goal: pressure ventilation mode guarantees a peak inspired airway pressure at the expense of a variable tidal volume, while volume ventilation mode guarantees flow and the set volume at the expense of inspiratory pressures.

Pressure ventilation has an almost unlimited ability to deliver flow and possesses a decelerating flow profile that tends to improve the distribution of ventilation in a lung with heterogeneous disease. With comparable settings in volume control, pressure-control ventilation will maintain a higher mean airway pressure. A potential disadvantage of pressure ventilation is that the tidal volume will depend on the compliance and resistance of the respiratory system. As lung compliance improves, the tidal volume will increase with the same inspiratory pressure. This type of ventilation will compensate for an air leak around an uncuffed endotracheal tube.

With volume-controlled ventilation, a preset tidal volume (the volume of gas to be moved in and out of the lungs with each breath) is delivered up to a maximum preset pressure limit. Tidal volume is controlled by a constant inspiratory flow rate and a set inspiratory time. A decrease in lung compliance or increase in airway resistance will be reflected by an increase in peak inspiratory pressures. For example, if an endotracheal tube becomes occluded, the airway resistance will increase, and the same tidal volume will now generate a higher inspiratory pressure. For healthy individuals, a normal tidal volume breath is 6 to 8 mL/kg. This volume is adjusted based on adequacy of chest rise in each patient.

In children with severe lung disease, such as ARDS, closing volume (the volume of gas in the lung after maximal exhalation at which the airways close) is increased above that of the functional residual capacity (FRC), causing diffuse atelectasis. Volume-controlled ventilation in ARDS allows for ventilation with lower tidal volumes (6 mL/kg) and is associated with decreased mortality, higher number of ventilator-free days, and a higher number of days without multiorgan failure[1].

Positive end-expiratory pressure (PEEP) increases FRC (the volume of gas in the lung after normal exhalation) above the closing volume. PEEP maintains alveolar volume, prevents atelectasis, and improves oxygenation by increasing the mean airway pressure (MAP). PEEP is set in both volume and pressure-controlled ventilation; it is the lowest expiratory pressure reached during mechanical ventilation. However, excess PEEP may cause lung hyperinflation, air trapping, or air leaks. PEEP will also increase intrathoracic pressure and may decrease systemic venous return to the heart (preload). On the other hand, PEEP improves cardiac output by decreasing afterload of the left ventricle. One of the major goals in mechanical ventilation is to find a balance between the good and bad effects of PEEP in each patient.

Advanced modes of mechanical ventilation used in pediatric patients include inverse-ratio ventilation, airway pressure release ventilation (APRV), and high-frequency ventilation. Inverse-ratio ventilation prolongs the inspiratory phase in excess of the expiratory phase during positive-pressure ventilation; this increases mean airway pressure and oxygenation during severe acute lung disease. Because it is a nonphysiologic pattern of breathing, these patients are administered heavy sedation and neuromuscular blockade. APRV is a form of inverse-ratio ventilation that utilizes a continuous gas flow circuit to allow the patient to breathe spontaneously throughout the ventilatory cycle, which is more comfortable and requires less sedation. High-frequency jet ventilation and high-frequency oscillatory ventilation combine small tidal volumes (smaller than calculated airway dead space) with increased frequencies (>1 Hz) to minimize the effects of elevated peak and mean airway pressures. High-frequency ventilation reduces the occurrence and treatment of air leak syndromes associated with neonatal and pediatric acute lung injury. High-frequency percussive ventilation (e.g., VDR) combines percussive ventilation with conventional ventilation, potentially improving ventilation, and secretion clearance.

Invasive Line Placement and Monitoring

Arterial Catheter Insertion

Arterial catheters are indicated when there is a need for precise beat-to-beat blood pressure monitoring or arterial blood gas monitoring and/or sampling. There are no absolute contraindications to placing an arterial catheter, but a risk/benefit analysis should be performed in patients with a hypercoagulable state or bleeding disorder.

The most favored site for arterial cannulation is the radial artery because it is easily accessible and there is collateral blood flow from the ulnar artery. Other possible sites include the ulnar, dorsalis pedis, posterior tibial, axillary, and femoral arteries. The brachial artery should be avoided because of the risk for median nerve damage and lack of collateral circulation in some patients. Before placement of a radial or ulnar arterial catheter, an Allen test should be performed to ensure adequate collateral blood flow. This test is performed by occluding both the radial and ulnar arteries until pallor of the hand occurs. Upon releasing pressure on the artery that is not planned for cannulation, the hand should reperfuse and pallor should subside. If this reperfusion is not established, alternative sites should be considered.

The artery can be cannulated either by inserting the catheter directly into the artery using a catheter-overneedle device or by using the Seldinger technique. The Seldinger technique involves entering the vessel with a needle, placing a guidewire through the needle after the vessel is entered, removing the needle, and then placing the catheter over the wire into the vessel. Aseptic technique should always be followed when placing an arterial line.

All arterial lines must be clearly identified to avoid accidental infusion of hypertonic solutions and sclerosing medications that would injure the artery. Arterial catheters are at risk for infection, disconnection causing significant blood loss, and arterial thrombus formation, which, in rare cases, can cause limb ischemia or loss. Ischemic necrosis may also occur from arteriolar spasm or emboli from air or clot.

Central Venous Catheter Insertion

Central venous catheters are useful to provide cardiac filling pressure measurements (i.e., CVP), and as a more efficient conduit for the administration of fluids, blood products, vesicant drugs to the central circulation, as well as high-concentration parenteral alimentation that would be sclerosing to peripheral veins. It can also be used as access for hemodialysis, plasmapheresis, right heart catheterization, and placement of a temporary transvenous pacemaker.

Common sites for central venous cannulation are the internal jugular, femoral, and subclavian veins. Contraindications are infection of the skin overlying the target vessel and thrombosis of the target vessel. All sites share the common complications of infection (site cellulitis, bacteremia), venous thrombosis with emboli, air embolism, catheter malfunction (occlusion, dislodgement, fractures), accidental arterial puncture, and bleeding. Additional complications are dysrhythmias (when the catheter tip is in the heart), pneumothorax, and hemothorax (more common with subclavian and internal jugular catheters). Universal precautions and sterile technique should be used when placing a central venous catheter.

The use of ultrasound to guide central venous catheter insertion is now the standard of care. Studies have shown decreased complications with the use of ultrasound guidance during procedure including decreased posterior hematoma, decreased arterial puncture, and increased efficiency with first attempt success. Ultrasound also helps measure the size of vessels to determine ideal catheter diameter and decrease risk for thrombosis. When choosing a vessel for cannulation, ultrasound can be used to identify thrombosed vessels which would not be ideal for cannulation. Finally, ultrasound use in real time with procedure can be used to troubleshoot difficulties with wire or catheter insertion such as identifying a wire going through the back wall of the vessel, wire curling up on itself, catheter abutting a valve, and so forth.

References

1. Tobias JD, Ross AK. Intraosseous Infusions: A Review for the Anesthesiologist with a Focus on Pediatric Use. *Anesth Analg.* 2010;110(2):391–401. https://doi.org/10.1213/ANE.0b013e3181c03c7f.

2. Glauser T, Shinnar S, Gloss D, et al. Evidence-Based Guideline: Treatment of Convulsive Status Epilepticus in Children and Adults: Report of the Guideline Committee of the American Epilepsy Society. *Epilepsy Curr.* 2016;16(1):48–61. https://doi.org/10.5698/1535-7597-16.1.48.

3. Kapur J, Elm J, Chamberlain JM, et al. Randomized Trial of Three Anticonvulsant Medications for Status Epilepticus. *N Engl J Med.* 2019;381:2103–2113. https://doi.org/10.1056/NEJMoa1905795.

4. Choong K, Kissoon N. Vasopressin in pediatric shock and cardiac arrest. *Pediatr Crit Care Med.* 2008;9(4):372–379. https://doi.org/10.1097/PCC.0b013e318172d7c8.

5. Topjian A, Raymond T, Atkins D, et al. Part 4: Pediatric Basic and Advanced Life Support: 2020 American Heart Association Guidelines for Cardiopulmonary Resuscitation and Emergency Cardiovascular Care. *Circulation.* 2020;142(16 2):S469–S523. doi:10.1161/CIR.0000000000000901.

Suggested Reading

Daigle C, Fiadjoe J, Laverriere E, et al. Difficult Bag-Mask Ventilation in Critically Ill Children Is Independently Associated With Adverse Events. Critical Care Medicine. 2020;48(9):e744–e752. doi:10.1097/CCM.0000000000004425.

The Pediatric Acute Lung Injury Consensus Conference Group. Pediatric Acute Respiratory Distress Syndrome: Consensus Recommendations From the Pediatric Acute Lung Injury Consensus Conference. Pediatric Critical Care Medicine. 2015;16(5):428–439. doi:10.1097/PCC.0000000000000350.

Index

Page numbers followed by "*f*" indicate figures, "*t*" indicate tables, "*b*" indicate boxes

As pediatric anesthesia is the subject of the book, all index entries refer to anesthesia in pediatric medicine unless otherwise indicated. Abbreviations: CHD – congenital heart disease